Practical Cardiology

Evaluation and Treatment of Common Cardiovascular Disorders

Practical Cardiology

Evaluation and Treatment of Common Cardiovascular Disorders

Editors

Kim A. Eagle, M.D.
Albion Walter Hewlett Professor of Internal Medicine
University of Michigan Medical School;
Chief of Clinical Cardiology
Division of Cardiology
Clinical Director, University of Michigan Cardiovascular Center
Ann Arbor, Michigan

Ragavendra R. Baliga, M.D.
Clinical Assistant Professor
Department of Internal Medicine, Division of Cardiology
University of Michigan Cardiovascular Center
Ann Arbor, Michigan

Section Editors

William F. Armstrong, M.D.
Department of Internal Medicine, Division of Cardiology
Eric R. Bates, M.D.
Department of Internal Medicine, Division of Cardiology
Robert J. Cody, M.D.
Department of Internal Medicine, Division of Cardiology
G. Michael Deeb, M.D.
Department of Surgery, Section of Cardiac Surgery
Fred Morady, M.D.
Department of Internal Medicine, Division of Cardiology
Richard L. Prager, M.D.
Department of Surgery, Section of Cardiac Surgery
James C. Stanley, M.D.
Department of Surgery, Section of Vascular Surgery
Mark R. Starling, M.D.
Department of Internal Medicine, Division of Cardiology
University of Michigan Cardiovascular Center
Ann Arbor, Michigan

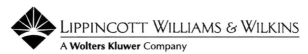
LIPPINCOTT WILLIAMS & WILKINS
A **Wolters Kluwer** Company

Philadelphia • Baltimore • New York • London
Buenos Aires • Hong Kong • Sydney • Tokyo

Acquisitions Editor: Ruth W. Weinberg
Developmental Editor: Julia Seto
Production Editor: Emmeline A. Parker
Manufacturing Manager: Ben Rivera
Cover Designer: Joan Greenfield
Compositor: TechBooks
Printer: Courier-Westford

Library of Congress Cataloging-in-Publication Data

Practical cardiology : evaluation and treatment of common cardiovascular disorders /
    editors, Kim A. Eagle, Ragavendra R. Baliga ; section editors, William F. Armstrong
    . . . [et al.].
       p. ; cm.
    Includes bibliographical references and index.
    ISBN 0-7817-3261-1
    1. Cardiology—Handbooks, manuals, etc. I. Eagle, Kim A.   II. Baliga, R. R.
    [DNLM: 1. Cardiovascular Diseases—diagnosis.   2. Cardiovascular
Diseases—therapy.   WG 141 P895 2003]
RC669.15 P73   2003
616.1′2—dc21   2002043091

Care has been taken to confirm the accuracy of the information presented and to describe generally accepted practices. However, the authors, editors and publisher are not responsible for errors or omissions or for any consequences from application of the information in this book and make no warranty, expressed or implied, with respect to the currency, completeness, or accuracy of the contents of the publication. Application of this information in a particular situation remains the professional responsibility of the practitioner.

The authors, editors and publisher have exerted every effort to ensure that drug selection and dosage set forth in this text are in accordance with current recommendations and practice at the time of publication. However, in view of ongoing research, changes in government regulations, and the constant flow of information relating to drug therapy and drug reactions, the reader is urged to check the package insert for each drug for any change in indications and dosage and for added warnings and precautions. This is particularly important when the recommended agent is a new or infrequently employed drug.

Some drugs and medical devices presented in this publication have Food and Drug Administration (FDA) clearance for limited use in restricted research settings. It is the responsibility of the health care provider to ascertain the FDA status of each drug or device planned for use in their clinical practice.

10 9 8 7 6 5 4 3 2 1

For more than 100 years, the University of Michigan has been a leader in cardiovascular care, education, and research. Experts in cardiology, cardiac surgery, vascular surgery, and hypertension and our partners in pediatric cardiovascular care, anesthesiology, radiology, pharmacology, and pathology have helped create the bases for the diagnosis and treatment of coronary, vascular, pericardial, valvular, and myocardial diseases. The institution has helped launch modern-day electrocardiography, electrophysiology, percutaneous coronary interventions, thrombolytic therapy, cardiac surgery, and clinical trials-based management of heart failure, acute myocardial infarction, stable coronary disease, and hypertension. Its programs have educated hundreds of cardiovascular specialists who have gone on to be leaders in their communities, hospitals, and medical schools. This book is dedicated to the men and women who preceded us, who laid the foundation of excellence in cross-disciplinary care, research, and education upon which we continue to build.

The Editors

Contents

G. Aortic and Major Vascular Diseases
Section Editors: G. Michael Deeb and James C. Stanley

H. Pulmonary Vascular Diseases
Section Editor: William F. Armstrong

I. Congenital Heart Disease in Adults
Section Editor: Ragavendra R. Baliga

Section III. Common Situations in Cardiovascular Care
Section Editor: Kim A. Eagle

Section IV. Other Issues in Cardiovascular Care
Section Editor: Ragavendra R. Baliga

Contributing Authors

Keith D. Aaronson, M.D., M.S.

Assistant Professor
Medical Director, Cardiac Transplant Program
Department of Internal Medicine
Division of Cardiology
University of Michigan Cardiovascular Center
Ann Arbor, Michigan

William F. Armstrong, M.D.

Professor
Department of Internal Medicine
Director, Echocardiography Laboratory
Associate Clinical Chief
Associate Chair for Network Development
Department of Medicine
Division of Cardiology
University of Michigan Cardiovascular Center
Ann Arbor, Michigan

David S. Bach, M.D.

Clinical Associate Professor
Department of Internal Medicine
Division of Cardiology
University of Michigan Cardiovascular Center
Ann Arbor, Michigan

Ragavendra R. Baliga, M.D., M.R.C.P. (UK)

Clinical Assistant Professor
Department of Internal Medicine
Division of Cardiology
University of Michigan Cardiovascular Center
Ann Arbor, Michigan

Eric R. Bates, M.D.

Professor
Department of Internal Medicine
Division of Cardiology
University of Michigan Cardiovascular Center
Ann Arbor, Michigan

John D. Bisognano, M.D., Ph.D.

Assistant Professor
Department of Internal Medicine
University of Rochester;
Director of Cardiac Rehabilitation
Cardiology Unit
Strong Memorial Hospital
Rochester, New York

Steven F. Bolling, M.D.

Professor
Department of Surgery
Section of Cardiac Surgery
University of Michigan Cardiovascular Center
Ann Arbor, Michigan

Eduardo Bossone, M.D., Ph.D.

Adjunct Assistant Professor
Department of Internal Medicine
Division of Cardiology
University of Michigan Cardiovascular Center
Ann Arbor, Michigan;
Director
Echocardiography Laboratory
National Research Council
Lecce, Italy

Edward L. Bove, M.D.

Professor and Head
Section of Cardiac Surgery
Director
Pediatric Cardiac Surgery
University of Michigan Cardiovascular Center
Ann Arbor, Michigan

Stanley Chetcuti, M.D.

Clinical Assistant Professor
Department of Internal Medicine
Division of Cardiology
University of Michigan Cardiovascular Center
Ann Arbor, Michigan

Robert J. Cody, M.D.

Professor
Associate Chief
Department of Internal Medicine
Division of Cardiology
University of Michigan Cardiovascular Center
Ann Arbor, Michigan

Sunil Das, M.D.

Professor
Department of Internal Medicine
Division of Cardiology
University of Michigan Cardiovascular Center
Ann Arbor, Michigan

G. Michael Deeb, M.D.

Professor
Department of Surgery
Section of Cardiac Surgery
University of Michigan Cardiovascular Center
Ann Arbor, Michigan

Claire Duvernoy, M.D.

Assistant Professor
Department of Internal Medicine
Division of Cardiology
University of Michigan Cardiovascular Center;
Director, Cardiac Catheterization Laboratory
Ann Arbor VA Health System
Ann Arbor, Michigan

David B. S. Dyke, M.D.

Clinical Assistant Professor
Department of Internal Medicine
Division of Cardiology
University of Michigan Cardiovascular Center
Ann Arbor, Michigan

Kim A. Eagle, M.D.

Albion Walter Hewlett Professor of Internal
*   Medicine*
University of Michigan Medical School;
Chief of Clinical Cardiology
Division of Cardiology
University of Michigan Cardiovascular Center
Ann Arbor, Michigan

William P. Fay, M.D.

Associate Professor
Department of Internal Medicine
Division of Cardiology
Medical Director
Department of Anticoagulation Service
University of Michigan Cardiovascular Center
Ann Arbor, Michigan

Lazar J. Greenfield, M.D.

Professor
Department of Surgery
University of Michigan
Ann Arbor, Michigan

Peter G. Hagan, M.D.

Clinical Assistant Professor
Department of Internal Medicine
Division of Cardiology
University of Michigan Cardiovascular Center
Ann Arbor, Michigan

Peter K. Henke, M.D.

Assistant Professor
Department of Surgery
Section of Vascular Surgery
University of Michigan Cardiovascular Center
Ann Arbor, Michigan

Susan L. Hickenbottom, M.D., M.S.

Clinical Assistant Professor
Director, Clinical Stroke Service
Department of Neurology
University of Michigan
Ann Arbor, Michigan

Kenneth A. Jamerson, M.D.

Associate Professor
Department of Internal Medicine
Division of Hypertension
University of Michigan Cardiovascular Center
Ann Arbor, Michigan

Bradley P. Knight, M.D.

Associate Professor
Director of Clinical Cardiac
*   Electrophysiology*
Department of Internal Medicine
Division of Cardiology
University of Chicago Hospitals
Chicago, Illinois

Todd M. Koelling, M.D.

Assistant Professor
Department of Internal Medicine
Division of Cardiology
University of Michigan Cardiovascular Center
Ann Arbor, Michigan

Theodore J. Kolias, M.D.

Clinical Assistant Professor
Department of Internal Medicine
Division of Cardiology
University of Michigan Cardiovascular Center
Ann Arbor, Michigan

William Kou, M.D.

Associate Professor
Department of Internal Medicine
Division of Cardiology
University of Michigan Cardiovascular Center;
Director of Cardiac Electrophysiology
Department of Internal Medicine
Ann Arbor VA Medical Center
Ann Arbor, Michigan

Julie A. Kovach, M.D.

Clinical Assistant Professor
Department of Internal Medicine
Division of Cardiology
Director, Adult Congenital Heart Disease Program
University of Michigan Cardiovascular Center
Ann Arbor, Michigan

Michael H. Lehmann, M.D.

Clinical Professor
Department of Internal Medicine
Division of Cardiology
Director of the Electrocardiography Laboratory
University of Michigan Cardiovascular Center
Ann Arbor, Michigan

Fernando J. Martinez, M.D., M.S.

Professor
Department of Internal Medicine
Division of Pulmonary and Critical Care Medicine
University of Michigan
Ann Arbor, Michigan

Rajendra H. Mehta, M.D.

Clinical Assistant Professor
Department of Internal Medicine
Division of Cardiology
University of Michigan Cardiovascular Center
Ann Arbor, Michigan

Fred Morady, M.D.

Professor of Medicine
Director, Adult Clinical Electrophysiology
   Laboratory
Division of Cardiology
Department of Internal Medicine
University of Michigan Cardiovascular Center
Ann Arbor, Michigan

Mauro Moscucci, M.D.

Associate Professor
Department of Internal Medicine
Division of Cardiology
University of Michigan Cardiovascular Center;
Director, Cardiac Catheterization Laboratory
University of Michigan Hospital
Ann Arbor, Michigan

Debabrata Mukherjee, M.D.

Assistant Professor
Department of Internal Medicine
Division of Cardiology
University of Michigan
Ann Arbor, Michigan

Thippeswamy H. Murthy, M.D.

Lecturer
Department of Internal Medicine
Division of Cardiology
University of Michigan Cardiovascular Center
Ann Arbor, Michigan

Hakan Oral, M.D.

Assistant Professor
Department of Medicine
Division of Cardiology
University of Michigan Cardiovascular Center
Ann Arbor, Michigan

Francis D. Pagani, M.D., Ph.D.

Associate Professor of Surgery
Department of Surgery
Section of Cardiac Surgery
University of Michigan Cardiovascular Center
Ann Arbor, Michigan

Frank Pelosi, Jr., M.D.

Assistant Professor
Department of Internal Medicine
Division of Cardiology
University of Michigan Cardiovascular Center
Ann Arbor, Michigan

Richard L. Prager, M.D.

Clinical Professor of Surgery
Section Head of Adult Cardiac
   Surgery
Section of Cardiac Surgery
University of Michigan Cardiovascular Center
Ann Arbor, Michigan

Sanjay Rajagopalan, M.D.

Assistant Professor
Department of Internal Medicine
Division of Cardiology
Co-Director
Section of Vascular Medicine
University of Michigan Cardiovascular Center
Ann Arbor, Michigan

Albert P. Rocchini, M.D.

Professor
Department of Pediatric Cardiology
Director
Mott's Children's Hospital
University of Michigan Cardiovascular Center
Ann Arbor, Michigan

Melvyn Rubenfire, M.D.

Professor
Department of Internal Medicine
Division of Cardiology
Director, Preventive Cardiology and
   Pulmonary Hypertension
University of Michigan Cardiovascular Center
Ann Arbor, Michigan

John T. Santinga, M.D.

Emeritus Assistant Professor of Internal Medicine
   and Geriatrics
Department of Internal Medicine
Division of Geriatric Medicine
University of Michigan Cardiovascular Center
Ann Arbor, Michigan

Michael J. Shea, M.D.

Professor
Department of Internal Medicine
Division of Cardiology
University of Michigan Cardiovascular Center
Ann Arbor, Michigan

Marshal Shlafer, Ph.D.

Professor
Department of Pharmacology
University of Michigan Medical School
Ann Arbor, Michigan

James C. Stanley, M.D.

Professor
Head, Section of Vascular Surgery
Department of Surgery
University of Michigan Cardiovascular Center
Ann Arbor, Michigan

Mark R. Starling, M.D.

Professor
Department of Internal Medicine
Division of Cardiology
University of Michigan Cardiovascular Center
Ann Arbor, Michigan

Gilbert R. Upchurch, Jr., M.D.

Assistant Professor
Department of Surgery
Section of Vascular Surgery
University of Michigan Cardiovascular Center
Ann Arbor, Michigan

Peter V. Vaitkevicius, M.D.

Assistant Professor
Division of Cardiology
University of Michigan Cardiovascular Center;
Research Scientist
Department of Veterans Affairs Ann Arbor
   Healthcare System
Ann Arbor, Michigan

Mani A. Vannan, M.B.B.S.

Professor
Drexel University College of Medicine;
Director of Echocardiography
Hahnemann University Hospital
Department of Medicine and Cardiology
Philadelphia, Pennsylvania

Thomas W. Wakefield, M.D.

S. Martin Lindenaves Professor
Department of Surgery
Section of Vascular Surgery
Staff Surgeon
Department of Surgery
Section of Vascular Surgery
University of Michigan Cardiovascular Center
Department of Veterans Affairs, Ann Arbor
   Healthcare System
Ann Arbor, Michigan

Sara L. Warber, M.D.

Lecturer
Department of Family Medicine
Co-Director, Complementary and Alternative
   Medicine Research Center
University of Michigan
Ann Arbor, Michigan

John G. Weg, M.D.

Professor Emeritus
Department of Internal Medicine
Division of Pulmonary and Critical Care Medicine
University of Michigan
Ann Arbor, Michigan

Steven W. Werns, M.D.

Professor of Medicine
Robert Wood Johnson Medical School
Cooper Hospital/University Medical Center
Camden, New Jersey

David M. Williams, M.D.

Professor
Department of Radiology
Director, Vascular and Interventional Radiology
University of Michigan Cardiovascular Center
Ann Arbor, Michigan

Preface

As the lifespan of the general population increases, the prevalence of cardiovascular disease is increasing, placing the burden of cardiovascular care on nurse practitioners, primary care physicians, and internists, in addition to cardiologists. This book is intended to serve practitioners involved primarily in preventive and general cardiac care of patients with cardiovascular disease: nurses, house officers, general practitioners, internists, and cardiovascular specialists. The main theme of this book is "how to manage or treat." The University of Michigan Cardiovascular Center physicians have an international reputation for rational and compassionate cardiovascular care because of their focus on the individual patient. The unique feature of this book is that it incorporates their best medical practices with the American College of Cardiology/American Heart Association guidelines and consensus documents to provide the reader a user-friendly but authoritative source of information in the practical aspects of cardiac disease. The reader-friendly features of this book include the standard format of the chapters in each section, and the liberal use of tables, figures, and algorithms in each chapter.

Practical Cardiology is divided into four parts: Section I covers the evaluation of common cardiovascular symptoms faced by clinicians. Each chapter has a standard order of subjects that include (a) definition, (b) principal causes, (c) keys to the history, (d) helpful signs on physical examination, (e) diagnostic tests, (f) when to refer, and (g) when to admit. Section II emphasizes the evaluation and management of common cardiovascular conditions. The chapters in this section also have a clinically relevant standard order of subjects that include usual causes, presenting symptoms and signs, helpful tests, differential diagnosis, complications, therapy, prognosis, and follow-up. Section III is unique in that it discusses management of common clinical challenges in cardiovascular care, including management of chronic anticoagulation, perioperative cardiovascular evaluation and care in noncardiac surgery, and management of the patient after cardiac surgery. In Section IV, Chapter 40 lists common cardiovascular drugs in a reader-friendly tabular format, and Chapter 41 provides a current perspective on alternative medical therapy in cardiovascular disease. Each chapter in the book also includes one final table summarizing practical points.

Like most first editions, this book has not met all of our goals, but we believe that we have been able to provide clinicians with information that will aid in the care of their patients. The royalties from this book will be used to enhance the missions of the University of Michigan Cardiovascular Center: world-class patient care, innovative research, and unending commitment to education.

At Lippincott Williams & Wilkins, we are grateful to our editor, Ruth Weinberg, for her patience and to Julia Seto for her diligence, which were critical to the preparation of this edition. We thank the many faculty members of our Cardiovascular Center for their contributions and their families who support them.

Kim A. Eagle, M.D.
Ragavendra R. Baliga, M.D.
Ann Arbor, Michigan

1

Chest Pain

Thippeswamy H. Murthy and Peter G. Hagan

DEFINITION AND SCOPE OF PROBLEM

Chest pain can be broadly defined as any discomfort in the anterior thorax occurring above the epigastrium and below the mandible. However, pain of cardiac origin may be felt primarily in the arms or jaw regions. Estimates of the number of Americans who experience significant chest pain range from 6.2 million (1) to 16.5 million (2). Patients frequently seek medical advice and treatment for chest pain, and over 5 million patients presented to emergency departments in 1997 for the evaluation of chest pain syndromes (3).

PRINCIPAL CAUSES

The principal causes of chest pain can be grouped as life-threatening and non–life-threatening (Table 1.1). The principal life-threatening causes are acute coronary syndromes, aortic dissection, and pulmonary embolism (PE). The principal non–life-threatening causes are stable angina, pericarditis, gastrointestinal reflux disease (GERD), esophageal spasm, musculoskeletal disorders, valvular heart disease, and hypertrophic cardiomyopathy.

Acute coronary syndromes comprise a broad range of clinical manifestations from acute myocardial infarction with cardiogenic shock to relatively "low-risk" unstable angina. The common pathophysiologic process involves rupture of an atherosclerotic plaque in an epicardial coronary artery with resultant platelet aggregation, activation of the coagulation cascade, and thrombus formation and dissolution with obstruction to coronary blood flow. Thus, treatment and management strategies are similar.

Aortic dissection is characterized by separation of intima and media and consequent prop-

agation as blood enters the intima/media space. The separation of the layers of the aorta with formation of a dissection flap can lead to ischemia of any of the branches of the aortic trunk, including the coronary arteries. Although much less common than acute coronary syndromes, dissection should be considered early in the evaluation of chest pain, in view of its divergent management and exceedingly high short-term mortality rate.

PE is a frequent cause of death. It generally results from the embolization of thrombotic material from lower extremity and deep pelvic veins. The thrombotic material can occlude any of the branches of the pulmonary artery and lead to hypoxia, pulmonary infarction, and acute right ventricular dysfunction. It is also critical to consider this diagnosis early in the evaluation of chest pain, because a recurrent pulmonary embolus may be fatal.

The great majority of patients with chest pain have a non–life-threatening cause. It is important to identify these patients early to provide effective treatment, allay patient concerns, and utilize health care resources appropriately.

HISTORY AND PHYSICAL EXAMINATION

History

The history is the most important component of the evaluation of chest pain. The history can be documented expeditiously for most patients and often leads to a clear diagnosis. In addition to detailed questioning about the nature of the chest pain, the physician should elicit a history of prior myocardial infarction, coronary revascularization [coronary artery bypass graft (CABG) or percutaneous transluminal coronary angioplasty (PTCA)], and congestive heart failure (CHF)

TABLE 1.1. *Principal causes of chest pain*

Life-threatening	Non–life-threatening
Acute coronary syndromes	Stable angina
	Pericarditis
Aortic dissection	GERD/esophageal spasm
Pulmonary embolism	Musculoskeletal
	Valvular heart disease
	Hypertrophic cardiomyopathy

GERD, gastroesophageal reflux disease.

symptoms. All patients should be queried about the major cardiovascular risk factors [diabetes, smoking, hypercholesterolemia, family history of premature coronary artery disease (CAD), and hypertension] and for a history or symptoms of peripheral vascular disease. Illicit drugs such as cocaine may cause chest pain and myocardial infarction more commonly in the younger population. All patients should be asked about the associated symptoms of dyspnea, diaphoresis, and nausea, as well as the response to nitroglycerin.

The interviewer should elicit the location, onset, duration, character, intensity, and radiation of the chest pain. When questioning the patient, the interviewer should use the term chest *"discomfort"* rather than chest *"pain,"* because many patients deny having a "pain." In fact, many patients emphatically point out to the interviewer that the discomfort is not a "pain." For the purposes of discussion, this chapter retains the traditional term chest *"pain."*

Chest pain that is cardiac in etiology is termed *angina.* Angina is defined as a clinical syndrome "characterized by discomfort in the chest, jaw, shoulder, back or arm" (2). Angina usually is provoked by physical exertion or emotional stress and is relieved with rest or nitroglycerin. Patients typically describe angina with adjectives such as "heavy," "dull," "pressure-like," "suffocating," or "squeezing," or they use phrases such as "like a heavy weight on my chest." Angina is classically substernal in location but can occur in the arm, shoulder, jaw, mandible, or upper back with or without radiation. Pain above the mandible, below the epigastrium, localized to an area less than one fingertip in size, or that radiates into the lower extremities is rarely angina. Angina usually lasts for a few minutes and is relieved by nitroglycerin within 5 minutes or less.

Continuous pain that lasts for several hours or fleeting pain that last for only a few seconds suggests an alternative diagnosis. Angina typically does not vary with respiration, position, or palpation.

Angina is termed *stable* when it occurs only with provocation, has been occurring for at least 2 months, and is symptomatically stable. According to the Canadian Cardiovascular Society Classification system (4), angina can be graded on the basis of the history (Table 1.2). Class I angina occurs only with strenuous exertion, Class II results in a slight limitation of ordinary activity and occurs only during moderate levels of exertion, Class III is associated with a marked reduction in ordinary activity and can occur with mild exertion, and Class IV angina causes limitations on activities of daily living and can occur even at rest.

Chest pain can be classified as noncardiac, atypical, or typical on the basis of the presence of three features: (a) substernal location, (b) provocation with exertion or emotional stress, and (c) relief with nitroglycerin or rest. If all three features are present, the chest pain is termed *typical angina;* if two are present, it is termed *atypical*

TABLE 1.2. *Grading of angina pectoris by the Canadian Cardiovascular Society Classification system*

Class I
Ordinary physical activity does not cause angina, such as walking, climbing stairs. Angina (occurs) with strenuous, rapid, or prolonged exertion at work or recreation.

Class II
Slight limitation of ordinary activity. Angina occurs on walking or climbing stairs rapidly, walking uphill, walking or stair climbing after meals, or in cold, or in wind, or under emotional stress, or only during the few hours after awakening.

Class III
Marked limitations of ordinary physical activity. Angina occurs on walking one or two blocks on the level and climbing one flight of stairs in normal conditions and at a normal pace.

Class IV
Inability to carry on any physical activity without discomfort—anginal symptoms may be present at rest.

From Campeau L. Letter: Grading of angina pectoris. *Circulation* 1976;54:522–523. Copyright 1976, American Heart Association, Inc. Reprinted with permission.

TABLE 1.3. *Principal presentations of unstable angina*

Rest angina	Angina occurring at rest and usually prolonged >20 minutes occurring within a week of presentation
New-onset angina	Angina of at least CCSC III severity with onset within 2 months of initial presentation
Increasing angina	Previously diagnosed angina that is distinctly more frequent, longer in duration or lower in threshold (i.e., increased by at least one CCSC class within 2 months of initial presentation to at least CCSC III severity).

CCSC, Canadian Cardiovascular Society Classification system.
From Braunwald E, Jones RH, Mark DB, et al. Diagnosing and managing unstable angina. Agency For Health Care Policy and Research. *Circulation* 1994;90:613–622.

angina; and if only one is present, it is considered *noncardiac chest pain.*

Unstable angina, which is an acute coronary syndrome, can be classified as rest angina, new-onset angina, or increasing angina (5) (Table 1.3). Rest angina occurs at rest without provocation for longer than 20 minutes within 1 week of presentation. New-onset angina is angina that is at least Class III in severity and presents within 2 months of initial presentation. Increasing angina is stable angina that is increasing in frequency or duration, has a decreasing threshold for provocation, or has increasing intensity.

Anginal pain from myocardial infarction classically is often described as "crushing" or "as if an elephant were standing on my chest" and is usually severe and unrelenting. For many patients, it is the sentinel episode of chest pain. Others may have a history of stable angina, unstable angina, or both in the preceding 2 weeks. It is not uncommon for patients to present several days after a myocardial infarction with congestive heart failure symptoms or postinfarction angina. Some patients are completely asymptomatic or able to recall only vague "gas pains."

Aortic dissection has classically been described as a severe and sudden "ripping" or "tearing" chest or back pain that radiates in a migratory fashion (6). A multicenter registry of almost 500 patients diagnosed with acute aortic dissection revealed that the pain of aortic dissection is more often sharp and typically of sudden and severe onset. The clinical manifestations of aortic dissection are quite varied, and thus the physician must have a high clinical index of suspicion in order to make the diagnosis.

The chest pain of PE can be pleuritic in nature and is associated with abrupt-onset dyspnea and apprehension. Many affected patients have risk factors for PE, such as previous deep vein thrombosis, recent surgery, prolonged immobilization, malignancy, hypercoagulability syndromes, advanced age, congestive heart failure, oral contraceptive use, or pregnancy.

Chest pain is a central complaint in acute pericarditis. The pain is typically located over the precordium with radiation to the trapezius ridge and neck. The pain is often "sharp" or "knife-like," is exacerbated by respiration and thoracic motion, is relieved by leaning forward, and is aggravated by recumbency. It is not related to exertion and can last for hours on end. Patients may complain of dyspnea, which is related to taking shallow respirations to avoid the pleuritic pain. Pericarditis is more common in men. Dyspnea on exertion and other symptoms of congestive heart failure should raise the suspicion for concomitant myocarditis.

Chest pain associated with GERD and esophagitis is often described as a "burning" sensation or simply as "heartburn" and occurs after meals or upon recumbency. The pain usually starts in the epigastric region, radiates superiorly across the entire chest, and does not radiate into the arms. However, the pain can also be retrosternal. The patient may also complain of hoarseness, a need to repeatedly clear the throat, or a deep pressure in the throat. A history of regurgitation or water brash supports the diagnosis. The chest pain of GERD is frequently exacerbated by maneuvers that increase intraabdominal pressure, such as bending, squatting, and coughing. Many patients have risk factors for GERD, such as excessive caffeine or alcohol use, cigarette smoking, and heavy meal consumption. The pain of esophageal spasm can be very severe, may last seconds to hours, radiates to the back, and is frequently indistinguishable from angina. It is important to query the patient about associated dysphagia, weight loss, or hematemesis. Of note, the pain of esophageal spasm and esophagitis may respond to nitroglycerin.

Musculoskeletal chest pain is commonly associated with a history of coughing, trauma, injury, or strenuous muscular exertion. The patient may relate a history of the pain's varying with physical position and being exacerbated by specific thoracic movements. The pain usually has a low intensity and a duration of several hours or days. Chest pain may be the presenting manifestation of severe valvular heart disease or hypertrophic cardiomyopathy. When present, it manifests as typical angina caused by a supply/demand imbalance in coronary blood flow that leads to myocardial ischemia or as chest discomfort caused by pulmonary congestion resulting from left atrial hypertension or volume overload. The symptoms are usually chronic and may be associated with CHF symptoms (dyspnea, fatigue, orthopnea, edema). If either valvular heart disease or hypertrophic cardiomyopathy is suspected, a history of syncope or aborted sudden cardiac death and a family history of sudden cardiac death should be sought. A history of rheumatic fever raises the possibility of rheumatic valvular disease.

Physical Examination

A focused physical examination should be performed expeditiously to rule out life-threatening causes. Bilateral arm blood pressures, heart rate, respiratory rate, and oxygenation saturation should ideally be measured in every patient with acute chest pain.

The physical examination of patients with acute coronary syndrome is particularly important. Both myocardial infarction and unstable angina can cause severe myocardial ischemia that manifests as acute left ventricular dysfunction. Patients may present with a low cardiac output state (e.g., hypotension, tachycardia, poor urine output, mental status changes, cool extremities), acute pulmonary edema (tachypnea, hypoxia, rales, elevated jugular venous pressure), or both. The cardiac examination may reveal a soft S1, an S3 gallop, or a displaced and/or enlarged apical impulse. A low-output state or pulmonary edema greatly increases the short-term mortality rate in patients with acute coronary syndrome, and physical examination findings of these are used to guide therapeutic decisions.

The classic findings of aortic dissection include hypertension, pulse deficits, and the murmur of aortic insufficiency. However, these findings occur in the minority of patients, and the physical examination is most often unhelpful in the diagnosis of aortic dissection (7). The murmur of aortic insufficiency is best heard at the lower left sternal border with the patient in the upright position, leaning forward, and at maximal expiration. Peripheral pulses should be evaluated and documented.

The most common physical examination finding in patients with PE is tachypnea (more than 16 respirations per minute) and is found in more than 90% of patients (8). With large pulmonary emboli, findings of acute cor pulmonale may be present (acute hypotension, accentuated pulmonic component of S2, elevated jugular venous pressures, and a right ventricular lift). Pulmonic auscultation findings, if present, include rales and evidence of consolidation or pleural effusion. As with aortic dissection, the physical examination is usually unrevealing; thus, clinical suspicion must be heightened in order to make the diagnosis.

The results of a characteristic physical examination of patients with chronic, stable angina are usually normal. There are no specific physical examination findings for chronic CAD. However, the findings of diminished peripheral pulses or carotid and femoral bruits greatly increase the probability of coexisting CAD. If the patient is examined during an episode of acute ischemia, it may be noted that the S1 is diminished and a soft mitral regurgitation murmur may be present. Both these findings are presumably caused by transient, ischemia-mediated left ventricular dysfunction. Patients with chronic CAD and left ventricular systolic dysfunction or those with a recent untreated myocardial infarction may have enlargement and displacement of the apical impulse, elevated jugular venous pressures, a soft S1, or an abnormal S3.

The pathognomonic sign of pericarditis is the friction rub. The friction rub has been classically described as a "scratchy," three-component (though frequently only one- or two-component) sound that is related to the cardiac motion. It is best heard when the patient is sitting upright at full expiration. Friction rubs are well known to be evanescent and vary from examination to examination. The most common physical examination finding is tachycardia. If a coexisting pericardial effusion is present, the heart sounds may be distant or muffled. If the patient is markedly dyspneic or distressed, pericardial tamponade should be considered, the jugular venous pressure inspected, and pulsus paradoxus measured.

The physical examination in patients with GERD or esophageal spasm is unrevealing. Patients with underlying scleroderma may present with calcinosis, sclerodactyly, and telangiectasias. The diagnosis is usually suspected from history alone or response to antacid therapy.

Reproduction of pain with palpation or with thoracic or extremity movement and costochondral joint tenderness or swelling are characteristic findings of patients with musculoskeletal chest pain. Prevesicular herpes zoster may produce intense chest pain and may be difficult to distinguish from angina; however, it usually has a dermatomal distribution and is constant in nature.

The physical examination of patients with chest pain is most useful in those with significant valvular heart disease or hypertrophic cardiomyopathy. Significant aortic stenosis is characterized by a loud, late-peaking, crescendo-decrescendo systolic ejection murmur, heard best over the base of the heart, which may radiate into the right carotid artery. An S4 is usually prominent. The S2 may become single, because of an inaudible A2 component, or paradoxically split. Carotid pulses may be slow to rise and small in amplitude (parvus and tardus) (9). Hypertrophic cardiomyopathy also manifests with a systolic murmur and an S4. The murmur is typically harsh in nature and heard best between the left sternal border and the apex without radiation to the carotid arteries. It is mostly midsystolic at the left sternal border and holosystolic at the apex (as a result of concomitant mitral regurgitation). In contrast to aortic stenosis, the murmur increases with Valsalva maneuvers (during strain) and with rising from squatting to standing (and other maneuvers that decrease preload); the carotid upstroke is brisk; and the S2 is normal (10).

DIAGNOSTIC TESTING

In all patients with chest pain, a 12-lead electrocardiogram (ECG) should be obtained. It may show evidence of acute ischemia or injury, previous myocardial infarction, left ventricular hypertrophy, left bundle branch block, pericarditis, acute right ventricular strain, or a variety of other disorders. The ECG should be obtained within 5 to 10 minutes of the patient's presentation.

Acute Coronary Syndromes

In patients suspected of having chest pain as a result of epicardial CAD, the physician should determine whether the patient is having an acute coronary syndrome with concomitant myocardial ischemia. The ECG should be compared with a previous ECG obtained during a pain-free episode. If significant ECG changes from the baseline ECG are present (ST segment elevation/depression, T wave abnormalities, Q waves, new left bundle branch block), myocardial ischemia is suggested. If an ECG is not available for comparison, a surface echocardiogram to assess wall motion may be helpful. Unfortunately, a normal ECG or an ECG unchanged from baseline does not necessarily exclude an acute coronary syndrome.

Chest radiographs are generally not first-line diagnostic tests for myocardial ischemia. However, if the patient is complaining of dyspnea or if the pulmonary examination findings are abnormal, a radiograph should be ordered. Occasionally, the chest radiograph may reveal uncommon chest pain causes such as pneumothorax or chest masses. A few centers (11–13) have reported on the use of resting nuclear scintigraphy in patients with acute chest pain; however, this is logistically challenging in the emergency department and is not widely available (14).

Simple bedside maneuvers may be tried if cautiously interpreted. Anginal pain typically abates completely less than 5 minutes after nitroglycerin administration. However, the pain of esophageal spasm and esophagitis is also relieved with nitroglycerin but may not completely resolve; there may be a residual dull ache in contrast to ischemic chest pain. A gastrointestinal (GI) "cocktail," a mixture of antacids and viscous lidocaine, is often employed as a diagnostic maneuver. Because of the variety of medications given with the "cocktail," the possibility of spontaneous, coincidental resolution of ischemic chest pain, and the lack of good data to support this maneuver, it cannot be recommended for the routine evaluation of chest pain. However, if a patient presents with symptoms that are strongly suggestive of gastrointestinal origin, relief of pain with antacids or a "GI cocktail" may support the clinical diagnosis.

Biochemical cardiac markers can be used to diagnose acute myocardial infarction and provide prognosis in unstable angina. The commonly available cardiac markers are creatine kinase (CK) and myocardial band (MB) fraction, myoglobin, and troponin I or T (TnI or TnT). Myoglobin is the enzyme most rapidly released after an acute coronary syndrome, its levels peaking within 4 to 6 hours and normalizing within 24 hours, but it is not very specific. CK-MB has traditionally been used to diagnose myocardial infarction; its levels become elevated within 12 hours of infarction, peak at 24 hours, and normalize by 72 hours. However, elevated levels of CK-MB can be found in normal individuals and in those with severe skeletal muscle injury. Troponin levels become elevated within 6 to 12 hours, peak by 48 hours, and can remain elevated for 10 to 14 days after the initial event. Because of their high cardiac specificity, troponins have rapidly become the biochemical cardiac markers of choice for diagnosing acute myocardial infarction. However, caution must be used in the interpretation of an elevated troponin level because it may represent a cardiac event that occurred in the preceding 14 days. In these cases, a myoglobin level can be checked. If it is elevated, the troponin elevation is probably a result of a recent cardiac event. However, normal troponin levels do not definitely rule out adverse cardiac outcomes in patients with chest pain. Patients with normal biochemical markers may be presenting without injury and thus will not have biochemical evidence of myocardial necrosis. When an acute coronary syndrome is suspected, acute myocardial infarction should be ruled out by serial troponin or CK-MB measurements. The first troponin measurement should be

drawn upon initial presentation, and a second test should be repeated 8 to 12 hours after the original symptom onset. If the patient has recurrent chest pain after the initial episode, or if the first two troponin measurements are indeterminate, further measurements of cardiac enzymes should be considered.

Aortic Dissection

When aortic dissection is suspected, diagnostic imaging should be performed without delay. There are no specific ECG findings for aortic dissection. The ECG may be normal, show nonspecific ST segment or T wave changes, or show evidence of acute myocardial ischemia. Chest radiography has a low sensitivity for aortic dissection, and at least 20% of patients with suspected aortic dissections do not have a widened mediastinum or altered aortic contours (7).

The most widely available and reliable imaging modalities for aortic dissection are contrast-enhanced computed tomography (CT) and transesophageal echocardiography (TEE). CT is generally more widely available than TEE, allows for visualization of the entire aorta, and provides information about extraaortic structures. The CT should be performed according to specific aortic dissection protocols that involve thinner tomographic slices to improve resolution and boluses of intravenous contrast instead of slow infusions to delineate the aortic lumen. We prefer TEE because it can be performed quickly at the patient's bedside with minimal risk to the patient. Overall, both tests have similar sensitivities and specificities, and the choice of test usually depends on availability and local expertise. If a strong clinical suspicion for aortic dissection exists even after a negative test result, a second modality should be utilized. Gadolinium-enhanced magnetic resonance imaging (MRI) is an excellent test for aortic dissection; however, few centers are able to provide this service for emergency diagnostic purposes.

Pulmonary Embolism

The ECG in PE is rarely diagnostic and is most likely to be normal or shows nonspecific changes. When present, ECG changes can be helpful. If a significant PE occurs, transient right bundle branch block, S_I Q_{III} T_{III} pattern, right axis deviation, or T-wave inversion in leads V_1 to V_3 can appear (15). The chest radiograph typically shows nonspecific findings. Specific findings on chest radiographs are exceedingly rare.

Most patients with PE have reduced arterial partial pressures of oxygen, an increased alveolar-arterial oxygen pressure gradient, or both. However, these findings are nonspecific and cannot be used alone to initiate therapy.

The most commonly available and widely used initial diagnostic test for PE is the ventilation/perfusion (V/Q) scan. The results should be reported as normal, indeterminate probability, low probability, intermediate probability, or high probability. If the result is normal, PE can almost always be ruled out. A high-probability result confirms the diagnosis. Patients with an intermediate- or indeterminate-probability result and those with a low-probability result and a high clinical suspicion should undergo pulmonary arteriography, which is considered to be the gold standard diagnostic test, to exclude the diagnosis.

D-Dimer levels have been shown to be elevated in patients with PE and are now rapidly available by enzyme-linked immunosorbent assay (ELISA) testing. One review (16) revealed that the ELISA D-dimer assay has an overall sensitivity of 90% to 95% but is not specific for the diagnosis of PE. However, negative D-dimer findings in a stable outpatient with a low clinical suspicion of PE can be used to exclude the diagnosis (16). Helical CT has been proposed as an alternative to V/Q scanning because it can noninvasively diagnose pulmonary emboli. The overall sensitivity is around 85% (16); however, this excludes subsegmental pulmonary emboli, which helical CT may fail to diagnose. MRI is promising in preliminary studies (17) but has not been thoroughly evaluated and is limited by longer diagnostic times.

Echocardiography is potentially helpful in the diagnosis of PE because its portability and safety make it ideal for critically ill patients. One study (18) revealed the sensitivity and specificity of echocardiography to be only 51% and 87%, respectively. Thus, a negative echocardiogram should not be used to exclude the diagnosis. However, echocardiography may be useful in predicting the short-term prognosis after acute PE. One study revealed that normotensive patients with acute PE and right ventricular dysfunction documented by echocardiography had a 10% rate of PE-related shock and a 5% in-hospital mortality rate and often required thrombolytic therapy, whereas similar patients with normal right ventricular function had a benign prognosis (19).

Stable Angina

If, on the basis of the history and physical examination, the physician determines that the patient is clinically stable and unlikely to be having an acute coronary syndrome, then an evaluation for chronic epicardial CAD should be undertaken. The ECG in chronic stable angina can be normal, can show evidence of prior myocardial infarction, or can show nonspecific ST segment and T wave changes. The chest radiograph is usually unrevealing and only rarely shows coronary artery calcifications. The definitive diagnostic test for epicardial coronary stenoses is coronary angiography. However, because of cost and safety considerations, it is not feasible to perform this test in every patient with chest pain and suspected CAD.

Therefore, stress testing is routinely performed primarily as a decision aid in estimating the probability of significant coronary artery disease. It is important to realize the principles of Bayes' theorem (20) when interpreting the results of stress testing. Briefly stated, the posttest probability of CAD is a function of the pretest probability of disease. In patients with a very low pretest probability of CAD, an abnormal stress test result can just as likely be a false-positive as a true-positive finding. Similarly, in a patient with a very high pretest probability of CAD, a negative test result does not rule out significant CAD. Patients with an intermediate pretest probability of CAD have the greatest benefit from stress testing, because a positive or negative result will result in a posttest probability that is significantly different from the pretest probability.

In a landmark study, Diamond and Forrester (21) showed that the pretest probability of CAD can be estimated solely on the basis of the patient's age, gender, and type of chest pain

TABLE 1.4. *Pretest likelihood of CAD in symptomatic patients according to age and sex*[a] *(combined Diamond/Forrester [21] and CASS [22] data)*

Age (years)	Nonanginal chest pain		Atypical angina		Typical angina	
	Men	Women	Men	Women	Men	Women
30–39	4	2	34	12	76	26
40–49	13	3	51	22	87	55
50–59	20	7	65	31	93	73
60–69	27	14	72	51	94	86

CAD, coronary artery disease; CASS, coronary artery surgery study.
[a] Each value represents the percent with significant CAD on catheterization.
From Gibbons RJ, Chatterjee K, Daley J, Douglas JS, Fihn SD, Gardin JM, Grunwald MA, Levy D, Lytle BW, O'Rourke RA, Schafer WP, Williams SV. ACC/AHA/ACP-ASIM guidelines for the management of patients with chronic stable angina: Executive summary and recommendations. A report of the American College of Cardiology/American Heart Association Task Force on Practice Guidelines (Committee on Management of Patients with Chronic Stable Angina). *Circulation* 1999;99:2829–2848. Copyright 1999, American Heart Association and the American College of Cardiology. Reproduced with permission.

(noncardiac, atypical, and typical), as shown in Table 1.4 [data combined with the CASS (22) trial]. In view of the pretest probability and the sensitivity and specificity of the specific stress employed, the posttest probability of significant CAD can be determined with reasonable accuracy.

Currently, there are five widely available stress tests: exercise treadmill testing (ETT), ETT with nuclear scintigraphy, ETT with echocardiography, vasodilator (dipyridamole or adenosine) nuclear scintigraphy, and inotropic (dobutamine) echocardiography. The tests can be divided into two groups: exercise (ETT, ETT-echocardiography, ETT-nuclear) and pharmacologic (dobutamine echocardiography, adenosine

or dipyridamole nuclear scintigraphy). The relative characteristics (23) of the various stress tests are summarized in Table 1.5.

In general, exercise tests are preferred over pharmacologic stress testing (e.g., dobutamine, adenosine, dipyridamole), because exercise is physiologic and provides important prognostic information. Furthermore, exercise testing objectively demonstrates whether the chest pain is exercise induced and at what level of exertion the chest pain is provoked. However, in order for an exercise test to have acceptable sensitivity for detecting significant CAD, the patient must be exercised to a workload of 6 metabolic equivalents of oxygen consumption (METS) and attain 85% of the maximum age-predicted heart rate. Exercise

TABLE 1.5. *Relative characteristics of*

Test	Sensitivity	Specificity	Sensitivity in single vessel disease	Sensitivity in multivessel disease	Relative cost	Assessment of LV ejection fraction
ETT	67	72	+	++	+++	No
ETT SPECT	89	76	++++	+++	−	Yes[a]
Adenosine SPECT	90	70	++++	+++	−	Yes[a]
ETT echocardiography	85	86	+++	++++	++	Yes
Dobutamine echocardiography	82	85	+++	++++	++	Yes

ECG, electrocardiogram; ETT, exercise treadmill testing; LV, left ventricular; SPECT, single photon emission computed tomography.
[a] Only if gated acquisitions available.
From Murthy TH, Bach DS. Comparative Review of Stress Tests. *Clinics in Family Practice* (in press). Copyright 2001, WB Saunders. Reproduced with permission.

tests are further divided into nonimaging (ETT) and imaging (ETT-echocardiography and ETT-nuclear). Imaging is generally indicated when the patient has an abnormal baseline ECG (resting ST segment depression, left bundle branch block, preexcitation, paced rhythm, and left ventricular hypertrophy), is taking digoxin, or has a history of previous coronary revascularization.

Pharmacologic stress testing is indicated for the evaluation of chest pain when the patient is unable to exercise adequately. In the United States, the choices for pharmacologic stress testing are either dobutamine echocardiography or vasodilator (adenosine or dipyridamole) nuclear scintigraphy. In general, the two tests have comparable sensitivities and specificities when performed in experienced laboratories. The choice of which type of test to order (echocardiography vs. nuclear scintigraphy) is largely a matter of physician's preference. However, each test has its own unique advantages and disadvantages. The advantages of echocardiography are its better specificity in hypertensive patients, better accuracy in women, lower cost, greater feasibility in the outpatient setting, faster turnaround times, and the ability to obtain concomitant anatomic and hemodynamic cardiovascular information. The disadvantages are the reduced feasibility and sensitivity in patients with poor echocardiographic image quality (caused by obesity and pulmonary disease) and reduced sensitivity for left circumflex artery disease. The advantages of nuclear scintigraphy are its superior resolution in predicting the location of a coronary artery stenosis and its greater availability and collective experience. The main disadvantage of nuclear scintigraphy is the decreased sensitivity for detecting balanced three-vessel and left main coronary artery disease. Ultimately, the decision of which type of imaging stress test to order (echocardiography vs. nuclear scintigraphy) is based on local expertise, test availability, and the patient's characteristics.

The evaluation of chest pain with stress testing requires the physician to temper the results of the stress test with the pretest probability of CAD. In patients with a high pretest probability of CAD, a negative stress test result should not lead the physician to falsely conclude that the patient does not have significant CAD. Instead, an alternative stress testing strategy or cardiac catheterization should be considered. Likewise, in patients with a very low pretest probability of CAD who have positive stress tests, the results should be interpreted in light of the known disadvantages of the particular stress test ordered and the overall cardiovascular status of the patient.

Pericarditis

The most important diagnostic test for pericarditis is the ECG. The diagnosis can be confirmed by serial ECGs demonstrating four classical stages. In Stage I, the ECG demonstrates ST segment elevation, which is concave upward and usually

various stress test modalities

Assessment of cardiac anatomy and function	Feasibility in outpatient	Feasibility in obese patients	Feasibility in severe pulmonary disease	Accuracy in women	Accuracy with hypertension	Appropriate with abnormal baseline ECG	Appropriate with concomitant digoxin therapy
No	+++	+++	+++	+	+	No	No
No	+	+++	+++	++	++	Yes	Yes
No	+	+++	++	++	++	Yes	Yes
Yes	+++	+	+	+	+++	Yes	Yes
Yes	++	++	++	+++	+++	Yes	Yes

present in all leads except V_1 and aV_R. The T waves are usually upright. The ST segment changes of acute pericarditis differ from acute myocardial infarction in that the ST segment elevation is concave upward, does not fit any particular coronary artery distribution, and lacks associated reciprocal ST segment depression. The first stage typically lasts for a few days before the Stage II changes evolve. In Stage II, the ST segments return to baseline and the T waves flatten. In contrast to acute myocardial infarction, the ST segments return to baseline before the T waves flatten. Stage III involves T wave inversion, and Stage IV represents normalization of the T waves. In addition to these changes, pericarditis is characterized by PR segment depression, which may be seen in Stages I and II. However, this classical evolution pattern is found in fewer than 50% of patients, and most patients present with some variant of the pattern just described.

The chest radiograph in pericarditis is usually unrevealing. If a significant pericardial effusion is present, cardiomegaly and a "water bottle" heart may also be present. An ECG should be obtained to quantify the pericardial effusion, rule out pericardial tamponade, and assess for concomitant myocarditis. The absence of a pericardial effusion does not rule out pericarditis.

Laboratory tests can be useful to confirm the presence and diagnose the cause of pericarditis. The erythrocyte sedimentation rate is typically elevated. Cardiac enzyme levels are usually normal, and elevation in troponin levels should suggest myocarditis. Causes of pericarditis and suggested laboratory tests include systemic lupus erythematosus [antinuclear antibodies (ANA), complements, and anti–double-stranded DNA antibodies], uremia [blood urea nitrogen (BUN)], and tuberculosis [purified protein derivative (PPD) and control skin tests].

Gastroesophageal Reflux Disease and Esophageal Spasm

A reasonable initial approach in patients with uncomplicated GERD or esophageal spasm (no dysphagia, weight loss, or hematemesis) is empirical therapy as a diagnostic modality. Empirical therapy should consist of behavioral modification (avoiding alcohol, cigarettes, caffeine, chocolate, heavy meals, or meals within a few hours before sleep) and drug therapy (H_2 blockers or proton pump inhibitors). Patients with complicated, severe, or unresponsive GERD and esophageal spasm should be referred to a gastrointestinal specialist.

Musculoskeletal Disorders

Diagnostic testing is generally not useful in this group. If trauma is suspected, then plain films specific to area of injury (e.g., rib fracture) should be considered.

Valvular Heart Disease and Hypertrophic Cardiomyopathy

Patients with significant aortic stenosis or hypertrophic cardiomyopathy probably have evidence of left ventricular hypertrophy on the ECG. The chest radiograph is rarely beneficial. All patients should undergo transthoracic echocardiography with Doppler examination.

In aortic stenosis, the echocardiogram allows for the anatomic assessment of the valve, which may be senile, calcific, congenital, or bicuspid. The peak, instantaneous, and mean gradients through the aortic valve can be assessed by Doppler echocardiography. The mean gradient by Doppler has been shown to have an excellent correlation with invasive measurements (24,25), except for a tendency to underestimate the valve area by Doppler echocardiography in mild aortic stenosis (24). However, the peak gradients obtained by the two techniques differ because echocardiography measures the peak, instantaneous gradient through the aortic valve, whereas cardiac catheterization measures a "peak-to-peak" gradient. Echocardiography is also useful for evaluating concomitant valve disease and left ventricular systolic function and hypertrophy. With the continuity equation, valve area can be calculated. If the aortic valve is poorly visualized by transthoracic imaging, transesophageal echocardiography may be used to obtain the aortic valve area by planimetry and Doppler gradients.

Echocardiography may be useful in diagnosing hypertrophic cardiomyopathy. Findings include systolic anterior motion of the anterior leaflet of the mitral valve into the left ventricular outflow tract, potentially causing a dynamic outflow tract obstruction, asymmetric or concentric left ventricular hypertrophy, and mitral regurgitation. However, the absence of the characteristic echocardiographic findings of hypertrophic cardiomyopathy does not rule out the diagnosis. ECG typically shows left ventricular hypertrophy.

INITIAL MANAGEMENT SCHEME

Management of chest pain is complicated by the broad range of origins and the need to rule out life-threatening causes. The physician needs to have a comprehensive and efficient plan for evaluating patients with chest pain. A suggested but not exhaustive chest pain evaluation scheme is presented in Figure 1.1. More detailed management strategies for unstable angina, stable angina, acute myocardial infarction, aortic dissection, pericarditis, and valvular heart disease are discussed in later chapters.

The first step in evaluating patients with chest pain is to take an expeditious history, perform a focused physical examination, and obtain an ECG. If a life-threatening cause (such as PE, aortic dissection, or acute coronary syndrome) is suspected, the patient should be transferred to an emergency room, placed on a cardiac monitor, and have initial laboratory tests, including measurements of cardiac enzymes.

If PE is suspected, a V/Q scan or helical CT should be ordered. If aortic dissection is suspected, anticoagulants should be avoided and a diagnostic test (CT, TEE, or MRI) ordered. If an acute coronary syndrome is suspected, aspirin should be administered unless contraindicated and an initial risk assessment performed. According to the American College of Cardiology/American Heart Association guidelines for the management of unstable angina (26), high-risk features of acute coronary syndrome include prolonged (more than 20 minutes) rest pain, age greater than 75 years, concomitant pulmonary edema, hypotension, transient ST segment changes (more than 0.05 mV), ventricular tachycardia, or markedly elevated cardiac enzymes. Intermediate risk factors include history of myocardial infarction, CABG, peripheral vascular obstructive disease, cerebrovascular obstructive disease, aspirin use, age greater than 70 years, prolonged but resolved ischemic chest pain (more than 20 minutes), T wave inversions, pathological Q waves, or slightly elevated cardiac enzyme levels. Patients who are at low risk and in whom acute myocardial infarction has been ruled out by cardiac enzyme measurements can safely undergo cardiac stress testing. Those at intermediate or high risk require ongoing management, which is discussed in later chapters.

If a clear, non–life-threatening cause of chest pain can be established by history, physical examination, and ECG, appropriate evaluation and treatment can be electively initiated. Patients with noncardiac chest pain can be monitored conservatively, depending on the cause. In those with pericarditis, serial ECGs (over days and weeks) may be obtained to follow the ECG course of the disease, and initial laboratory studies (e.g., erythrocyte sedimentation rate, troponin measurements) conducted. If myocarditis is suspected on the basis of either echocardiography or elevated cardiac enzyme levels, exercise should be proscribed and hospitalization considered. Patients with significant valvular heart disease, such as aortic stenosis, should undergo echocardiography to assess the anatomy, severity of disease, chamber sizes, and ventricular function. Patients with stable angina and without any recent history of unstable angina can be managed electively as well. If there is a high pretest probability of CAD and no need for risk assessment or prognostication, then empirical CAD therapy can be initiated without a stress test. Otherwise, stress testing should be electively performed to either confirm the diagnosis or provide risk assessment.

A challenging group of patients consists of those in whom a life-threatening cause of chest pain is not suspected and no clear diagnosis is established by history, physical examination, and ECG. This group comprises a large percentage of patients presenting for chest pain evaluation. The physician must balance the consequences

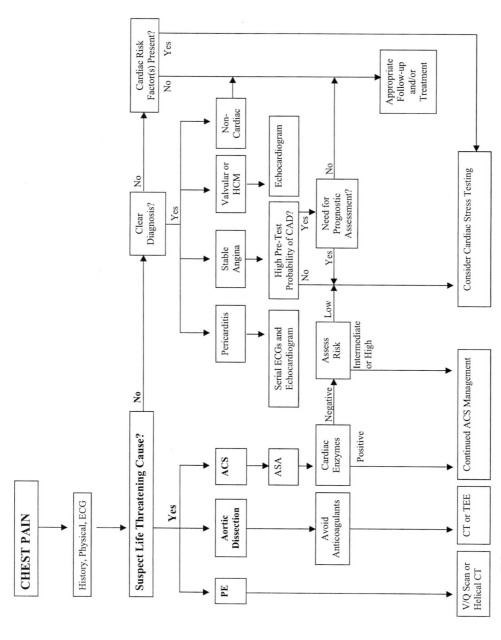

FIG. 1.1. Proposed algorithm for managing chest pain. The major branch point in decision-making is the clinical suspicion of a life-threatening cause of chest pain. ACS, acute coronary syndrome; ASA, aspirin; CAD, coronary artery disease; CT, computed tomography; ECG, electrocardiogram; HCM, hypertrophic cardiomyopathy; PE, pulmonary embolism; TEE, transesophageal echocardiogram; V/Q, ventilation perfusion.

TABLE 1.6. *Key points and recommendations for exercise testing in chest pain centers*

Which patients?	Acceptably safe in chest pain centers when they have been identified as "low risk/low likelihood" (by Goldman criteria) for having an acute coronary syndrome.
Clinical protocol	Must include serial clinical assessments, two negative cardiac enzymes drawn at 4-hour intervals, resting ECGs.
ECG	Exercise ECG testing can be used as first-line noninvasive testing when resting ECG is normal and the patient is not taking digoxin therapy.
Facility requirements	Should adhere to the guidelines of the American Heart Association. Exercise testing can safely performed by properly trained nurses, exercise physiologists, physical therapists, or medical technicians working directly under the supervision of a properly trained physician.
Supervision	A properly trained physician should be in the immediate vicinity and be available for emergencies. For higher risk patients, exercise testing should be directly supervised by the physician.
Exercise protocol	A Bruce treadmill protocol can be used. Elderly or deconditioned patients can be tested with less vigorous protocols such as Cornell, Naughton, ACIP, Balke, and ramp.
Adequacy of stress	The patient should attain 85% of the maximum age-predicted heart rate and accomplish at least 6 METS of workload (for patients >75 years of age, 4–5 METS is acceptable).
Prognosis	A negative test result will indicate a low probability of disease and good 30-day outcome in patients who initially have a low pretest probability of disease.
Limitations	Even with a negative exercise test result, a small number of low- to intermediate-risk patients will present in the next 30 days with acute myocardial infarction or a need for coronary revascularization.

ACIP, Advisory Committee on Immunization Practices; ECG, electroencephalogram; METS, metabolic equivalents (of oxygen consumption).

Adapted from Fletcher GF, Balady GJ, Amsterdam EA, Chaitman B, Eckel R, Fleg J, Froelicher VF, Leon AS, Pina IL, Rodney R, Simons-Morton DA, Williams MA, Bazzarre T. Exercise standards for testing and training: a statement for healthcare professionals from the American Heart Association. *Circulation* 2001;104:1694–1740.

of missing the diagnoses of acute myocardial infarction, PE, or aortic dissection against the need to utilize health care resources appropriately in managing a group of patients with an overall low risk of adverse outcomes. To advise physicians who manage patients in chest pain centers, the American Heart Association has published guidelines for performing exercise ECG testing in chest pain centers (27). The key points of the guidelines are summarized in Table 1.6. In general, patients without any cardiac risk factors and in whom the cause of the chest pain is not clear from history, physical examination, and ECG are at low risk for adverse cardiovascular outcomes and can be conservatively managed.

In summary, the initial management of chest pain patients involves ruling out life-threatening causes, establishing readily apparent diagnoses, determining prognosis, and determining which patients need evaluation for CAD. A systematic approach is necessary to avoid missing life-threatening causes while still efficiently utilizing vital health care resources. Although numerous clinical guidelines have been developed, ultimately the physician's individual judgment always remains the most important factor in managing chest pain.

PRACTICAL POINTS

- Many patients deny having "chest pain" on initial questioning but admit to "chest discomfort" upon further questioning.
- All patients with acute onset chest pain should undergo 12-lead ECG and be evaluated within 5 to 10 minutes of presentation.

(continued)

- A positive response to a "GI cocktail" should not routinely be used to rule acute coronary syndromes as an origin of chest pain.
- The principal life-threatening causes of chest pain are acute coronary syndromes, aortic dissection, and PE.
- The principal non–life-threatening causes of chest pain are stable angina, pericarditis, GERD, esophageal spasm, musculoskeletal disorders, valvular heart disease, and hypertrophic cardiomyopathy.
- The chest pain of acute coronary syndromes has a broad overlap with the chest pain of non–life-threatening causes of the pain.

- The most common characteristic of chest pain in aortic dissection is its sudden onset.
- Aortic dissection has an extremely high mortality rate, and its diagnosis requires a high degree of clinical suspicion on the physician's part.
- The initial management of acute chest pain involves performing ECG, obtaining a focused history and physical examination, deciding whether the patient may have a life-threatening cause, and evaluating the patient for high-risk features.
- A positive stress test result in a patient with a low pretest probability of CAD may just as likely be a false positive as a true positive result.

REFERENCES

1. American Heart Association. *1999 Heart and stroke statistical update.* Dallas: American Heart Association, 1999.
2. Gibbons RJ, Chatterjee K, Daley J, et al. ACC/AHA/ACP-ASIM guidelines for the management of patients with chronic stable angina: executive summary and recommendations. A Report of the American College of Cardiology/American Heart Association Task Force on Practice Guidelines (Committee on Management of Patients with Chronic Stable Angina). *Circulation* 1999;99:2829–2848.
3. Nourjah P. *National Hospital Ambulatory Medical Care Survey: 1997 emergency department summary.* [Advance data no. 304] Hyattsville, MD: National Center for Health Statistics, 1999:1–24.
4. Campeau L. Letter: Grading of angina pectoris. *Circulation* 1976;54:522–523.
5. Braunwald E, Jones RH, Mark DB, et al. Diagnosing and managing unstable angina. Agency for Health Care Policy and Research. *Circulation* 1994;90:613–622.
6. Slater EE, DeSanctis RW. The clinical recognition of dissecting aortic aneurysm. *Am J Med* 1976;60:625–633.
7. Hagan PG, Nienaber CA, Isselbacher EM, et al. The International Registry of Acute Aortic Dissection (IRAD): new insights into an old disease. *JAMA* 2000;283:897–903.
8. Bell WR, Simon TL, DeMets DL. The clinical features of submassive and massive pulmonary emboli. *Am J Med* 1977;62:355–360.
9. Braunwald E. Valvular heart disease. In: Braunwald E, ed. *Heart disease: a textbook of cardiovascular medicine,* 5th ed. Philadelphia: WB Saunders, 1997:1007–1076.
10. Wynne J, Braunwald E. The cardiomyopathies and myocarditides. In: Braunwald E, ed. *Heart disease: a textbook of cardiovascular medicine,* 5th ed. Philadelphia: WB Saunders, 1997:1404–1463.
11. Varetto T, Cantalupi D, Altieri A, et al. Emergency room technetium-99m sestamibi imaging to rule out acute myocardial ischemic events in patients with nondiagnostic electrocardiograms. *J Am Coll Cardiol* 1993;22:1804–1808.
12. Weissman IA, Dickinson CZ, Dworkin HJ, et al. Cost-effectiveness of myocardial perfusion imaging with SPECT in the emergency department evaluation of patients with unexplained chest pain. *Radiology* 1996;199:353–357.
13. Hilton TC, Fulmer H, Abuan T, et al. Ninety-day follow-up of patients in the emergency department with chest pain who undergo initial single-photon emission computed tomographic perfusion scintigraphy with technetium 99m-labeled sestamibi. *J Nuclear Cardiol* 1996;3:308–311.
14. Mather PJ, Shah R. Echocardiography, nuclear scintigraphy, and stress testing in the emergency department evaluation of acute coronary syndrome. *Emerg Med Clin North Am* 2001;19:339–349.
15. Nielsen TT, Lund O, Ronne K, et al. Changing electrocardiographic findings in pulmonary embolism in relation to vascular obstruction. *Cardiology* 1989;76:274–284.
16. Indik JH, Alpert JS. Detection of pulmonary embolism by D-dimer assay, spiral computed tomography, and magnetic resonance imaging. *Progr Cardiovasc Dis* 2000;42:261–272.
17. Meaney JF, Weg JG, Chenevert TL, et al. Diagnosis of pulmonary embolism with magnetic resonance angiography [see comments]. *N Engl J Med* 1997;336:1422–1427.
18. Grifoni S, Olivotto I, Cecchini P, et al. Utility of an integrated clinical, echocardiographic, and venous ultrasonographic approach for triage of patients with suspected pulmonary embolism. *Am J Cardiol* 1998;82:1230–1235.
19. Grifoni S, Olivotto I, Cecchini P, et al. Short-term clinical

outcome of patients with acute pulmonary embolism, normal blood pressure, and echocardiographic right ventricular dysfunction. *Circulation* 2000;101:2817–2822.

20. Todhunter I. *A history of the mathematical theory of probability.* London: Macmillan, 1865.

21. Diamond GA, Forrester JS. Analysis of probability as an aid in the clinical diagnosis of coronary-artery disease. *N Engl J Med* 1979;300:1350–1358.

22. Chaitman BR, Bourassa MG, Davis K, et al. Angiographic prevalence of high-risk coronary artery disease in patient subsets (CASS). *Circulation* 1981;64:360–367.

23. Murthy TH, Bach DS. Comparative review of stress tests. *Clin Family Pract* (in press).

24. Danielsen R, Nordrehaug JE, Vik-Mo H. Factors affecting Doppler echocardiographic valve area assessment in aortic stenosis. *Am J Cardiol* 1989;63:1107–1111.

25. Oh JK, Taliercio CP, Holmes DR, et al. Prediction of the severity of aortic stenosis by Doppler aortic valve area determination: prospective Doppler-catheterization correlation in 100 patients. *J Am Coll Cardiol* 1988;11:1227–1234.

26. Braunwald E, Antman EM, Beasley JW, et al. ACC/AHA guidelines for the management of patients with unstable angina and non–ST-segment elevation myocardial infarction. A report of the American College of Cardiology/American Heart Association Task Force on Practice Guidelines (Committee on the Management of Patients With Unstable Angina). *J Am Coll Cardiol* 2000;36:970–1062.

27. Fletcher GF, Balady GJ, Amsterdam EA, et al. Exercise standards for testing and training: a statement for healthcare professionals from the American Heart Association. *Circulation* 2001;104:1694–1740.

2

Dyspnea

Fernando J. Martinez and Keith D. Aaronson

DEFINITION

Dyspnea has been variously described as the sensation of breathlessness or of difficult or uncomfortable breathing. One consensus statement defined dyspnea as "... a term used to characterize a subjective experience of breathing discomfort that consists of qualitatively distinct sensations that vary in intensity. The experience arises from interactions among multiple physiological, psychological, social, and environmental factors and may induce secondary physiological and behavioral responses" (1). Some degree of dyspnea is normal at high altitude or in the context of vigorous exercise; dyspnea is abnormal when it occurs at levels of activity and in environmental circumstances for which normal individuals would not be breathless. The severity of dyspnea that an individual experiences for a given activity appears to be related to the level of ventilation required for that activity in relation to the ventilatory capacity of the individual.

Breathlessness is an extremely common complaint. In one large study of medical outpatients, it was the third most frequent complaint, following only fatigue and back pain (2). Dyspnea is the usual presenting symptom for some of the most common chronic conditions afflicting Americans, including chronic obstructive lung disease (14 million people), asthma (10 million individuals), and heart failure (5 million Americans). It is a prominent symptom in nearly all other pulmonary disorders and may be the presenting symptom in patients with coronary artery disease.

USUAL CAUSES

Dyspnea can be divided into acute and chronic dyspnea. Acute dyspnea develops over minutes to days. It usually results from an acute cardiovascular or pulmonary process and, as such, mandates urgent diagnostic evaluation and treatment. Cardiovascular conditions precipitating acute dyspnea include myocardial or valvular abnormalities that cause pulmonary edema (e.g., myocardial ischemia or infarction, acute mitral or aortic regurgitation), hypertensive urgency or emergency, pericardial tamponade, and pulmonary artery thromboembolism. Pulmonary abnormalities include pneumonia, asthma or other reactive airway disease, pneumothorax, upper airway obstruction, or diffuse lung injury as a manifestation of the systemic inflammatory response syndrome. Overdoses of aspirin or ethylene glycol may cause dyspnea by direct stimulation of the respiratory center. Fortunately, the cause of acute dyspnea can usually be determined from a history, a physical examination, basic laboratory studies, a chest radiograph, and an electrocardiogram, with other testing as indicated [e.g., cardiac enzyme levels for myocardial infarction, ventilation/perfusion lung scanning for pulmonary embolism, transesophageal echocardiography for proximal aortic dissection with aortic insufficiency, and peak flow for acute airway disease (3)]. The evaluation and management of the cardiovascular disorders are discussed elsewhere in this text.

Chronic dyspnea (symptoms present for at least a month) often represents a greater diagnostic challenge and is the focus of the remainder of this chapter. Table 2.1 provides a pathophysiologic framework for the causes of chronic dyspnea, along with specific examples. The causes can be conveniently divided into those characterized by impaired cardiovascular function, by impaired pulmonary function, or by abnormally altered central ventilatory drive or perception.

TABLE 2.1. *Pathophysiologic framework for chronic dyspnea, with specific examples*

Category	Example
Impaired cardiovascular function	
Myocardial disease	
Systolic dysfunction	Ischemic cardiomyopathy
	Nonischemic cardiomyopathies
Diastolic dysfunction	Hypertensive heart disease
	Coronary artery disease
	Hypertrophic cardiomyopathy
	Restrictive cardiomyopathy
Valvular disease	Aortic or mitral regurgitation
	Aortic or mitral stenosis
Pericardial disease	Constrictive pericarditis
Pulmonary vascular disease	Pulmonary thromboembolism
	Primary pulmonary hypertension
Congenital anomalies	Cyanotic heart diseases (right-to-left shunts)
Impaired pulmonary function	
Airflow obstruction	
Diffuse	Asthma
	COPD
Focal	Vocal cord dysfunction or paralysis
	Tracheal stenosis
	Endobronchial tumor
Restriction of lung mechanics	
Interstitial lung disease	Idiopathic pulmonary fibrosis
	Pneumoconioses
	Lymphangitic carcinomatosis
Extrapulmonary thoracic restriction	Kyphoscoliosis
	Pleural effusion or fibrosis
Neuromuscular weakness	Phrenic nerve paralysis
	Spinal cord injury
	Amyotrophic lateral sclerosis
Abnormal gas exchange	
Abnormal alveoli/capillary interface	Eosinophilic pneumonia
Right to left shunting	Pulmonary arteriovenous malformations
Altered central ventilatory drive or perception	
Systemic or metabolic disorders	
Increased metabolic requirements	Hyperthyroidism
	Obesity
Decreased oxygen-carrying capacity	Anemias
Metabolic acidosis	Renal failure
	Mitochondrial myopathies
Direct stimulation of respiratory center	Aspirin or ethylene glycol overdose
Physiologic processes causing dyspnea	
Vigorous exercise	
Pregnancy	
Hypoxic breathing at high altitude	
Deconditioning	

COPD; chronic obstructive pulmonary disease.
Adapted from Sietsema K: Approach to the patient with dyspnea. In Humes HD (ed) *Kelley's Textbook of Medicine,* 4th ed. Philadelphia, Lippincott Williams & Wilkins, 2000.

Impaired Cardiovascular Function

Any condition that increases left atrial pressure results in a concomitant rise in pulmonary venous pressure, with vascular congestion and decreased pulmonary compliance. Left atrial pressure rises in patients with elevated left ventricular end-diastolic pressure, whether the latter results from systolic dysfunction (e.g., ischemic or nonischemic cardiomyopathies), diastolic dysfunction (e.g., hypertensive heart disease with left ventricular hypertrophy, hypertrophic cardiomyopathy, or restrictive cardiomyopathy), or an obstruction to left atrial emptying (e.g., mitral stenosis). More profound or acute elevations in pulmonary venous pressure lead to alveolar filling with impaired gas exchange and arterial hypoxemia. Bronchial hyperresponsiveness (i.e., "cardiac asthma") occurs in some individuals in this setting. If the ability to increase cardiac output with exercise is reduced (e.g., left ventricular systolic dysfunction, aortic stenosis), oxygen delivery is compromised and lactic acidosis occurs prematurely. Ventilation must increase to eliminate the excess acid, and this may result in dyspnea, even in the absence of pulmonary congestion.

Coronary artery disease (CAD) is an important and often unrecognized cause of dyspnea in patients with *normal* left ventricular systolic function at rest. Chest pain may be absent in such patients (e.g., many diabetics), for whom dyspnea is the "anginal equivalent." Transient ischemia resulting from increased metabolic demand, heightened coronary vascular tone, or coronary microthrombi may cause papillary muscle dysfunction with acute mitral regurgitation, systolic dysfunction, or diastolic dysfunction.

Dyspnea is a prominent symptom in patients with pericardial and pulmonary vascular disease, even when oxygenation and lung mechanics are normal. The mechanism underlying dyspnea in these settings probably is related to activation of stretch receptors or baroreceptors in the central circulation.

Congenital cardiac anomalies may also manifest with dyspnea. Anatomic abnormalities resulting in right-to-left shunts cause hypoxemia. This stimulates arterial chemoreceptors, which in turn activate respiratory control centers to increase ventilation. Left-to-right shunts, if sufficiently large, will over time result in left ventricular volume overload and progressive systolic dysfunction. In some patients, increased flow though the pulmonary vasculature results in adverse pulmonary vascular remodeling and consequent pulmonary hypertension.

Impaired Pulmonary Function

Conditions that obstruct airflow, whether diffuse [e.g., asthma, chronic obstructive pulmonary disease (COPD)] or focal (e.g., vocal cord paralysis, tracheal stenosis, endobronchial tumor), result in dyspnea. Increased work of breathing is typically noted in these conditions. Heterogenous reduction of airflow, when present, results in regional ventilation/perfusion mismatching, with consequent hypoxemia and increased ventilatory requirements. However, ventilatory muscle fatigue and air trapping reduce ventilatory capacity.

Restriction of lung mechanics may result from abnormalities of the lung parenchyma (e.g., idiopathic pulmonary fibrosis), pleural disease, skeletal abnormalities (e.g., kyphoscoliosis), or neuromuscular disorders. The reduction in ventilatory capacity may be exacerbated by an increase in ventilatory requirements that results from ventilation/perfusion mismatching. Abnormal gas exchange may result from abnormalities of the alveolar/capillary interface or from pulmonary right-to-left shunting.

**Altered Central Ventilatory Drive
or Perception**

Hyperthyroidism and obesity increase respiratory drive because of increased metabolic requirements. Anemic patients have reduced oxygen-carrying capacity, which, when severe, raises the respiratory rate. The lactic acidosis accompanying renal failure and mitochondrial myopathies results in compensatory respiratory alkalosis. Respiratory drive is directly stimulated in aspirin toxicity and is a response to the metabolic acidosis that occurs in this setting, as well.

The prevalence of the aforementioned conditions in patients presenting for evaluation of dyspnea probably depends on the patient sample, physician type, and practice setting. Three studies (4–6) have catalogued the causes of chronic dyspnea and their frequencies in referral samples (Table 2.2). It is evident that airway diseases, such as asthma or COPD, represented the majority of cases, followed by cardiac disease, interstitial lung disease, deconditioning, psychogenic disorders, gastroesophageal reflux, neuromuscular disease, and pulmonary vascular disease. Referral bias may have influenced these studies, inasmuch as they all originated from pulmonary referral clinics. Cardiologists would probably identify a higher proportion of cardiovascular disease in their practices. Unfortunately, similar data are not available for cardiology or primary care practices.

KEYS TO HISTORY

An evaluation of the patient should always begin with a detailed history, which in turn begins with the timing of symptoms. An intermittent, acute onset may suggest bronchoconstriction, pulmonary embolism, cardiac ischemia, or airway obstruction caused by foreign body or secretion. In contrast, chronic dyspnea is more likely to reflect slowly progressive disorders such as COPD, congestive heart failure (CHF), or interstitial lung disease.

Precipitating factors, such as the type of activities that causes exertional breathlessness, may provide diagnostic value. Because patients frequently reduce their activity level as disease severity progresses, it is important to inquire about both past and present activity levels.

Positional dyspnea may be a useful historical feature. Orthopnea (dyspnea in the supine position) is most common in patients with CHF, severe COPD, ascites, obesity, anterior mediastinal masses, and respiratory muscle weakness. Trepopnea (dyspnea in one lateral position but not in the other) can be seen with patients with unilateral lung disease, unilateral pleural effusion, and unilateral obstruction of the airway. Platypnea (dyspnea in the upright position, which may be relieved by recumbence) can be seen in patients with an intracardiac shunt, parenchymal lung shunts, or hepatopulmonary syndrome.

Associated symptoms, such as cough or wheezing, can provide additional information in the differential diagnosis. The presence of cough may support a diagnosis of airway disease, interstitial lung disease, gastroesophageal reflux disease, or CHF. Similarly, wheezing may suggest airway disease, COPD, or CHF. Inquiries about past medical history, concurrent conditions, previous surgical procedures, social information (including cigarette smoking, previous and current occupations, family or living status),

TABLE 2.2. *Etiology of chronic dyspnea in three series of patients studied in tertiary pulmonary clinics*

Study	Number (%) of patients
Pratter et al. (4)	
Asthma	25 (29)
COPD	12 (14)
Interstitial lung disease	12 (14)
Cardiomyopathy	9 (11)
Upper airway disease	7 (8)
Psychogenic disorders	4 (5)
Deconditioning	4 (5)
Gastroesophageal reflux	3 (4)
Extrapulmonary disease	3 (4)
Miscellaneous	5 (6)
DePaso et al. (5)	
Asthma	12 (17)
Interstitial lung disease	2 (3)
Chronic obstructive disease	3 (4)
Pulmonary vascular disease	4 (6)
Neuromuscular disease	3 (4)
Cardiac disease	10 (14)
Hyperventilation syndrome	14 (19)
Thyroid disease	2 (3)
Gastroesophageal reflux	3 (4)
Deconditioning	2 (3)
Upper airway disease	2 (3)
Miscellaneous	1 (1)
Unexplained	14 (19)
Martinez et al. (6)	
Asthma	12 (24)
Interstitial lung disease	4 (8)
Cardiac disease	7 (14)
Deconditioning	14 (28)
Psychogenic disorders	9 (18)
Gastroesophageal reflux	1 (2)
Unexplained	7 (14)
Miscellaneous	1 (2)

COPD, chronic obstructive pulmonary disease.

and medication history are essential and equally important.

The patient should also be questioned about the quality of the respiratory discomfort. Studies have shown that different descriptors of dyspnea exist in patients with various cardiopulmonary diseases (7,8). Table 2.3 demonstrates the clustering of such descriptors with varying cardiopulmonary disorders from one such study (8). A preliminary report about 11 patients suggested benefit from the use of such a descriptor model in determining the origin of dyspnea (9). The value of this form of evaluation in the assessment of patients presenting with breathlessness requires further prospective validation.

PHYSICAL EXAMINATION

A detailed and directed physical examination, with special attention to the cardiovascular and pulmonary system, is essential. The "view from the door" should take in the extent of respiratory distress (e.g., tachypnea, use of accessory muscles, fatigue). The vital signs may give additional diagnostic clues. A paradoxical pulse is seen with airway obstruction and pericardial tamponade. A weak or alternans pulse suggests severe heart failure. A wide pulse pressure with a bounding, "water-hammer" pulse is associated with aortic insufficiency, whereas a *bisferiens* pulse is seen with the obstructive variant of hypertrophic cardiomyopathy.

The jugular veins should be assessed for elevation (e.g., heart failure, pericardial disease), contours (e.g., V waves of tricuspid regurgitation), and response to the respiratory cycle (e.g., Kussmaul's sign in constrictive pericarditis, pericardial tamponade, or right-sided heart failure). Carotid bruits may be evidence of associated CAD.

Respiratory excursions should be examined for symmetry and adequacy. Rapid, shallow breathing may suggest interstitial lung disease or neuromuscular disease. A fixed level of asymmetric dullness with decreased breath sounds in a patient who has undergone recent coronary bypass surgery suggests phrenic nerve injury or a persistent postoperative pleural effusion. Auscultation may reveal wet (e.g., as in CHF) or

TABLE 2.3. *Relation between the description of the sensation of dyspnea and the etiology of the breathlessness*

Descriptions	Pathologic condition
My breathing requires effort. My breathing is heavy. My breathing requires more work. I feel a hunger for more air. I feel out of breath. I cannot get enough air. I am gasping for breath.	COPD
My breathing requires more work. I feel a hunger for more air. I feel out of breath. I cannot get enough air. I am gasping for breath. My breathing does not go out all the way.	Asthma
My breathing requires effort. I feel out of breath. My breathing requires work. I am gasping for breath. My breathing is shallow.	Interstitial lung disease
My breathing requires effort. My breathing is heavy. I feel a hunger for more air. I feel out of breath. I cannot get enough air. I feel that I am smothering. I feel that I am suffocating. I feel that my breathing is rapid.	Congestive heart failure
My breathing does not go in all the way. My breathing requires effort. My breathing is heavy. I am gasping for breath. My breathing require more work. My breathing is shallow.	Neuromuscular disease
My breathing does not go in all the way. I feel that my breathing is rapid.	Pulmonary vascular disease
I feel that I am breathing more.	Deconditioning

COPD, chronic obstructive pulmonary disease.
Data from Simon PM, Schwartzstein RM, Weiss JW, et al. Distinguishable types of dyspnea in patients with shortness of breath [see comments]. *Am Rev Respir Dis* 1990;142:1009–1014.

dry (e.g., as in interstitial lung disease) crackles, wheezing (as in intrathoracic airway obstruction), or stridor (as in extrathoracic airway obstruction).

In an examination of the heart, the physician should seek evidence of left or right ventricular enlargement. Rhythm abnormalities heighten suspicion for cardiac disease, although atrial premature complexes and multifocal atrial tachycardia are common in patients with severe COPD (reflecting the impact of the latter on the right side of the heart). Special attention should be paid to the intensity of the second heart sound: if it is louder than the first heart sound at the left lower sternal border, the pulmonary artery systolic pressure is at least 45 mm HG; if it is louder than the first heart sound over the left ventricular apex, the pressure is at least 60 mm HG. A fourth heart sound may be evidence of diastolic dysfunction from hypertensive heart disease. Patients with severe heart failure often have a palpable and audible third heart sound, but patients with mild or moderate heart failure rarely do. The reader is directed to the appropriate sections of this text for a discussion of dynamic auscultation for murmurs of valvular heart disease.

Other organ systems pertinent to the history should also be investigated with equal sensitivity.

HELPFUL DIAGNOSTIC TESTS

Blood Testing

Simple blood tests, including a basic metabolic panel, complete blood cell count, and thyroid function tests, are helpful in evaluating basic systemic disorders related to dyspnea. A complete blood cell count is used to identify the presence of anemia. Renal dysfunction should prompt consideration of the connective tissue diseases and vasculitides that affect the lungs and kidneys. Thyroid function testing may uncover hyperthyroidism or hypothyroidism. Hyperthyroid individuals have excessive ventilation with exercise (10), hypothyroid patients may experience reversible diaphragmatic dysfunction (11), and either condition may reduce cardiac contractility. Dyspnea can be seen with either form of thyroid disease.

Chest Radiography

Chest radiography is an important part of the initial workup. It reveals evidence of pneumothorax, hyperinflation, interstitial fibrosis, or pulmonary edema. Cardiac enlargement, enlarged pulmonary arteries (e.g., pulmonary hypertension), and elevated hemidiaphragms (e.g., respiratory muscle weakness or phrenic nerve palsies) may be seen. However, the insensitivity of the technique should be kept in mind. Fibrotic lung disease, for example, may be "invisible" on chest radiographs but clearly manifest on pulmonary function tests and high-resolution computed tomography (CT) (12,13). Therefore, the absence of prominent changes on chest radiographs should not be used alone to rule out the presence of a disorder.

Further Diagnostic Testing

Because of the prevalence of respiratory disease in patients with dyspnea, limited pulmonary function testing [e.g., spirometry with a flow-volume loop and measurement of diffusion capacity (DL_{CO})] has a major role in the evaluation of dyspnea. Most authors suggest that this is an essential test for all dyspneic patients, in view of the predominance of respiratory disorders in the published series. However, we temper this recommendation with the knowledge that all these series originated from pulmonary referral centers and reflect an inherent referral bias. Certainly, patients in whom there is a high index of suspicion for cardiac disorders (e.g., older patients with CAD risk factors or those with exertional chest pain, electrocardiographic evidence of acute or chronic coronary disease, or obvious physical findings of heart failure) can undergo testing and therapeutic trials directed at these processes, with pulmonary function tests reserved for patients with inconclusive test results or inadequate therapeutic responses. In the absence of a high index of suspicion for a cardiac disorder or when pulmonary disease is suspected, pulmonary function testing is the next logical step.

High Suspicion for Cardiovascular Disease

Surface echocardiography with Doppler studies is indicated for evaluation of possible systolic or diastolic heart failure, valvular heart disease, or pericardial disease. In general, this test is preferable to radionuclide ventriculography (it provides more information about valvular, pericardial, and diastolic abnormalities) and radionuclide single photon emission CT (SPECT) perfusion imaging (see later discussion).

If CAD is suspected, stress testing is warranted. Treadmill testing without imaging certainly confirms an early onset of exertional dyspnea, if present, but many affected patients fail to achieve an adequate double product [i.e., (peak systolic blood pressure × peak heart rate)/100], which renders this test's sensitivity and specificity inadequate for detection of CAD in this setting. Therefore, most patients in whom CAD is suspected as the cause of dyspnea require pharmacologic stress testing with echocardiographic or radionuclide perfusion imaging. Both techniques have excellent sensitivity and specificity in most patients when performed in experienced laboratories, and the choice of modalities is often guided by local expertise. Echocardiography allows concomitant evaluation of left ventricular function, valvular abnormalities, pulmonary hypertension, and pericardial disease and is preferable in patients with left bundle branch block. Radionuclide imaging with sestamibi (but not with thallium) also affords an evaluation of left ventricular function (i.e., gated SPECT) and is preferable in patients in whom echocardiographic images are likely to be of poor quality(e.g., severely obese patients).

Echocardiography can be combined with dobutamine imaging as the initial test to evaluate CAD as the cause of systolic or diastolic dysfunction when the suspicion for CAD is high. Another option would be surface echocardiography, followed by coronary angiography, or coronary angiography combined with contrast-enhanced left ventriculography in patients with obvious coronary disease.

It is important to be aware of the high prevalence of heart failure in older individuals. In an ambulatory practice and inpatient service of a Department of Family Medicine in a university setting, the frequency of CHF increased with age (14). In fact, 74% of the patients were older than 65 years. Interestingly, 40% of the patients had preserved systolic function; this was more common in women. Diastolic heart failure is particularly more common in the presence of hypertension, diabetes mellitus, obesity, or valvular disease (15). Thus, older patients may be best evaluated with specific functional cardiac studies early in the evaluation process.

Further discussion of the relative merits and interpretation of echocardiography and radionuclide imaging studies, with and without exercise or pharmacologic "stress," is available in other chapters of this text.

Other Patients

Pulmonary function testing is the next diagnostic step in most patients with unexplained dyspnea. Spirometric tracings should be examined to make sure that they meet with the "acceptability" and "reproducibility" criteria suggested by the American Thoracic Society (1). Spirometric testing that does not adhere to these guidelines can lead to significant errors in diagnosis or choices of unnecessary diagnostic tests. Spirometry can be used to determine and define the functional type of respiratory abnormality. The diagnosis of airflow obstruction is confirmed by a decreased ratio of forced expiratory volume in 1 second (FEV_1) to forced vital capacity (FVC). Once a diagnosis of airflow obstruction is made, no further diagnostic evaluation is immediately warranted. During a therapeutic course for obstructive lung disease, further spirometric testing is helpful for assessing response to treatment. If dyspnea persists despite response to therapy, or if there is no objective response to therapy, then further diagnostic evaluation is required. A reduced FVC accompanied by a normal ratio of FEV_1 to FVC is suggestive, but not definitively diagnostic, of restrictive lung disease. Further pursuit of restrictive lung disease requires measurement of lung volumes (16).

Important information can also be obtained by examining the flow-volume curve. For example, in upper airway obstruction, a flattening of either inspiratory or expiratory flow-volume curve or of both may be noted. These flow-volume curves may also be helpful in determining patient effort and intent in the performance of the procedure.

Certain changes in the flow-volume loop and in the volume-time curve (such as short expiratory time or staggering of the expiratory loop) may suggest poor effort or potential malingering.

The DL_{CO} is measured to assess the ability of the alveolar-arterial interface to transfer gas without limitation (17). Decreases in DL_{CO} can reflect destruction of lung parenchyma, changes in the interface secondary to fibrosis or inflammation, loss of pulmonary vascular area, or anemia. Increases can reflect alveolar hemorrhage, polycythemia, or altitude adjustments. It may be useful to identify an isolated reduction in DL_{CO}, which may be suggestive of several possible causes of dyspnea (17).

The measurement of maximal inspiratory and expiratory pressures during pulmonary function testing is a useful tool in the screening of respiratory muscle function. In patients with neuromuscular disease, the earliest physiologic abnormalities are decreases in respiratory pressures measured at the mouth (18). Syndromes of respiratory muscle weakness may be uncovered with this simple test. Unfortunately, in the setting of dyspnea, the sensitivity and specificity of this test are unknown. The measurement of maximum voluntary ventilation can serve as an additional surrogate measurement of impaired respiratory muscle function (19). Some investigators have suggested that an isolated decrement in maximal ventilatory volume (MVV), in comparison with that expected for a measured FEV_1, can identify patients with mitochondrial myopathy (20). Unfortunately, the effort dependence of MVV measurement limits the diagnostic accuracy of this diagnostic study.

Subsequent Diagnostic Testing

Unfortunately, the initial evaluation of dyspnea may not lead to a specific single diagnosis, and the findings will suggest a course for further evaluation. Figure 2.1 demonstrates a potential subsequent approach to the patient with dyspnea. If the initial evaluation suggests a cardiac cause, then further cardiac testing is warranted. Similarly, if initial testing demonstrates pulmonary abnormalities, then further pulmonary function

testing can be devised. For example, the evaluation of a decreased MVV should include assessment of upper airway abnormalities (21) and potential neuromuscular disease (19). A suspicion of restriction shown on spirometry is best evaluated by the evaluation of lung volume by body plethysmography or by gas dilution techniques (16). These procedures also give a clear assessment of the severity of the disorder.

An isolated decrease in DL_{CO} can be evaluated with cardiac testing (echocardiography for pulmonary hypertension) (22), diagnostic imaging for parenchymal disease (high-resolution CT for fibrotic or emphysematous lung disease) (23,24), or imaging for recurrent pulmonary emboli. The most appropriate diagnostic approach in a dyspneic patient with an isolated reduction in DL_{CO} is debatable; in part, modification tailored to the expertise of the evaluating institution is required.

If this initial evaluation does not suggest a clear-cut cardiac or respiratory disorder, further testing is probably required. This can proceed with pulmonary function testing or specific cardiovascular testing, depending on the clinical scenario. For example, in a young individual, particularly in the setting of intermittent breathlessness and normal initial pulmonary testing, bronchoprovocation challenge (BPC) is probably the best approach, because of the increased likelihood of hyperactive airway disease in this setting (5). BPC is very sensitive for airway hyperreactivity but is not specific for the diagnosis of asthma (25); disorders such as sinusitis and recent viral or pulmonary infections can cause a positive result on a methacholine challenge test (26,27). However, in the series of Martinez et al. (6), BPC testing was helpful in identifying airway hyperreactivity in patients with a median age of 54 years. Further research is necessary to better define the role of BPC in the evaluation of unexplained dyspnea.

Cardiopulmonary Exercise Testing (CPET)

Cardiopulmonary exercise testing is a diagnostic modality in which the examiner utilizes the measurement of oxygen uptake, carbon dioxide

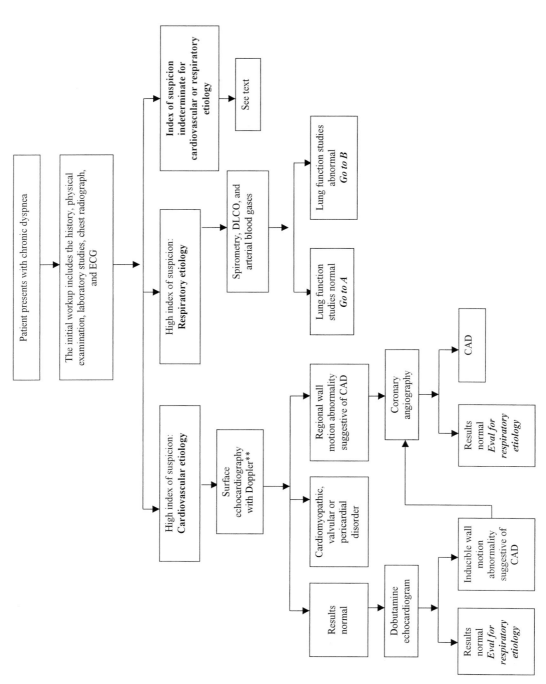

FIG. 2.1. Evaluation for patients presenting with chronic dyspnea. If there is a high index of suspicion for coronary artery disease, a dobutamine echocardiogram may be the initial test.

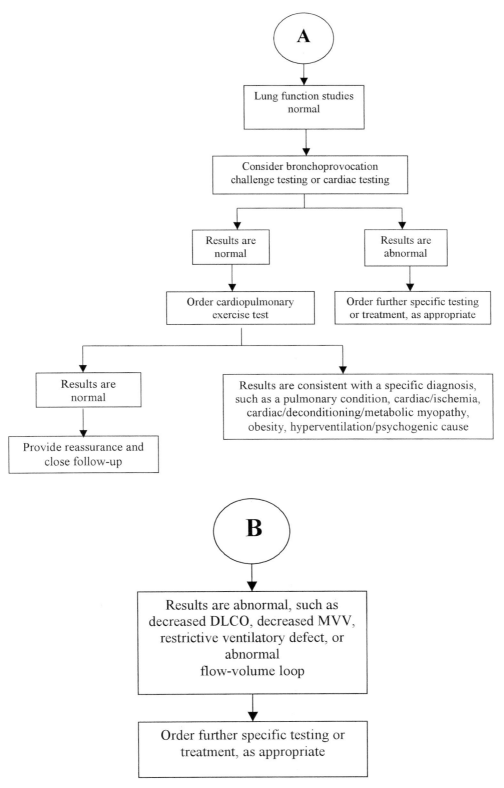

FIG. 2.1. *Continued.*

output, and minute ventilation while also monitoring electrocardiography, pulse oximetry, and symptoms during a maximal symptom-limited exercise tolerance test (28). Appropriate analysis of the patterns of response can suggest various disorders that can contribute to the sensation of breathlessness. A detailed discussion of the interpretation of these studies is out of the scope of this chapter. Readers are referred to excellent reviews of the topic (28,29). Figure 2.2 demonstrates possible diagnostic categories derived from CPET in patients evaluated for dyspnea, which makes it a key diagnostic study in the evaluation of patients with unexplained dyspnea (30,31). A completely normal study finding does not exclude early disease but should serve to reassure the patient that a major disorder is probably not present.

Most patients with psychogenic dyspnea have a normal response to exercise, although an erratic pattern of ventilation may be suggestive (31). Similarly, a hyperventilation syndrome (32) may be suggested during CPET, although this diagnosis is generally one of exclusion. Abnormal electrocardiographic tracings can suggest the presence of ischemic heart disease, although other findings on CPET are nonspecific. For example, one prospective study has demonstrated the similar responses of patients with deconditioning and those with nonischemic heart disease (6). In addition, data suggest a similar hyperdynamic and hyperventilatory response in patients with histologically or enzymatically confirmed mitochondrial disease (20,33).

CPET can be used to identify potential pulmonary disorders in patients with dyspnea. Measurement of arterial blood gases can provide useful information in identifying parenchymal lung disease (changes in PaO_2 and $P(A-a)O_2$) (34,35) or pulmonary vascular disease [pulmonary dead space (V_D/V_T) abnormality] (28). A low DL_{CO} appears to identify a group of patients more likely to demonstrate abnormal gas exchange during CPET (36). Those patients may be best assessed with collection of arterial blood samples during exercise testing.

Additional data collected during or after CPET may provide valuable diagnostic information. Measurement of pleural and diaphragmatic pressures can identify unexpected respiratory muscle dysfunction (37). Serial spirometry after exercise may identify patients with exercise-induced bronchospasm, although its sensitivity is clearly less than that of other forms of bronchoprovocation testing (38). Nevertheless, in view of its simplicity, spirometry should be performed routinely after maximal exercise testing. The addition of tidal flow-volume loop analysis may improve diagnostic accuracy, although specific data are lacking (39). Examination of vocal cord function during exercise or of flow-volume loops during and after exercise may identify patients with vocal cord dysfunction. One report identified vocal cord dysfunction in 5 of 33 young military personnel evaluated for exertional dyspnea (40). Because many patients present with multiple disorders that may contribute to their sensation of dyspnea, CPET can been useful in determining which disorders are the predominant source of limitation (6,41,42).

WHEN TO REFER?

The initial evaluation and diagnostic testing of a patient with dyspnea can be performed by a family physician, internist, pulmonologist, or cardiologist, according to the approach outlined in this chapter. Subsequent diagnostic testing, if needed, often requires specific pulmonary or cardiology expertise. Specialized multidisciplinary clinics for the evaluation of patients with unexplained dyspnea are increasingly available at academic medical centers.

CONCLUSION

Dyspnea is a common diagnostic problem, and its evaluation can be challenging. A logical, stepped diagnostic approach can lead to a successful diagnosis in a majority of patients. Further research is necessary to establish the optimal cost-effective diagnostic algorithm in the evaluation of this frequent complaint.

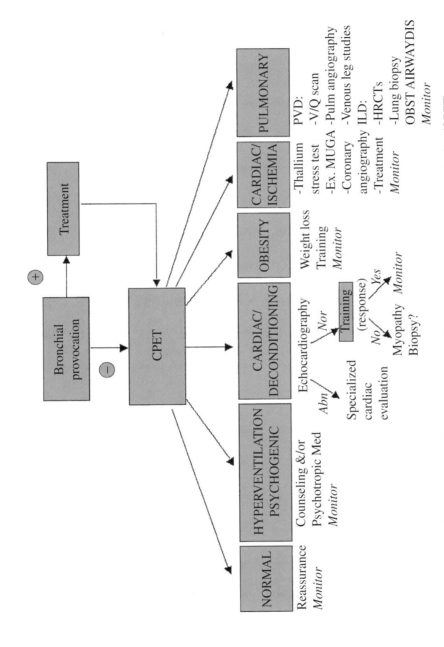

FIG. 2.2. Diagnostic categories derived from cardiopulmonary exercise testing (CPET).

PRACTICAL POINTS

- The severity of dyspnea that an individual experiences for a given activity appears to be related to the level of ventilation required for that activity relative to the ventilatory capacity of the individual.
- CAD is an important and often unrecognized cause of dyspnea in patients with normal LV systolic function at rest.
- A detailed and directed physical examination, with special attention to the cardiovascular and pulmonary system, is essential.
- In the evaluation of dyspnea the insensitivity of chest radiography should be kept in mind. Fibrotic lung disease, for example, may be "invisible" on chest x-ray but clearly manifest on pulmonary function tests and high resolution CT scanning.

- It is important to be aware of the high prevalence of heart failure in older individuals—diastolic heart failure is particularly more likely in the presence of hypertension, diabetes mellitus, obesity or valvular disease
- The initial evaluation of dyspnea may not lead to a specific single diagnosis and the findings will suggest a course for further evaluation
- A completely normal cardiopulmonary stress test does not exclude early disease but should serve to reassure the patient that a major disorder is not likely present.
- Most patients with psychogenic dyspnea will have a normal response to exercise during cardiopulmonary stress test although an erratic pattern of ventilation may be suggestive.

REFERENCES

1. American Thoracic Society. Standardization of spirometry, 1994 update. American Thoracic Society. *Am J Respir Crit Care Med* 1995;152:1107–1136.
2. Kroenke K, Arrington ME, Mangelsdorff AD. The prevalence of symptoms in medical outpatients and the adequacy of therapy [see comments]. *Arch Intern Med* 1990;150:1685–1689.
3. Ailani RK, Ravakhah K, DiGiovine B, et al. Dyspnea Differentiation Index: A new method for the rapid separation of cardiac vs pulmonary dyspnea. *Chest* 1999;116:1100–1104.
4. Pratter MR, Curley FJ, Dubois J, et al. Cause and evaluation of chronic dyspnea in a pulmonary disease clinic. *Arch Intern Med* 1989;149:2277–2282.
5. DePaso W, Winterbauer R, Lusk J, et al. Chronic dyspnea unexplained by history, physical examination, chest roentgenogram, and spirometry. Analysis of a seven-year experience. *Chest* 1991;100:1293–1299.
6. Martinez FJ, Stanopoulos I, Acero R, et al. Graded comprehensive cardiopulmonary exercise testing in the evaluation of dyspnea unexplained by routine evaluation. *Chest* 1994;105:168–174.
7. Elliott M, Adams L, Cockcroft A, et al. The language of breathlessness. Use of verbal descriptions by patients with cardiopulmonary disease. *Am Rev Respir Dis* 1991;144:826–832.
8. Simon PM, Schwartzstein RM, Weiss JW, et al. Distinguishable types of dyspnea in patients with shortness of breath [see comments]. *Am Rev Respir Dis* 1990;142:1009–1014.
9. Scott JA, Mahler DA. Prospective evaluation of a descriptor model to diagnose the etiology of dyspnea. *Chest* 1995;108(Suppl 3):188S.
10. Small D, Gibbons W, Levy R, et al. Exertional dyspnea and ventilation in hyperthyroidism. *Chest* 1992;101:1268–1273.
11. Martinez FJ, Bermudez-Gomez M, Celli BR. Hypothyroidism. A reversible cause of diaphragmatic dysfunction. *Chest* 1989;96:1059–1063.
12. Epler GR, McLoud TC, Gaensler EA, et al. Normal chest roentgenograms in chronic diffuse infiltrative lung disease. *N Engl J Med* 1978;298:934–939.
13. Orens J, Kazerooni E, Martinez F, et al. The sensitivity of high-resolution CT in detecting idiopathic pulmonary fibrosis proved by open lung biopsy: a prospective study. *Chest* 1995;108:190–215.
14. Diller P, Smucker D, David B, et al. Congestive heart failure due to diastolic or systolic dysfunction: frequency and patient characteristics in an ambulatory setting. *Arch Fam Med* 1999;8:414–420.
15. Vasan R, Benjamin E, Levy RD. Prevalence, clinical features and prognosis of diastolic heart failure: an epidemiologic prespective. *J Am Coll Cardiol* 1995;26:1565–1576.
16. Irvin C. Lung volumes. *Semin Respir Med* 1998;19:325–334.
17. Crapo R. Carbon monoxide diffusing capacity (transfer factor). *Semin Respir Crit Care Med* 1998;19:335–347.
18. Demedts M, Beckers J, Rochette F, et al. Pulmonary

function in moderate neuromuscular disease without respiratory complaints. *Eur J Respir Dis* 1982;63:62–67.

19. Celli BR, Grassino A. Respiratory muscles: functional evaluation. *Semin Respir Med* 1998;19:367–382.
20. Flaherty K, Wald J, Weisman K, et al. Unexplained exertional limitation: characterization of patients with a mitochondrial myopathy. *Am J Respir Crit Care Med* 2001;164:425–432.
21. Martinez FJ. Pulmonary function testing in the evaluation of upper airway obstruction. In: Norton M, ed. *Atlas of the difficult airway.* St. Louis: Mosby, 1996:125–133.
22. Rubin L. Primary pulmonary hypertension. *N Engl J Med* 1997;336:111–117.
23. Hansell D. High-resolution computed tomography in the evaluation of fibrosing alveolitis. *Clin Chest Med* 1999;20:739–760.
24. Klein JS, Gamsu G, Webb WR, et al. High-resolution CT diagnosis of emphysema in symptomatic patients with normal chest radiographs and isolated low diffusing capacity. *Radiology* 1992;182:817–821.
25. Sterk P. Bronchoprovocation testing. *Semin Respir Med* 1998;19:317–324.
26. Hallett J, Jacobs R. Recurrent acute bronchitis: the association with undiagnosed bronchial asthma. *Ann Allergy* 1985;55:568–570.
27. Boldy D, Skidmore S, Ayres J. Acute bronchitis in the community: clinical features, infective factors, changes in pulmonary function and bronchial reactivity to histamine. *Respir Med* 1990;84:377–385.
28. Wasserman K, Hansen J, Sue D, et al. *Principles of exercise testing and interpretation. Including pathophysiology and clinical applications.* Philadelphia: Lippincott Williams & Wilkins, 1999.
29. Weisman I, Zeballos R. An integrated approach to the interpretation of cardiopulmonary exercise testing. *Clin Chest Med* 1994;15:421–445.
30. Weisman I, Zeballos R. A step approach to the evaluation of unexplained dyspnea: the role of cardiopulmonary exercise testing. *Pulm Persp* 1998:8–11.
31. Weisman I, Zeballos R. Clinical evaluation of unexplained dyspnea. *Cardiologia* 1996;41:621–634.
32. Gardner W. The pathophysiology of hyperventilation disorders. *Chest* 1996;109:516–534.
33. Hooper R, Thomas A, Kearl R. Mitochondrial enzyme deficiency causing exercise limitation in normal-appearing adults. *Chest* 1995;107:317–322.
34. Risk C, Epler G, Gaensler E. Exercise alveolar-arterial oxygen pressure difference in interstitial lung disease. *Chest* 1984;85:69–74.
35. Keogh B, Lakatos E, Price D, et al. Importance of the lower respiratory tract in oxygen transfer. Exercise testing in patients with interstitial and destructive lung diseases. *Am Rev Respir Dis* 1984;129(Suppl):S76–S80.
36. Mohsenifar Z, Collier J, Belman MJ, et al. Isolated reduction in single-breath diffusing capacity in the evaluation of exertional dyspnea. *Chest* 1992;101:965–969.
37. Knobil K, Becker F, Harper P, et al. Dyspnea in a patient years after severe poliomyelitis. The role of cardiopulmonary exercise testing. *Chest* 1994;105:777–781.
38. Eliasson A, Phillips Y, Rajagopal K. Sensitivity and specificity of bronchial provocation testing. An evaluation of four techniques in exercise-induced bronchospasm. *Chest* 1992;102:347–355.
39. Johnson BD, Weisman IM, Zeballos RJ, et al. Emerging concepts in the evaluation of ventilatory limitation during exercise: the exercise tidal flow-volume loop. *Chest* 1999;116:488–503.
40. Morris MJ, Deal LE, Bean DR, et al. Vocal cord dysfunction in patients with exertional dyspnea. *Chest* 1999;116:1676–1682.
41. Palange P, Carlone S, Forte S, et al. Cardiopulmonary exercise testing in the evaluation of patients with ventilatory vs circulatory causes of reduced exercise tolerance. *Chest* 1994;105:1122–1126.
42. Messner-Pellenc P, Ximenes C, Brasileiro CF, et al. Cardiopulmonary exercise testing. Determinants of dyspnea due to cardiac or pulmonary limitation. *Chest* 1994;106:354–360.

3

Palpitations

Michael H. Lehmann

DEFINITIONS

Palpitations refer to a subjective awareness of one's heartbeat, often with the perception of some type of heart rhythm irregularity, acceleration, or both. Patients use a variety of terms to describe the symptoms (Table 3.1). Although an awareness of strong or rapid heartbeats is universal under states of sympathetic stimulation (exercise, anxiety, or stress), patients complaining of palpitations are usually bothered by their symptoms under resting conditions or perceive an exaggerated accelerated heart rate in the setting of physical activity.

Approximately 15% of the general population experiences palpitations in a given year (1). Palpitations are typically encountered in outpatient settings, reportedly ranking among the top 10 symptom complaints of patients attending a general internal medicine clinic (2). However, patients may seek emergency room care when their palpitations are especially prolonged, frightening, or associated with other symptoms such as lightheadedness, chest pain, or shortness of breath.

PRINCIPAL CAUSES

Palpitations often reflect the occurrence of atrial or ventricular extrasystoles but may also be caused by nonsustained or sustained episodes of supraventricular or, less commonly, ventricular tachycardia. A common mechanism for symptom production in a number of these arrhythmias [e.g., ventricular extrasystoles and atrioventricular (AV) nodal-dependent reentrant paroxysmal supraventricular tachycardias (PSVT)] is an alteration in the normal mechanical systolic AV sequence, such that the atria are contracting simultaneously during or shortly after contraction of the ventricles. Because of the greater intracavitary pressures prevailing in the ventricles, the AV valves cannot open, and regurgitant canon A waves are transmitted to central and pulmonary venous structures. This phenomenon, especially when occurring in the context of tachycardia, can give rise to dyspnea or a pounding sensation in the neck, or both.

Another mechanism of symptom production involves the pause occurring in the wake of an extrasystole. Independent of whether there is an altered AV sequence associated with the premature beat, the inotropic potentiation associated with a post-extrasystolic ventricular contraction, especially in contrast to the possibly reduced stroke volume accompanying the extrasystolic beat (reflecting reduced filling time), contributes to a perception of intermittent skipped beats or of the heart pounding. A similar mechanism may be operative in the uncommon scenario in which palpitations are experienced in association with second-degree AV block. In high cardiac output states, increased force of ventricular contractions, as well as accompanying sinus tachycardia, may be perceived as palpitations.

Along with palpitations, there may be attendant symptoms of lightheadedness, weakness, and near syncope or syncope, depending on the extent of reduced cardiac output that may accompany the reduced cardiac mechanical efficiency occurring during an arrhythmia. Such compromised cardiac output is expected to be more marked in patients with structural heart disease. AV dyssynchrony may contribute to symptoms of chest pain and, in the occasional patient, an urge to cough.

TABLE 3.1. *Palpitations and related symptoms*

Spectrum of descriptions
   Heart flips or flip-flops
   Skipped beats
   Strong beats
   Irregular beats
   Heart thumping
   Bubble sensation in chest/heart
   Heart fluttering
   Racing or rapid heart beats
   Pounding in chest or neck
   Heart jumping out of chest
   Chest or whole body shaking
Potential ancillary symptoms
   Dyspnea, chest pain, lightheadedness, altered
     mental status, visual disturbance, diaphoresis,
     syncope
   Anxiety, jitteriness, feeling shaky
   Polyuria

KEYS TO THE HISTORY

Characterization of the Palpitations

In addition to documenting the patient's description of his or her symptoms (Table 3.1), it is important for the physician to define certain characteristic features of the palpitations:

- *Duration of the Problem*–Have the palpitations been occurring for some time (weeks, months, years), or did they begin very recently (hours to days)? Whereas the former suggests chronically recurring primary arrhythmias, the latter should raise the possibility of a causative acute or subacute cardiopulmonary process (especially if there are premonitory or ancillary symptoms, such as shortness of breath or chest pain).
- *Circumstances at Onset*–Do the palpitations occur at rest or more typically during physical activity? The latter suggests a catecholamine-facilitated arrhythmia. Do the palpitations cluster in a certain portion of a 24-hour period? Patients commonly become aware of ectopic beats at night when they are trying to fall asleep and there is a paucity of distracting external stimuli. Tachyarrhythmias consistently occurring in the middle of the night, interrupting sleep, may represent episodes of vagally mediated atrial fibrillation (3). Palpitations that

chronically recur with assumption of the upright position are suggestive of sinus tachycardia; most commonly, this phenomenon is secondary to "postural orthostatic tachycardia syndrome," a type of dysautonomic response typically seen in younger (usually female) patients (4).

- *Mode of Onset/Offset*–For tachycardia-type symptoms, does the rapid heart rhythm begin and end abruptly, as if activated by a switch (consistent with a pathologic tachyarrhythmia), or does the heart rate accelerate and decelerate more gradually (typical of sinus tachycardia)? There may be an overlap between the two types of symptom onset/offset patterns. For example, PSVT may develop suddenly, but the abruptness of tachycardia offset may be partly masked by a sinus tachycardia that reflects an arrhythmia-related catecholamine surge. Analogously, abruptness of tachycardia onset may be difficult for a patient to appreciate if the tachyarrhythmia arises in the setting of exertional sinus tachycardia.
- *Rhythm Regularity versus Irregularity.* An attempt should be made to determine whether the rhythm feels regular or irregular, particularly when patients complain of episodic rapid heart rates. Asking the patient to tap out the rhythm may clarify not only this issue but give the physician a sense of whether the palpitations truly seem to be rapid and, if so, how fast. If the patient describes or taps out a fairly irregular rhythm, that might prompt consideration of frequent supraventricular or ventricular beats, or an atrial tachyarrhythmia with an irregular ventricular response.
- *Episode Duration*–Does an episode of palpitations last seconds, minutes, or hours? Fleeting symptoms are much less likely to warrant consideration for treatment, especially in the absence of organic heart disease.
- *Symptom Frequency*–It is important to ascertain whether symptoms occur at intervals of hours to days versus weeks to months. Besides its clinical relevance, this information has bearing on the type of diagnostic modality best suited for detecting a culprit arrhythmia.

Attendant Symptoms

As discussed previously, arrhythmias may also give rise to symptoms of dyspnea, light-headedness, weakness, dizziness, and near syncope or syncope, depending on the extent of hemodynamic embarrassment. On the other hand, palpitations preceded by symptoms of angina or dyspnea might suggest that an arrhythmia or sinus tachycardia is occurring on a secondary basis (owing to ischemia, left-sided heart failure, pulmonary hypertension, or pulmonary embolism).

When patients describe symptoms suggestive of tachycardia, inquiries should be made regarding the occurrence of polyuria during a protracted spell, a phenomenon that may result from an atrial neurohormonal response to supraventricular tachyarrhythmias (5). Anxiety-type responses may accompany palpitations. In fact, for some patients, the frightening nature of PSVT symptoms may so dominate their subjective experience as to contribute to a misdiagnosis of "panic attacks," especially when episodes are self-terminating in the absence of organic heart disease (6).

Cardiac History

Central to the evaluation and management of patients with palpitations is the determination of presence or absence of underlying heart disease. This assessment begins during the history with inquiries regarding any known current or prior cardiac conditions. The presence of ischemic heart disease (especially prior myocardial infarction) should certainly prompt suspicion of premature ventricular beats or ventricular tachyarrhythmias. Such arrhythmias may also be considered in the setting of congestive heart failure (either known or suspected on the basis of predisposing conditions such as hypertension). At the same time, it is important to appreciate that patients with sustained supraventricular (especially atrial) tachyarrhythmias, even at relatively low rates of 110 to 140 beats per minute, may over time secondarily acquire symptoms of congestive heart failure—so called tachycardia-induced cardiomyopathy (7). Careful questioning may help to distinguish between these different

cause-and-effect scenarios. Atrial dilatation in the setting of left or right ventricular dysfunction, or both, or resulting from mitral valve disease can lead to symptomatic atrial tachyarrhythmias. In the absence of organic heart disease, isolated palpitations may be either atrial or ventricular in origin, but sustained rapid-rhythm episodes may well represent reentrant PSVT (especially in younger or middle-aged adults) or paroxysmal atrial fibrillation or flutter (more so in middle-aged and elderly patients).

Arrhythmia History

Knowing that a patient has a history of a specific arrhythmia increases the likelihood that recurrent symptoms are more of the same. Of course, the physician must always be open to the possibility that a new arrhythmia has developed [e.g., paroxysmal atrial fibrillation in a patient with known left ventricular systolic dysfunction and prior symptomatic premature ventricular complexes (PVCs)]. A history of recent (within a few weeks to months) radiofrequency ablation should prompt consideration of recurrence of the treated tachyarrhythmia, although palpitations are common after even successful procedures (8).

It is also important to determine whether the patient has a pacemaker or implantable cardioverter defibrillator. Ventricular pacing through either of these devices is capable of giving rise to PVC-like symptoms, especially when there is 1:1 retrograde (ventriculoatrial) conduction; the attendant palpitations and other symptoms reflecting the reversed AV sequence are collectively referred to as *pacemaker syndrome*. In patients with dual-chamber pacemakers or defibrillators, palpitations may reflect the occurrence of pacemaker-mediated "endless-loop tachycardias." When these devices employ internal sensors to modulate pacing rate, overly sensitive rate-responsive ventricular pacing during minimal activity may produce a sensation of inappropriately rapid heart beating.

Family History

For patients with a family history of sudden death, the physician should maintain a high index of suspicion that palpitations may be caused by an inherited arrhythmogenic disorder, such as long QT Syndrome (Chapter 18), Brugada's syndrome (Chapter 18), or familial catecholamine-mediated polymorphic ventricular tachycardia (9). With these conditions, palpitations may reflect the occurrence of non-sustained ventricular tachycardia. Clinical concern deepens when there are ancillary symptoms of lightheadedness, near syncope, or syncope. There is also growing recognition of the existence of certain families that harbor an inherited predisposition to atrial fibrillation (10); inquiries about such a family history may prove informative.

Possible Endocrinologic Disorders

A history of symptoms consistent with hyperthyroidism (on an endogenous or iatrogenic basis) may imply that sinus tachycardia or paroxysmal atrial fibrillation is responsible for the palpitations. Patients with pheochromocytoma may come to attention because of palpitations secondary to sinus tachycardia; this diagnosis may be suspected when there are associated symptoms of headache, diaphoresis, and pallor.

Drug Use

Supraventricular and ventricular tachyarrhythmias may be precipitated by bronchodilator therapy or various over-the-counter sympathomimetic agents taken for cold symptoms. It is important to determine whether patients are taking cardiac or noncardiac QT-prolonging medications, which would raise the possibility of life-threatening polymorphic ventricular tachycardia (torsades de pointes). (A list of the most common QT-prolonging drugs may be found in Chapter 17, Table 17.2; a more complete listing is available on the World Wide Web at www.torsades.org). The examiner should inquire about possible excessive consumption of caffeine or alcohol, certain herbal agents (ephedra), or other stimulatory substances (e.g., cocaine and amphetamines), all of which are capable of causing supraventricular and ventricular arrhythmias. Symptomatic arrhythmias associated with hyper-

thyroidism may occur in patients taking thyroid replacement medication on a therapeutic or surreptitious basis.

HELPFUL SIGNS ON PHYSICAL EXAMINATION

In a patient with palpitations, the physical examination should focus primarily on possible evidence of organic heart disease: hypertension; stigmata of congestive heart failure (rales, elevated jugular venous pressures or positive hepatojugular reflux, displaced point of maximum impulse, S3 gallop, and peripheral edema); or murmurs that might suggest valvular or congenital heart disease or hypertrophic obstructive cardiomyopathy. Evidence of chronic obstructive pulmonary disease might point to culprit atrial tachyarrhythmias; so too would peripheral stigmata of Graves' disease. Often, however, especially in young adults, the physical examination yields uninformative findings regarding the origin of the patient's palpitations.

DIAGNOSTIC TESTS

Various diagnostic tests are available for evaluating patients with palpitations. Each has certain advantages and limitations, knowledge of which aids the physician in choosing the tests that are most suitable for a particular patient.

The Resting Electrocardiogram

This test should be performed in all patients. Obviously, a palpitation is not likely to be "caught" during the brief recording period of an electrocardiogram (ECG). However, the resting ECG provides important clues as to the presence or absence of underlying structural heart disease, which can provide a substrate for arrhythmias. A completely normal ECG cannot absolutely exclude coronary artery disease, but it tends to imply preserved left ventricular systolic function (11). Impaired left ventricular systolic function may be suspected in middle-aged and older patients who exhibit left bundle branch block, nonspecific intraventricular block, or prior myocardial infarction (especially when multiple). ECG evidence of left ventricular hypertrophy, whether associated with abnormal left ventricular systolic function or not, raises the possibility of not only PVCs but also atrial tachyarrhythmias, secondary to elevated mean left atrial filling pressure. Increased susceptibility to atrial tachyarrhythmias can also be suspected in patients in whom the ECG shows signs consistent with chronic obstructive pulmonary disease or mitral stenosis.

In the absence of stigmata of organic heart disease, the ECG should be scrutinized for the possible presence of a delta wave (slurred QRS upstroke with short PR interval). The latter indicates ventricular preexcitation (Wolff-Parkinson-White syndrome) and suggests the possibility that palpitations are being caused by AV reentrant tachycardias and/or paroxysmal atrial fibrillation with rapid conduction via an accessory pathway. Delta waves on an ECG can thus be a useful clue to the origin of palpitations; when this ECG sign is overlooked, misdiagnosis can result (6). In this regard, it should be noted that the delta wave may be quite subtle (and with PR interval sometimes greater than 0.12 seconds) in patients with a left lateral accessory pathway, owing to the relatively long intraatrial conduction time from sinus node to the accessory pathway, in comparison with sinus impulse propagation to the ventricles via the normal AV conduction system.

An ECG lacking the aforementioned abnormalities should also be examined for the possible presence of a prolonged rate-corrected QT interval (longer than 0.45 seconds in men and longer than 0.46 seconds in women) and/or "bifid" or "notched" T waves or other ST-T wave morphologic abnormalities, which may suggest long QT syndrome (12). "Coved"-type ST elevation in the right precordial leads, with concomitant T wave inversion, and often incomplete or complete bundle branch block pattern in V_1, points to a diagnosis of Brugada's syndrome (Chapter 18, Figure 18.1) (13). Finally, low-amplitude notching early in the ST segment of the right precordial leads, with associated T wave inversions, suggests a diagnosis of arrhythmogenic right ventricular dysplasia (13).

Echocardiography

If the history, physical examination, or ECG raises any question about possible cardiac pathol-ogy, an echocardiogram can be very useful in ruling in or ruling out overt structural heart disease. For several decades, there has been a widely held belief in some association between mitral valve prolapse and various cardiac symptoms, including palpitations. According to more recent echocardiographic observations, however, the prevalence of this valvular abnormality in a community-based population is low (1% to 2% range), and frequencies of various cardiac symptoms and arrhythmias are no different from those found in individuals without evidence of mitral valve prolapse (14). Thus, except perhaps in patients with significant attendant mitral regurgitation, mitral valve prolapse, per se, should not be considered a likely explanation for palpitations.

Exercise Testing

In patients with palpitations who also have chest pain symptoms suggestive of angina, exercise stress testing may help in uncovering evidence of ischemic heart disease, which, in turn, might be contributing to the patient's symptoms. Above and beyond such diagnostic utility, exercise testing represents a noninvasive modality for inducing suspected arrhythmias in patients with palpitations. This approach is most relevant in individuals with palpitations that are consistently brought on by exercise, if there are no contraindications to stress testing. For patients without organic heart disease but with exercise-associated palpitations, exercise testing may aid in inducing and thereby diagnosing PSVT, right ventricular outflow tract tachycardia, or polymorphic (in some cases, bidirectional) ventricular tachycardia, in the absence of QT prolongation—a possible marker of a genetically based disorder that confers an increased risk of syncope and sudden cardiac death (9).

24-Hour Ambulatory Electrocardiographic (Holter) Recording

For patients who experience their palpitations at least once (and, ideally for monitoring, multiple times) per day, a Holter monitor can be helpful in trying to identify a culprit arrhythmia. ECG signals are recorded continuously on two or more channels via chest electrodes, facilitating identification of P waves and potential discrimination of supraventricular from ventricular origin of wide QRS complexes. ECG recordings stored on a tape cartridge or digital memory card are scanned by a technician through a computerized interactive program that enables every beat to be classified into a supraventricular or ventricular category; the number of beats in these categories and the characteristics (rate and duration) of tachycardia episodes, if any, are then tabulated in a summary report.

During the 24-hour recording period, the patient is also provided with a diary into which he or she is instructed to log various symptoms and times of their occurrence. Because the Holter recorder has a real-time channel, it may be possible to determine a possible correspondence between palpitations (or other symptoms) and specific arrhythmias detected contemporaneously on the Holter recording.

Event Monitor ECG

When palpitations occur not daily but rather with a frequency ranging from once every few days to once every 1 to 4 weeks, a 24-hour Holter monitor is not likely to be diagnostically helpful. For this common scenario of only modestly frequent palpitations, an event monitor—which allows for on-demand ambulatory ECG recording, synchronous with the patient's symptoms—is the most appropriate diagnostic modality. The event monitor can be worn for weeks at a time (but is removable periodically, as per patient preference), permitting arrhythmias to be "ambushed" and electrocardiographically captured. In general, this approach has a much higher yield than does Holter monitoring for detecting and diagnosing an arrhythmic etiology for palpitations (15,16).

There are two basic event recorder ECG storage systems utilized in event monitors. The first is called a *memory-loop recorder,* in which there is a buffer memory that is continually updated with single-channel ECG signals recorded from two chest electrodes. Upon experiencing palpitations or other cardiac-related symptoms, the patient can press a "Record" button on the beeper-size, waist-worn device (Fig. 3.1). This serves to freeze the immediately preceding 30 to 60 sec-onds (a programmable duration) of ECG signals stored in the buffer memory, as well as a programmable duration of subsequent ECG signals (typically 30 seconds). Current devices are capable of storing several such events. A stimulus artifact coincident with the patient's manual triggering of event storage is indicated directly on the ECG recording channel (Fig. 3.2). A loop recorder is best suited for patients with fleeting symptoms, because the buffer memory affords the patient sufficient time to freeze the corresponding ECG signals.

In patients with more prolonged palpitations (lasting at least 1 to 2 minutes), a non–memory-loop event recorder may suffice. This type of device records only forward in time from the point of activation by the patient. The inconvenience of continually worn chest electrodes can be avoided because electrode introduction is needed only with the onset of symptoms. One way of accomplishing this is by applying directly to the chest a small hand-held recorder that has exposed electrode contacts. A more popular version of the non–memory-loop type of event recorder is one that is worn on the wrist. This so-called *wrist recorder* (Fig. 3.3) has an electrode on its undersurface that is in contact with the skin. When the patient experiences palpitations or related symptoms, he or she can begin to record the cardiac rhythm by pressing the thumb and forefinger of the opposite hand against two opposing electrodes on the recording device. With electrode contact now spanning the two upper extremities, the wrist device essentially records limb lead I ECG signals.

Regardless of the type of event recorder utilized, all the devices have in common the ability to transmit to a central monitoring station via transtelephonic module the most recent stream or streams of stored ECG signals (Fig. 3.4). The central monitoring station is staffed 24 hours a day, 7 days a week, by technicians or nurses who render an initial interpretation of the transmitted rhythm and notify the referring physician in the event that potentially clinically significant tachyarrhythmias or bradyarrhythmias (defined by prespecified criteria) are observed. Final overreading and official interpretation of the transmitted ECG recordings can subsequently be performed by either the referring physician

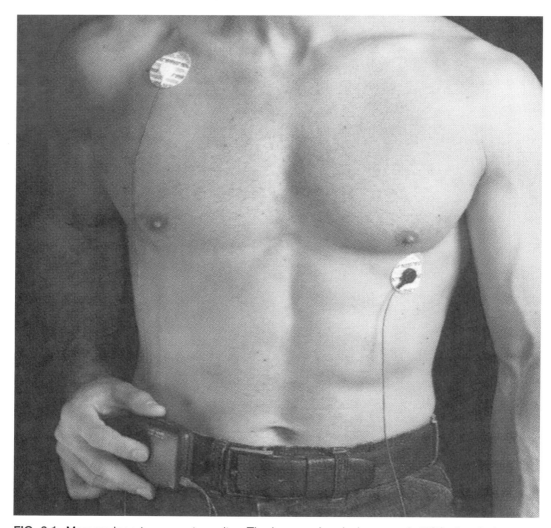

FIG. 3.1. Memory-loop type event monitor. The beeper-size device records ECG signals from two chest electrodes and stores them into a continuously updated buffer memory. When the patient presses the "Record" button on the device, a stream of ECG signals stored beforehand plus a variable length afterward goes into permanent storage, available for subsequent transtelephonic uploading to a central monitoring station. (Permission being sought)

FIG. 3.2. Segment of supraventricular tachycardia captured on an event monitor of the memory-loop type. *Asterisk* denotes stimulus artifact, indicating manual activation of the "Record" function in response to symptoms of "heart pounding." Note that the tachycardia terminates after the third QRS complex on the bottom strip. Although this abnormal rhythm starts and stops before the patient's activation of the "Record" function, these signals are retrievable from the event monitor's buffer memory.

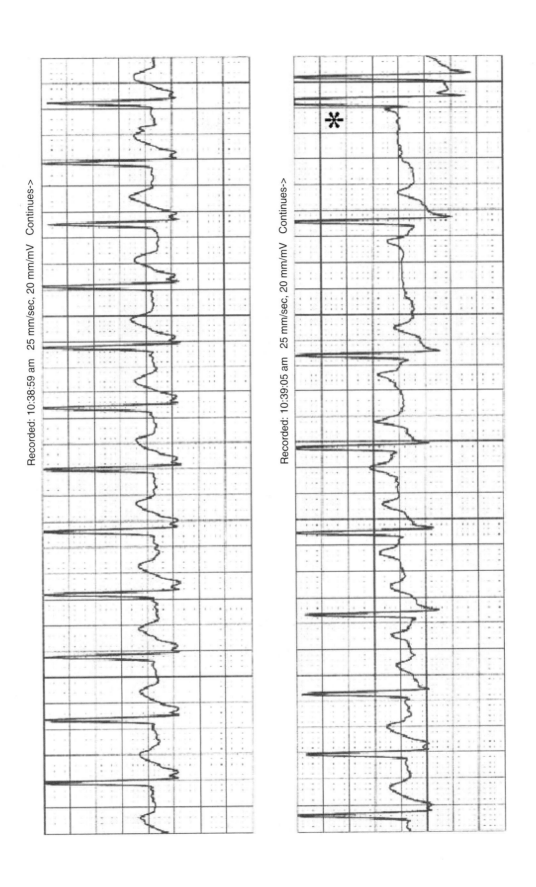

Recorded: 10:38:59 am   25 mm/sec, 20 mm/mV   Continues->

Recorded: 10:39:05 am   25 mm/sec, 20 mm/mV   Continues->

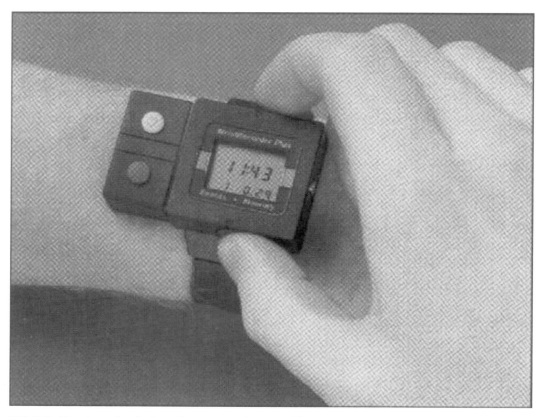

FIG. 3.3. Event monitor that can be worn on the wrist. This non–memory-loop device starts to record upper extremity ECG signals beginning from the time that the patient grasps the device with finger and thumb of the opposite hand. (Permission being sought)

or a cardiologist employed by the monitoring company.

Electrophysiologic Testing

With an intracardiac electrophysiologic (EP) study, electrical pacing techniques make it possible to provoke tachyarrhythmias, thereby facilitating diagnosis. In patients with palpitations, this invasive procedure is usually not undertaken until a tachyarrhythmia has first been documented by one of the noninvasive tests (Table 3.2) (17). Exceptions to this rule may be made for individuals in high-risk occupations, such as competitive athletes, airplane pilots, or bus drivers, or when there are associated symptoms of lightheadedness, near-syncope, or syncope, which occur relatively infrequently (decreasing the likeli-

hood of arrhythmia capture by an event recorder), particularly in patients with underlying heart disease.

Implantable Loop Recorder

For palpitations that are too infrequent even for an event recorder, a small continuous recording device can be implanted subcutaneously in the infraclavicular area. The device is capable of storing ECG signals typically for 10 minutes at a time (8 minutes before and 2 minutes after activation); storage of signals can be initiated by the patient (through application of a magnet) or can be accomplished automatically through the use of preprogrammed rate limit parameters (see also Chapter 5). This diagnostic modality, however, is usually reserved for patients whose symptoms

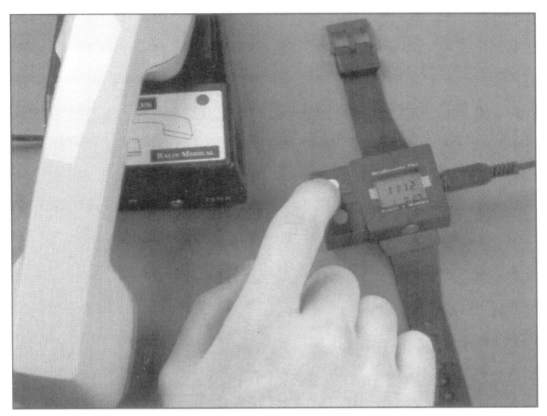

FIG. 3.4. Transtelephonic transmission of stored ECG signals from an event monitor (wrist recorder) to a central monitoring station.

TABLE 3.2. *ACC/AHA Recommendations for electrophysiologic (EP) study in patients with unexplained palpitations*

Class I: There is evidence and/or general agreement that EP testing is useful and effective
1. Patients with palpitations who have a pulse rate documented by medical personnel as inappropriately rapid and in whom ECG recordings fail to document the cause of the palpitations
2. Patients with palpitations preceding a syncopal episode

Class II: There is conflicting evidence and/or a divergence of opinion about the usefulness/efficacy of EP testing
Patients with clinically significant palpitations, suspected to be of cardiac origin, in whom symptoms are sporadic and cannot be documented. Studies are performed to determine the mechanisms of arrhythmias, direct or provide therapy, or assess prognosis

Class III: There is evidence and/or general agreement that EP testing is not useful and in some cases may be harmful
Patients with palpitations documented to be due to extracardiac causes (e.g., hyperthyroidism)

ACC/AHA, American College of Cardiology/American Heart Association; ECG, electrocardiographic.
From Zimetbaum PJ, Josephson ME. The evolving role of ambulatory arrhythmia monitoring in general clinical practice. *Ann Intern Med* 1999;130:848–856.

include syncope or near syncope, rather than palpitations alone.

Holter/Event Monitor Data: Interpretational Issues

Arrhythmia-Symptom Correlation

It is extremely important to confirm reproduction of palpitation symptoms coincident with the detected arrhythmia, as a prerequisite for labeling the arrhythmia as etiologic. Such a diagnostic requirement is necessitated by the high prevalence of atrial or ventricular extrasystoles and occasional occurrence of "complex" PVCs (e.g., multifocal, couplets, or longer runs) in the general population (see later discussion). On the other hand, documenting a consistent lack of correlation between the symptoms and arrhythmias—especially when no arrhythmias are ever recorded in association with documented palpitations—helps exclude an arrhythmic origin for the patient's symptoms.

Premature Ventricular Complexes

Ventricular arrhythmias detected on Holter and event monitor recordings, even when asymptomatic, continue to be a source of anxiety for physicians. Patients commonly become more symptomatic with their PVCs once they sense their physician's heightened concern, which possibly prompts fear that these arrhythmias may lead to a "heart attack." Such anxieties can be minimized if physicians are aware of the spectrum of PVC frequency and complexity in the general population.

Table 3.3 summarizes PVC-related observations from nine Holter studies involving 962 healthy young and middle-aged adults (18–24) and 156 predominantly healthy elderly individuals (75 years of age or older) (25,26). Over a given 24-hour period, on average, at least one PVC is recorded in 57% of such a broad population sample; PVC prevalence increases with age but does not differ significantly by sex. In the approximate ninety-fifth percentile for PVC frequency, the average is 65 PVCs per 24 hours in young adults and 300 PVCs per 24 hours in middle-aged adults; thus, some 5% of healthy nonelderly sub-

jects may exhibit even more frequent PVCs (as high as 1,000 or more per 24 hours). Complex PVCs are not so rare: multiform PVCs can be found in 9.7%, ventricular couplets in 2.4%, and runs of ventricular tachycardia in 1.3% of healthy nonelderly adults, on average. When observed, ventricular tachycardia episodes typically occur no more than once during a given 24-hour period and are *not* sustained, consisting of only three to eight consecutive PVCs at rates usually of less than 200 (rarely up to 300) beats per minute. Elderly individuals tend to have more frequent and complex PVCs.

In the absence of organic heart disease or genetic arrhythmogenic disorders, frequent or complex PVCs (including isolated episodes of nonsustained ventricular tachycardia) do not carry an increased risk of life-threatening sustained ventricular tachyarrhythmias or sudden death (27).

Sinus Tachycardia

Not uncommonly, the only arrhythmia documented in association with symptoms is commonly sinus tachycardia. Of course, the examiner must clarify that this is occurring at rest, in the absence of external sources of stress or excitement. The sinus tachycardia that may be observed on Holter or event monitor recordings in such a scenario has a rate typically in the range of 100 to 120 beats per minute, although rates up to 140 to 150 beats per minute are sometimes observed. When the physician fails to uncover more serious arrhythmias, there is a natural tendency to consider the monitor test "negative," with attribution of symptoms to "anxiety," especially in young or middle-aged patients (often women) with no underlying organic heart disease. An anxiety disorder may well be present in a subset of these cases. However, the physician should also be mindful of the possibility that patients whose palpitations are associated with sinus tachycardia may be suffering from some type of dysautonomia or intrinsic disturbance of sinus nodal function. Assuming that the physician is not dealing with situations of acute or subacute blood loss, he or she may suspect *postural orthostatic tachycardia syndrome* if the heart rate increases by 30 or more beats per

TABLE 3.3. *Prevalence of PVCs in the general adult population[a] on 24-hour ambulatory electrocardiograms*

Study	No. subjects	Males	Age [range (mean)]	At least one PVC	PVC Frequency for ≈ 95% of Population (no./24 hr)	"Complex" PVCs		
						Multifocal	Couplets	VT
Young								
Brodsky et al. (18)	50	100%	23–27 (NA)	50%	≤30	12%	2%	2%
Sobotka et al. (19)	50	0%	22–28 (NA)	54%	≤100	10%	0%	2%
Middle-aged								
Kostis et al. (20)	101	50%	16–68 (49)	39%	≤500	4%	0%	0%
Bjerregaard et al. (21)	260	65%	40–79 (54)	69%	≤200	23%	8%	2%
Bethge et al. (22)	170	69%	18–70 (42)	41%	≤240[b]	10%	3%	2%
Rasmussen et al. (23)	111	51%	20–79 (50)	61%	≤500	NA	2%	1%
Takada et al. (24)	220	69%	20–79 (47)	44%	≤50[c]	9%	2%	0%
Elderly								
Camm et al. (25)	106	NA	75–95 (NA)	69%	≤2,400[d]	22%	4%	4%
Kantelip et al. (26)	50	12%	81–100 (NA)	96%	≤2,400	18%	8%	2%

NA, information not available; PVC, premature ventricular complex; VT, ventricular tachycardia (≥3 consecutive PVCs at rate >100 beats/minute)

[a] All deemed to be "healthy" (by history, physical examination, and 12-lead electrocardiogram) except for a subset of the active elderly subjects studied by Camm et al. (25).

[b] Applied to 90% of population.

[c] Applied to 93% of population.

[d] Applied to 88% of population.

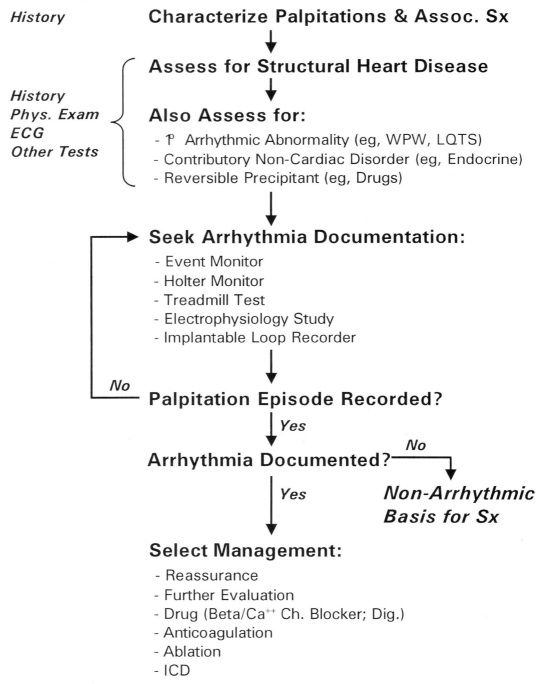

FIG. 3.5. Summary algorithm for diagnostic evaluation of a patient with palpitations. See text for details. Assoc, associated; Ch, channel; Dig, digoxin; LQTS, long QT syndrome; Phys, physical; Sx, symptoms; WPW, Wolff-Parkinson-White syndrome.

minute (in the absence of significant hypotension) within 5 minutes of changing from a supine to a standing position (4). *Inappropriate sinus tachycardia* should be considered in patients with an average heart rate of over 90 beats per minute throughout a 24-hour Holter ECG recording, once an endocrine disorder has been excluded.

MANAGEMENT CONSIDERATIONS

The overall diagnostic approach to a patient with palpitations is summarized in the schema of Fig. 3.5. At any point along this evaluation process, various findings may warrant referral of the patient to the emergency room (Table 3.4) or to a cardiologist (Table 3.5).

It is important to ascertain whether the patient has organic heart disease, because this factor

TABLE 3.4. *Palpitations: when to refer to the emergency room*

Palpitations with
  New-onset syncope
  New-onset or worsening chest pain or dyspnea
Recent onset palpitations (especially with any
    suggestion of lightheadedness) in patients with
  Possible drug-induced long QT syndrome
  Known or family history of long QT syndrome,
    Brugada's syndrome, catecholamine-induced
    polymorphic VT, or arrhythmogenic right
    ventricular dysplasia
Sustained regular SVT, especially with associated
    hypotension, lightheadedness, chest pain, or
    dyspnea
Atrial fibrillation or flutter with
  Hypotension, lightheadedness, chest pain, or
    dyspnea
  Average ventricular response >120 beats/minute
  Onset clearly within 48 hours, regardless of rate,
    potentially amenable to acute cardioversion
  Onset of uncertain duration but known history of
    TIA, stroke, or other thromboembolic event in a
    patient not currently receiving anticoagulation
    therapy
Sustained VT
Nonsustained VT in association with unexplained
    syncope, new-onset or worsening chest pain, or
    dyspnea, especially in patients with known
    organic heart disease
Asymptomatic polymorphic VT with
  Underlying organic heart disease
  Prolonged QT interval
  Brugada's syndrome
  Induction by exercise
  Rate ≥120 beats/minute

SVT, supraventricular tachycardia; TIA, transient ischemic attack; VT, ventricular tachycardia.

TABLE 3.5. *Palpitations: when to refer to a cardiologist*

Patients with Wolff-Parkinson-White syndrome,
    particularly if atrial fibrillation or flutter or other SVT
    has previously been documented
Atrial fibrillation, atrial flutter or regular SVT in patients
    with
  Syncope
  Impaired left ventricular systolic function
  Hypertrophic cardiomyopathy
  Suboptimal response or intolerance to AV nodal
    blocking medication
Nonsustained VT in patients with organic heart disease
Frequent, symptomatic PACs or PVCs not responsive
    to beta or calcium channel blockers

AV, atrioventricular; PAC, premature atrial complex; PVC, premature ventricular complex; SVT, supraventricular tachycardia; VT, ventricular tachycardia.

has a significant impact on prognosis and therapeutic decision making. Besides information gleaned from the history and physical examination, noninvasive tests, particularly echocardiography, can be very helpful in more definitively establishing the presence or absence of underlying structural heart disease. The advisability of cardiac catheterization should be based on conventional indications for this invasive procedure, ordinarily not warranted by a complaint of palpitations alone. The therapeutic options depicted in Fig. 3.5 must be tailored to the arrhythmia and to the patient's cardiovascular diagnoses.

For the majority of patients, whose palpitations are occurring in the absence of organic heart disease and without associated syncope or near syncope, PVCs, even short runs of nonsustained ventricular tachycardia, are generally thought to carry a benign prognosis (27), and the patient can be reassured accordingly; this is also the case for patients who are found to have premature atrial complexes, including short runs. (The analogy between cardiac extrasystoles and muscle twitches elsewhere in the body, such as hiccups and facial tics, is conceptually satisfying to most patients.) Use of medical therapy in these cases should be discouraged, unless the patient remains considerably symptomatic even after he or she verbalizes understanding of the benign nature of the condition. For such individuals, empirical therapy is typically limited to beta-adrenergic blockers or calcium channel blockers, in view of concerns about serious adverse effects (especially proarrhythmia) with other antiarrhythmic agents.

When palpitations are accompanied by syncope, near syncope, or other manifestations of compromised cardiac function, or when detected arrhythmias are occurring in the setting of organic heart disease, more aggressive therapeutic interventions are warranted. These include AV nodal blocking medication with oral anticoagulation for patients with atrial fibrillation or atrial flutter; consideration of radiofrequency ablation procedures for various symptomatic sustained supraventricular tachyarrhythmias (Chapters 16 and 17); ablation for certain sustained ventricular tachycardias; and, less commonly, automatic defibrillator implantation for sustained ventricular tachyarrhythmias (spontaneous or induced) in patients with various cardiomyopathic processes or in symptomatic high-risk patients with primary ventricular tachyarrhythmias (e.g., long QT syndrome and Brugada's syndrome).

PRACTICAL POINTS

- In the history, characterize duration of palpitations, circumstances surrounding occurrence, rapidity of onset/offset, whether regular or irregular, episode duration, and frequency.
- Paroxysmal supraventricular tachycardia may masquerade as "panic attack," leading to misdiagnosis.
- Search for evidence of structural heart disease by history, physical examination, ECG, and, if indicated, noninvasive tests.
- In the absence of significant mitral regurgitation, mitral valve prolapse is *not* a plausible explanation for palpitations.
- The ECG may point to an arrhythmic etiology (e.g., Wolff-Parkinson-White syndrome).
- A 24-hour recording by Holter monitor is useful only if symptoms are occurring at least daily.
- An event monitor (with memory loop), worn for days to weeks, is the higher yield ambulatory ECG test for detecting arrhythmias associated with palpitations.
- For either Holter or event monitor recordings, a given arrhythmia must be strongly correlated with palpitations to be considered etiologic.
- Premature ventricular complexes are fairly common in the general population and should be of prognostic concern only if associated with organic heart disease.
- Sinus tachycardia recorded during palpitations—in the absence of exertion—should not be presumed a "negative" finding (or automatically attributed to "anxiety"); the patient could be suffering from postural orthostatic tachycardia syndrome or inappropriate sinus tachycardia.
- Management of palpitations is guided by the nature of the detected arrhythmia, the severity of associated symptoms (e.g., syncope), and the presence and extent of underlying heart disease.

REFERENCES

1. Lochen M-L, Snaprud T, Zhang W, et al. Arrhythmias in subjects with and without a history of palpitations: the Tromso study. *European Heart J* 1994;15:345–349.
2. Kroenke LTCK, Arrington ME, Mangelsdorff AD. The prevalence of symptoms in medical outpatients and the adequacy of therapy. *Arch Intern Med* 1990;150:1685–1689.
3. Coumel P. Neural aspects of paroxysmal atrial fibrillation. In: Falk RH, Podrid PJ, eds. *Atrial fibrillation: mechanism and management.* New York: Raven Press, 1992:109–125.
4. Sandroni P, Opfer-Gehrking TL, McPhee BR, et al. Postural tachycardia syndrome: clinical features and follow-up study. *Mayo Clin Proc* 1999;74:1106–1110.
5. Zullo MA. Atrial regulation of intravascular volume: observations on the tachycardia-polyuria syndrome. *Am Heart J* 1991;122:188–194.
6. Lessmeier TJ, Gamperling D, Johnson-Liddon V, et al.

Unrecognized paroxysmal supraventricular tachycardia: potential for misdiagnosis as panic disorder. *Arch Intern Med* 1997;157:537–543.

7. Shinbane JS, Wood MA, Jensen DN, et al. Tachycardia-induced cardiomyopathy: a review of animal models and clinical studies. *J Am Coll Cardiol* 1997;29:709–715.

8. Mann De, Kelly PA, Adler SW, et al. Palpitations occur frequently following radiofrequency catheter ablation for supraventricular tachycardia, but do not predict pathway recurrence. *Pacing Clin Electrophysiol* 1993;16:1645–1649.

9. Swan H, Piippo K, Viitasalo M, et al. Arrhythmic disorder mapped to chromosome 1q42-q43 causes malignant polymorphic ventricular tachycardia in structurally normal hearts. *J Am Coll Cardiol* 1999;34:2035–2042.

10. Brugada R, Tapscott T, Czernuszewicz GZ, et al. Identification of a genetic locus for familial atrial fibrillation. *N Engl J Med* 1997;336:905–911.

11. O'Keefe JH Jr, Zinsmeister AR, Gibbons RJ. Value of normal electrocardiographic findings in predicting resting left ventricular function in patients with chest pain and suspected coronary artery disease. *Am J Med* 1989;86:658–662.

12. Zhang L, Timothy KW, Vincent GM, et al. Spectrum of ST–T-wave patterns and repolarization parameters in congenital long-QT syndrome: ECG findings identify genotypes. *Circulation* 2000;102:2849–2855.

13. Marcus FI. Electrocardiographic features of inherited diseases that predispose to the development of cardiac arrhythmias, long QT syndrome, arrhythmogenic right ventricular cardiomyopathy/dysplasia, and Brugada syndrome. *J Electrocardiol* 2000;33(Suppl):1–10.

14. Freed LA, Levy D, Levine RA, et al. Prevalence and clinical outcome of mitral valve prolapse. *N Engl J Med* 1999;341:1–7.

15. Kinlay S, Leitch JW, Neil A, et al. Cardiac event recorders yield more diagnoses and are more cost-effective than 48-hour Holter monitoring in patients with palpitations: a controlled clinical trial. *Ann Intern Med* 1996;124:16–20.

16. Zimetbaum PJ, Josephson ME. The evolving role of ambulatory arrhythmia monitoring in general clinical practice. *Ann Intern Med* 1999;130:848–856.

17. Zipes DP, DiMarco JP, Gillette PC, et al. Guidelines for clinical intracardiac electrophysiological and catheter ablation procedures. *J Am Coll Cardiol* 1995;26:555–573.

18. Brodsky M, Wu D, Denes P, et al. Arrhythmias documented by 24 hour continuous electrocardiographic monitoring in 50 male medical students without apparent heart disease. *Am J Cardiol* 1977;39:390–395.

19. Sobotka PA, Mayer JH, Bauernfeind RA, et al. Arrhythmias documented by 24-hour continuous ambulatory electrocardiographic monitoring in young women without apparent heart disease. *Am Heart J* 1981;101:753–759.

20. Kostis JB, McCrone K, Moreyra AE, et al. Premature ventricular complexes in the absence of identifiable heart disease. *Circulation* 1981;63:1351–1356.

21. Bjerregaard P. Premature beats in healthy subjects 40–79 years of age. *Eur Heart J* 1982;3:493–503.

22. Bethge KP, Bethge D, Meiners G, et al. Incidence and prognostic significance of ventricular arrhythmias in individuals without detectable heart disease. *Eur Heart J* 1983;4:338–346.

23. Rasmussen V, Jensen G, Schnohr P, et al. Premature ventricular beats in healthy adult subjects 20 to 79 years of age. *Eur Heart J* 1985;6:335–341.

24. Takada H, Mikawa T, Murayama M, et al. Range of ventricular ectopic complexes in healthy subjects studied with repeated ambulatory electrocardiographic recordings. *Am J Cardiol* 1989;63:184–186.

25. Camm AJ, Evans KE, Ward DE, et al. The rhythm of the heart in active elderly subjects. *Am Heart J* 1980;99:598–603.

26. Kantelip JP, Sage E, Duchene-Marullaz P. Findings on ambulatory electrocardiographic monitoring in subjects older than 80 years. *Am J Cardiol* 1986;57:398–401.

27. Kennedy HL, Whitlock JA, Sprague MK, et al. Long-term follow-up of asymptomatic healthy subjects with frequent and complex ventricular ectopy. *New Engl J Med* 1985;312:193–197.

4

Edema

Peter V. Vaitkevicius and Ragavendra R. Baliga

DEFINITIONS

Edema is an increase in the interstitial fluid volume and is typically first noted in the lower extremities. Often more than 4 kg of excess total body fluid may be present before the development of edema. Therefore, it is typical to have a weight gain of several kilograms before the overt findings of swelling on the physical examination. The distribution of edema is generally proportional to the extent of collected interstitial fluid and may be diffuse or localized. *Anasarca,* or *dropsy,* defines a large and generalized accumulation of edema fluid. Depending on the mechanisms, both anasarca and smaller amounts of lower extremity edema may be associated with *ascites* (accumulation of fluid in the peritoneal cavity) or a *pleural effusion* (accumulation of fluid in the pleural cavity). *Dependent edema* is the collection of fluid at specific sites in response to the hydrostatic effects of gravity and often first appears in the feet and ankles of ambulatory patients. Dependent edema in bed-bound patients in best assessed by examination of the posterior surfaces of the calves and sacrum. *Pitting edema* is demonstrated when the thumb is pressed into the skin against a bony surface—for example, over the tibia, fibula, or sacrum. When pressure is removed, an indentation persists, the depth of which should be estimated in millimeters as a means to score its severity. *Lymphedema* results from the obstruction of lymphatic channels and is often indistinguishable from edema produced by other mechanisms. When chronic, lymphedema is often nonpitting. *Brawny edema* defines a nonpitting fibrotic thickening of the subcutaneous tissues, which results from chronic tissue swelling (1).

PRINCIPLES OF EDEMA FORMATION (STARLING FORCES)

One third of the total body water is confined to the extracellular space (Fig. 4.1). The plasma volume constitutes 25% of the extracellular volume, and the remaining 75% is made up of the interstitial fluid volume. The *hydrostatic pressure* within the vascular system and the *colloid oncotic pressure* within the interstitial fluid facilitate the movement of fluid out of the vascular compartment and into extravascular space. The *tissue tension* (plasma colloid oncotic pressure and interstitial hydrostatic pressure) promotes the movement of fluid from the extravascular space into the vascular compartment. These forces are usually balanced, but if the oncotic or hydrostatic pressures are adversely altered, then the movement of fluid into the interstitial space or a body cavity occurs (2,3).

An increase in the capillary pressure may result from an elevation of venous pressure caused by a local obstruction in venous drainage. The increased venous pressure may be generalized, as with congestive heart failure (CHF), or localized, as with a deep venous thrombosis (DVT) (4). The plasma colloid oncotic pressure may be altered by hypoalbuminemia from malnutrition, liver disease, urinary protein loss, or a severe catabolic state. The reduction in oncotic pressure lessens the movement of interstitial fluid into the vascular compartment.

A fall in the cardiac output (e.g., as in CHF) reduces the effective arterial blood volume and systolic blood pressure (hypotension) and decreases renal blood flow. Compensatory activation of the sympathetic nervous system and renin-angiotensin system promotes renal

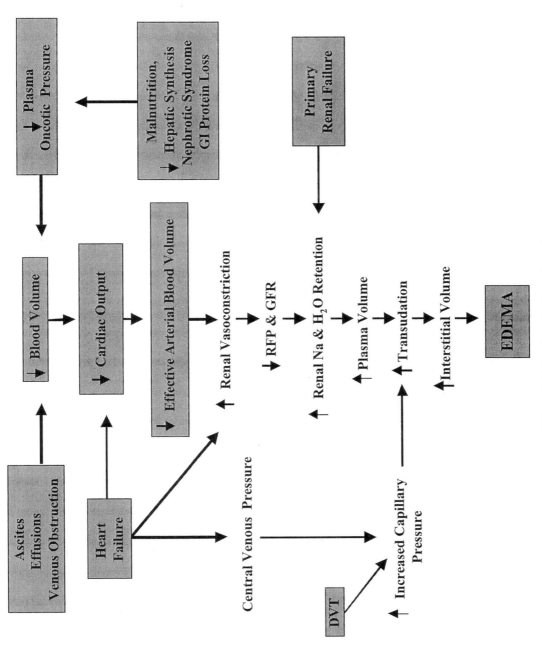

FIG. 4.1. Principles of edema formation.

vasoconstriction, a reduction in renal salt and water excretion, and an expansion of the extracellular volume with edema formation. In addition, the mechanisms responsible for maintaining a normal serum osmolality are activated promoting thirst and secretion of antidiuretic hormone. If the increase in total body salt and water is insufficient to restore and maintain an appropriate effective arterial volume, then the stimuli promoting renal salt retention are not turned off and the severity of the edema is progressive.

The nephrotic syndrome and hepatic cirrhosis are associated with a severe reduction in serum albumin by either an increase in the loss of protein or a reduction in protein synthesis. The reduction in the plasma colloid oncotic pressure reduces plasma volume and the effective arterial blood volume, further promoting renal salt and water reabsorption (5).

Damage to the capillary endothelium increases vascular permeability and the movement of fluid and protein into the interstitial space. The vascular injury is often the result of infection, drugs, hypersensitivity reactions, or thermal or mechanical damage. This manner of vascular damage usually results in a nonpitting edema with associated inflammation. In addition, an occlusion of the lymphatic drainage of a specific site results in edema.

KEYS TO THE HISTORY

Distribution

Unilateral edema (Table 4.1) is a common clinical complaint, particularly of the lower extremities, and is routinely seen in the outpatient setting. Most patients with unilateral lower extremity edema should be considered for venous

Doppler assessment to screen for the presence of a Deep Venous Thrombosis (DVT), regardless of whether it is associated with pain or not (Chapter 32). Rectal, pelvic, and regional lymph node examinations should be conducted if a malignancy is suspected (6–8).

Besides a DVT, mechanisms for a painful unilateral swelling may include the following. The postphlebitic syndrome commonly follows a DVT (9). A ruptured popliteal (Baker's) cyst produces posterior knee tenderness and occasionally petechiae and may clinically resemble a DVT (10). A tear or rupture of the gastrocnemius muscle is often acute and can be confused with a DVT (11). Soft tissue infections (cellulitis and fasciitis) can initially present with swelling and pain, before the development of erythema or warmth. A psoas muscle hematoma or abscess can also produce unilateral swelling and may be associated with flank or hip pain as well as a painful leg lift test result (psoas sign).

Bilateral lower extremity or *generalized edema* (Table 4.2) is the primary result of three mechanisms: an increase in central venous pressure, such as in pulmonary hypertension; renal sodium and water retention, as with a primary renal disease; or a reduction in cardiac output

TABLE 4.1. *Unilateral edema*

Deep venous thrombosis
Postphlebitic syndrome
Baker's cyst rupture
Gastrocnemius rupture
Cellulitis
Trauma
Insect stings
Venous insufficiency
Varicosities
Lymphatic obstruction

TABLE 4.2. *Generalized edema*

Deep venous thrombosis
Left ventricular systolic and diastolic dysfunction
Valvular heart disease
Right ventricular volume and pressure overload.
  Chronic lung disease
  Sleep apnea
  Pulmonary embolism
  Primary pulmonary hypertension
Hepatic dysfunction
Renal disease
Venous insufficiency/varicosities
Constrictive pericardial disease
Drug induced
Loss of venous tone secondary to lack of exercise
High-output cardiac failure
  Thyrotoxicosis, beriberi, AV malformations
Hypothyroidism
Idiopathic cyclic edema
Exercise edema
High-altitude edema
Tropical edema
Lymphedema
Malnutrition

AV, arteriovenous.

with activation of the sympathetic nervous system and the renin-angiotensin system, as seen with CHF. The distribution of the edema is influenced by the hydrostatic effects of gravity (dependent edema) and by the limitation in venous and lymphatic return, and the edema often accumulates in dependent structures such as the scrotum or the abdominal pannus in obese patients. Generalized edema limited primarily to above the diaphragm can result from infection, dermal irritants, or compression or obstruction of the superior vena cava and mediastinal vasculature, as is seen with chest neoplasms (12).

Chronic right ventricular failure may be the result of left ventricular dysfunction, pulmonary hypertension, or chronic lung disease. It produces marked bilateral edema, often with ascites, as a result of an increase in central venous pressure. Acute right-sided heart failure secondary to a large pulmonary embolism or a myocardial infarction also produces elevated central venous pressures. A careful review of the history to seek evidence of chest pains consistent with angina or a prior cardiac history (myocardial infarction or angina) should be completed early in the evaluation of generalized edema. CHF resulting from left ventricular systolic or diastolic dysfunction, or both, is one of the most common mechanisms for bilateral edema and is often associated with pleural effusion or ascites. Hepatic cirrhosis is the end point of chronic liver disease (e.g., viral hepatitis, alcoholic liver disease). Edema of hepatic origin is primarily in the lower extremities and abdominal cavity and is proportional to the elevation in portal venous pressure. A history of a change in urinary frequency, hematuria, or foamy urine supports a renal process for the edema. The edema associated with the nephrotic syndrome (urinary protein loss of more than 3.0 g per day) is the result of a marked reduction in serum albumin and occasionally by venous thrombosis that results from the associated hypercoagulable state. Minimal change disease, membranous glomerulopathies, diabetic renal disease, human immunodeficiency virus infection, glomerulosclerosis, and myeloma kidney are common causes of the nephrotic syndrome (13).

Idiopathic cyclic edema is an episodic swelling, often with abdominal distention, noted primarily in women, and is unrelated to the menstrual cycle. Many of these patients may have used diuretics extensively in the past. *Exercise edema* is occasionally noted as facial and ankle edema in healthy subjects performing strenuous exercise. *High-altitude edema* is a lower limb and facial edema typically noted in persons hiking at altitudes above 2,400 meters. It is augmented by a high-salt diet and resolves with the return to lower altitudes. *Tropical edema* is a pitting edema of the ankles that often occurs abruptly in normal adults within 48 hours after traveling from a temperate climate to the heat of the tropics. It spontaneously resolves within a few days of acclimatization. *Carcinoma,* most significantly cervical, colorectal, prostate, or *lymphomas,* can result in edema by local extension and obstruction of venous and lymphatic drainage.

Lymphedema (Table 4.3) can have several causes (14). Primary or congenital lymphedema manifesting at or soon after birth is rare. Most forms of primary lymphedema manifest after puberty with lower extremity swelling and more often affect women. Secondary lymphedema manifesting with the onset of swelling in a single limb suggests proximal lymphatic obstruction. Pelvic causes of venous or lymphatic obstruction such as tumors or thrombosis should be sought in evaluation of lower extremity swelling. Prior treatments for cancer, such as a lymph node dissection for breast cancer or radiotherapy, are common causes. Relapsing tumors should always be considered when limb swelling develops after a cancer treatment. Worldwide, filariasis is a secondary cause of lymphedema and should be considered in a patient who has traveled or lived in an endemic area. Characteristic skin changes are swelling in the subcutaneous layers, thinning, hyperkeratosis, and occasionally elephantiasis.

TABLE 4.3. *Causes of lymphatic obstruction*

Metastatic carcinoma or lymphoma
Radiotherapy or chemotherapy
Retroperitoneal fibrosis
Sarcoidosis
Filariasis
Milroy's disease
Meige's syndrome
Klippel-Trenaunay syndrome

Drugs Associated with Edema

Nonsteroidal antiinflammatory drugs (NSAIDs) are an extremely common mechanism for drug-related lower extremity swelling (15) (Table 4.4). As a class, they promote salt and water retention via renal microvascular constriction and a diminished glomerular filtration rate. These drugs may adversely limit the therapeutic effects of antihypertensive medications and diuretics. They are often found to frustrate the management of excessive volume in conditions such as CHF. As a class, cyclooxygenase-2 (COX-2) inhibitors are also associated with edema formation. Antihypertensive medications that are direct arterial or arteriolar dilators have a high rate of producing edema. Alpha-adrenergic antagonists have become popular medications because of their role in reducing symptoms of prostatic obstruction, but they have also been implicated in causing lower extremity edema. Adrenal corticosteroids and estrogens are implicated in edema formation caused by salt and water retention, primarily by their effects on the aldosterone-sensitive sodium channel in the cortical collecting ducts of the nephron. Corticosteroids are occasionally associated with a metabolic alkalosis and mild degrees of hypokalemia.

TABLE 4.4. *Drugs associated with edema*

NSAIDs & COX 2 inhibitors
Antihypertensives
  Minoxidil
  Hydralazine
  Clonidine
  Methyldopa
  Guanethidine
  Calcium channel blockers
  Alpha-adrenergic antagonists
Steroids
  Corticosteroids
  Anabolic steroids
  Estrogens
  Progestins
Cyclosporine
Growth hormone
Immunotherapies
  IL-2
  OKT3

COX-2, cyclooxygenase 2; IL-2, interleukin-2; NSAID, nonsteroidal antiinflammatory drug; OKT3, anti-CD3 monoclonal antibody.

Helpful Signs on Physical Examination

The physical characteristics of the edema should be assessed carefully to provide insight in to the process responsible for it. Skin changes, such an erythema and blanching associated with an infection, or rubor (hemosiderin staining of the skin) in venous insufficiency, are helpful in defining its mechanism and chronicity. Concerns for a unilateral swelling in the lower extremities are still initially best assessed by the measurement of the calf's circumference with a tape measure around the bilateral calves at the same level below the patella. Clinical signs supportive of a DVT are inconsistent but should be reviewed—for example, Homans' sign (calf pain with dorsiflexion of the foot). Regional lymph nodes should be palpated. Muscle rupture is typically associated with local tenderness and pain with movement. The clinical signs of thyroid disease, both hyperthyroidism and hypothyroidism, should also be reviewed.

In evaluating cardiac mechanisms for edema, the physical examination should focus on the following. Elevation of jugular venous pressure, which is a direct measure of central venous pressure, is best assessed in supine position with the head elevated to approximately 30 to 45 degrees. The detection of a right ventricular heave is indicative of pressure or volume overload. Dilation of the left ventricle with displacement of the maximal impulse is best assessed with careful palpation of the anterior chest. Auscultation of the heart should be performed with attention to murmurs suggestive of significant valvular disease, gallops (S3) suggestive of left ventricular congestion, and pericardial rubs or a knock. The chest examination should also be focused to evaluate the presence of inspiratory rales, which suggest CHF, or the finding of chronic lung disease, such as increased anteroposterior diameter, flattened diaphragms, poor air movement, prolonged expiration, wheezing, coarse rales, or rhonchi.

Hepatic causes of edema often have the following physical findings. The presence of ascites is demonstrated by an increase in the abdominal girth, shifting dullness, a puddle sign, or a fluid wave. In primary hepatic disease, the jugular venous pressure is normal or low, although gross volume expansion (anasarca) can exist. If there is associated cardiac dysfunction, then the jugular venous pressure is likely to be elevated. Signs of chronic liver disease may include jaundice, palmar erythema, spider angiomata, male gynecomastia, testicular atrophy, caput medusa, asterixis, an enlarged liver, a small nodular liver, and central nervous system changes suggestive of an encephalopathy.

Renal disease is typically associated with systemic hypertension, diabetic end-organ disease (retinopathy or neuropathy), and clinical signs of uremia (fetor of the breath, periorbital edema, a pericardial rub).

Diagnostic Tests

DVT is best evaluated with the use of Doppler ultrasound examination of the venous system. D-Dimers, used in a serologic test of fibrin degradation, are also helpful in screening for venous clot (Chapter 32). The postphlebitic syndrome should be differentiated from an acute DVT by appropriate testing. A popliteal cyst rupture is best evaluated with ultrasonography, magnetic resonance imaging (MRI), or arthrogram of the knee. Gastrocnemius muscle rupture is best assessed with MRI. A cellulitis is evaluated with measurements of the white blood cell counts, cultures, and other markers of inflammation.

Measurements of serum sodium, potassium, blood urea nitrogen (BUN), creatinine, BUN/ creatinine ratio, uric acid, liver enzymes, serum albumin, and cholesterol are helpful in assessing specific organ function. The selection of appropriate tests should be directed by findings in the history and physical examination. Hyponatremia may occur with CHF, cirrhosis, or hypothyroidism. Hepatic disease is best assessed by the measurement of liver enzymes and bilirubin. When significant liver injury is present, abnormal laboratory test results may include hypokalemia, hypoalbuminemia, respiratory alkalosis, low magnesium and phosphorus levels, the presence of ethanol, macrocytosis, and a low serum folate level. Markers of renal disease include elevated creatinine and BUN levels, hyperkalemia, metabolic acidosis, hyper-

phosphatemia, hypocalcemia, an anemia that is typically normocytic, an active urinary sedimentation rate, a low serum albumin level (less than 2.0 g per deciliter with a nephrotic syndrome), and proteinuria that is typically more than 3+ on dipstick testing or greater than 500 mg per deciliter in a 24-hour urine collection. Thyroid-stimulating hormone and thyroid hormone levels should be reviewed when indicated.

Noninvasive testing is often needed. The use of a two-dimensional cardiac echocardiogram is very useful for assessing left ventricular function, valvular disease, or significant pericardial disease. Right ventricular function (ejection fraction) is often best assessed by means of a nuclear ventriculogram. Liver ultrasonography rapidly evaluates the presence of regenerative nodules or frank cirrhosis. Renal ultrasonography is helpful in measuring the size of the kidneys and in screening for obstruction (hydronephrosis).

Investigation of the causes of lymphedema may include lymphoscintigraphy. After the injection of a radiolabeled colloid into the dorsum of the foot, tracer uptake within the lymph nodes is assessed after a defined interval and distinguishes lymphedema from edema of nonlymphatic origin. The appearance of tracer outside the main lymph routes, particularly the skin, indicates lymph reflux and suggests proximal obstruction. Poor transit of the isotope from the injection site suggests hypoplasia. Lymphangiography injection of tracer directly into a peripheral lymphatic vessel, usually in the dorsum of the foot, is a means for diagnosing obstruction. Computed tomography or MRI can be used to detect a characteristic honeycomb pattern in the subcutaneous compartment that is not seen with other causes of edema. The muscle compartment deep to the fascia is enlarged in DVT but is unchanged with lymphedema.

TREATMENT

Dietary intervention, specifically the restriction of sodium intake, regardless of the cause of the edema, is essential for the successful management of excessive interstitial fluid. Typically, a diet restricting sodium intake to less than

3 g per day is the first goal and is readily achieved by avoiding the addition of salt to prepared foods. Elimination of added salt during food preparation and avoidance of canned and processed food can further reduce sodium intake to approximately 1.5 g per day. A restriction in water intake is typically limited to patients with severe diseases that have led to the edema, particularly CHF and cirrhosis. Limiting water intake to 2 L per day is moderately restrictive and can be achieved with appropriate patient education. More stringent restrictions, to approximately 1 L per day, are difficult to achieve in ambulatory patients.

Diuretic therapy is the primary means of reducing excessive volume via the kidney. These compounds belong to three principal groups (Table 4.5). Thiazides are well absorbed, have a late onset and peak in action, and are conveniently taken once a day. Thiazides' primary site of action is the distal renal tubule. As a group, they are less effective in patients with renal insufficiency and are associated with hyponatremia. Loop diuretics inhibit sodium reabsorption by the ascending limb of the loop of Henle. They can be given orally or intravenously and typically have a potent and rapid onset of action. The duration of action, however, is short, and twice-a-day dosing may be required. When renal impairment is present, they are more effective than thiazides. When a patient's condition becomes refractory to their action, the addition of a distal tubule agent can be synergistic in promoting a more aggressive diuresis. The additional use of a low-dose dopamine infusion with intravenous loop

diuretic has been considered a means of stimulating volume reduction in refractory disease, although randomized trials evaluating this practice are not fully supportive of the proposed benefit.

Potassium-sparing diuretics also act at the distal renal tubule and, as a class, are weak agents. Their ability to mitigate potassium loss during chronic diuretic therapy makes them useful in treatment of chronic conditions such as CHF. Spironolactone, an inhibitor of aldosterone-sensitive sodium transport, has been demonstrated to have marked mortality benefits for patients with significantly symptomatic CHF (16). When first prescribed, they should be given in lower doses with a gradual increase in dose to mitigate the potential for significant hyperkalemia.

A poor response to diuretic therapy is often noted in specific individuals. Mechanisms for diuretic resistance include excessive dietary sodium intake, chronic use of loop diuretics, and the development of hypertrophy of the distal nephron, which facilitates renal sodium retention, severe renal hypoperfusion secondary to a loss of effective arterial blood volume (CHF, cirrhosis) or to progressive arterial occlusions, and diminished gastrointestinal tract absorption because of progressive bowel wall edema (17). These patients often improve after a course of intravenous diuretics to decrease wall edema and demonstrate improved responses to oral agents. The presence of hypoalbuminemia and the use of NSAIDs, including newer COX-2 inhibitors, and steroids, such as prednisone, contribute to

TABLE 4.5. *Diuretic therapy*

Diuretic class	Name	Dose range (mg)	Half-life	Potency	Class effects and adverse reactions
Thiazide	Chlorthalidone	50–100	~3 days	++	Hypokalemia, hypomagnesemia,
	Hydrochlorothiazide	25–200	10–12 hr	++	hypercalcemia, hyponatremia,
	Metolazone	2.5–20	8–14 hr	+++	hyperuricemia, increased blood
					glucose and lipid levels
Loop	Bumetanide	0.5–2	1–1.5 hr	+++	Hypokalemia, hypomagnesemia,
	Ethacrynic acid	25–100	1.4 hr	+++	hypochloremia, metabolic alkalosis,
	Furosemide	20–100	1 hr	+++	hypocalcemia, hyperuricemia,
	Torasemide	5–100	>3 hr	+++	increased blood glucose
					and lipid levels
Potassium sparing	Amiloride	25–20	6–9 hr	+	Hyperkalemia, metabolic acidosis;
	Spironolactone	12.5–100	1–1.5 hr	+	spironolactone: antiandrogen/
	Triamterene	50–100	1–6 hr	+	gynecomastia

diuretic resistance. The addition of amiloride, spironolactone, hydrochlorothiazide, chlorthalidone, or metolazone to a loop agent may facilitate improved volume reductions but confer a higher risk of hypokalemia (18).

Electrolytes and acid-base status should be monitored regularly. With the increasing use of spironolactone for CHF, the incidence of symptomatic hyperkalemia is increasing. Continuous infusions of loop diuretics have been limited to patients with refractory CHF and advanced renal failure, and, if carefully managed, it can be an effective means of decreasing volume. In patients with the nephrotic syndrome or cirrhosis who demonstrate a severe reduction in albumin and plasma colloid oncotic pressure, the administration of albumin is associated with improved diuresis.

Management of lymphedema includes the following. Promoting exercise and its dynamic muscle contraction encourages both passive and active increase in lymphatic drainage. Compression stockings, which act as a force to counter muscle contraction, and generate greater interstitial pressure. Manual lymphatic drainage by a form of massage that stimulates lymph flow is potentially effective in more proximal, normally draining lymphatic areas. Multilayer bandaging, pneumatic compression, elevation of the limbs, and the prevention of infection with good skin care, good hygiene, and antiseptic dressing for minor wounds are paramount in lymphedema. Diuretics are of limited benefit. Surgery is occasionally needed if the weight of the limb inhibits it use, and the aim is either to remove excessive tissue or to bypass local lymphatic defects (19).

WHEN TO REFER

The majority of patients with edema can be managed in an outpatient primary care setting with little difficulty or risk. Referrals should be made when the underlying diseases promoting the collection of fluid are severe or are unclear. Individuals with CHF require a systematic evaluation of the mechanisms of its onset and severity and a determined effort to find a potential cause that may be addressed by medications or surgery. Such a comprehensive approach can beneficially affect the morbidity and mortality associated with heart failure and is often best directed by a cardiologist. The development of renal failure or the nephrotic syndrome should also be considered appropriate indications for consultation. In addition, the treatment of significant hepatic dysfunction, which causes a generalized edema, is often benefited by consultation with a specialist.

Individuals with a DVT generally do not require a referral unless it is associated with a prothrombic state (protein C or S deficiency, antithrombin III deficiency, lupus anticoagulant, or factor V Leiden mutation). In this scenario a review by a hematologist is appropriate. Finally, when a malignancy or a recurrence is thought to play a role, the advice of an oncologist is essential.

WHEN TO ADMIT

A study evaluating the use of low molecular heparin in the outpatient management of a DVT has been published; but as a group, these patients should be considered candidates for hospitalization particularly if they are at high risk (Chapter 32).

Factors that indicate the benefits of hospitalization are related more to the severity and symptoms of the underlying disease that precipitated the edema. The need to administer intravenous medications is the most common reason to admit—for example, cellulitis, diuretic resistance, or the acute need for cardiac medications.

Symptomatic heart failure, unstable angina, a potential myocardial infarction, syncope, the need to remove a large volume of fluid, a poor response to maximal oral diuretic, the associated metabolic complications of CHF (hyponatremia, hypokalemia, progressive renal insufficiency), and the need to remove fluid from the pleural or abdominal cavity are common reasons to hospitalize patients with cardiac edema.

Uremic symptoms, the need for dialysis, hyperkalemia, severe hypertension, volume overload, a marked metabolic acidosis, and the need of invasive testing to diagnose or treat the mechanisms of a primary cause of renal failure are common reasons to hospitalize patients with edema related to renal failure.

Hepatic encephalopathy, a coagulopathy, anasarca, marked ascites, suspected subacute bacterial peritonitis, gastrointestinal bleeding, and severe anemia are examples of the adverse complications of hepatic disease that often precipitate admissions.

PRACTICAL POINTS

- Most patients with unilateral lower extremity edema should be considered for venous Doppler assessment to screen for the presence of a DVT, regardless of whether it is associated with or pain or not.

- Bilateral lower extremity or generalized edema is the primary result of three mechanisms: an increase in central venous pressure, such as in pulmonary hypertension; renal sodium and water retention, as with a primary renal disease; or a reduction in cardiac output.

- NSAIDs are an extremely common mechanism for drug-related lower extremity swelling.

- Clinical signs supportive of a DVT are inconsistent.

- Dietary intervention, specifically the restriction of sodium intake, regardless of the cause of the edema, is essential for the successful management of excessive interstitial fluid.

- The majority of patients with edema can be managed in an outpatient primary care setting with little difficulty or risk. Referrals should be made when the underlying diseases promoting the collection of fluid are severe or are unclear.

REFERENCES

1. Braunwald E. Edema. In: Fauci AS, Braunwald E, Isselbacher KJ, et al., eds. *Harrison's principles of internal medicine,* 14th ed. New York: McGraw-Hill, 1998:212.
2. Starling EH. Physiologic forces involved in the causation of dropsy. *Lancet* 1896;1:267–270.
3. Hammel HT. Role of colloid proteins in Starling's hypothesis and in returning interstitial fluid to the vasa recta. *Am J Physiol* 1995;268:H2133–H2144.
4. Gorman WP, Davis KR, Connelly R. ABC of arterial and venous disease: swollen lower limbs—2: general assessment and deep vein thrombosis. *BMJ* 2000;320:1453–1456.
5. Schrier RW. Pathogenesis of sodium and water retention in high-output and low-output cardiac failure, nephrotic syndrome, cirrhosis and pregnancy. *N Engl J Med* 1989;319:1127–1134.
6. Kearon C, Julian JA, Math M, et al. Non-invasive diagnosis of deep venous thrombosis. *Ann Intern Med* 1998;128:663–677.
7. Lensing WA, Prandoni P, Prins MH, et al. Deep vein thrombosis. *Lancet* 1999;353:479–485.
8. Merlin GJ, Spandorfer J: The outpatient with unilateral leg swelling. *Med Clin North Am* 1995;79:435–477.
9. Johnson BF, Manes RA, Bergen RO, et al. Relationship between changes in the deep venous system and the development of the post-thrombotic syndrome after an acute episode of lower limb deep vein thrombosis: a one to six year follow-up study. *J Vasc Surg* 1995;21:307–313.
10. Brady HR, Quigley CL, Stafford FJ, et al. Popliteal cyst rupture and the pseudothrombophlebitis syndrome. *Ann Emerg Med* 1987;16:1151–1154.
11. McLure J. Gastrocnemius musculotendinous rupture: a condition confused with thrombophlebitis. *South Med J* 1984;77:1143–1145.
12. Diskin CJ, Stokes TJ, Dansby LM, et al. Education and debate: towards an understanding of oedema. *BMJ* 1999;318:1610–1613.
13. Cannann-Kuhl S, Venkatramen ES, Ernst SI, et al. Relationships among proteins and albumin concentration in nephrotic plasma. *Am J Physiol* 1993;264:F1052–F1059.
14. Mortimer PP. ABC of arterial and venous disease: swollen lower limb—2: lymphoedema. *BMJ* 2000;320:1527–1529.
15. Pope JE, Anderson JJ, Felson DT. A meta-analysis of the effects of nonsteroidal anti-inflammatory drugs on blood pressure. *Arch Intern Med* 1993;153:477.
16. Pitt B, Zannad F, Remme WJ, et al. The effect of spironolactone on morbidity and mortality in patients with severe heart failure. *N Engl J Med* 1999;341:709–717.
17. Inoue M, Okajima K, Itoh K, et al. Mechanism of furosemide resistance in analbuminemic rats and hypoalbuminemic patients. *Kidney Int* 1987;32:198–203.
18. Black WD, Shiner PT, Roman J. Severe electrolyte disturbances with metolazone and furosemide. *South Med J* 1978;71:380–381.
19. Ko DA, Lerner R, Klose G, et al. Effective treatment of lymphedema of the extremities. *Arch Surg* 1998;133:452–458.

5

Syncope

Ragavendra R. Baliga and Michael H. Lehmann

DEFINITION

Syncope (from the Greek *Syn* with *koptein,* meaning to cut off) is the sudden, transient loss of consciousness and postural tone with subsequent spontaneous recovery. Before syncope, the patient may experience a variety of prodromal symptoms, typically including the awareness of an impending faint. The latter "near-syncopal" or "presyncopal" state may not progress to frank loss of consciousness, if the underlying pathophysiologic disturbances that would otherwise culminate in syncope are aborted (either spontaneously or via countermaneuvers, such as assuming the recumbent position). Hypotension with cerebral hypoperfusion distinguishes true syncope from other syndromes with which it may be confused.

Most individuals with the "common faint" (vasovagal syncope, described later) do not consult a doctor, and hence the prevalence of syncope is difficult to determine. About one third of adults experience at least one episode of syncope in their lifetime, and syncope accounts for about 3% of emergency room visits and up to 6% of general hospital admissions in the United States (1). The recurrence rate is as high as 34% on 3-year follow-up (2).

The range of prognoses in syncope is wide and the main task of the clinician, therefore, is to determine whether the patient has a benign or a life-threatening cause for syncope (3,4). One must be concerned about the possibility that the syncopal event actually represents a self-aborted cardiac arrest, with a potentially catastrophic outcome the next time around. Yet even when syncope is not a harbinger of sudden death, it may incur serious secondary morbidity consequent to trauma.

An important caveat to bear in mind for a patient with syncope is recognition that that the ac-

tual event has come and gone, leaving the physician to, in effect, "reconstruct" what transpired. Even when abnormalities are uncovered in the course of various diagnostic procedures, it is not immediately evident that the physician has determined the true cause. The physician must integrate all available information, with focused use of diagnostic tests, and then apply sound clinical judgment to arrive at the most reasonable working diagnosis, which will guide therapy selection. Often, only with the passage of time is the accuracy of the hypothesized cause borne out (suppression of further events) or refuted (syncope recurrence)—in which case diagnostic reevaluation is required.

PRINCIPAL CAUSES (TABLE 5.1)

Neurally Mediated Syncope

Patients with these conditions have in common the paroxysmal occurrence of peripheral vasodilatation, bradycardia, or both, which reflects sympathetic withdrawal and hypervagotonia (5).

Vasovagal, vasodepressor, or *neurocardiogenic* syncope—also called the "common faint"—is often caused by a precipitating event such as prolonged standing, hypovolemia (commonly dehydration), fear, severe pain, the sight of blood, strong emotion, or instrumentation; however, it can also occur without obvious cause. In a typical episode of the common faint, there is a prodrome in which the patient may feel unsteady, "feel bad," be confused, yawn, or experience ringing in the ears or visual disturbances (dimming, blurring, or seeing spots). Often there is associated warmth and nausea, sometimes with vomiting; facial pallor and diaphoresis are common. These presyncopal features (typically lasting from 30 to 60 seconds) are not seen in

TABLE 5.1. *Principal causes of syncope*

Neurally mediated syncope
  Vasovagal
  Situational
  Carotid sinus
Orthostatic syncope (drugs, autonomic
  insufficiency, volume depletion)
Cardiac syncope
  Arrhythmic
  Structural
Metabolic disturbances
Neurologic, psychiatric disorders
Unexplained etiology

all patients; the faint may occur suddenly without warning, not allowing time for protection against injury. At the onset of syncope, there is hypotension, often (but not necessarily) accompanied by bradycardia. With protracted hypotension, there may be attendant seizurelike activity (involuntary muscle jerking). On recovery, along with return of consciousness, color returns to the face, blood pressure increases, and bradycardia resolves. Characteristically, consciousness is regained rapidly after the individual is in the supine position, although there is commonly a feeling of postevent fatigue. In patients who have minimal presyncopal warning, telltale symptoms and signs of vasovagal syncope—nausea, warmth, diaphoresis, and pallor—sometimes become apparent only during the recovery phase. The long-term prognosis in neurocardiogenic syncope is generally excellent; however, in some patients, recurrences are frequent and are a major cause for seeking medical attention.

Situational or *reflex* syncope is loss of consciousness during or immediately after coughing, micturition, swallowing, or defecation. Alcohol has been implicated in micturition-related syncope.

Carotid sinus syncope is induced by carotid sinus stimulation, resulting in hypotension, bradycardia, or both. Sensitive individuals, typically elderly men, may develop carotid sinus syncope with tight shirt collars or while shaving the neck.

Orthostatic Syncope

This type of syncope results from orthostatic hypotension, diagnosed by documentation of a 20 mm Hg or more fall in systolic blood pressure during the initial 5 minutes after the patient is in upright position; the associated heart rate either remains unchanged or increases (in contrast to vasovagal syncope). Orthostatic hypotension is a common cause of syncope in the elderly and is exacerbated by medications (as discussed later). Detection of orthostatic hypotension should trigger an investigation for fluid depletion and blood loss, particularly with syncope of new onset. A major intraabdominal hemorrhage (e.g., gastrointestinal or from ectopic pregnancy) can precipitate syncope before overt signs of bleeding are apparent. Autonomic insufficiency is a cause of orthostatic hypotension in diabetic patients, patients with Parkinson's disease, and the elderly.

Cardiac Syncope

A cardiac cause of syncope is seen in about one fifth of patients. Syncope associated with cardiovascular disease portends a much higher risk of mortality than is the case in the absence of underlying structural heart disease. Patients with cardiac syncope are at highest risk of dying within 1 to 6 months (6). The 1-year mortality rate is 18% to 33%, in comparison with that of syncope with noncardiac causes (0% to 12%) or syncope in patients with no etiology (6%) (7). The incidence of sudden death in patients with a cardiac cause is substantially higher than in the other two groups. Cardiac causes of syncope include the following:

Arrhythmic syncope results from tachyarrhythmias (ventricular or supraventricular) and bradyarrhythmias. Specific examples include sinus arrest; atrial fibrillation with very rapid conduction over an accessory pathway in patients with Wolff-Parkinson-White syndrome; and sustained monomorphic ventricular tachycardia (VT). Patients with complete heart block may develop self-limiting syncopal episodes in which there is no effective cardiac output as a result of transient asystole or ventricular tachyarrhythmias (Stokes-Adams attacks).

Torsades de pointes is a polymorphic VT that occurs in patients with prolonged ventricular repolarization [long QT syndrome (LQTS)] but otherwise structurally normal hearts. LQTS may occur either on a congenital or acquired basis (e.g., hypokalemia or exposure to certain drugs, as described later). Torsades de pointes can readily progress to ventricular fibrillation (Fig. 5.1). Thus, individuals with LQTS are at risk not only for syncope but also for "seizures" (from transient cerebral hypoxia) and sudden death. Other congenital, potentially lethal arrhythmic disorders include Brugada's syndrome (ST segment elevation in precordial leads V_1, V_2, and V_3, often with incomplete or complete right bundle branch block) (8), familial catecholaminergic polymorphic VT (9), and arrhythmogenic right ventricular dysplasia with associated ventricular arrhythmias (10). In some variants of hypertrophic cardiomyopathy, patients may exhibit minimal, if any, cardiac hypertrophy, and yet affected individuals may be predisposed to sudden death, presumably from sustained ventricular tachyarrhythmias. Another explanation for syncope in hypertrophic cardiomyopathy is the obstructive type in which there is an intraventricular gradient (see Chapter 15).

Pacemaker and implantable cardiac defibrillator (ICD) malfunction may be a cause of syncope in patients with these devices. With ICDs, however, it should be appreciated that even when a rapid ventricular tachyarrhythmia is successfully treated by the device, syncope may nonetheless occur, depending on the duration of hypotension preceding the termination of tachyarrhythmia. ICD interrogation can provide information about possible tachyarrhythmia occurrence and therapy delivery/outcome coincident with the syncopal event in question.

Structural syncope is caused by valvular stenosis (aortic, mitral, pulmonic), prosthetic valve dysfunction or thrombosis, hypertrophic cardiomyopathy, pulmonary embolism, pulmonary hypertension, cardiac tamponade, and anomalous origin of the coronary arteries. Syncope in aortic stenosis occurs during exertion when the fixed valvular obstruction prevents an increase in cardiac output into the dilated vascular bed of the exercising skeletal muscles. The syncope can occur during exertion or immediately afterward. Syncope can also occur at rest in aortic stenosis when paroxysmal tachyarrhythmias or bradyarrhythmias accompany this valvular abnormality. Aortic dissection, subclavian steal, severe left ventricular dysfunction, and my-

ocardial infarction are other important causes of cardiac syncope. In elderly patients, syncope may be the presenting feature in acute myocardial infarction (11). Left atrial myxomas or ball-valve thrombi that fall into the mitral valve during diastole can result in the obstruction of ventricular filling and in syncope.

Metabolic Disturbance

Syncope due to hypoglycemia is the loss of consciousness that accompanies a blood glucose level of less than 40 mg per deciliter and is preceded by tremors, confusion, salivation, hyperadrenergic state, and hunger. Hypoglycemic syncope should be suspected in diabetic patients who take insulin or oral hypoglycemic agents. In contrast to true syncope, the loss of consciousness caused by hypoglycemia is not associated with hypotension, persists even when the patient is in the supine position, and usually does not resolve until the blood glucose level is restored to normal. Hypoadrenalism, which can cause postural hypotension as a result of inadequate cortisol secretion, is an important treatable cause for syncope and should be suspected when long-term steroid therapy is suddenly discontinued or when there are other stigmata of adrenal insufficiency.

Neurologic Disease

Neurologic conditions can mimic syncope by causing impairment or loss of consciousness; these conditions include transient cerebral ischemia (usually in the vertebrobasilar territory), migraines (basilar artery territory), temporal lobe epilepsy, atonic seizures, and unwitnessed grand mal seizures. Disorders resembling syncope, but without loss of consciousness, include drop attacks (sudden loss of postural tone), cataplexy, and transient ischemic attacks of carotid origin. In neurologic conditions associated with severe pain, such as trigeminal or glossopharyngeal neuralgia, the loss of consciousness is usually caused by vasovagal syncope.

Psychiatric Disorder

Syncope or syncopelike syndromes associated with psychiatric conditions are not associated

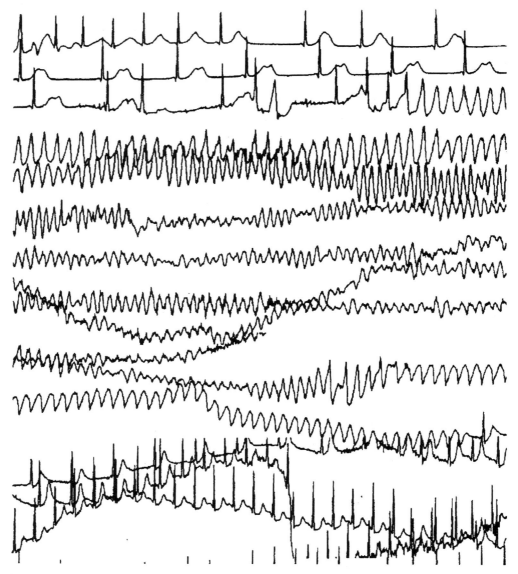

FIG. 5.1. A 25-year-old woman who had had a single syncopal episode 2 years earlier was hospital-ized after a 2-minute episode of syncope during an argument with a police officer over a traffic ticket. A 12-lead electrocardiogram obtained on admission showed sinus rhythm, 52 beats per minute, with a markedly prolonged QT interval of 0.68 second. Twenty-four-hour Holter monitoring in the hospital revealed recurrent asymptomatic, mostly short, episodes of torsades de pointes. One such episode, beginning with bradycardia-related further QT prolongation, occurred during sleep and degenerated into ventricular fibrillation that lasted one and half minutes and terminated spontaneously. [From: Ben-horin J, Medina A. Congenital long QT syndrome (images in medicine). *N Engl J Med* 1997;336:1568.]

with increased rates of mortality but have high 1-year recurrence rates (up to 50%) (12). The association between syncope and psychiatric disorders may be complicated. First, psychiatric disorders may represent comorbidity in a patient with syncope and have no role in syncope occurrence. Second, psychiatric disorders may cause syncope-like states, often involving a conversion reaction. Psychiatric conditions associated with syncope include generalized anxiety and panic disorders (in which hyperventilation leads to cerebral vasoconstriction and possible loss of consciousness), major depression, alcohol and substance abuse, and somatization disorders. Third, there may be a complex interaction between syncope and the psychiatric condition. Stress, depression, and psychosocial disorders are capable of provoking arrhythmias and myocardial infarction. It is possible that all these factors may, in turn, precipitate syncope, although the magnitude of this problem is unclear. Finally, it is possible that recurrent syncope itself may secondarily give rise to psychiatric conditions such anxiety and panic attacks. A diagnosis of syncope resulting from psychiatric disorders is usually made after organic causes have been excluded. Diagnosis may be difficult when patients have both organic and psychogenic seizures.

Unexplained Etiology

Earlier studies reported that, in about half of the patients with syncope, no cause could be determined. However, with the wider use of tilt testing, event monitoring, electrophysiologic studies, and more aggressive investigation of elderly patients and those with suspected psychiatric causes, the proportion of syncope cases in which the cause can be determined has increased.

KEYS TO THE HISTORY

A meticulously documented history is critical in the assessment of syncope. For new-onset syncope, the examiner focuses primarily on ruling out underlying structural heart disease and other life-threatening conditions as such as acute myocardial infarction and upper gastrointestinal hemorrhage, which necessitates evaluation in the emergency department. In contrast, the diagnostic assessment of recurrent syncope involves a broader consideration of causes and is often undertaken in an ambulatory setting. The history and physical examination should identify a cause of syncope in about 45% of patients (13). These basic elements of a medical evaluation can lead to recognition of ischemic heart disease, heart failure, aortic stenosis, hypertrophic cardiomyopathy, and pulmonary embolism; neurologic causes such as seizure disorder and subclavian steal syndrome; and familial conditions such as long QT syndrome. Emphasis should be placed on the circumstances surrounding the syncopal event, the nature of prodromal and associated symptoms, characterization of the recovery period, medications and drugs, the presence of known cardiac disease, family history (e.g., cardiomyopathy or LQTS), and psychiatric history. Observations from witnesses or a family member may be helpful. In documenting the history, the examiner should focus on the relation of syncopal events to posture, exertion, and palpitations. The examiner should determine the number and chronicity of prior syncopal and near-syncopal episodes; the latter may be more frequent (albeit of shorter duration) than full-blown syncopal events and may provide an opportunity for diagnostic electrocardiographic monitoring to capture a clinically relevant event. Inquiry also should be made into whether the patient has sustained any trauma in association with the symptoms; serious secondary injury warrants a more aggressive diagnostic and treatment strategy aimed at preventing subsequent morbidity.

Circumstances Surrounding Onset

Painstaking attention should be paid to the chronology of symptoms: sudden onset without a prodrome may suggest arrhythmias, whereas protracted autonomic symptoms (pallor, diaphoresis, nausea) in association with a precipitating factor such as pain, extreme heat or emotion, viewing an unpleasant sight, or prolonged standing suggest vasovagal syncope. Loss of consciousness after prolonged standing at attention suggests vasovagal syncope, whereas that which occurs immediately on standing is caused by orthostatic hypotension. Situational syncope occurs during or immediately after swallowing, coughing, defecation, and micturition. Alcohol ingestion may be the most important predisposing factor in micturition syncope. Alcohol ingestion has also been implicated in about 10% of syncope cases in young adults, and the syncope in those cases has been attributed to orthostatic stress because of impaired vasoconstriction (14). Carotid syncope occurs with head rotation while the person is wearing tight collars. Exertional syncope suggests possible structural heart disease such as aortic stenosis, hypertrophic cardiomyopathy, or exercise-induced tachycardias. In highly competitive athletes, vasovagal syncope documented by history and head-up tilt testing has been shown to occur during as well as after exertion (15). Syncope associated with arm exercise is a feature of subclavian steal syndrome. A history of exertional chest pain, as well as exertional syncope, in an adolescent or young adult raises the possibility of anomalous origin of a coronary artery (16). Syncope in patients with LQTS may occur in association with physical exertion (particularly swimming), during emotional stress, or in response to sudden, unexpected acoustic stimuli (e.g., sound of an alarm clock or telephone) (17).

Posture at the Onset of Attack

Vasodepressor syncope typically occurs in the upright position; once the patient is horizontal, the autonomic derangements begin to reverse. In some instances, if the patient returns to the upright position too soon, there can be a recurrent faint. Syncope resulting from arrhythmias and other causes of loss of consciousness that resembles syncope, such as hypoglycemia and hyperventilation, can occur independently of posture. Moreover, syncope caused by pain or emotion-related vasovagal syncope (e.g., after a needlestick or on the sight of blood or injury) need not occur while the patient is upright. By definition, syncope caused by orthostatic hypotension occurs soon (within seconds to minutes) after the patient assumes an upright posture from the recumbent or sitting position.

Associated Symptoms

Associated symptoms are not always present and depend on the cause of syncope. The peri-event symptoms typically associated with neurally mediated syncope have been discussed. Of note, recovery from cardiac syncope is often rapid (within 30 seconds). Palpitations preceding syncope, especially an awareness of rapid heart beating, suggests an arrhythmic origin (see Chapter 3). Features of neurologic syncope include brainstem findings (vertigo, dysarthria, ataxia, visual disturbances), whereas postevent confusion is more likely to be caused by seizures. Loss of consciousness associated with headache indicates migraine or seizures, whereas that associated with throat or facial pain suggests glossopharyngeal or trigeminal neuralgia.

Differentiating Syncope from Seizures

This distinction can be clinically challenging (Table 5.2), and eyewitness accounts are often helpful in discriminating between the two conditions. Both phenomena involve loss of consciousness. As a further confounding factor, myoclonic jerking may occur during the course of true syncope secondary to transient cerebral hypoxia (18). The best discriminatory features between syncope and seizures are sensorium of the patient after the episode and the patient's age. When a patient older than 45 years is disorientated after

TABLE 5.2. *Characteristics of syncope versus seizures*

Clinical features	Syncope	Seizures[a]
Loss of consciousness precipitated by pain, micturition, exercise, pain, defecation, or stressful events	+	−
Sweating and nausea before or during the event	+	−
Aura	−	+
Tongue biting	−	+
Clonic or myoclonic jerks or rhythmic movements	+/−	++
Disorientation after the event	−	+
Slowness in returning to consciousness	−	+
Unconscious >5 min	−	+

an episode, seizures are five times more likely than syncope to have occurred (19). Older individuals with prolonged disorientation after an episode of loss of consciousness are therefore more likely to have had a seizure. An exception would be arrhythmic syncope with a prolonged hypotensive episode, which may secondarily cause transient cerebral hypoxic injury and postevent disorientation. Other clinical features suggestive of a seizure include cyanotic facial appearance, as opposed to pallor, during the episode; frothing at the mouth; unconsciousness lasting more than 5 minutes; feeling sleepy after the episode; aching muscles; and tongue biting along the lateral aspect of the tongue. Seizures are also suggested by an aura before the event, horizontal eye movement during the event, and a headache after the episode. Fecal and urinary incontinence can occur in both syncope and seizures but is far more common with seizures. Tonic-clonic movements suggest grand mal seizures. Syncope caused by cerebral ischemia can be accompanied by rigidity and clonic movements of the arms and legs. In petit mal epilepsy, the lack of responsiveness is associated with preserved postural tone. Temporal lobe seizures can easily be mistaken for syncope because they usually lack tonic-clonic movements and are associated with autonomic changes such as flushing and fluctuating changes in the level of consciousness. Vertebrobasilar insufficiency should be suspected when the patient has features of brainstem ischemia such as tinnitus, diplopia, vertigo, dysarthria, and focal sensory loss or weakness.

Age at Onset

In younger individuals (younger than 30 years), common causes (Table 5.3) include neurally mediated syncope, undiagnosed seizures, Wolff-Parkinson-White syndrome and other supraventricular tachycardias, hypertrophic cardiomyopathy, LQTS, and congenital coronary anomalies (16).

In middle-aged individuals, typical causes of syncope are neurally mediated and cardiac (arrhythmic, mechanical/obstructive) in origin.

TABLE 5.3. *Causes of syncope by age*

Age	Causes

Youth (<30 years)	Neurally mediated syncope
	Situational
	Alcohol
	Undiagnosed seizures
	Cardiac syncope:
	    Hypertrophic cardiomyopathy
	    Coronary artery anomalies
	    WPW syndrome, other SVT
	    Long QT syndrome

Middle-aged (30–65 years)	Neurally mediated syncope Cardiac (arrhythmic, mechanical/obstructive)
Elderly (>65 years)	Neurally mediated syncope Cardiac (arrhythmic, mechanical/obstructive) Drugs: antihyperhypertensive medications, antidepressants (see text for list) Orthostatic hypotension

SVT, Supraventricular tachycardia; WPW, Wolff-Parkinson-White.

Syncope in the elderly (older than 65 years) may be overlooked when the episode is described by the patient simply as a "fall," owing to postsyncope retrograde amnesia (4). In the elderly, the cause of syncope is often multifactorial, and older patients tend to have serious arrhythmias (sustained VT in the setting of cardiomyopathy), orthostatic hypotension, or neurologic disorders that are contributory (3). Elderly patients are also prone to neurally mediated syncope related to known triggers, such as micturition, defecation, coughing, laughing, swallowing, and eating. Postprandial hypotension (secondary to splanchnic vascular volume shifts) can result in syncope during or after a meal. Another confounding factor in this age group is polypharmacy: Many medications at therapeutic doses cause postural hypotension. Aortic stenosis, myocardial infarction, and carotid sinus hypersensitivity are other conditions that predispose to syncope in the elderly. Carotid sinus hypersensitivity has been suggested to be responsible for syncope or "falls" in the elderly, and the bradycardia documented in these patients has been successfully managed by dual-chamber pacing (4). The multifactorial nature of syncope in older patients often necessitates a management approach aimed at correcting many of these factors simultaneously.

Other Historical Clues

Cardiac syncope must be kept in mind in patients with structural heart disease, particularly ischemic heart disease with left ventricular dysfunction. A family history of sudden death (including accidental drownings) or seizures is a feature of hypertrophic cardiomyopathy, LQTS, and Brugada's syndrome. A history of LQTS is particularly important in syncope precipitated by medications (to be described).

Features of the history that suggest syncope caused by VT or atrioventricular (AV) block (odds ratio greater than 5) are male gender, age older than 54 years, three or fewer episodes of syncope, and a 6-second or shorter duration of warning before syncope (20). The same study found that features of clinical history that suggest that the syncope is *not* caused by VT or AV block (odds ratio less than 0.2) are palpitations, nausea, blurred vision, warmth, diaphoresis, or lightheadedness before syncope and the sensation of warmth, nausea, fatigue, or diaphoresis after syncope (features that point instead to a vasovagal mechanism).

Drugs

Drugs can frequently cause syncope, particularly in the elderly. Antihypertensive and antidepressant medications are the most commonly implicated agents. Culprit antihypertensive agents include doxazosin, clonidine, hydralazine, prazosin, and angiotensin-converting enzyme inhibitors. Other drugs associated with syncope are morphine, nitroglycerin, phenothiazines, perioperative amiodarone, calcium channel blockers (e.g., nifedipine), citrated blood, aggressive diuretic therapy, interleukin-2, protamine, and quinidine. Documentation of drug-induced syncope may require ambulatory monitoring of blood pressure.

Drug history is also important in patients with syncope who are suspected of having LQTS. After exposure to drugs that prolong ventricular repolarization, even previously asymptomatic gene carriers may suddenly develop syncope or cardiac arrest caused by torsades de pointes. A detailed list of QT-prolonging drugs can be found

at *www.torsades.org.* A partial list of such drugs known to precipitate syncope caused by torsades de pointes include (a) *cardiac drugs,* such as quinidine, procainamide, sotalol, disopyramide, amiodarone, and dofetilide, and (b) *noncardiac drugs,* such as macrolide antibiotics, tricyclic antidepressants, phenothiazines, some antihistamines, and cisapride. Of note, QT-prolonging drugs are prone to induce torsades de pointes more frequently in women than in men (21,22).

Pregnancy

Syncope is relatively common in pregnancy (3), but its exact mechanism and prognosis remain unclear. In the third trimester, syncope can occur even in the supine position as a result of compression of the aorta and inferior vena cava in the abdomen by the enlarged uterus. Pregnant women with known cardiac disease, palpitations or arrhythmias, exertional syncope, or pathologic murmur merit further evaluation.

HELPFUL SIGNS ON PHYSICAL EXAMINATION

Clinical signs are not readily apparent, and findings depend on the underlying cause of syncope. Clinical examination should be targeted to identify underlying causes suspected from the history. Physical examination is most useful in diagnosing syncope caused by postural hypotension, cardiovascular conditions, and neurologic diseases. Preliminary assessment includes the following:

- Recording of the heart rate: Severe bradycardia may suggest second- or third-degree heart block, whereas tachycardia should trigger an investigation of ventricular or supraventricular tachyarrhythmia. "Postural orthostatic tachycardia syndrome," with associated symptoms of near syncope, may overlap with the clinical picture of vasovagal syncope (23). Postural orthostatic tachycardia should be suspected when there is an increase of 30 beats per minute within 5 minutes of standing, accompanied by symptoms of orthostatic intolerance (lightheadedness, dizziness, near syncope).
- Recording of supine and erect blood pressure for orthostatic hypotension: Erect blood

pressure should be recorded at least 3 minutes after the patient stands upright. Orthostatic hypotension should be suspected when there is a 20-mm Hg fall in systolic blood pressure or a 10-mm Hg fall in diastolic blood pressure within 5 minutes after the patient stands upright. Patients with autonomic insufficiency typically lack a compensatory sinus tachycardia.

- Assessment of pulse deficit and blood pressures in the arms when aortic dissection is suspected.
- Auscultation of the heart for ejection systolic murmur of aortic stenosis and hypertrophic cardiomyopathy and for gallops.
- Pulmonary examination includes assessment of respiratory rate and other chest findings to help exclude pulmonary embolus, congestive heart failure, and chronic obstructive pulmonary disease.
- Carotid sinus massage is useful in elderly patients with suspected carotid sinus syncope. It is best performed with a cardiac monitor but should be deferred in a patient with carotid bruits; in the setting of a recent myocardial infarction, stroke, or transient ischemic attacks; or in patients with a history of VT. Before massaging the carotid sinus, the physician should ensure that there are no carotid bruits and then massage one side at a time, 5 seconds per attempt. The massage should be performed with the patient both supine and erect. An abnormal test result is associated with a pause of greater than 3 seconds with or without prolonged hypotension. The test result is more meaningful if the patient's symptoms of presyncope are reproduced. The reproducibility of the test is enhanced when the symptoms are elicited with the patient in both the supine and erect positions, usually with a tilt table.
- Neurologic examination and auscultation for carotid bruit should be performed when a stroke or focal neurologic deficits are suspected.

DIAGNOSTIC TESTS

The investigation of syncope is limited by fact that there are no diagnostic gold standards against which the diagnostic tests can be assessed. For example, the detection of coronary artery disease in a patient who has fainted does not necessarily imply that such a pathologic process is the cause of syncope.

- **Baseline Laboratory Tests:** Routine laboratory testing is not warranted, and these tests should be performed only if suggested by the history or clinical examination findings. Useful measurements include blood glucose to exclude hypoglycemia and hematocrit to exclude blood loss. Hypokalemia and hypomagnesemia should be ruled out if QT prolongation is observed. Pregnancy testing should be considered in women of childbearing age, particularly before head-up tilt testing or electrophysiologic testing.
- **Twelve-Lead ECG** should be recorded in all patients with syncope, and rhythm strips recorded by paramedics should be reviewed. Although yield of the ECG is low, there is no risk, and the test is relatively inexpensive. Moreover, abnormalities such as previous myocardial infarction, nonsustained VT, or bundle branch block may guide further evaluation. These findings, however, do not necessarily point to a unique cause. For example, a patient with bifascicular block and prior myocardial infarction may turn out to have VT rather than AV block as the cause of syncope (4). Left ventricular hypertrophy may suggest underlying cardiomyopathy. A completely normal ECG implies a more favorable prognosis and tends to reduce (but does not absolutely exclude) the likelihood of a ventricular tachyarrhythmic origin. The ECG is particularly useful in identifying acute ischemia; sinoatrial conduction disturbances; bundle branch/bifascicular blocks; second- or third-degree heart block; supraventricular tachycardia; nonsustained VT; accessory pathways with ventricular preexcitation [e.g, Wolff-Parkinson-White syndrome, with short PR interval and slurred QRS upstroke ("delta wave")]; prolonged QT interval; ST segment elevation in the right precordial leads (V_1, V_2, and V_3), possibly with incomplete/complete right bundle branch block (Brugada's syndrome; Chapter 18, Fig. 18.6); and, on occasion, the "epsilon waves" of arrhythmogenic

right ventricular dysplasia, with associated T wave inversions, in the right precordial leads (Fig. 5.2).

- For diagnosing LQTS, a rate-corrected QT (QTc) of more than 0.44 seconds (in the absence of bundle branch block) has traditionally been considered prolonged. However, it should be recognized that in normal persons, the upper 95% confidence limit for QTc is 0.46 seconds in women and 0.45 seconds in men (24). Thus, although longer intervals are probably truly abnormal, QTc values of 0.42 to 0.46 seconds are diagnostically equivocal, because both LQTS gene carriers and noncarriers may exhibit QTc intervals in that normal/borderline range (25). The QTc is calculated as $QT/\sqrt{RR}$,

where the QT (traditionally measured in lead II) and RR intervals are measured in seconds. Because computerized ECG measurements are not always reliable, manual assessment of QTc in patients with syncope is advisable. Care should be taken to avoid inclusion of the U wave in the measurement of QT interval (26). Certain T wave morphologic features, particularly "notches"/"humps" (Fig. 5.3), may also be present in LQTS patients even with borderline or normal QTc intervals (26,27).

- **Exercise Stress Testing** is useful for diagnosing underlying myocardial ischemia when an ischemic substrate is suspected to be the cause of arrhythmogenic syncope. In addition, it may be useful in the detection of rate-dependent

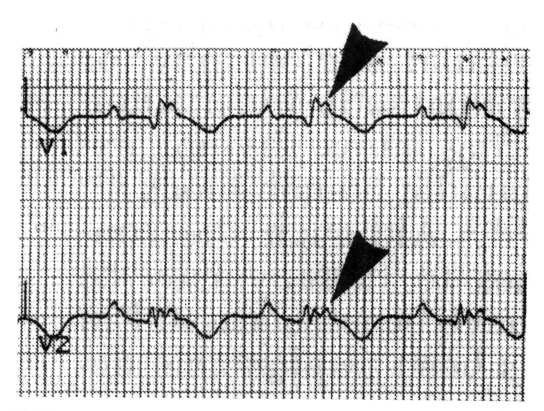

FIG. 5.2. Epsilon waves on electrocardiographic leads V_1 and V_2 of a patient with arrhythmogenic right ventricular dysplasia. Note deflection early in the ST segment (*arrows*) just after the QRS complexes. Typical right precordial T wave inversion is also seen. (From Zipes DP. Specific arrhythmias: diagnosis and treatment. In: Braunwald E, ed. *Heart disease: a textbook of cardiovascular disease,* 5th ed. Philadelphia: WB Saunders, 1997:640–704.)

AV block, exercise-induced tachyarrhythmias (such as familial catecholaminergic polymorphic VT (9)], or exercise-associated syncope (15). Before exercise testing, all patients with exertional syncope must have an echocardiogram to rule out aortic stenosis or hypertrophic cardiomyopathy (or, in young patients and athletes, congenital anomalous coronary arteries).

- **Echocardiogram:** The ECG is particularly useful when structural heart disease, such as aortic stenosis, hypertrophic cardiomyopathy, left ventricular dysfunction, right ventricular dysplasia, or pulmonary hypertension, is suspected (28) (Table 5.4). Right ventricular wall motion and function should be explicitly assessed when the examiner tries to exclude right ventricular dysplasia by echocardiography; if any question about this diagnosis remains, computed tomographic scan and/or cardiac magnetic resonance imaging should be considered.
- **Head-up tilt table testing** (Table 5.5) is useful in patients suspected of having neurally mediated syncope. Patients are tilted passively to an angle of 60 to 70 degrees for 20 to 45 minutes, depending on the protocol utilized, with frequent or continuous monitoring of vital signs (Fig. 5.4). The procedure may involve the use of a provocative agent, such as isoproterenol, to augment the sensitivity of the test, when initial results are negative. It is generally accepted that occurrence of hypotension (*vasodepressor* response)—often, but not necessarily accompanied by, bradycardia (*cardioinhibitory* response)—during head-up tilt is akin to spontaneous vasovagal syncope.

About half of the patients with unexplained syncope have a positive test result with passive tilt; after the administration of isoproterenol, the overall response rate increases to 64% (29). The exact mechanism of enhanced response with isoproterenol remains to be determined but probably involves vasodilatation as well as stimulation of afferent myocardial mechanoreceptors. The sensitivity of the tilt test is 67% to 83%, whereas the overall specificity is about 75%. A "negative" tilt test result can occur even in the presence of an obvious case of neurally mediated syncope, and a "positive" test result can occur when syncope is clearly due to other causes (1).

The procedure is not advisable for pregnant women and the elderly because hypotension is especially detrimental to these patients. Hypertrophic cardiomyopathy and aortic stenosis should also be excluded before head-up tilt testing. The test is not indicated for individuals who have had a single episode of syncope that is characteristic of vasovagal syncope and during which no injury was sustained. Older individuals (men older than 45 years and women older than 55 years) should undergo cardiac stress testing before tilt testing, because isoproterenol and the ensuing hypotension can exacerbate underlying ischemic heart disease. Head-up tilt testing is recommended for patients with recurrent syncope in the absence of cardiac cause.

- **Ambulatory Electrocardiographic (Holter) Monitoring for 24 to 48 Hours:** This type of monitoring (Table 5.6) is used to detect arrhythmogenic causes of syncope (30). The yield of this investigation is enhanced when a record is obtained during an episode of syncope (a rare, fortuitous occurrence). The optimal duration for monitoring is not known; however, several studies have suggested that it is not cost effective to monitor for periods longer than 48 hours (30). In general, culprit tachyarrhythmias or bradycardias are sporadic and transient, and continuous ambulatory recordings are thus often unrewarding. Nonetheless, Holter monitoring is recommended for patients with a high pretest probability of arrhythmias, such as patients with structural heart disease, an abnormal ECG, brief sudden loss of consciousness without a prodrome, or palpitations associated with syncope. Holter monitoring is most likely to be informative in patients with frequent (virtually daily) episodes of presyncopal symptoms. Nondiagnostic arrhythmias found during Holter monitoring (i.e., those not correlated with symptoms of presyncope or syncope) usually do not require treatment; this issue frequently arises with regard to

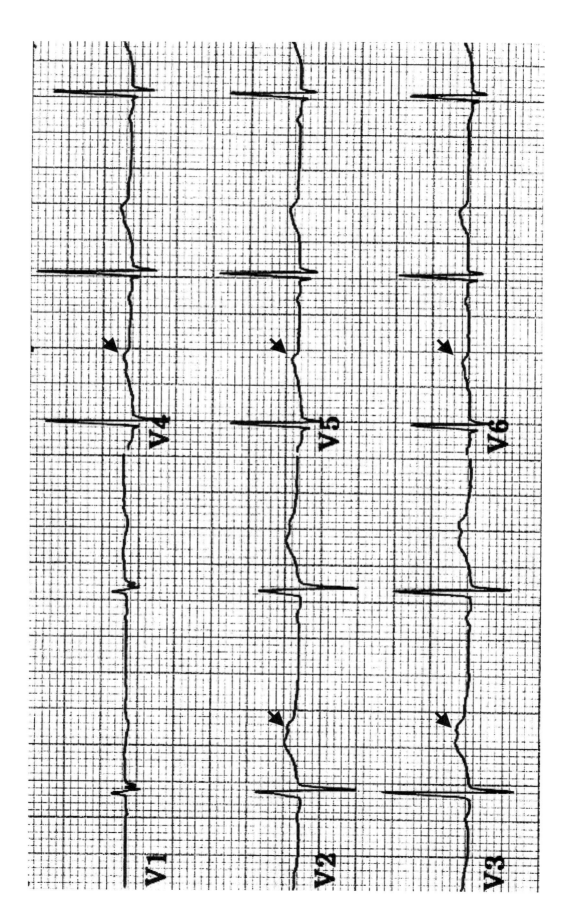

TABLE 5.4. *ACC/AHA recommendations for echocardiography*

Class I: There is evidence and/or general agreement that echocardiography is useful and effective
Syncope in a patient with clinically suspected heart disease
Periexertional syncope
Class IIa: The weight of evidence/opinion is in favor of usefulness/efficacy
Syncope in a patient in a high-risk occupation (e.g., a pilot)
Class IIb: Usefulness/efficacy is less well established by evidence/opinion
Syncope of occult etiology with no findings of heart disease on history or physical examination
Class III: There is evidence and/or general agreement that echocardiography is not useful and in some cases may be harmful
Recurrent syncope in a patient in whom previous echocardiographic or other testing was demonstrated as a cause of syncope
Syncope in a patient for whom there is no clinical suspicion of heart disease
Classic neurogenic syncope

ACC/AHA, American College of Cardiology/American Heart Association.
Modified from Cheitlin MD, Alpert JS, Armstrong WF, et al. ACC/AHA guidelines for the clinical application of echocardiography. *Circulation* 1997;95:1686–1744.

TABLE 5.5. *ACC recommendations for tilt-table testing*

Class I: tilt-table testing is warranted
Recurrent syncope or single syncopal episode in a high-risk patient whether the medical history is suggestive of neurally mediated (Vasovagal) origin or not and
    No evidence of structural or cardiovascular disease or
    Structural cardiovascular disease is present but other causes of syncope have been excluded by appropriate testing
Further evaluation of patients in whom an apparent cause has been established (e.g., asystole, atrioventricular block) but in whom demonstration of susceptibility to neurally mediated syncope would affect treatment plans
Part of the evaluation of exercise-induced or exercise-associated syncope
Class II: conditions in which reasonable differences of opinion exist regarding tilt table testing
Differentiating convulsive syncope from seizures
Evaluating pateints (especially the elderly) with recurrent unexplained falls
Assessing recurrent dizziness or presyncope
Evaluating unexplained syncope in the setting of peripheral neuropathies or dysautonomias
Follow-up evaluation to assess therapy of neurally mediated syncope
Class III: conditions in which tilt-table testing is not warranted
Single syncopal episode, without injury and not in a high-risk setting, with clear-cut vasovagal clinical features
Syncope in which an alternative specific cause has been established and in which additional demonstration of a neurally mediated susceptibility would not alter treatment plans
Relative contraindications to tilt-table testing
Syncope with clinically severe left ventricular outflow obstruction
Syncope in the presence of critical mitral stenosis
Syncope in the setting of known critical proximal coronary artery stenoses
Syncope in conjunction with known critical cerebrovascular stenoses

---

ACC, American College of Cardiology.
Modified from Benditt DG, Ferguson DW, Grubb BP, et al. Tilt table testing for assessing syncope: ACC expert consensus document. *J Am Coll Cardiol* 1998;28:263–275.

FIG. 5.3. Precordial electrocardiographic leads from a healthy asymptomatic young woman who has family members with long QT syndrome. Rate-corrected QT (QTc) varies from 0.43 seconds (long RR intervals) to 0.49 seconds (short RR intervals). "Notched" or "bifid" T waves are seen, with secondary T wave "humps" (*arrows*), distinct from subsequent low-amplitude U waves. These morphologic changes, particularly when seen in the left precordial or limb leads [Lehmann et al., 1994 (26)], are believed to reflect asynchronous ventricular repolarization. In the absence of structural heart disease or electrolyte abnormalities, bifid T waves should suggest a long QT syndrome mutation of the LQT2 type [Zhang et al., 2000 (27)].

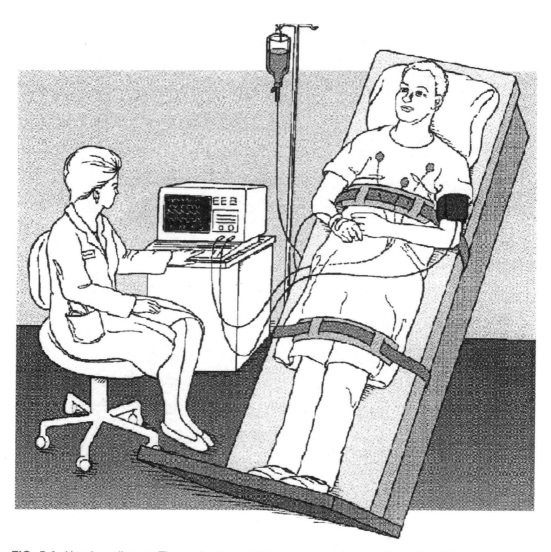

FIG. 5.4. Head-up tilt test. The patient's weight is supported by a footboard, which allows the leg muscles to relax. The resultant blood pooling in the lower extremities and contraction of central vascular volume may stimulate neurally mediated reflex vasodilatation and bradycardia. Restraints prevent the patient from falling in the event of syncope. The patient is being continuously monitored, and an intravenous line is in place for possible administration of isoproterenol, if the control tilt is negative for induction of hypotension/bradycardia. With permission from Health Trend Publishing, Menlo Park, CA.

TABLE 5.6. *ACC/AHA recommendations for ambulatory electrocardiography*

Class I: There is evidence and/or general agreement that ambulatory electrocardiography is useful and effective
Patients with unexplained syncope, near syncope or episodic dizziness in whom the cause is not obvious
Class IIb: Usefulness/efficacy is less well established by evidence/opinion
Patients with symptoms such as syncope, near syncope, episodic dizziness or palpitation in whom a probable cause other than an arrhythmia has been identified but in whom symptoms persist despite treatment of this other cause
Class III: There is evidence and/or general agreement that the ambulatory electrocardiography is not useful and in some cases may be harmful
Patients with symptoms such as syncope, near syncope, episodic dizziness, or palpitation in whom other causes have been identified by history, physical examination or laboratory tests

ACC/AHA, American College of Cardiology/American Heart Association.
Modified from Crawford MH, Bernstein SJ, Deedwania PC, et al. ACC/AHA guidelines for ambulatory electrocardiography. *Circulation* 1999;100:886–893.

premature ventricular complexes, which are commonly seen in the normal population (see Chapter 3).

- **Event Monitors** (see Chapter 3) are useful when patients have presyncopal symptoms every few days to weeks. The devices commonly utilize a "memory loop" to store ongoing ECG signals, which can be "frozen" into memory by patient activation (in response to symptoms) and subsequently retrieved for transtelephonic transmission and analysis (Fig. 5.5). Event monitors are typically used for 2- to 4-week periods at a time and are therefore more likely than the Holter monitors to capture an arrhythmia. Loop-type monitors are especially valuable for detecting fleeting arrhythmias (Figs. 5.5 and 5.6). In about 8% to 20% of patients, event monitors detect arrhythmias with symptoms; in an additional 27%, symptoms are present without arrhythmias (31). Patients who use event monitors must be capable of activating the device and performing the transtelephonic transmissions. This diagnostic modality is particularly useful when syncope is associated with palpitations, dizziness, or presyncope. Event monitors have a limited role when syncope occurs suddenly, preventing the patient from activating the device.
- **Implantable Loop Recorders** are helpful in recurrent syncope that is undiagnosed after initial investigations including Holter monitoring and electrophysiologic testing (32). These subcutaneous implantable recorders (Fig. 5.7) allow electrocardiographic monitor-

ing for periods up to 18 months. The devices are single-lead ECG systems and, when activated by patients, can store rhythms recorded for several minutes before and after the device is activated. Newer generation devices can be programmed to record rhythms automatically, on the basis of prespecified upper and lower rate thresholds. As with pacemakers and ICDs, the stored recordings can be retrieved by radiotelemetry-based interrogation of the device (Fig. 5.8). A limitation of relying on the implantable loop recorder before selecting a therapy is that the physician must wait for the patient to experience another episode of syncope, which may carry some risk of being fatal; such a risk is considered low, however, in patients without structural heart disease or known familial arrhythmic disorders. More important, implantable loop recordings can lead to a correct diagnosis, thereby avoiding misdirected therapy that is based on a presumed, but erroneous, cause of syncope.

- **Signal-Averaged Electrocardiogram** Patients showing ventricular "late potentials" in the setting of underlying structural heart disease, particularly from myocardial infarction, are likely to have a ventricular tachyarrhymogenic cause of syncope and should undergo electrophysiologic testing. This test may be somewhat useful for risk stratification and for diagnosis of VT when the latter is a suspected cause of syncope. It is not useful when bundle branch block is present. There are no studies regarding the utility of signal-averaged

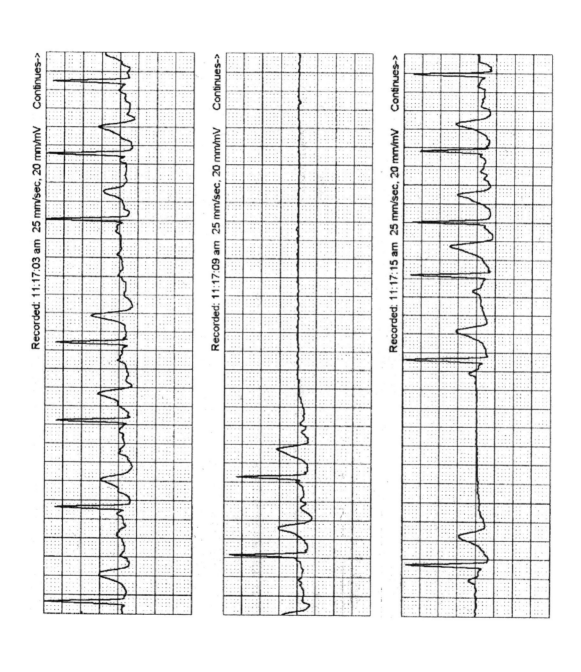

Recorded: 11:17:03 am   25 mm/sec, 20 mm/mV   Continues->

Recorded: 11:17:09 am   25 mm/sec, 20 mm/mV   Continues->

Recorded: 11:17:15 am   25 mm/sec, 20 mm/mV   Continues->

ECG in a large, unselected population of patients with unexplained syncope (3). It is also unclear whether it is prudent to avoid electrophysiologic testing in all patients with a negative signal-averaged ECG, particularly those with underlying structural heart disease. Therefore, the routine use of signal-averaged ECG is not recommended until further studies are available regarding the utility of this diagnostic modality.

- **Electrophysiologic Testing:** Electrophysiologic (EP) testing (Table 5.7) can aid in uncovering as yet undocumented arrhythmic propensities that may give rise to syncope (33). EP testing involves intracardiac electrical stimulation and monitoring of electrophysiologic parameters to detect bradyarrhythmias and tachyarrhythmias. Most protocols, for induction of tachyarrhythmias, consist of delivery of up to three extrastimuli at one or two sites in the ventricle. Isoproterenol is used to increase the sensitivity for detecting tachyarrhythmias, but it reduces specificity. Parameters that are usually evaluated include sinus node function, AV conduction, and the inducibility of supraventricular and ventricular arrhythmias. Sustained VT is an important abnormality identified in patients with syncope and structural heart disease (34). Other abnormalities that can be detected include His-Purkinje block and sinus node dysfunction. It is recommended that caution be used in interpreting the induction of certain arrhythmias, such as atrial flutter, atrial fibrillation, nonsustained VT, polymorphic VT, and ventricular fibrillation during aggressive stimulation protocols, because these may represent "nonclinical" responses. In patients with structural heart disease, such as coronary artery disease, cardiomyopathy, and valvular or congenital heart disease, the diagnostic yield of this procedure is as high as 50%, whereas in the absence of structural heart conditions, the yield is about 10% (35).

Limitations of EP testing include the possibility of not identifying an arrhythmic cause; lack of informativeness for all patient populations, with poor negative predictive value in patients with reduced left ventricular function (36); and possible detection of multiple abnormalities, with difficulty in proving which is etiologic for syncope. A negative EP test result (with no demonstrable induction of sustained VT or ventricular fibrillation) is generally predictive of a low risk of sudden death (37). However, unexplained syncope in nonischemic dilated cardiomyopathy may still reflect an occult propensity to ventricular tachyarrhythmias despite a negative EP study result; indeed, prophylactic implantable defibrillators have been shown to reduce mortality rates in this setting (38,39). For patients with structural heart disease and nondiagnostic Holter or event monitoring, EP testing is recommended if clinical assessment suggests an arrhythmogenic cause for syncope. Although EP tests are relatively safe in the assessment of syncope, fewer than 3% of the patients may develop significant morbid conditions, including cardiac perforation, arteriovenous fistula, pulmonary embolism, and myocardial infarction (35). Patients whose hearts appear normal clinically, with normal ECG and normal echocardiogram, should rarely undergo EP testing, whereas patients with structural heart disease, such as myocardial infarction or congestive heart failure, or those with other anatomic abnormalities that might predispose to arrhythmic syncope (e.g., Wolff-Parkinson-White syndrome) should be considered for the procedure early in the diagnostic cascade. Conduction system disease in patients susceptible to morbidity because of syncope—particularly the elderly,

---

FIG. 5.5. Event monitor (loop-type) recording from a patient with recurrent near syncope. The continuous electrocardiographic tracing shows atrial fibrillation, abruptly ceasing in the *middle strip,* causing an approximately 5-second asystolic pause, followed (in *bottom strip*) by two complexes of marked sinus bradycardia, and, after one more sinus complex, resumption of atrial fibrillation. The patient hit the "Record" button 12 seconds after end of bottom strip.

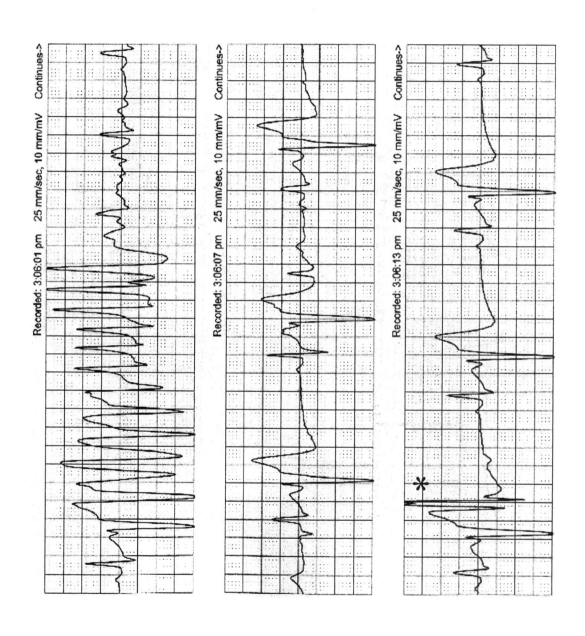

Recorded: 3:06:01 pm   25 mm/sec, 10 mm/mV   Continues->

Recorded: 3:06:07 pm   25 mm/sec, 10 mm/mV   Continues->

Recorded: 3:06:13 pm   25 mm/sec, 10 mm/mV   Continues->

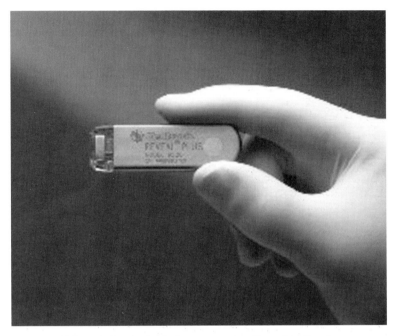

FIG. 5.7. Implantable loop recorder. From Medtronic.

who are prone to significant sequelae (such as hip fractures)—should be considered for inpatient evaluation.

- **Pacemakers and Implantable Cardiac Defibrillators:** These devices must be tested when device malfunction is suspected.
- **Routine Nonselective Neurologic Testing:** These types of tests, such as head-computed tomography, electroencephalogram, and carotid Doppler studies, are all too often performed routinely. These laboratory evaluations rarely provide diagnostic information unless clinical features suggest a neurologic condition; therefore, they should be selectively performed as directed by clinical data.
- **Psychiatric assessment** is usually made only after other investigations have excluded struc-

tural heart disease. In such cases, the hyperventilation maneuver (open-mouthed deep respiration for 2 to 3 minutes for possible precipitation of syncope) and other screening instruments for mental disorders may be useful (40).

WHEN TO ADMIT, WHEN TO REFER, AND TO WHOM

The threshold for admitting a patient with syncope is relatively low (Table 5.8). All patients with a first episode of syncope—other than perhaps a classic case of vasovagal syncope in a young patient with history and physical examination findings negative for any acquired or familial cardiac disorder and with a normal ECG—should be referred to the emergency room to

←————————————————————————————————————

FIG. 5.6. Event monitor (loop-type) recording during an episode of "dizziness and fluttering," occurring at rest, showing a run of rapid polymorphic ventricular tachycardia (in the absence of QT prolongation), as well as frequent premature ventricular complexes. Stimulus artifact on bottom strip (*asterisk*) indicates the point at which the patient activated the recorder to store the electrocardiographic recordings.

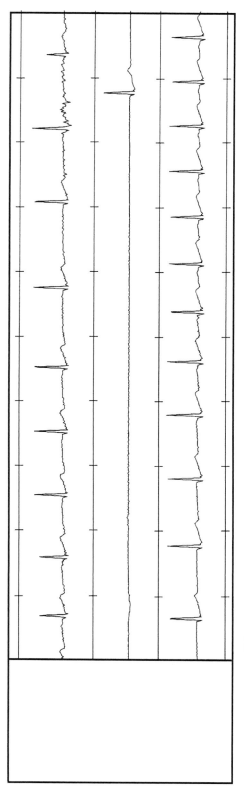

FIG. 5.8. Stored intracardiac electrocardiographic (ECG) recording from implantable loop recorder (ILR) in a patient with unexplained recurrent, drug-resistant "seizures." Within 6 months, the ILR captured a syncopal episode, with stored ECG signal showing sinus rhythm/sinus bradycardia (*top strip*), followed by a 25-second asystolic pause (portion of which shown in *middle strip*, terminated by a junctional complex) and then resumption of sinus rhythm/sinus bradycardia (*bottom strip*). After dual-chamber pacemaker implantation, there were no recurrences of syncope. From Medtronic.

TABLE 5.7. *ACC/AHA recommendations for electrophysiologic testing*

Class I: There is evidence and/or general agreement that electrophysiologic testing is useful and effective
Patients with suspected structural heart disease and syncope that remains unexplained after appropriate evaluation
Class II: There is conflicting evidence and/or a divergence of opinion about the usefulness/efficacy of electrophysiologic testing
Patients with recurrent unexplained syncope without structural heart disease and a negative head-up tilt test
Class III: There is evidence and/or general agreement that the electrophysiologic testing is not useful and in some cases may be harmful
Patients with a known cause of syncope for whom treatment will not be guided by electrophysiologic testing

ACC/AHA, American College of Cardiology/American Heart Association.
From Zipes DP, Di Marco JP, Gillette PC, et al. Guidelines on clinical intracardiac electrophysiologic and catheter ablation procedures. *J Am Coll Cardiol* 1995;26:555–573.

exclude life-threatening cardiopulmonary conditions (acute myocardial infarction, pulmonary embolism), hypoglycemia, orthostatic hypotension (acute severe fluid loss, as in, e.g, severe gastrointestinal hemorrhage) and life-threatening arrhythmias, including drug-induced torsades de pointes. Patients with recurrent syncope may also require hospitalization for a variety of reasons— for example, if their syncope has not previously been evaluated or treated, especially if cardiopulmonary disease is suspected or there is an untreated known or suspected arrhythmic cause; if there is a family history of sudden death; if there is a history of or concern regarding possible secondary injury; if the recent clinical events represent failure of treatment for syncope (especially of cardiac origin); or if pacemaker or ICD malfunction is suspected (4). Patients with recurrent syncope that remains unexplained after initial medical evaluation or with syncope of known or suspected cardiac origin, should be referred to a cardiologist or electrophysiologist to aid in the in the diagnosis and management of the patient.

SYNCOPE AND DRIVING

Although the incidence of syncope-related motor vehicle accidents is low (4,41), syncope can have devastating consequences on the patient and others involved in such an accident. Therefore, when a patient is undergoing evaluation for syncope, the physician must carefully consider the implications regarding driving restrictions, taking into account pertinent laws of the relevant state or country, the chances of recurrent syncope, whether syncope occurs when the patient is standing up or on sitting down, and the presence of a prodrome (which might give the patient time to avoid injury). Guidelines for determining length of driving restrictions, if any, are available (41).

TABLE 5.8. *ACP indications for hospital admission in patients with syncope*

Indicated (associated with such adverse outcomes as myocardial infarction, stroke, or arrhythmias)
History of coronary artery disease, congestive heart failure, or ventricular arrhythmia
Accompanying symptoms of chest pain
Physical signs of significant valve disease, congestive heart failure, stroke, or focal neurologic disorder
Electrocardiographic findings: ischemia, arrhythmia (serious bradycardia or tachycardia), increased QT interval or bundle branch block
Often indicated
Sudden loss of consciousness with injury, rapid heart action, or exertional syncope
Frequent spells, suspicion of coronary disease or arrhythmia (for example, use of medications associated with torsades de pointes)
Moderate to severe hypotension
Older than 70 years of age

ACP, American College of Physicians.
From Linzer M, Yang EH, Estes M, et al. Diagnosing syncope: part 2: Unexplained syncope. *Ann Intern Med* 1997;127:76–86.

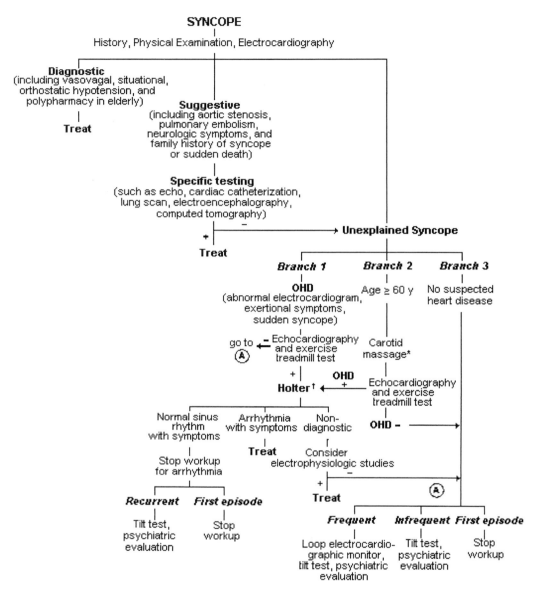

FIG. 5.9. Diagnostic algorithm for the patient with syncope, as proposed by___. Algorithm for diagnosing syncope. *Carotid massage can be performed in an office setting only in the absence of bruits, ventricular tachycardia, recent stroke, or recent myocardial infarction. Carotid hypersensitivity should be diagnosed only if clinical history is suggestive and massage is diagnostically positive (asystole ≥ 3 seconds, hypertension, or both). †May be replaced by inpatient telemetry if there is concern about serious arrhythmia. Echo, echocardiography; OHD, organic heart disease.

CONCLUSIONS

The approach to syncope requires that both the science and art of medicine come together. A major challenge in the evaluation of syncope is that it is a transient symptom, not a disease, with causes ranging from benign to life-threatening. There is rarely an opportunity to capture a spontaneous episode during diagnostic evaluation, and there is no gold standard test for establishing the diagnosis. Syncope in the elderly is especially problematic, in view of its multifactorial causation. However, with the appropriate use of history, physical signs, and diagnostic tests (Fig. 5.9), patients with life-threatening syncope can be identified with a high degree of accuracy, and a diagnosis can be established, overall, in about 75% of patients with syncope (42). This allows appropriate treatment to be initiated in these patients. For those in whom syncope recurs without clear explanation, especially after institution of what initially appears to be appropriate therapy based on thorough evaluation, further observation and investigation over time (e.g., through use of an implantable loop recorder) may reveal the underlying cause.

PRACTICAL POINTS

- Patients with a first episode of syncope should be referred to the emergency room to assess for life-threatening conditions.
- The multifactorial origin of syncope in the elderly often necessitates management approaches aimed at correcting many of these factors simultaneously.
- Key questions during initial evaluation include the following: (a) Is the loss of consciousness attributable to syncope or another cause? (b) Is cardiac disease absent or present? (c) Are there clues in the history suggesting the diagnosis? (Brignole et al., 2001) (4).
- After return of consciousness, rapid restoration of normal sensorium is the rule in syncope, whereas persistent confusion (more than 5 minutes) suggests a seizure.
- Ventricular arrhythmias should be suspected in those with underlying structural heart disease, particularly ventricular involvement.
- ECG findings suggestive of an arrhythmic cause of syncope include sinoatrial dysfunction; second- or third-degree AV block; bifascicular block; Q waves (priormyocardial infarction); delta wave; prolonged QTc; Brugada's sign (ST elevation, especially with T wave inversion, in the right precordial leads, often with right bundle branch block pattern); and right precordial T wave inversion with epsilon wave.
- Evaluation for LQTS should include manual measurement of QTc and a search for T wave morphologic abnormalities (e.g., "notches" in left precordial or limb leads or both).
- Event monitors have a higher yield than do Holter monitors for identifying possible arrhythmic causes of near syncope.
- Electroencephalogram, head computed tomographic scan, and carotid ultrasonography should be reserved for cases of syncope in which clinical features suggest a neurologic etiology.
- Patients with clinically normal hearts and with normal ECG and echocardiogram should rarely undergo EP testing, whereas patients with structural heart disease, such as myocardial infarction, congestive heart failure, or ventricular preexcitation, should be considered for the procedure early in the diagnostic cascade.
- Implantable loop recorders are helpful in documenting recurrent but infrequent syncope that is undiagnosed after initial investigations, including Holter monitoring and electrophysiologic testing.

REFERENCES

1. Benditt DG, Ferguson DW, Grubb BP, et al. Tilt table testing for assessing syncope: ACC expert consensus document. *J Am Coll Cardiol* 1996;28:263–275.

2. Kapoor WN, Peterson JR, Wieand HS, et al. The diagnostic and prognostic implications of recurrences in patients with syncope. *Am J Med* 1987;83:700–708.

3. Linzer M, Yang EH, Estes M, et al. Diagnosing syncope: part 1: value of history, physical examination and electrocardiography. *Ann Intern Med* 1997;126:989–996.

4. Brignole M, Alboni P, Benditt D, et al. Guidelines on management (diagnosis and treatment) of syncope. *Eur Heart J* 2001;22:1256–1306.

5. Abboud FM. Neurocardiogenic syncope. *N Engl J Med* 1993;328:1117–1120.

6. Eagle KA, Black HR, Cook EF, et al. Evaluation of prognostic classifications for patients with syncope. *Am J Med* 1985;79:455–460.

7. Kapoor W. Evaluation and outcome of patients with syncope. *Medicine* 1990;69:160–175.

8. Brugada J, Brugada R, Antzelevitch C, et al. Long-term follow-up of individuals with the electrocardiographic pattern of right bundle-branch block and ST-segment elevation in precordial leads V1 to V3. *Circulation* 2002;105:73–78.

9. Swan H, Piippo K, Viitasalo M, et al. Arrhythmic disorder mapped to chromosome 1q42-q43 causes malignant polymorphic ventricular tachycardia in structurally normal hearts. *J Am Coll Cardiol* 1999;34:2035–2042.

10. Fontaine G, Fontaliran F, Frank R. Arrhythmogenic right ventricular cardiomyopathies: clinical forms and main differential diagnoses. *Circulation.* 1998;97:1532–1535.

11. Uretsky BF, Farquhar DS, Berezin AF, et al. Symptomatic myocardial infarction without chain pain: prevalence and clinical course. *Am J Cardiol* 1977;40:498–503.

12. Kapoor WN, Fortunato M, Hanusa BH, et al. Psychiatric illnesses in patients with syncope. *Am J Med* 1995;99:505–512.

13. Eagle KA, Black HR. The impact of diagnostic tests in evaluating patients with syncope. *Yale J Biol Med* 1983;56:1–8.

14. Narkiewicz K, Cooley RL, Somers VK. Alcohol potentiates orthostatic hypotension. *Circulation* 2000;101:398–402.

15. Calkins H, Seifert M, Morady F. Clinical presentation and long-term follow-up of athletes with exercise-induced vasodepressor syncope. *Am Heart J* 1995;129:1159–1164.

16. Basso C, Maron BJ, Corrado D, et al. Clinical profile of congenital coronary artery anomalies with origin from the wrong aortic sinus leading to sudden death in young competitive athletes. *J Am Coll Cardiol* 2000;35:1493–1501.

17. Schwartz PJ, Priori SG, Spazzolini C, et al. Genotype-phenotype correlation in the long-QT syndrome: gene-specific triggers for life-threatening arrhythmias. *Circulation* 2001;103:89–95.

18. Lempert T, Bauer M, Schmidt D. Syncope: a videometric analysis of 56 episodes of transient cerebral hypoxia. *Ann Neurol* 1994;36:233–237.

19. Hoefnagels WAJ, Padberg GW, Overweg J, et al. Transient loss of consciousness: the value of history for distinguishing seizure from syncope. *J Neurol* 1991;238:39–43.

20. Calkins H, Shyr Y, Frumin H, et al. The value of clinical history in the differentiation of syncope due to ventricular tachycardia, atrioventricular block and neurocardiogenic syncope. *Am J Med* 1995;98:365–373.

21. Makkar RR, Fromm BS, Steinman RT, et al. Female gender as a risk factor for torsades de pointes associated with cardiovascular drugs. *JAMA* 1993;270:2590–2597.

22. Lehmann MH, Hardy S, Archibald D, et al. Sex difference in risk of torsade de pointes with d,l-sotalol. *Circulation* 1996;94:2535–2541.

23. Schondorf R, Low PA. Idiopathic postural orthostatic tachycardia syndrome: an attenuated form of acute pandysautonomia? *Neurology* 1993;43:132–137.

24. Moss AJ, Robinson J. Clinical features of the idiopathic long QT syndrome. *Circulation* 1992;85(Suppl I):I-140–I-144.

25. Vincent GM, Timothy KW, Leppert M, et al. The spectrum and QT intervals in carriers of the gene for the long QT syndrome. *N Engl J Med* 1992;327:846–852.

26. Lehmann MH, Suzuki F, Fromm BS, et al. T wave "humps" as a potential electrocardiographic marker of the long QT syndrome. *J Am Coll Cardiol* 1994;24:746–754.

27. Zhang L, Timothy KW, Vincent GM, et al. Spectrum of ST–T-wave patterns and repolarization parameters in congenital long-QT syndrome: ECG findings identify genotypes. *Circulation* 2000;102:2849–2855.

28. Cheitlin MD, Alpert JS, Armstrong WF, et al. ACC/AHA guidelines for the clinical application of echocardiography. *Circulation* 1997;95:1686–1744.

29. Kapoor WN, Smith M, Miller NL. Upright tilt testing in evaluating syncope: a comprehensive literature review. *Am J Med* 1994;97:78–88.

30. Crawford MH, Bernstein SJ, Deedwania PC, et al. ACC/AHA guidelines for ambulatory electrocardiography. *Circulation* 1999;100:886–893.

31. Linzer M, Pritchett ELC, Pontinen M, et al. Incremental diagnostic yield of loop electrocardiographic recorders in unexplained syncope. *Am J Cardiol* 1990;66:214–219.

32. Krahn AD, Klein GJ, Yee R, et al. Randomized assessment of syncope trial: conventional diagnostic testing versus a prolonged monitoring strategy. *Circulation* 2001;104:46–51.

33. Zipes DP, DiMarco JP, Gillette PC, et al. Guidelines on clinical intracardiac electrophysiologic and catheter ablation procedures. *J Am Cardiol* 1995;26:555–573.

34. Militianu A, Salacata A, Seibert K, et al. Implantable cardioverter defibrillator utilization among device recipients presenting exclusively with syncope or near-syncope. *J Cardiovasc Electrophysiol* 1997;8:1087–1097.

35. Linzer M, Yang EH, Estes M, et al. Diagnosing syncope: part 2: unexplained syncope. *Ann Intern Med* 1997;127:76–86.

36. Middlekauff HR, Stevenson WWG, Saxon LA. Prognosis after syncope: impact of left ventricular function. *Am Heart J* 1993;125:121–127.

37. Kushner HA, Kou WH, Kadish AH, et al. Natural history of patient with unexplained syncope and a

non-diagnostic electrophysiologic study. *J Am Coll Cardiol* 1989;14:391–396.

38. Knight BP, Goyal R, Pelosi F, et al. Outcome of patients with nonischemic dilated cardiomyopathy and unexplained syncope treated with an implantable defibrillator. *J Am Coll Cardiol* 1999;33:1964–1970.

39. Fonarow GC, Feliciano Z, Boyle NG, et al. Improved survival in patients with nonischemic advanced heart failure and syncope treated with an implantable cardioverter-defibrillator. *Am J Cardiol* 2000;85:981–985.

40. Spitzer RL, Williams JB, Kroenke K, et al. Utility of a new procedure for diagnosing mental disorders in primary care. The PRIME-MD 1000 study. *JAMA* 1994; 272:1749–1756.

41. Epstein AE, Miles WM, Beniditt DG. Personal and public safety issues related to arrhythmias that may affect consciousness: implications for regulation and physician recommendations. *Circulation* 1996;94:1147–1166.

42. Calkins H. Syncope. in eds. Zipes DP, Jalife J. Cardiac Electrophysiology, 3rd ed. WB Saunders 2000:873–881.

6

Approach to Claudication

Sanjay Rajagopalan and Thomas W. Wakefield

PREVALENCE

Lower extremity atherosclerotic peripheral artery disease (PAD) is commonly encountered in clinical practice. Although prevalence figures vary widely, noninvasive testing (typically assessing the ankle/brachial index) indicates that prevalence increases sharply to rates in excess of 20% after 75 years. The vast majority of these are, however, asymptomatic; only 3% to 6% experience claudication at the age of 60 in most large population studies (1).

RISK FACTORS FOR CLAUDICATION

The risk factors for claudication are the same as those for atherosclerosis in general and are outlined in Fig. 6.1. Smoking and hyperhomocystinemia seem to have particularly strong associations with lower extremity atherosclerosis (1). In view of the commonality of risk factors and the systemic nature of atherosclerosis, it is not surprising that peripheral vascular disease is closely associated with coronary artery and cerebrovascular disease. Cardiac disease accounts for the majority of deaths in patients with peripheral vascular disease, in whom the relative risk of death from cardiac causes is increased more than fivefold (1).

PRESENTATION

Lower extremity occlusive disease is asymptomatic in the majority of patients, in whom it is commonly detected only by noninvasive screening. When it does manifest, lower extremity vascular occlusive disease typically causes intermittent claudication (derived from the Latin word for "limp"). Intermittent claudication is classically described as cramping pain or weakness that occurs with exercise and is relieved by rest, although atypical manifestations are well described (2). The pain is caused by inadequacy of the blood supply to contracting muscles and is therefore localized to muscle groups, including those of the buttocks, thigh, or, most commonly, the calf. The amount of exercise producing pain is usually reproducible, and patients can typically quantify their exercise capacity in terms of walking distance or time. Because endothelial function is an important determinant of symptoms, factors such as time of day, meals, and medications may influence symptoms. The pain of intermittent claudication is relieved, usually within 5 minutes, by rest and is sometimes relieved by slowing the pace of walking.

The examiner may deduce the level and extent of disease by considering the location and severity of discomfort. The amount of exercise required to precipitate pain is approximately inversely related to the severity of the narrowing of the vessel, and pain is usually manifested one segment below the area of stenosis. In other words, aortic disease is manifested by buttock pain; iliac disease, by thigh muscle pain; and superficial femoral arterial disease (in the most commonly affected artery), by calf claudication (Fig. 6.2). Because calf muscles may be more metabolically active than other muscle groups, calf symptoms often predominate in patients irrespective of the level of disease. Although exercise-induced calf discomfort is usually readily recognized as claudication, it is important to appreciate that aortoiliac disease may also produce aching discomfort in the hips and thighs along with a sensation of weakness in the lower extremity. As arterial insufficiency progresses, rest pain becomes a prominent

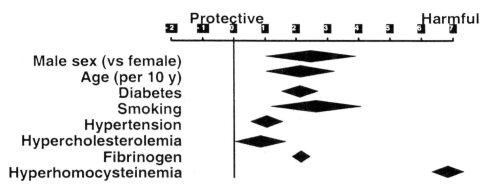

FIG. 6.1. Risk factors for claudication.

feature as blood flow becomes insufficient to supply the basal needs of the sensory nerves. Rest pain is classically defined as severe nocturnal pain or a burning sensation that begins over the metatarsal heads and is relieved by dependency. Rest pain is a sign of very severe ischemia and suggests impending limb loss if no intervention is undertaken.

DIFFERENTIAL DIAGNOSIS

Vascular Causes

Apart from atherosclerotic involvement of the lower extremity vasculature, other vascular causes, such as peripheral embolization (heart or proximal vasculature, especially aneurysmal disease), coarctation of the aorta, and Buerger's disease, must be considered.

Nonvascular Causes

Various nonvascular disorders mimic intermittent claudication. Of particular importance in the differential diagnosis are the following:

1. Neurogenic claudication (pseudoclaudication): This occurs secondary to impingement of the spinal cord by osteophytes or spinal stenosis. The pain characteristically occurs

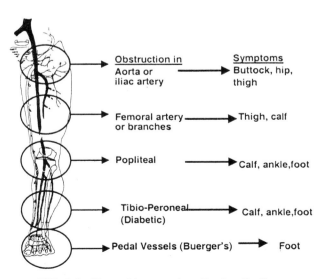

FIG. 6.2. Sites of lower extremity claudication.

simply with assumption of the upright posture, although some patients think it is related to exertion. The pain is often described as an ache in the thighs, hips, and buttocks that may be associated with some numbness and is often relieved by stopping and changing posture (particularly by forward flexion of the lumbar spine or sitting). Patients with neurogenic claudication often find that whereas walking may produce symptoms, riding a bicycle (with forward flexion of the lumbar spine) will not cause the same symptoms at an equivalent amount of exertion.

2. Venous claudication: This condition is often accompanied by signs of chronic venous insufficiency. Absence of such findings helps exclude the condition from the diagnosis. Venous claudication is often described as a "bursting" discomfort in the limb with activity that is relieved with elevation of legs and with rest.

3. Compartment syndrome: This results from impaired venous outflow in the limb secondary to hypertrophied muscles. This condition is often described in athletes with hypertrophied muscles, and a fairly high level of effort is characteristically necessary to induce the discomfort.

4. Neuropathic pain: Such pain follows the distribution of the dermatome and may be aggravated by exercise. It is often present at rest and is relieved by changes in posture that relieve pressure on a peripheral nerve.

DIAGNOSIS

The approach should be individualized according to the severity of symptoms and the functional status of the patient. A strict algorithmic approach as outlined in Fig. 6.3, although valuable in streamlining an approach to diagnosis, is seldom likely to be applicable in all patients. For instance, even moderately severe claudication could be an indication to proceed with contrast-enhanced angiography, especially if it involves an active individual whose lifestyle requires mobility. Severe symptoms in an elderly individual with a limited lifestyle may also compel the physician to continue aggressive medical management. In general, the resting ankle/brachial index (ABI), segmental pressures, and Doppler waveform analysis may be obtained in all patients with claudication. These measurements may help identify patients with predominantly aortoiliac disease who may benefit from early percutaneous intervention. This is in view of the excellent long-term patency rates of this procedure (more than 85% at 5 years) in

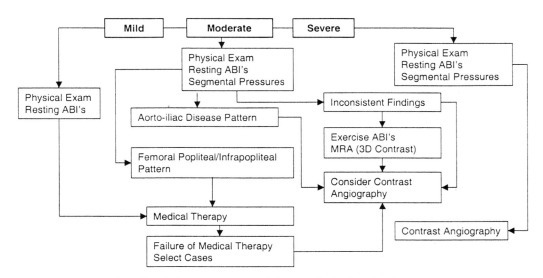

FIG. 6.3. Diagnostic approach to a patient with claudication.

selected patients with focal iliac artery disease. Patients with predominantly femoropopliteal or infrapopliteal disease who have moderate symptoms may be managed medically. In selected cases (failure of medical treatment or very active lifestyle), contrast-enhanced angiography with the possibility of intervention (surgical/percutaneous) may be considered early on. For the patient with severe symptoms, proceeding to contrast-enhanced angiography directly is justified in order to assess the suitability of the patient for surgical or percutaneous options.

PHYSICAL EXAMINATION OF THE PATIENT WITH CLAUDICATION

Careful physical examination of the pulses, combined with accurate delineation of the history, can enable the physician to localize arterial disease in close to 90% of patients (3). Because of the systemic nature of atherosclerosis, the examiner should carefully assess the entire cardiovascular system. Asymptomatic bruits over the carotid arteries, epigastrium (renal or aortic), lower abdomen, or femoral regions may signify concomitant disease in these locations. In addition to pulse deficits, chronic ischemia is characterized by loss of hair, atrophic skin changes, and thickening of nails.

Pitfalls

The dorsalis pedis and, to a lesser extent, posterior tibial pulses may be congenitally absent in a small number of normal patients. In these cases, noninvasive studies are of help. Detection of arterial pulses does not rule out severe ischemia in cases of very distal occlusions that may occur as part of the cholesterol embolization syndrome or in a few diabetic patients.

LABORATORY TESTING IN THE PATIENT WITH CLAUDICATION

The following tests should be routinely performed in all patients with claudication: complete blood cell count with platelets, fasting blood glucose (HbA1c) measurement, renal function measurements (creatinine and blood urea nitrogen), fasting lipid profile, urinalysis

(for microalbuminuria), and homocysteine level measurements. In the atypical patient (premature disease, personal or family history of thrombosis, early failure of intervention graft failure), the physician should consider a comprehensive hypercoagulable screen (1).

Noninvasive Testing

The noninvasive tests that are commonly used in the laboratory at the University of Michigan are summarized in Table 6.1.

Resting Ankle/Brachial Indices by Doppler Ultrasonography

Blood pressure by Doppler flow is determined at levels distal to a pneumatic compression cuff. The cuff (which is placed proximal to the vessel interrogated) is inflated until blood flow distal to the cuff stops. The cuff is then deflated, and the pressure when flow resumes is noted. This pressure is then compared with the brachial artery pressure, and a ratio is calculated. At the level of the ankle, this ratio is the ABI (Fig. 6.4). Although the level of the resting ABI correlates approximately with that of clinical presentation, considerable overlap exists. In the presence of a single chronic occlusion, the ABI usually is greater than 0.50, whereas multilevel occlusions often result in ABIs of less than 0.50.

Pitfalls

In patients with calcified vessels, such as in diabetics and patients with renal failure, the calcification may prevent the pneumatic cuff from being able to adequately compress the vessel and stop blood flow, which leads to a falsely elevated ABI. In these circumstances, measuring the blood flow at the toe level [resulting in a toe/brachial index (TBI)] by Doppler study or

TABLE 6.1. *Noninvasive testing for claudication*

Doppler study–derived resting ankle/brachial indices
Segmental arterial pressure analysis
Exercise ankle/brachial indices
Arterial duplex examination
Magnetic resonance imaging

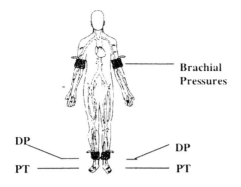

Rest ABI	Interpretation
0.90-1.30	Normal
0.70-0.89	Mild
0.40-0.69	Moderate
<0.40	Severe
>1.30	Non-Compressible Vessels

Pointers in Rest ABI Measurement
- Use higher of two brachial pressures if different
- Use higher of two ABI's (at DP or PT levels) if different
- Request a Toe Brachial Index if vessels non- compressible

FIG. 6.4. Interpreting resting ankle/brachial indices.

pulse velocity recording will be more accurate in assessing the limb blood flow. The TBI usually is greater than 0.70 in the nondiseased situation.

Segmental Arterial Pressure Analysis

Noninvasive tests can help distinguish patients with predominantly aortoiliac disease from those with infrainguinal disease by measuring pressures at different levels along the lower extremity. Blood pressure cuffs are placed along the lower extremity with Doppler assessment of one of the pedal arteries to give an idea of the extent of disease. Usually two cuffs are placed on the thigh (upper and lower), one below the knee and the other above the ankle. Between adjacent levels there should be less than a 20-mm Hg drop. A gradient of more than 40 mm Hg suggests occlusive disease. The accuracy of this test alone in localizing disease, in comparison with angiography, is 85% (4).

Pitfalls

In practice, two small cuffs are usually applied to the thigh for the separation of iliac from femoral disease. The use of small cuffs can lead to overestimation of pressures at the upper thigh level and consequent underestimation of the hemodynamic severity of iliac and proximal femoral lesions.

Doppler Velocity Waveform Analysis

Patterns of arterial flow may be recorded by a continuous Doppler monitor over the femoral, popliteal, posterior tibial, and the dorsalis pedis arteries in conjunction with segmental limb pressures. This analysis complements segmental limb pressures in assessing the extent and location of disease. The normal waveform is triphasic and includes forward and reverse components. With progression of disease, the reverse component is lost, and the waveform becomes biphasic. When forward flow becomes continuous, the waveform is considered monophasic. With severe disease, the waveform amplitude is attenuated (Fig. 6.5).

Pitfalls

Pulse waveforms are qualitative indices of disease and cannot provide information about the severity of stenosis. Pulse velocity recordings are used by some laboratories instead of Doppler waveforms because they tend to be less operator dependent than Doppler recordings.

Provocative Testing (Exercise Ankle/Brachial Index)

In this test, the ABI is measured after exercise. This test allows a noncritical stenosis at rest to

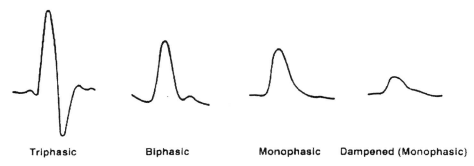

Triphasic   Biphasic   Monophasic   Dampened (Monophasic)

FIG. 6.5. Doppler arterial waveform analysis.

become evident with exercise (5). The normal response to exercise is a slight increase or no change in the ankle systolic pressures in comparison with resting pressures. If ankle systolic pressure decreases by at least 15 mm Hg, the test result is considered positive. Both constant grade (usually at 2 mph up to a 10% grade) and variable grade testing are acceptable. In Gardner's graded test, treadmill speed is kept constant while the incline is varied (2% change every 2 minutes) to increase workload. Exercise ABIs are extremely helpful in making the diagnosis in unclear cases in which resting ABIs are borderline or in the midrange. Two components of the response to exercise are evaluated: (a) the magnitude of the immediate decrease in ankle systolic pressure and (b) the time for recovery to resting pressure. The examiner can also determine both the peak walking time as well as the claudication onset or pain-free walking time as objective indices of disease progression, to monitor these patients.

Pitfalls

Other associated conditions such as angina or arthritis may limit a patient's ability to exercise, and it is therefore important to note the degree of drop in pressures in addition to the actual duration of exercise.

Duplex Ultrasonography

Duplex ultrasonography incorporates real-time B-mode testing in addition to pulsed and color Doppler scanning. B-mode testing gives anatomic detail of the vessel; Doppler measurements provide an estimate of the degree of stenosis. Analyses based on these tests include comparison of the spectral characteristics of the waveform as well as the peak velocities generated. The main disadvantages of color Doppler scanning are that it requires considerable training and that scanning of the entire arterial tree is impractical. Duplex scanning is particularly valuable in graft surveillance and should be used in this situation in lieu of ABIs that have low sensitivity in this situation. Graft failure secondary to atherosclerosis accounts for 80% of graft failures within 5 years; only one third of patients with failing grafts have symptoms, which supports the argument for graft surveillance. It has been recommended that intervention thresholds after ultrasonography should be a velocity ratio of more than 3.5, a peak systolic velocity of more than 300 cm per second, and a low flow velocity (less than 45 cm per second) (6).

Pitfalls

Precise quantitation of stenoses in the range of 50% to 99% is currently not possible with Doppler and flow parameters.

Magnetic Resonance Angiography

This method offers good resolution at the aortoiliac level but currently lacks the resolution to distinguish between varying grades of stenosis in more distal vessels. Advances in magnetic resonance angiography, including improved spatial resolution and the development of tests of vascular function, are expected to greatly enhance its utility in the diagnosis and management of peripheral vascular disease.

Pitfalls

Magnetic resonance angiography appears to overestimate the degree of stenosis associated with atherosclerotic plaques. Variations in the quality of magnetic resonance angiograms that are related to the magnet strength may also degrade image quality.

Invasive Testing

Contrast-Enhanced Angiography

This test should be performed in patients with claudication only if a decision has been made to intervene, because it is not risk free. In the patient with critical limb ischemia, it is the procedure of choice because it guides therapy, whether percutaneous or surgical. In patients with contraindications to receiving contrast media owing to advanced renal insufficiency or contrast media allergy, alternative modalities such as gadolinium- or CO_2-enhanced angiography may be considered, although these rarely provide the same high level of resolution seen with conventional angiography.

Pitfalls

Peripheral angiography is limited in some sense because it merely provides a "luminogram" and, because it gives no information about the arterial wall, it may underestimate the degree of stenosis. In addition, because angiographic views are often obtained in only one anatomic plane, they may either overestimate or underestimate stenosis severity.

APPROACH TO TREATMENT

The treatment approaches are covered in detail in Chapter 33. In general, all patients with claudication, irrespective of severity of symptoms, should undergo aggressive risk factor modification. In patients with debilitating symptoms, prompt referral to a vascular specialist after appropriate workup will expedite patient care (Fig. 6.6). In patients with moderate symptoms, a formal

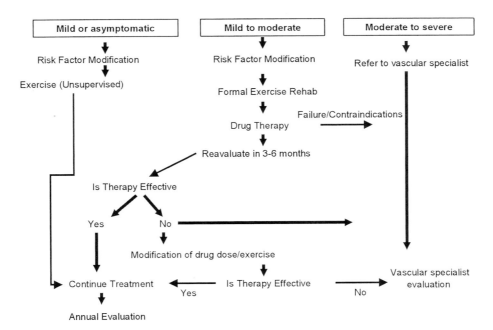

FIG. 6.6. Treatment approach to the claudicant.

exercise rehabilitation program has tremendous benefit that may rival that observed with interventional therapy or with supervised exercise alone (7,8). Justifying supervised programs for the asymptomatic or minimally symptomatic individual in this era of increasing health care costs is more difficult. Appropriate risk factor modification is of pivotal importance in all patients, irrespective of symptom severity. In the moderately symptomatic patient, additional use of drugs as outlined in Chapter 33 is well jus-

tified. These patients may then be evaluated at the end of a 3- to 6-month period to assess efficacy of drugs, risk factor intervention, and supervised exercise rehabilitation. In patients who seem to be benefiting, drugs may be continued; patients who show no improvement or evidence of deterioration may be referred to a vascular specialist. In the minimally symptomatic or asymptomatic patient, risk factor modification and exercise may be all that is required.

PRACTICAL POINTS

- Intermittent claudication is classically described as cramping pain or weakness that occurs with exercise and is relieved by rest.
- Careful physical examination of the pulses, combined with accurate delineation of the history, can enable the physician to localize arterial disease in close to 90% of patients.
- Aortic disease is manifested by buttock pain; iliac disease, by thigh muscle pain; and superficial femoral arterial disease, by calf claudication. Calf claudication, however, predominates, irrespective of level of disease.
- Resting ABIs, segmental pressures, and

- Doppler waveform analysis may be obtained as initial studies in all patients with claudication.
- Exercise ABIs are extremely helpful in making the diagnosis in unclear cases in which resting ABIs are borderline or in the midrange and as a measure of monitoring progress in patients.
- Claudication irrespective of severity of symptoms should receive aggressive risk factor modification.
- In patients with debilitating symptoms, prompt referral to a vascular specialist after appropriate workup expedites patient care.

REFERENCES

1. Dormandy JA, Rutherford RB. Management of peripheral arterial disease (PAD). TASC Working Group. Transatlantic Inter-society Consensus. *J Vasc Surg* 2000;31(1, pt 2):S1–S296.
2. McDermott MM, Mehta S, Greenland P. Exertional leg symptoms other than intermittent claudication are common in peripheral arterial disease. *Arch Intern Med* 1999;159:387–392.
3. Baker WH, String ST, Hayes AC, et al. Diagnosis of peripheral occlusive disease: comparison of clinical evaluation and noninvasive laboratory. *Arch Surg* 1978;113:1308–1310.
4. Rutherford RB, Lowenstein DH, Klein MF. Combining segmental systolic pressures and plethysmography to diagnose arterial occlusive disease of the legs. *Am J Surg* 1979;138:211–218.
5. Wolf EA Jr, Sumner DS, Strandness DE Jr. Correlation between nutritive blood flow and pressure in limbs of patients with intermittent claudication. *Surg Forum* 1972; 23:238–239.
6. Bandyk D. Appropriateness of non-invasive follow-up for vascular procedures. In: Yao J, Pierce W, eds. *Practical vascular surgery.* Stamford, CT: Appleton & Lange, 1999:55–68.
7. Creasy TS, McMillan PJ, Fletcher EW, et al. Is percutaneous transluminal angioplasty better than exercise for claudication? Preliminary results from a prospective randomised trial. *Eur J Vasc Surg* 1990;4:135–140.
8. Gardner AW, Poehlman ET. Exercise rehabilitation programs for the treatment of claudication pain. A meta-analysis [see comments]. *JAMA* 1995;274:975–980.

7

Primary Prevention of Coronary Artery Disease

Melvyn Rubenfire and Eric R. Bates

Despite dramatic advances in the detection and management of cardiovascular diseases (CVDs) since the 1960s, nearly 1 million men and women in the United States died of CVD in 1998 (1). An estimated 12 million people in the United States have established coronary heart disease (CHD), and more than 650,000 experience a first myocardial infarction (MI) each year (1). The majority of patients with newly diagnosed CHD present with an acute coronary event (unstable angina, MI, or sudden death), and half of the events occur in previously asymptomatic people.

Observational studies and randomized trials provide evidence that lifestyle changes and drug therapies can reduce coronary events and mortality rates in asymptomatic men and women (2). Clearly, if CHD can be detected in the preclinical stage and a high percentage of those destined for an acute event can be identified by risk stratification, a considerable amount of the related disability and death is preventable.

Effective coronary disease prevention requires five major steps: (a) a society willing to pay for prevention, (b) accurate knowledge of the pathobiology of atherosclerosis, (c) an understanding of the contributing risk factors and risk markers, (d) a method of reliable risk stratification or early detection, and (e) safe and effective therapy for risk factors and preclinical disease.

COST AND BENEFIT TO SOCIETIES AND INDIVIDUALS

There is general agreement that societal health care costs can be reduced by prevention and possibly by early detection. It is difficult to measure the cost and relative value of prevention, particularly in CVD. In contrast to preventing communicable diseases such as smallpox and polio,

the rationale for using government resources to prevent diseases (e.g., CHD or stroke) that do not threaten the life of others, that may never be manifest, and that, if manifest, do so only in old age requires a considerably different mindset.

Health care costs can be expressed as cost per quality-of-life (QOL) year saved. In the United States, a treatment costing up to $40,000 per QOL year saved, which is the annual cost for hemodialysis in end-stage renal disease, is considered reasonable and more than $75,000 excessive. Although this is a reasonable way to compare the cost of the care provided, known as "direct care," the method sorely underestimates the value of prevention of clinical atherosclerosis. Equally important are the indirect societal costs of disability from MI, angina, heart failure, and stroke, including lost wages, the cost of medical disability, and the decrease in business productivity. The direct costs of CVD care are in excess of $180 billion dollars, but the total annual economic burden for CVD exceeds $286 billion (1).

The cost expressed as QOL year saved is influenced by the cost of the drug or treatment, by age, and by the probability of an event's occurring without treatment. The cost per QOL year saved by using statins to lower cholesterol levels varies from $15,000 cost saving in persons with established CVD to $150,000 for primary prevention, depending on the expected clinical event rate, age, and gender. The cost of treating healthy men and women who have an estimated annual risk of CHD of 1.5% (intermediate risk) with pravastatin is about $32,000 for each QOL year saved (3). In comparison, the cost of CHD prevention with aspirin is about $3,000 for each QOL year saved; for detection and treatment of elevated homocysteine levels, about $3,500; and for treatment of hypertension in middle-aged men and women, from less than $5,000 to over $300,000, depending on the drug (4). Regardless of the cost and who pays (patient, third party, health maintenance organization), guidelines are needed to provide a method of selecting who would benefit from treatment according to an estimate of individual risk of the disease being prevented, the likelihood of success of the treatment, and a cost-benefit assessment.

PATHOBIOLOGY OF ATHEROSCLEROSIS

Atherosclerosis is a systemic vascular disease involving the aorta and the coronary, carotid, and peripheral arteries. It is the result of inflammation in response to endothelial injury by one or more risk factors, such as hypertension, oxidized low-density lipoprotein (LDL), homocysteine, and infection (5). The earliest lesions, fatty streaks, are found in some children and in all men and women between the ages of 15 and 34 years who die of noncardiac causes. Diffuse nonocclusive coronary plaque has been found in 25% to 50% of young people at postmortem examination and by intravascular ultrasonography (6,7), and the amount of fatty streaks and plaque correlates with the prevalence of classic coronary risk factors (6).

At least six major processes occur in the development of atherosclerotic plaque (atheroma), and each is a potential therapeutic target: (a) injury of the endothelial lining, which facilitates entry of monocytes and adherence of platelets and microthrombi that release growth factors; (b) active and passive transport of LDL and very low density lipoprotein (VLDL) remnant particles into the subendothelial space, followed by lipid peroxidation; (c) conversion of monocytes to macrophages that ingest oxidized LDL and transform to lipid-engorged foam cells that coalesce into fatty streaks; (d) inflammatory T lymphocyte response and release of cytokines and chemotactic proteins that stimulate smooth muscle cells to migrate to the intimal layer and convert from contractile to secretory function; (e) smooth muscle cells and fibroblasts, which provide a matrix skeleton of collagen, fibrin, and calcification; and (f) spontaneous death or digestion of foam cells with release of cholesterol and other lipids to form a lipid pool (5,8).

Histologic evidence suggests that plaque growth may be gradual over years with bursts of growth from periodic intraplaque hemorrhage and repair. The predominant type of plaque in individuals is a major determinant of risk of acute coronary events (8,9). Figure 7.1 demonstrates the two extremes of plaque morphology. Angina

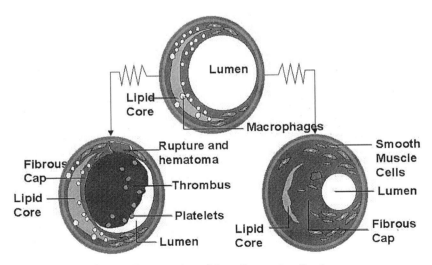

FIG. 7.1. Progression of the atherosclerotic plaque.

pectoris and stress-induced ischemia are usually caused by flow-limiting, partially occlusive, stable coronary stenoses (greater than 70% narrowing) composed of fibrocalcific plaque abundant in smooth muscle and fibrous tissue with or without a lipid pool. There is both clinical and pathologic evidence that most acute coronary events are the result of an occluding or partially occluding thrombus at the site of a vulnerable plaque in nonocclusive (less than 70% of vessel diameter) coronary segments (9). The vulnerable plaque has a large lipid pool and a thin fibrous cap that can rupture, often at the junction of the plaque and normal wall, which results in unstable angina, MI, and sudden death (9).

Calcification is uniformly present in early and mature plaque and begins in the second and third decades (10). The calcium is present as a hydroxypatite identical to that found in bone. There is a highly significant relationship between calcium plaque area and atherosclerotic plaque area as measured histologically, and calcium accumulation is more prevalent in complex plaques that may have undergone rupture and healing (11). As with other factors associated with atherosclerosis and the response to injury hypothesis, it is highly likely that the amount of calcification of plaque is regulated or influenced by several related and unrelated genes.

The arterial *endothelium* provides a protective vascular barrier and produces a wide variety of peptides involved in regulating vascular tone, thrombosis, and cellular adhesion, migration, and growth. Nitric oxide (NO·) and prostacyclin are released in response to wall shear stress and autonomic tone (12). Prostacyclin, acting through the cyclic adenosine monophosphate (AMP) pathway, and NO·, acting through the cyclic guanidine monophosphate pathway, are vasodilators with antithrombotic, antiplatelet, and antioxidant functions. The formation and release of prostacyclin and NO· by the endothelium is impaired in all stages of coronary atherosclerosis in conduit vessels with or without plaque and in the intramyocardial resistance vessels. Impairment of endothelial function is not merely a surrogate for preclinical atherosclerosis. It occurs at all ages simply in the presence of risk factors. Impairment of brachial endothelial function

is found in young healthy people with a family history of CHD, in smokers, and in patients with depression and can be reversed with simple measures (13–16).

Coronary artery plaque appears focal on angiography but appears diffuse when assessed with intravascular ultrasonography (17). Coronary arteriograms are luminograms and often appear normal in patients with significant arterial wall plaque. The normalization of the lumen in the segments with plaque is the result of arterial enlargement and remodeling (Glagov's effect), which has been demonstrated on pathologic specimens and by intravascular ultrasonography (18,19).

RISK FACTORS AND RISK MARKERS

Coronary risk factors are defined as factors whose presence is associated with or is correlated with an increased likelihood that disease will be present at a later time (20,21). The test of whether a given factor is independent of others and causative generally requires a graded response [e.g., LDL cholesterol (LDL-C), tobacco], time exposure (decades), and a response to treatment in placebo-controlled trials (hypertension, cholesterol). However, controlled trials are not always possible or necessary. Observational studies provide adequate evidence of the benefits of smoking cessation, exercise, and weight control.

Family history of premature CHD is a major risk factor, but the mechanism is often illusive or multifactorial. Seventy-five percent of the CHD risk attributed to family history may relate to lifestyle factors, including smoking, diet, obesity, and physical inactivity. There is also evidence for a strong interaction between genetic polymorphisms and the risk attributable to lifestyle. An example is the gene encoding for aldosterone synthase, in which the C allele is associated with increase in left ventricular mass. Although the C allele has only a modest effect on MI risk, its presence markedly increases the relative risk of MI among smokers and persons with low levels of high-density lipoprotein cholesterol (HDL-C) (22). The weight or contribution of the established major risk factors (particularly LDL-C and

HDL-C) creates difficulty in establishing causality for other putative risk factors, which may not have adequate prevalence for detection.

Coronary risk factors can be divided into three major categories: (a) causal, (b) conditional, and (c) predisposing (21). The major clinically useful risk factors are listed in Table 7.1.

Causal risk factors include smoking, hypertension, diabetes mellitus, high total cholesterol (TC) and LDL-C, and low HDL-C. Each factor

TABLE 7.1. *Established and putative coronary risk factors and markers*

Predisposing risk factors related to and increasing causal risk
Age: duration of exposure to LDL-C, hypertension, diabetes
Male gender: decrease in HDL-C in comparison with women
Menopause: loss of protective effect of estrogens
Family history of premature CHD
   First-degree relative: male < 55 years, female < 65 years
Socioeconomic: hypertension, poor diet, physical inactivity, less than high school education, low income
Physical inactivity: low HDL-C, hypertension
Overweight–abdominal fat deposition: low HDL-C, hypertension, ↑ CRP, ↑ cytokines, ↑ insulin
Psychologic: hypertension, stress/depression/anxiety, hostility, low self-esteem

Causative independent risk factors: categorical and graded response by severity
Blood pressure: threshold 120/80 mm Hg; hypertension—categorical ≥140/90 mm Hg
Glycemic control: threshold 100 mg/dL; diabetes—fasting glucose >126 mg/dL
Smoking: ever, categorical—current
Increased LDL-C: threshold >100 mg/dL, 2 fold when ≥160 mg/dL or increased apo B-100.
   Low HDL cholesterol: <40 mg/dL in men and 45 mg/dL in women

Conditional: enhanced risk of causative classic risk factors; may be causal
Lipoprotein (a)
Homocysteine
Triglycerides and VLDL remnant particles
Small LDL particles
Elevated insulin
CRP
Increased platelet count
Fibrinogen
Increased WBC
High levels of PAI-1
Factor VIIa

Other possible causative or contributing factors
Dental hygiene: increase systemic inflammation, bacteria flora in plaque
Chronic infection: enhance plaque growth, local T cell activity, endothelial damage
   Chlamydia pneumonia
   Herpes simplex
   Cytomegalovirus
Collagen vascular diseases: endothelial dysfunction, systemic inflammation
Radiation therapy: endothelial damage

Related risk factors whose association increases risk
Metabolic or insulin resistance syndrome: three or more of the following
   Increased abdominal girth: men >40, women > 35 inches
   Increased triglycerides: > 150 mg/dL
   HDL-C: < 40 mg/dL in men and < 50 mg/dL in women
   Systolic pressure ≥ 130 mm Hg, diastolic ≥ 85 mm Hg
   FBS ≥ 110 mg/dL
Increased triglycerides
   Low HDL-C
   Increase PAI-1 and decrease t-PA
   Increase factor VIIa

CHD, coronary heart disease; CRP, C-reactive protein; FBS, fasting blood glucose; HDL-C, high-density lipoprotein cholesterol; LDL-C, low-density lipoprotein cholesterol; PAI-1, plasminogen activator inhibitor–1; t-PA, tissue plasminogen activator; VLDL, very low density lipoprotein; WBC, white blood cell count.

can be considered to have a continuum of risk from an optimal value (e.g., LDL-C less than 100 mg per deciliter and blood pressure lower than 120/80 mm Hg with risk increasing for every unit, quartile, or decile), can be considered a categorical risk (e.g., smoking or not), or can be defined by a cut point (e.g., LDL-C higher than 160 mg/dL or blood pressure higher than 140/90 mm HG). The incremental risk for a factor varies across a wide range of values and is markedly affected by years of exposure and associated risk factors. For example, the risk attributable to LDL-C increases twofold when the triglyceride levels exceed 200 mg per deciliter. The presence of each major risk factor increases the probability of developing CHD about twofold. When several factors are present, the risk may increase 15- or 20-fold. Observational studies suggest that clinically relevant atherosclerosis is unlikely to occur with very low levels of LDL-C, but once the level of LDL-C reaches a "permissive" level and plaque formation begins, the other risk factors independently accelerate plaque formation and instability (21). Diabetes is a particularly strong risk factor, possibly because of its association with other risk factors such as hypertension, low HDL-C, and increasing triglyceride levels. The risk for coronary events in diabetic patients without CHD is equivalent to that in men and women with a history of MI (2% or higher annually) (23).

Conditional risk factors [e.g., homocysteine, lipoprotein (a), and insulin] are associated with an increased risk for CHD, but the causal link to CHD is uncertain. The uncertainty may be due to their having less influence than the major risk factors, their low frequency, or a required interaction with other factors that is yet unknown. There is strong evidence in support of the conditional risk factors listed in Table 7.1.

Predisposing risk factors generally intensify causal risk factors or conditional risk factors and may be independent and causal but in unidentified ways (e.g., family history, ethnicity, socioeconomic factors).

Risk markers identify a person as being at increased risk for coronary events, but they may or not be risk factors for atherosclerosis. For example, the risk of coronary events is increased with higher levels of C-reactive protein (CRP), an acute-phase reactant produced in the liver in response to inflammatory cytokines, but there is also evidence that CRP itself may influence plaque stability and growth and may be a risk factor for acute events (24).

RISK STRATIFICATION

The physician, the patient, and the payer need guidelines that provide a balance among efficacy, safety, and cost of each diagnostic tool or treatment. Individual *risk stratification* has been at the heart of guidelines for lipid-lowering and antihypertensive therapies for the prevention of CVD in the United States (25,26).

The significance of individual or multiple risk factors is expressed with the following terms: *absolute risk, relative risk* or *odds ratio, attributable risk, number needed to treat* (NNT), *relative risk reduction,* and *categorical risk.*

Absolute risk is the probability of an individual's developing a defined endpoint (i.e., coronary event) over a finite period, such as 150/1,000 over 10 years, or 1.5% annually. For example, using the Framingham risk score in Table 7.2, the 10-year risk of a coronary event in a 50-year-old man with a cholesterol level of 250 mg per deciliter and no other risk factors is 6%, or 0.6% annually (27).

Relative risk or *odds ratio* is the ratio of absolute risk in a patient with one or more risk factors in comparison with a person with standard risk. For example, the relative risk for development of CHD over 10 years in a 50-year-old man with a cholesterol level of 249 mg per deciliter in comparison with 199 mg per deciliter is 1.5 (odds ratio, 1.5), or 50% greater (27). The relative risk appears high, but the absolute risk for both men is relatively low: 0.6% versus 0.4% annually.

Attributable risk is the additional probability an individual with a risk factor will have an event over time in comparison to the standard risk. In the previous example, the attributable risk of the added 50 mg per deciliter in the 50-year-old man is 20/1000, or 2% for 10 years and 0.2% annually.

Number needed to treat is the number of patients with a given risk factor needed to treat (NNT) to prevent one event over a given period of time; for example, treating 25 subjects for 5 years will prevent one event. This is estimated after a clinical trial in which there are a treatment

TABLE 7.2. *Global risk score by Framingham risk estimates*

Estimate of 10-year risk for men (Framingham point scores)		Estimate of 10-year risk for women (Framingham point scores)	
Age (years)	Points	Age (years)	Points
20–34	−9	20–34	−9
35–39	−4	35–39	−4
40–44	0	40–44	0
45–49	3	45–49	3
50–54	6	50–54	6
55–59	8	55–59	8
60–64	10	60–64	10
65–69	11	65–69	11
70–74	12	70–74	12
75–79	13	75–79	13

Total cholesterol (mg/dL)	Points					Total cholesterol (mg/dL)	Points				
	Age 20–39 y	Age 40–49 y	Age 50–59 y	Age 60–69 y	Age 70–79 y		Age 20–39 y	Age 40–49 y	Age 50–59 y	Age 60–69 y	Age 70–79 y
<160	0	0	0	0	0	<160	0	0	0	0	0
160–199	4	3	2	1	0	160–199	4	3	2	1	1
200–239	7	5	3	1	0	200–239	8	6	4	2	1
240–279	9	6	4	2	1	240–279	11	8	5	3	2
≥280	11	8	5	3	1	≥280	13	10	7	4	2

	Points						Points				
	Age 20–39 y	Age 40–49 y	Age 50–59 y	Age 60–69 y	Age 70–79 y		Age 20–39 y	Age 40–49 y	Age 50–59 y	Age 60–69 y	Age 70–79 y
Nonsmoker	0	0	0	0	0	Nonsmoker	0	0	0	0	0
Smoker	8	5	3	1	1	Smoker	9	7	4	2	1

HDL (mg/dL)	Points	HDL (mg/dL)	Points
≥60	−1	≥60	−1
50–59	0	50–59	0
40–49	1	40–49	1
<40	2	<40	2

Systolic BP (mm HG)	If untreated	If treated	Systolic BP (mm HG)	If untreated	If treated
<120	0	0	<120	0	0
120–129	0	1	120–129	1	3
130–139	1	2	130–139	2	4
140–159	1	2	140–159	3	5
≥160	2	3	≥160	4	6

Point total	10-year risk (%)	Point total	10-year risk (%)
<0	<1	<9	<1
0	1	9	1
1	1	10	1
2	1	11	1
3	1	12	1
4	1	13	2
5	2	14	2
6	2	15	3
7	3	16	4
8	4	17	5
9	5	18	6
10	6	19	8
11	8	20	11
12	10	21	14
13	12	22	17
14	16	23	22
15	20	24	27
16	25	≥25	≥30
≥17	≥30		

BP, blood pressure; HDL, high-density lipoprotein.

From executive summary of the third report of the National Cholesterol Education Program (NCEP) Expert Panel on Detection, Evaluation, and Treatment of High Blood Cholesterol in Adults (Adult Treatment Panel III). *JAMA* 2001;285:2486–2497.

group and a control group. Values are entered as events per 100 or per 1,000 (expressed as a decimal fraction) in the placebo or standard treatment and new treatment groups [NNT = 1 ÷ (control − treated)]. For example, assume that the hypothetical drug "Atherobloc" reduced the 5-year coronary event rate by 50% in comparison with placebo in a high-risk group. The Atherbloc event rate was 500/5,000, or 2% per year; in comparison, the placebo event rate was 250/5,000, or 1% per year. Twenty persons with comparable risk would need to be treated for five years in order to prevent one event.

Relative risk reduction (RRR) is the reduction of adverse events or endpoints in the treated group versus placebo group in a trial [RRR = (placebo − treated) ÷ placebo].

Categorical risk, or categories of risk, can be expressed in several forms but differ principally from risk when it is expressed as a continuum. A classic categorical risk method would stratify an individual by a single parameter, such as present or absent; high, intermediate, and low risk; or above or below a cut point (e.g., age, LDL cholesterol, and blood pressure). Several levels of categorical risk were used in the 1993 Adult Treatment Panel II (ATP-II) guidelines for cholesterol management (25). The decision for diet, drug therapy, and the LDL-C target goal was based on fasting LDL-C level (greater than 190, 160 to 189, 130 to 159, and less than 130 mg per deciliter), the presence of major risk factors (none, one, two, or more), and age and gender.

Prevention decision trees and guidelines have been primarily developed from the results of longitudinal cohort studies and large randomized clinical trials. The Framingham Heart Study, a prospective single community study of 5,075 people 30 to 74 years of age and without CHD who were monitored for 12 years, provided the evidence for causal risk factors and a framework for categorical risk stratification and more complex CHD prediction models (28). The Framingham Risk Score (Table 7.2) provides a 10-year estimate of risk for CHD, defined as angina, coronary insufficiency, and fatal or nonfatal MI (27). The weight attributable to the causal independent risk factors in the Framingham Heart Study are similar for white and black men and women

(29). For Japanese American men, Hispanic men, and Native American women, the Framingham risk score systematically overestimates the risk of CHD, and over-weights the importance of cholesterol in elderly men and women (29). In secondary prevention, short-term risk may encompass 30 days to 6 months, and long-term risk may encompass 5 years. In contrast, in primary prevention, short-term risk encompasses 10 years and long-term risk encompasses 20 years or a lifetime. The probability of a CHD event occurring in the lifetime of a 40-year-old man is about 40%, and that in a 40-year-old woman is about 25% (30).

Risk models are particularly useful in distinguishing high-risk (more than 2% annually) and low-risk (less than 0.6% annually) subsets for which the treatment decisions are clear, but further characterizing the large intermediate-risk group (0.6% to 2% annually) is problematic (31). Applying the Framingham Risk Score to the U.S. population as measured by National Health and Nutrition Examination Survey (NHANES) III, Greenland et al. (32) estimated 25% of adults in the US are at high risk, 35% are at low risk, and 40% are at intermediate risk for CHD. Patients at high-risk should be treated aggressively, and those at low risk may not require any intervention. The ATP-III guidelines (33) recommend using the Framingham Risk Score, the number of classic risk factors, and the LDL-C cut point to decide when to prescribe drugs and the intensity of treatment in the intermediate-risk group (Table 7.2).

All models ignore the 30% of patients with subsequent CHD who have an LDL-C level less than 130 mg per deciliter and the conditional risk factors, including family history of premature CHD. The ATP-III guidelines do suggest consideration of the conditional risk factors (Table 7.1) to enhance treatment decisions. The triad of increased fasting insulin levels (higher than 12 to 15 μmol per milliliter), increased apolipoprotein B (apoB) levels (higher than 110 mg per deciliter), and small LDL particle size (phenotype B) may be a better predictor of CHD than is the lipid profile when laboratory standards become available (34). In preclinical or established CHD in which the standard lipid profile is relatively normal, levels of apoB and measurement of HDL and LDL particle by gradient gel electrophoresis or nuclear magnetic resonance spectroscopy can be used to determine targets and specific treatment strategies (35).

C-REACTIVE PROTEIN

There is a robust correlation between high-sensitivity C-reactive protein (hs-CRP) and coronary risk, but the clinical role for measuring the hs-CRP in coronary risk stratification is not clear (36,37). CRP is an acute-phase reactant produced in the liver in response to inflammatory cytokines (interleukins 1 and 6 and tumor necrosis factor α) and is a marker or barometer of systemic inflammation at a given point in time. It can be influenced by acute or chronic infections, but the level in healthy persons is relatively stable over years (37). The standard CRP measurement is not capable of distinguishing coronary risk. The high-sensitivity method, for which laboratory standards have been developed, has a range of normal (0.01 to 0.8 mg per deciliter; median, about 0.16 mg per deciliter; fiftieth percentile, 0.21 mg per deciliter; seventy-fifth percentile, 0.375 mg per deciliter), and the measurement is similar in ethnic groups throughout the world (36,38). It is increased by obesity, female gender, estrogens, smoking, any infection or inflammation (including those dental), and diabetes. There is a good correlation between the quartile of hs-CRP (first vs. fourth) and subsequent risk of CHD in both men and women, including the elderly. At least some of the benefit of aspirin and the statins (e.g., lovastatin) in primary prevention may be mediated by their antiinflammatory effects (38,39). Further studies are needed to determine whether a low hs-CRP identifies a population for whom aspirin or statins therapy could be avoided.

NONINVASIVE DETECTION OF ATHEROSCLEROSIS

An accurate and sensitive noninvasive test that could determine the presence or absence of preclinical or subclinical coronary or other atherosclerosis would be very useful in the large group characterized as being at intermediate risk by the Framingham Risk Score. Such testing could potentially convert the patient at intermediate risk (0.6% to less than 2% annual event rate) to one at high risk (higher than 2% or coronary disease equivalent) in whom treatment is necessary and very cost effective or low risk (0.5% or lower) for whom expensive therapies may be avoided.

The American Heart Association (AHA) Prevention Conference V expert panel concluded that there was insufficient evidence to justify the cost of screening asymptomatic patients for CHD risk with carotid ultrasonography, exercise electrocardiographic testing, exercise or pharmacologic echocardiography, radionuclide myocardial perfusion imaging, or ambulatory electrocardiographic monitoring (40). However, the exercise treadmill test may be used in asymptomatic men and women at high risk, in order to identify those who might benefit from other testing and interventions (41).

Carotid ultrasonography is invaluable for the noninvasive assessment of cerebral vascular disease. A finding of carotid plaque is an indication for treatment as a CHD equivalent; however, carotid plaque is a relatively insensitive marker of preclinical CHD. In contrast, there is a good correlation between carotid intima-media thickness by high-resolution ultrasonography and CHD, coronary events, and stroke (42). The normal range is 0.5 to 0.8 mm, and the thickness increases with age (42). Carotid ultrasonography is more demanding than routine ultrasonography and requires special skill and equipment but, in expert centers, can help guide therapy. In asymptomatic men and women older than 50 years, a significant increase in carotid intima-media thickness is associated with a risk of coronary events comparable to "high risk" or coronary disease equivalent of 2% or more annually (43).

Brachial artery endothelial function reflects systemic and coronary endothelial function and has been recommended as a surrogate marker of preclinical disease (14). The change in brachial artery diameter in response to flow-mediated wall shear stress, cold, and exercise is correlated with coronary risk factors as well as with the presence of CHD (14,44). Normal vessels dilate by 5% to 15% in response to wall shear stress. The technique has been useful for characterizing risk factors that affect endothelial function and response to various therapies in small cohorts, but the lack of biologic and technical reproducibility is a serious limitation for clinical application in individuals.

The *ankle/brachial index* (ABI) is a simple tool that can be used effectively by all physicians to detect atherosclerotic disease in men and women older than 55 to 60 years (32). Considering that peripheral vascular occlusive disease (PVOD) correlates highly with CHD and mortality, it is not surprising an abnormal ABI in men and women older than 60 years is highly correlated with coronary events (45), and it can provide prognostic value beyond the Framingham risk score. The ABI is the ratio of the posterior tibial or dorsalis pedis artery pressure by pulse Doppler measurement on each foot to the Doppler pressure average of both arms. The normal value is 1 to 1.3, and PVOD is defined by an ABI of less than 0.9. The test is easy to perform with minimal training by medical assistants. Patients with an ABI of less than 0.9 should be treated as a CHD risk equivalent (the coronary event rate in established CHD, which is at least 20% over ten years or 2% annually) (33).

Electron beam computed tomography (EBT) and multidetector computed tomography of the chest can detect small amounts of coronary artery calcification present in the very early stage of atherosclerosis. Coronary artery calcium score (CACs) correlates with the number and severity of major risk factors, and the CACs is predictive of future coronary events independent of risk factors in asymptomatic men and women (46). The location of calcium does not reflect the severity of stenosis, but EBT may provide prognostic information beyond that of coronary arteriography (47).

Table 7.3 is a summary of the American College of Cardiology/American Heart Association Expert Consensus statements regarding EBT (48). Although there is insufficient evidence to support use of EBT for "routine" coronary risk stratification, the evidence that it can be used to characterize asymptomatic middle-aged men and women at intermediate and high risk has been consistent and compelling. Arad et al. (46) reported the long-term follow-up of a group of "worried well" men and women who underwent EBT screening for coronary artery calcium. A CACs of 80 or higher had an 85% sensitivity, 75% specificity, and an odds ratio of 16.1 (95% confidence interval, 6.7 to 38.9) for identifying who among the 1,172 men and women would have a CHD event during the following 4 years (18 fatal and nonfatal MI and 21 coronary revascularizations). EBT significantly improved upon the predictive value of the Framingham risk score in this intermediate-risk group.

A guideline for the clinical use of EBT incorporating the results of recent studies and the recommendations published by Rumberger et al. (49) in 1999 is presented in Table 7.4. The value of EBT and the relevance of results are influenced considerably by age and gender. EBT calcium scores cannot be used casually or as a single definitive tool. Patients with scores exceeding 80 to 100 or above the ninetieth percentile at any age should be treated as a CHD risk equivalent. The presence of significant coronary calcium disproportionate to standard risk analysis infers the

---

TABLE 7.3. *ACC/AHA expert consensus statement regarding EBT*

A negative EBT test result makes the presence of atherosclerotic plaque, including unstable plaque, very unlikely
A negative EBT test result is highly unlikely in the presence of significant lumenal obstructive disease
Negative test results occur in the majority of persons who have angiographically normal coronary arteries
A negative test result may be consistent with a low risk of a cardiovascular event in the next 2 to 5 years
A positive EBT test result confirms the presence of atherosclerotic plaque
The greater the amount of calcium, the greater the likelihood of occlusive coronary heart disease, but there is not a 1-to-1 relationship, and findings may not be site specific
The total amount of calcium correlates best with the total amount of atherosclerotic plaque, although the true "plaque burden" is underestimated
A high calcium score may be consistent with moderate to high risk of a cardiovascular event within the next 2 to 5 years

ACC/AHA, American College of Cardiology/American Heart Association; EBT, electron beam computed tomography.

TABLE 7.4. *Clinical guidelines for EBT in asymptomatic persons 45–75 years by Framingham Risk Score*

EBT coronary calcium score	Estimated annual CHD event risk	Recommendations
0	Very low (<0.2%)	Reassure, treat LDL > 160 mg/dL, repeat EBT in 3 years in middle-aged and elderly
1–10	Low (<0.5%)	Reassure, lipid treatment if CACs at 50th percentile; repeat EBT in 2–3 years
11–100	Moderate (0.5%–2%)	ATP-III guidelines; if CACs >80th or 90th percentile, treat as CHD equivalent
101–400	Moderately high (>2%)	Treat as CHD equivalent with secondary prevention; consider stress ECG
>400	High (2%–5%)	Treat as CHD equivalent with secondary prevention; obtain stress nuclear or echocardiogram

ATP-III, Adult Treatment Panel III; CAC, coronary artery calcium (score); CHD, coronary heart disease; EBT, electron beam computed tomography; ECG, electrocardiography; LDL, low-density lipoprotein.

presence of one or more conditional risk factors that could be investigated as possible treatment targets.

There has been concern that widespread use of EBT would trigger further unnecessary testing for ischemia. Stress imaging (echocardiographic or nuclear) studies should be considered in men and women with a CACs exceeding 400. A CACs exceeding 400 in asymptomatic men and women identifies a group of which a large percentage (nearly 50%) have demonstrable ischemia (50). Conversely, fewer than 7% of those with scores less than 400 have a defect on exercise single photon emission computed tomography (radionuclide), and more than 99% of such defects are small (less than 15% by perfusion defect size) (50).

RISK FACTOR MODIFICATION

Risk factor modification by lifestyle changes and drug therapies can reduce the risk of CHD and stroke by more than 50% in men and women, regardless of age. An estimated 75% of coronary risk is modifiable by lifestyle changes. Each of the major modifiable causal and conditional coronary risk factors is influenced by lifestyle and behavior. The evidence-based coronary prevention strategies can best be summarized and remembered by patients, nurses, physicians, and other health care professionals as the *ABCs of coronary prevention*, which are outlined in Table 7.5.

The National Cholesterol Education Program ATP-III guidelines (33) strongly recommend at-

tention to identifying adverse lifestyle patterns and institution of therapeutic lifestyle change (TLC) that addresses diet, exercise, weight management, and control of stress.

Smoking

Cigarette smoking increases the risk of MI threefold in men and sixfold in women and has an attributable risk more than double that of other risk factors. It is the most important modifiable coronary risk factor and the most preventable cause of mortality from cardiovascular and other diseases. The effects are dose dependent acutely and over decades and are greater from high-tar than from low-tar cigarettes. Approximately 30% of CHD deaths are attributable to smoking. Smoking tobacco can increase the risk of atherosclerosis, coronary events, and stroke by one or more of several mechanisms, including (a) impairment of endothelial function; (b) decrease in HDL-C and increase in triglyceride levels; (c) increase in catecholamine release with increase in heart rate and vasoconstriction; (d) hypertension; (e) increase in CRP, (f) chronic oral or respiratory infection and inflammation; (g) increase in fibrinogen, platelet aggregation, plasminogen activator inhibitor–1 (PAI-1), and thrombosis; (h) increase in oxidation of lipoproteins; and (i) increase in homocysteine levels. Both active and passive cigarette smoking leads to increased plaque, rate of plaque progression, plague rupture, and acute events (51). Smoking cessation results in immediate benefit in people of all ages.

TABLE 7.5. *The spectrum of the ABCs of primary coronary prevention*

Treatment	Mechanism of benefit	Benefit
Aspirin: 81–160 mg/day	Antiplatelet and antiinflammatory effects	Reduce CHD by 30%–45% in intermediate- and high-risk men and women, including the elderly with hypertension
Blood pressure control: targeting to <135/85 mm Hg with most cost-effective agents, beginning with diuretic, then ACEI; use combination drugs to reduce costs	Improves endothelial function, inhibits renin-angiotensin system, reduces arterial wall stress, reduces LVH	Reduce CHD events by 15%, hypertensive heart disease and CHF by 50%, and stroke risk by 50%
Cholesterol/lipids: risk stratification and target lipids by ATP-III guidelines	Improves endothelial function, reduces new lesion and CHD progression and plaque rupture	Decrease CHD events, stroke, revascularization, and mortality by 25%–35%
Diet as per ATP-III guidelines targeted to ideal body weight, LDL, and triglyceride goals	Reduces total and LDL-C by about 10% and can eliminate components of the metabolic syndrome	High-fiber, cold-water fish, and low-fat diets reduce coronary event rates and, when combined with exercise, can delay the onset of diabetes in the metabolic syndrome
Exercise: about 20–30 minutes of moderate aerobic activity at least three times weekly, with light weight training to increase muscle strength and tone	Reduces BP, increases HDL-C, reduces insulin resistance, reduces thrombosis, and increases thrombolysis	About a 50% reduction in CHD in fit men and women of all ages, particularly in events occurring during and after strenuous activity
Folic acid: about 400 μg/day in persons with homocysteine >12 μmol/L	Reduces effects of homocysteine on endothelial function and thrombosis	Not established as beneficial, but epidemiologic evidence is strongly supportive
Infection and inflammation: influenza vaccine for intermediate and high risk and early treatment of all infections	Reduces inflammatory cytokines and CRP that are associated with plaque instability and CHD events	Routine screening with CRP and early treatment of infection is not an evidence-supported recommendation, but good dental hygiene and early treatment of infection have other benefits
Smoking cessation: using behavior change and drug therapies	Improves endothelial function; decreases BP, inflammation, and procoagulation; increases HDL-C; reduces adverse neurohumoral effects	Reduced CHD event rate, strokes, and PVOD by 20%–50%
Stress reduction: by awareness, counseling, meditation, drugs, and referral to behaviorist	Reduces BP and adverse neurohumoral effects	Not established, but improvement in quality of life

ACEI, angiotensin-converting enzyme inhibitor; ATP-III, Adult Treatment Panel III; BP, blood pressure; CHD, coronary heart disease; CHF, congestive heart failure; CRP, C-reactive protein; HDL-C, high-density lipoprotein cholesterol; LDL-C, low-density lipoprotein cholesterol; LVH, left ventricular hypertrophy; PVOD, peripheral vascular occlusive disease.

The clinical approach to smoking cessation is summarized in Table 7.6.

Lipids and the Adult Treatment Panel III Guidelines

The major primary prevention trials designed to test the value of lipid-lowering treatment are summarized in Table 7.7. Statins, bile resins, and fibrates have been shown to reduce coronary event rates by 20% to 40% (52–54). The benefit of statins and bile resins has been considered to be primarily a result of a decrease in TC and LDL-C. However, statins decrease CHD events more than is attributable to their effect on LDL-C (55). This may reflect the modest increase in HDL-C

TABLE 7.6. *Physician-assisted patient stepwise approach to smoking cessation*

Provide the rationale for and give an unequivocal message to quit smoking

Determine whether the patient is willing to quit

Describe proven alternatives and have patient choose his or her quitting method of choice

Describe the potential problems associated with withdrawal and develop a plan for coping with each

Have the patient set a quit date and sign a contract in the medical record

Make sure that the patient can articulate how to cope with urges to smoke

Assure the patient of your support and that of your office staff

Follow up by telephone call or visit

Develop a plan for dealing with failure

(3–6%) or antiinflammatory and antithrombotic effects and the enhancement of endothelial function.

The importance of a low HDL-C as a risk marker and possible target was confirmed in two of the studies whose entry criteria included an HDL-C below the mean for healthy populations. The Helsinki Heart Study (52) used gemfibrozil, and the Air Force/Texas Coronary Atherosclerosis Prevention Study (AFCAPS/TexCAPS) (56) used lovastatin (Table 7.7), and each study found treatment benefit greatest in patients with lower HDL-C levels.

TABLE 7.7. *Summary of primary coronary prevention studies with lipid-lowering drugs*

Study (year)	Population	Design lipid results	Outcome
Lipid Research Clinic–Coronary Primary Prevention Trial (LRC-CPPT) (1984)	3,806 middle-aged men with hypercholesterolemia; mean cholesterol, 292 mg/dL, and LDL-C, 216 mg/dL	Randomized after diet to 24 g/d of cholestyramine vs. placebo and followed for 3 years. Average 12% reduction in LDL-C vs. placebo	A 19% reduction in CHD risk compared to placebo; in patients with a 35% reduction in LDL-C, a 50% reduction in CHD; no reduction in overall mortality
Helsinki Heart Study (HHS) (1987)	4,081 middle-aged men with non-HDL cholesterol >200 mg/dL	Randomized after diet to 600 mg of gemfibrozil BID vs. placebo and followed for 5 years. Average 10% reduction in cholesterol, 14% in non–HDL-C, 11% in LDL-C, and 35% in triglycerides; 11% rise in HDL-C	34% reduction in CHD events over 5 years with no reduction in overall mortality, suggesting increased non-CHD mortality; benefit predominantly in those with mixed elevated LDL-C and triglycerides and particularly with low HDL-C and obesity
West of Scotland Coronary Prevention Study (WOSCOPS) (1995)	6,595 middle-aged men with hypercholesterolemia; 10% angina but no MI; and mean LDL-C, 172 mg/dL	Randomized after diet to 40 mg/d pravastatin vs. placebo, followed for 5 years. 26% reduction in LDL-C compared to placebo	31% reduction in non-fatal MI and in CHD deaths, and 22% reduction in all-cause mortality at 5 years; maximum benefit seen with 25% reduction in LDL-C, suggesting a non–lipid-lowering effect
Air Force/Texas Coronary Artery Prevention Study (AFCAPS/TexCAPS) (1998)	6,605 subjects with 15% women and 20% over 65 years; mean cholesterol, 220 mg/dL; LDL, 150 mg/dL; HDL-C, 38 mg/dL for men and 40 mg/dL in women entry criteria: LDL-C, >110 mg/dL; HDL, <45 mg/dL for men and <47 mg/dL for women; and triglycerides, <400 mg/dL	Randomized after diet to 20 mg/day of lovastatin or placebo, titrated to 40 mg if LDL-C > 110 mg/d, and followed for 5 years. Average reduction in LDL was 25%, HDL-C increased by 6%, and triglycerides decreased 15%	37% reduction in CHD events, 40% reduction in fatal or nonfatal MI, and 33% reduction in revascularization at 5 years; benefit similar in men vs. women and older vs. younger than 60 years; subjects were average risk, on basis of U.S. population

BID, twice a day; CHD, coronary heart disease; HDL-C, high-density lipoprotein cholesterol; LDL-C, low-density lipoprotein cholesterol; MI, myocardial infarction.

TABLE 7.8. *Classification of lipids by the ATP-III guideline*

Classification	Level (mg/dL)
LDL Cholesterol	
Optimal	<100
Near or above optimal	100–129
Borderline high	130–159
High	160–189
Very high	≥190
Total Cholesterol	
Desirable	<200
Borderline high	200–239
High	≥240
HDL cholesterol	
Low	<40
High	≥60
Triglycerides	
Normal	<150 mg/dL
Borderline high	150–199 mg/dL
High	200–499 mg/dL
Very high	≥500 mg/dL

ATP-III, Adult Treatment Panel III; HDL, high-density lipoprotein; LDL, low-density lipoprotein.

The ATP-III classification of TC, HDL-C, LDL-C, and triglyceride level is provided in Table 7.8 (33). The risk factors that alter LDL goals are listed in Table 7.9, and the information on the Framingham Risk Score and 10-year estimate of CHD events for men and women is provided in Table 7.2. Table 7.10 summarizes the salient features of the ATP-III guidelines (33).

Risk screening with a fasting lipid (lipoprotein) profile, including TC, HDL-C, triglyceride level, and estimated LDL-C, is recommended for all adults (older than 19 years) and should be repeated in about 5-year intervals if results are

TABLE 7.9. *Major risk factors that modify LDL goals other than LDL cholesterol*

Cigarette smoking
Hypertension, defined as blood pressure ≥140/90 mm Hg, or on antihypertensive therapy
Low HDL cholesterol (<40 mg/dL)
Family history of premature CHD in a first-degree relative (male, <55 years, and female, <65 years)
Age (men, ≥45 years, and women, ≥55 years)

Diabetes is a CHD risk equivalent. HDL-C ≥ 60 mg/dL is a negative risk factor, and its presence removes one risk factor from the count.

CHD, coronary heart disease; HDL, high-density lipoprotein; LDL, low-density lipoprotein.

within the acceptable range. Screening should begin earlier in children and adolescence when first-degree relatives have premature atherosclerosis or dyslipidemia. If in a nonfasting patient the cholesterol level is higher than 200 mg per deciliter or the HDL-C is lower than 40 mg per deciliter, a fasting lipoprotein profile should follow. Patients with risk factors at any age should undergo appropriate counseling regarding diet, optimal weight, and exercise, collectively known as therapeutic lifestyle change (Table 7.10) (33).

LDL-cholesterol is the primary target for reducing coronary events, on the basis of epidemiologic and placebo-controlled trial evidence in healthy men and women with high and relatively normal lipid levels. The effect of beginning treatment with diet should not be underestimated. The average reduction in LDL-C with the AHA diet of 25% to 30% fat with less than 7% saturated fat is about 5% to 10%, a magnitude similar to doubling the dose of each of the statin drugs. Patients willing to tolerate a vegetarian diet with less than 10% fat and no saturated fat may reduce the LDL-C by as much as 50%. The severe restriction in fat and compensatory increase in dietary carbohydrates, however, is associated with a 10% to 30% increase in triglyceride levels and a 10% to 20% decrease in HDL-C. Restriction in saturated fat usually results in a decrease in HDL-C. The significance of these trade-offs is not clear but is probably positive and can be offset with exercise and an increase in monounsaturated fats from foods such as olive oils and walnuts.

The average doses, responses, and complications of the lipid-lowering drugs are listed in Table 7.11. By blocking hepatic 3-hydroxy-3-methylglutaryl coenzyme A (HMG-CoA) reductase, the rate-limiting enzyme in cholesterol synthesis, the statins induce an increase in the number and activity of hepatic LDL-receptors and promote clearance of cholesterol-rich LDL particles. The range of LDL-C reduction by the starting dose of the statins varies from 25% to 35%, but the individual response can vary considerably. Doubling the dose of each of the statins reduces the LDL-C by an additional 6%

TABLE 7.10. *Summary of the Adult Treatment Panel III, (ATP-III) guidelines for treating lipids*

Focus on risk stratification, estimate of coronary event rate, and multiple risk factors

Complete lipid profile (fasting cholesterol, HDL-C, triglycerides, and calculated LDL-C) for all persons 20 years and older

Framingham Risk Score (FRS) to predict the 10-year absolute coronary event rate in persons with two or more CHD risk factors

Target those with at least a 2% annual event rate for more intense treatment as a CHD equivalent

Raise diabetics to the level of a CHD risk equivalent

Identify persons with multiple metabolic risk factors (the metabolic syndrome) as candidates for more intensive therapeutic lifestyle change (TLC)

In intermediate-risk persons and low-risk persons with a family history of CVD, consider preclinical atherosclerosis screening by EBT, carotid ultrasonography, ABI, and conditional risk factors such as Lp(a), hs-CRP, homocysteine, metabolic syndrome, and LDL particle size to modify treatment intensity

TLC modified from ATP-III[a]

Diet 25%–35% fat, <7% saturated fat, up to 10% polyunsaturated and 20% monounsaturated fatty acids, 50%–60% carbohydrate, 15% protein, <200 mg/d cholesterol

Encourage consumption of plant stanols and soluble fiber to lower LDL cholesterol

Increase use of monounsaturated fats, increase in complex carbohydrates, and reduced simple sugars, particularly in obesity, diabetes, and the metabolic syndrome

Regular aerobic exercise

Smoking cessation[a]

Recognition and control of stress[a]

Risk category	LDL-C goal mg/dL	LDL-C to consider drug therapy (mg/dL)	Non-HDL cholesterol goal (mg/dL)
CHD and CHD risk equivalent as diabetes or FRS 10-year risk ≥20%	<100	≥130 100–129 optional	<130
Multiple (2+) risk factors and FRS 10-year risk <20%	<130	10-year risk 10%–19%, ≥130 10-year risk <10%, ≥160	<160
0–1 Risk factor	<160	≥190 (160–189; LDL lowering optional)	<190

[a] Not from ATP-III.

ABI, ankle/brachial index; CHD; coronary heart disease; CVD, cardiovascular disease; EBT, electron beam computed tomography; HDL-C, high-density lipoprotein cholesterol; hs-CRP, high-sensitive C-reactive protein; LDL-C, low-density lipoprotein cholesterol; Lp(a), lipoprotein a.

to 7%. The statins have an excellent safety profile. Mild to moderate elevation in liver enzyme levels [alanine aminotransferase (ALT)] is not an indication for discontinuation of statins. If the ALT level rises by more than twofold, drug or food (grapefruit) cytochrome P-450 interactions should be considered, and the statin should be withheld for 2 to 3 weeks. When the ALT level returns to normal, the same drug at half dosage or another statin can be tried.

A good alternative or adjunctive treatment with the statins is the plant stanols (2- to 3-g-per-day decrease in LDL-C by 10%) and the bile acid sequestrants. By preventing reabsorption of bile, these agents enhance LDL receptor activity and lower LDL-C by 5% to 30%. Fenofibrate lowers LDL-C modestly when triglyceride levels are increased, but as a single agent, it is not as potent as the statins or resins. Nicotinic acid (vitamin B_6) in low doses has little effect on LDL-C, but in high doses (3 to 5 g per day) may reduce LDL-C by 25% and, when combined with statins, may decrease LDL-C by more than 50%.

Non-HDL cholesterol (TC − HDL-C = LDL-C + VLDL-C) is recommended as a secondary treatment target in the ATP-III guidelines in persons with triglyceride levels exceeding 200 mg per deciliter. This is based on the epidemiologic and trial evidence that the level of triglycerides, which reflects the number and cholesterol content of VLDL and VLDL remnant particles, is correlated highly with coronary event rates, particularly when LDL-C is elevated. The cholesterol content of VLDL particles or VLDL-C can be estimated by Friedewald's equation as 20% of the fasting triglyceride level if the triglyceride

TABLE 7.11. Drugs affecting lipid metabolism

Drug class, agents, and daily doses	Lipid/lipoprotein effects	Safety and efficacy with combinations	Side effects	Contraindications
HMG-CoA reductase inhibitors (statins) Double dose ↓ LDL 6%	LDL: ↓ 18%–55% HDL: ↑ 5%–15% TG: ↓ 7%–30%	Safe with resins and probably with nicotinic acid Do not use lovastatin or atorvastatin with fibrates	Myopathy; increased liver enzymes; monitor ALT 6–12 wk then annually	Absolute: active or chronic liver disease Relative: concomitant use of certain drugs,[a] reduce dose in renal disease
Bile acid sequestrants[b]	LDL: ↓ 15%–30% HDL: ↑ 3%–5% TG: No change or increase	Resins decreased absorption of other drugs, including warfarin and thyroid. Take 1 hr before or 4 hr after; safe with nicotinic acid	Gastrointestinal distress; constipation; decreased absorption of fat-soluble vitamins	Absolute: dysbetalipoproteinemia; TG >400 mg/dL Relative: TG >200 mg/dL
Cholesterol absorption inhibitor	LDL: decrease 15–18% HDL: increase 4% TG: no significant change	Additive and safe with statins better than resins in statin intolerance reduced cost in lieu at doubling statin dose		Not tried with cyclosporines
Nicotinic acid[c]	LDL: ↓ 5%–25% HDL: ↑ 10%–35% TG: ↓ 10%–25%	Established safety with lovastatin and pravastatin Advicor: combination of niacin and lovastatin	Flushing; hyperglycemia; hyperuricemia (or gout); upper gastrointestinal distress; hepatotoxicity	Absolute: chronic liver disease; severe gout Relative: diabetes; hyperuricemia; peptic ulcer disease
Fibric acids[d]	HDL: ↑ 10%–20% TG: ↓ 20%–50% LDL: ↓ 5%–25% (may increase in patients with high TG)	Relatively safe with pravastatin, and possibly simvastatin; screen with CK at 6 weeks or with any muscle ache; can be used with nicotinic acid	Dyspepsia; gallstones; myopathy; unexplained non-CHD deaths in WHO study	Absolute: severe renal disease; severe hepatic disease

ALT, alanine aminotransferase; CHD, coronary heart disease; CK, creatine phosphokinase; HDL, high-density lipoprotein; HMG-CoA, 3-hydroxy-3-methylglutaryl coenzyme A; LDL, low-density lipoprotein; TG, triglycerides; WHO, World Health Organisation.

Lovastatin (20–80 mg), pravastatin (20–80 mg), fluvastatin (20–80 mg), atorvastatin (10–80 mg), simvastatin (10–80 mg).

[a] Cyclosporine, macrolide antibiotics, various antifungal agents, and other cytochrome P-450 inhibitors, including grapefruit juice. Pravastatin is relative safe with other drugs as it is not metabolized via the P-450 system. Fibrates and niacin should be used with appropriate caution and monitoring of liver function.

[b] Cholestyramine (4–16 g), colestipol (5–20 g) and colesevelam (2.6–3.8 g). About 4% reduction in LDL-C per initial dose equivalent.

[c] Immediate-release (crystalline) nicotinic acid (1.5–3 g), extended-release nicotinic acid (1–2 g), and sustained-release nicotinic acid (1–2 g).

[d] Gemfibrozil (600 mg twice daily), fenofibrate (160 mg daily), and clofibrate (1,000 mg twice daily). Before using combinations of statins and fibrates, consider consultation with a lipid specialist.

level is less than 400 mg per deciliter (e.g., if triglyceride level is 300 mg per deciliter, the VLDL-C is 60 mg per deciliter).

Because of associated risk factors, it has been difficult to establish the significance of triglyceride levels as an independent causal risk factor. Increased triglyceride levels are associated with highly atherogenic small LDL particles, low HDL-C, increased PAI-1 levels, and activated factor VII levels. Familial combined hyperlipidemia and familial dysbetalipoproteinemia are two inherited dyslipidemias with elevated TC, LDL-C, and triglyceride levels that are highly associated with CHD. Factors contributing to increased fasting levels of serum triglycerides include a high-carbohydrate diet, obesity, alcohol, diabetes, chronic renal failure, nephrotic syndrome, and drugs, particularly steroids and estrogens.

Lowering non-HDL cholesterol and triglyceride levels requires an emphasis on diet and exercise. The diet should be limited in fat, particularly restrictive in simple sugars and white flours, targeted to near an ideal body weight, and accompanied by regular aerobic exercise. These measures result in decreased VLDL particle formation, increased removal of triglycerides from VLDL particles to form VLDL remnants, increased clearance of remnant particles, and increased insulin sensitivity necessary to metabolize triglycerides through capillary endothelial lipoprotein lipase. Diet and exercise can reduce triglyceride and VLDL levels by 20% to 80%.

Lowering of VLDL cholesterol generally occurs with drugs that lower triglyceride levels (Table 7.11). The coronary prevention strategy requires first reducing the LDL-C to target level, preferably with a statin. If the non-HDL cholesterol target is not reached, the most effective drug class for decreasing triglyceride level and the associated increase in VLDL-C is the fibrates. Gemfibrozil is particularly effective and may lower triglyceride level by 20% to 50%. The benefit is augmented markedly by proper diet, weight loss, and exercise. Fenofibrate is less effective at lowering triglyceride level but, in mixed lipid disorders, may also decrease LDL-C by as much as 20% to 25%. Fenofibrate has not yet been shown to be effective for primary preven-

tion in nondiabetic patients. Fibrates can be combined with certain statins safely (pravastatin in particular), but liver function must be monitored at intervals. Patients should be warned to discontinue the lipid-lowering drugs, particularly the combinations of statins and fibrates, with the onset of muscle aches or weakness, which may indicate rhabdomyolysis. Nicotinic acid is considerably less effective than the fibrates for reducing triglyceride level but is relatively safe when combined with statins. The combination of high doses of statins and niacin may reduce the LDL-C by more than 40% to 50% and may increase HDL-C by more than 25%. Caution is needed when lipid-lowering drugs are used with all other drugs, and the combination of lovastatin and gemfibrozil must be avoided.

Low HDL-C is an independent causal risk factor for CHD. Low HDL-C can be inherited as isolated hypoalphalipoproteinemia and is often found in association with hypertriglyceridemia or mixed hyperlipidemia. It can also be secondary to physical inactivity, obesity, smoking, a diet low in fat and high in carbohydrates, high triglyceride level, and such drugs as beta blockers, androgens, and progestational agents. At least part of the decrease in event rate found with gemfibrozil in the Helsinki Heart Study (52) and with lovastatin in AFCAPS/TexCAPS (56) is attributable to a modest 6% to 8% increase in HDL-C. Nevertheless, there is no direct evidence in support of targeting a low HDL-C with drugs for primary prevention. Patients with low HDL-C should be encouraged to exercise and achieve ideal weight. Emphasis should be on targeting LDL-C and non-HDL cholesterol. Should patients with a family history of premature atherosclerotic disease be found to have significant preclinical coronary or carotid disease and an isolated low HDL-C, there is evidence that gemfibrozil and possibly niacin would be of value. In the Veterans Affairs High-Density Lipoprotein Cholesterol Intervention Trial (VA-HIT), gemfibrozil reduced coronary event rates and coronary mortality (57).

Younger adults (men aged 20 to 35 years and women aged 20 to 45 years) need special attention (33). About 15% to 25% of younger adults require diet counseling and recommendations for reassessment more frequently than the general recommendation of every 5 years. If diet is not effective, drug treatment with a statin or resin is generally indicated in anyone with a LDL-C level exceeding 190 mg per deciliter and in men who smoke or have a family history of premature CHD and a LDL-C level of 160 to 189 mg/dL. Statins have been shown to be safe during and after puberty but should be avoided during pregnancy and by women planning to become pregnant. There have been no reports of effects of statins on male fertility or teratogenicity, but, like all drugs, the statins should be used with caution and with proper informed consent. Severe forms of hypercholesterolemia in younger persons can be safely treated with bile resins as well as combinations of resins and statins, preferably by experts in lipid management.

The guidelines for lipid management in the general population of middle-aged adults in the United States are applicable to minorities and specific ethnic groups as well as to the elderly who are otherwise relatively healthy and expected to live at least 5 years.

Hypertension

Hypertension is present in about 50 million adults in the United States and is a major causal risk factor for CHD, hypertensive heart disease and heart failure, and stroke (26). A considerable percentage of adults with hypertension have associated obesity and glucose intolerance. The major benefit of antihypertensive therapy is a reduction in stroke and in the consequences of hypertensive heart disease. The reduction of coronary events is less than that anticipated from coronary risk models. For this reason, the Joint National Committee (JNC) VI panel recommended a more comprehensive approach by treating hypertension as a part of targeting the total cardiovascular risk profile (26).

Treatment of hypertension requires that the arm blood pressure be obtained in a standardized manner. This includes (a) an appropriate sized cuff; (b) sitting with the arm supported at the level of the heart; (c) inflating the cuff to at least 50 mm Hg above expected pressure or 200 mm Hg; (d) measuring the pressure in each arm at least once, the final pressure being the higher of the two; (e) repeating the measurement in 2 minutes and, if there is a significant systolic difference of more than 10 mm Hg, repeating again 5 minutes later; and (f) averaging the second and third measurements. The systolic pressure is the first audible sound heard when the occluding pressure is slowly reduced, and the change in sound identifies the diastolic pressure. A continuous increase in CVD risk is attributable to systolic pressures exceeding 120 mm Hg and diastolic pressures exceeding 80 mm Hg. The definition of hypertension is at 140/90 mm Hg or higher. A pressure of 160/80 mm Hg would be characterized as isolated systolic hypertension. An increase in pulse pressure higher than 75 mm Hg in the elderly is more highly correlated with CHD and stroke than are the systolic, diastolic, or mean pressures and is a target for therapy. *White-coat hypertension* is the term used to characterize persons in whom the pressure is elevated in the doctor's office but not at home. It was once considered innocent, but the evidence suggests that white-coat hypertension is associated with abnormal peripheral vascular resistance, left ventricular hypertrophy, and other coronary risk factors and is a risk factor for stroke and hypertensive heart disease (58). Before the diagnosis of hypertension is confirmed, elevated pressures should be documented on three separate occasions. Both 24-hour ambulatory pressure monitoring and home blood pressure measurement are effective in assessing average pressures and guiding treatment decisions, with the understanding that the office pressure has significant implications.

The JNC VI guidelines (26) characterize and treat hypertension by stage and association with other coronary risk factors, presence of diabetes, CVDs, and target organ damage. The JNC VI guidelines for risk stratification and treatment are listed in Table 7.12, and an algorithm for drug therapy is summarized in Fig. 7.2. The pharmacoeconomics of antihypertensive therapy depend on several factors, including age, severity, comorbid conditions, and cost of single or combinations of drugs. Diuretics and beta blockers are less costly than angiotensin-converting enzyme (ACE) inhibitors, angiotensin receptor blockers, and calcium channel blockers. The cost of preventing one major cardiovascular event in

TABLE 7.12. *Joint National Committee VI risk stratification and treatment of hypertension*

Blood pressure stages (mm Hg)	Risk group		
	A No risk factors No TOD or CCD[b]	B At least 1 risk factor, no diabetes, TOD or CCD[b]	C TOD or CCD and/or diabetes
High-normal: 130–139/85–89	Lifestyle modification	Lifestyle modification	Drug therapy[c]
Stage 1: 140–159/90–99	Lifestyle modification (up to 12 months)	Lifestyle modification[d] (up to 6 months)	Drug therapy
Stages 2 and 3: ≥160/≥100	Drug therapy	Drug therapy	Drug therapy

[a] Lifestyle modification for all patients treated with drugs.
[b] TOD includes stroke, transient ischemic attack, nephropathy, and retinopathy; CCD includes left ventricular hypertrophy, coronary heart disease, CABG, congestive heart failure, peripheral vascular occlusive disease, and aortic aneurysm.
[c] For heart failure, renal disease, and diabetes.
[d] For patients with multiple risk factors, consider early drug treatment and adjustment later.
CABG = coronary artery bypass graft; CCD, clinical cardiovascular disease; TOD, target organ damage.

middle-aged men and women is estimated at about $4,700 for hydrochlorothiazide, $156,000 for an ACE inhibitor, and $345,000 for long-acting nifedipine (4).

Diabetes Mellitus

Diabetes is a major risk factor whose very presence indicates CHD. The relative risk of MI is 50% higher in diabetic men and 150% greater in diabetic women than in age-matched nondiabetic persons (59). Similarly, sudden cardiac death is 50% more frequent in diabetic men and 300% more frequent in diabetic women than in age-matched nondiabetic persons. In addition to the increased prevalence of CHD among diabetic patients, the extent of the disease is greater at autopsy (60). In comparison with nondiabetic patients, diabetic men and women have a higher incidence of two- and three-vessel disease (e.g., 83% vs. 17%). For these reasons, the ATP-III guidelines and the American Diabetic Association guidelines recommend treating diabetic patients as CHD equivalents for each of the prevention therapies.

The *metabolic syndrome,* or the insulin resistance syndrome, is a very common inherited or acquired metabolic trait in which there is insulin receptor insensitivity of all tissues, which results in increasing levels of circulating insulin and an "atherogenic lipid phenotype" of low HDL-C, high triglyceride levels, increase in LDL-C and apoB levels, and small LDL particles (35). The ATP-III guidelines emphasize the importance of the metabolic syndrome and provide diagnostic criteria, summarized in Table 7.13. Persons with any three of the five criteria are characterized as having the metabolic syndrome. A family history of diabetes, hypertension, high triglyceride levels, and abdominal obesity should be considered risk factors for the metabolic syndrome. One or more clinical features of atherosclerosis and hypertension in the form of CHD, stroke, PVOD, hypertensive heart disease, diabetes, and chronic renal insufficiency are essentially certain to be present in patients with unrecognized metabolic syndrome who live into their seventh or eighth decades and very often occur in men younger than 55 years and women younger than 65 years. The metabolic syndrome predisposes to accelerated atherosclerosis, MI, and stroke by the interaction between several associated risk factors, endothelial dysfunction, and a prothrombotic state. The features of the metabolic syndrome are present in diabetic persons 5 to 15 years before carbohydrate intolerance. The characteristic phenotype of the metabolic syndrome may be acquired through long-term obesity, and men with a waist larger than 37 inches should be counseled that they could be genetically predisposed. The importance of early identification of the traits of the syndrome cannot be overemphasized. Regular exercise increases insulin sensitivity and, when combined with weight loss and

***Aggressive life style modification** for all patients including salt restriction and diet to ideal body weight, exercise, and stress control with referral for nutrition, behavior, and exercise consultation as necessary.*

First line drugs or initial choices

Uncomplicated hypertension
- Diuretic – hydrochlorthiazide or dyrenium/HCTZ,
- Beta blocker – single daily dose, selective or non-selective
- Generic angiotensin converting enzyme inhibitor

Specific compelling indications for specific drugs

Diabetes with or without microscopic proteinuria
- ACE inhibitor – first choice
- Angiotensin receptor blocker – second choice

Myocardial infarction
- Beta-blocker and ACE inhibitor

Congestive heart failure
- ACE inhibitor –first choice
- Angiotensin receptor blocker
- Diuretic
- Long acting nitrates

Systolic hypertension of the elderly
- Diuretics
- Beta blockers
- Long-acting calcium channel blockers, dihydropyridines

Other possible selections
- Alpha blocker peripheral or central
- Beta blocker with alpha blocking properties

Prefer once daily drugs, and initiation with a starting dose. For step 2 or second drug, can reduce cost and side effects by adding a diuretic or combination ACEi-diuretic or beta-blocker-diuretic.

Target blood pressure in mm Hg	
Healthy middle aged and elderly	<135/85
CHF, renal failure	120–130/80
Diabetes	<130/80

FIG. 7.2. Algorithm for selecting drug treatment for hypertension as modified from the Joint National Committee VI.

TABLE 7.13. *Features of the metabolic syndrome of insulin resistance*

Risk factor	Defining level
Abdominal obesity	
Men	>40 inches or 102 cm
Women	>35 inches or 88 cm
Triglycerides	≥150 mg/dL
High-density lipoprotein cholesterol	
Men	<40 mg/dL
Women	<50 mg/dL
Blood pressure	≥130/≥80 mm Hg
Fasting blood glucose	≥110 mg/dL

reduction in body fat by appropriate number and selection of calories, can delay the onset of diabetes and reverse many of the risk factors, including low HDL-C, hypertension, and elevated triglyceride levels.

Other Considerations

Obesity is not a major independent risk factor, but it contributes significantly to a number of the causal factors (Table 7.14). Body mass index (BMI) is the body weight divided by the height squared (kg/m^2). Overweight is defined as a BMI over 25 kg/m^2; obesity is defined as a BMI exceeding 27.8 kg/m^2 for men and 27.3 kg/m^2; and morbid obesity is more than 50% above ideal body weight. The risk attributable to obesity is very high with a BMI higher than 40 kg/m^2.

Obesity is generally associated with excessive dietary calories, fat calories, saturated fat, and sugars in the diet and with physical inactivity (61). Contrary to common beliefs, the energy

TABLE 7.14. *Coronary risk factors influenced by obesity*

Metabolic syndrome of insulin resistance
Diabetes
Hypertension
Atherogenic lipid phenotype: increased triglycerides, low-HDL-C, shift to small LDL particles
Increased fibrinogen
Increased C-reactive protein
Abnormal endothelial function

HDL-C, high-density lipoprotein cholesterol; LDL, low-density lipoprotein.

imbalance leading to weight gain in middle-aged persons is relatively small. An estimated excess of 300 calories per day (15% increase) over 10 years will result in approximately 22 pounds of excess weight (600 calories will result in an extra 44 pounds, and so forth). The central distribution of body fat ("gut" fat vs. "butt" fat) is a classic coronary phenotype associated with a cluster of risk factors (hypertension, low HDL-C, small LDL particles, carbohydrate intolerance). Together they are the most virulent contributors to coronary events, stroke, PVOD, and end-stage renal disease. The waist circumference is an excellent measure of abdominal fat and is correlated highly with serum insulin level and insulin resistance. Insulin resistance or the metabolic syndrome should be suspected in a patient with a rapidly increasing abdominal girth without much change in weight, in a man with a waist circumference of more than 40 inches (102 cm), and in a woman with a waist circumference of more than 35 inches (88 cm). Weight loss requires restriction of total calories, proper selection of calories, limiting fat (9 calories per gram vs. 4 calories per gram for protein and carbohydrates) and simple sugars, and exercise. A weight loss goal of about 10% over 4 to 6 months is reasonable and achievable. Patients should be encouraged to set their own goals for caloric intake and distribution, snacking, and exercise. Severe calorie restrictions are not necessary or sustainable. Exercise should be part of every weight-loss program.

Physical inactivity is a risk factor for coronary disease, and a high level of fitness is associated with a 50% reduction in risk of CHD in men and women of all ages (62). A moderate amount of regular exercise reduces CHD risk in previously sedentary men and women. The benefits attributable to regular exercise include improved well-being, lower blood pressure, decreased body fat, increased HDL-C, lower triglyceride levels, improved carbohydrate tolerance and insulin sensitivity, improved endothelial function, enhanced fibrinolysis, and decreased thrombosis. Both leisure time and work energy expenditure contribute to decreasing CHD risk and improving metabolic parameters. Strenuous exercise is not necessary to obtain benefit and may increase the risk of injury and acute coronary events. Regular aerobic exercise such as walking, cycling, or aerobic sport for 25 to 30 minutes 3 to 5 days per week should be accompanied by some form of activity that enhances upper body muscle tone and strength (62).

Inflammation and infection are likely contributors to the pathogenesis of early atherosclerosis, progression of coronary and noncoronary heart disease, and acute coronary events (5,8,9). Chronic infections of all types (respiratory, dental, urinary tract) increase the risk of carotid atherosclerosis and seropositivity to infectious agents, and the CRP levels have independent and combined predictive value in CHD (36,37,63). It is not clear whether the infectious organisms (e.g., *Chlamydia pneumoniae, Helicobacter pylori,* dental flora) in the atheroma, the immune response to local or systemic infection, or both are the culprits (64). As yet, there is no evidence that treating any of the specific organisms with antibiotics is beneficial. Because some of the benefit of aspirin in primary coronary disease prevention is an antiinflammatory effect, it is prudent for physicians to encourage good oral hygiene, liberally administer flu vaccines to high-risk middle-aged patients and all elderly patients, and treat bacterial infections without delay.

ASPIRIN AND HORMONE REPLACEMENT THERAPY

Aspirin

Low-dosage aspirin [acetylsalicylic acid (ASA)] reduced the overall occurrence of MI by about 45% in the Physicians Health Study and by 33% in a metaanalysis of four large trials (65). ASA irreversibly inhibits platelet aggregation, which reduces thrombus formation at the site of ruptured coronary plaques. The effect is comparable across a dose range from 81 to 325 mg per day. Higher dosages of ASA, such as those used for arthritis, may increase platelet aggregation and thrombosis by inhibiting endothelium-derived prostacyclin, a powerful vasodilator and inhibitor of platelet aggregation. A second mech-

anism for the benefit of ASA may be its antiinflammatory effect.

The benefit of aspirin must be weighed against the risk of bleeding from the gastrointestinal tract and a potential increase in hemorrhagic stroke. A metaanalysis concluded that ASA reduced the incidence of first MI by 30% and that of all cardiovascular events by 15% but at the expense of a significant 69% increased risk of bleeding complications, including a 6% nonsignificant increase in hemorrhagic stroke (65). One guideline recommended treating persons at intermediate risk (3% five-year risk) and high risk (20% 10-year risk) with low-dosage ASA (66). Risk can be calculated from the Framingham Risk Score (Table 7.2).

Postmenopausal Estrogens

Estrogen or estrogen/progestin replacement therapy (collectively, hormone replacement therapy) has been shown to reduce cardiac events in observational studies, but benefit was not found in randomized trials. The present AHA recommendation is that hormone replacement therapy not be prescribed solely for coronary prevention, but it can be continued on the basis of established noncoronary benefits, including reduction of menopausal symptoms and of risk of osteoporosis (67). Although findings are encouraging, the role of selective estrogen receptor modulators in coronary disease prevention remains to be established.

NUTRIENT SUPPLEMENTS

Vitamins

Lipid peroxidation is clearly a significant contributor to endothelial dysfunction and the pathogenesis of atherosclerosis, but there is little to no evidence in support of the claims of cardiovascular benefit for supplements of vitamin E, vitamin C, or beta-carotene (68).

Marine Oils

Populations with a diet high in fish and omega-3 fatty acids have a decreased prevalence of CHD and stroke. Supplemental marine oil (850 mg per day of omega-3 fatty acids) reduced rates of recurrent MI by 22% and of sudden death by 45% in men and women after MI (69). The effects were independent of lipid-lowering medications and other secondary prevention therapy. There is ample information to encourage incorporating cold-water fish that is high in protein and marine oil into the average American diet.

Folic Acid

Supplemental B vitamins have been recommended for CHD prevention, but as yet there is no evidence of benefit. A homocysteine level above 10 to 12 μmol per liter is a *conditional* causal risk factor for CHD, PVOD, and stroke (70). Homocysteine is prothrombotic and a powerful prooxidant, and levels correlate with severity of CVD. Elevated levels of homocysteine are found in patients who smoke and in those with hypothyroidism, abnormal or deficient methylte-

trahydrofolate reductase and cystathionine beta synthase genes, chronic renal failure, niacin, dilantin, methotrexate, and a diet deficient in folic acid, pyridoxine, or vitamin B_{12}. About 400 μg of folic acid per day reduces homocysteine levels by an average of 3 to 4 μmol per liter. Placebo-controlled trials testing the value of reducing homocysteine levels with folic acid are ongoing.

SUMMARY

The concept of primary prevention for CHD and atherosclerosis is entrenched in evidence-based trials. Much is known, and there are many more possible targets for therapy according to the current understanding of the pathobiology of atherosclerosis. Clinical risk stratification with the Framingham Risk Score, supplemented by novel methods of assessing risk and preclinical disease, including EBT and magnetic resonance imaging in the future, may enhance the cost effectiveness of coronary prevention.

PRACTICAL POINTS

- Atherosclerosis is a systemic vascular inflammatory disease process present in nearly all adults and at least 25% of youths and is triggered by endothelial injury by one or more coronary risk factors.
- *Coronary risk factors* are factors whose presence are associated with or are correlated with an increased likelihood that atherosclerotic coronary disease will be present at a later time. *Coronary risk markers* are factors associated with acute coronary events and may also be risk factors, such as tobacco use and hs-CRP.
- The majority of acute coronary events result from rupture of a nonocclusive vulnerable plaque. Prevention strategies are intended to reduce the atherosclerotic burden and increase plaque stability.
- Primary prevention of coronary disease is

most cost effective when patient selection for drug therapy is made by careful risk stratification with age, gender, and the ATP-III guidelines supplemented by the AHA Global Risk Score, derived from the Framingham data base.
- Detection of coronary calcification by EBT, determination of carotid intima-media thickness and plaque volume by ultrasonography, and hs-CRP can be used to supplement risk stratification in the intermediate-risk group.
- Evidence-based primary prevention strategies include antiplatelet therapy with aspirin, blood pressure control, and lowering LDL-C with drugs and with diet, exercise, and smoking cessation. There is no role for postmenopausal estrogen therapy for coronary prevention.

REFERENCES

1. American Heart Association. *2001 Heart and Stroke Statistical Update.* Dallas, TX: American Heart Association, 2000.

2. Gotto AM. Primary prevention of coronary heart disease. Where do we go from here? *Arch Intern Med* 2001;161:922–924.

3. Shepard J. Economics of lipid lowering in primary prevention: Lesions from the West of Scotland Coronary Prevention Study. *Am J Cardiol* 2001;87:19B–22B.

4. Pearce KA, Furberg CD, Psaty BM, et al. Cost-minimization and the number needed to treat in uncomplicated hypertension. *Am J Hypertens* 1998;11:618–629.

5. Ross R. Atherosclerosis—an inflammatory disease. *N Engl J Med* 1999;340:115–126.

6. Strong JP, Malcom GT, McMahan CA, et al. Prevalence and extent of atherosclerosis in adolescents and young adults: implications for prevention from the Pathobiological Determinants of Atherosclerosis in Youth Study. *JAMA* 1999;281:727–735.

7. Tuzcu EM, Kapadia SR, Tutar E, et al. High prevalence of coronary atherosclerosis in asymptomatic teenagers and young adults: evidence from intravascular ultrasound. *Circulation* 2001;103:2705–2710.

8. Stary HC, Chandler AB, Dinsmore RE, et al. Definition of advanced types of atherosclerotic lesions in a histological classification of atherosclerosis: a report from the Committee on Vascular Lesions of the Council on Arteriosclerosis, American Heart Association. *Circulation* 1995;92:1355–1374.

9. Falk E, Shah PK, Fuster V. Coronary plaque disruption. *Circulation* 1995;92:657–671.

10. Stary HC. The sequence of cell and matrix changes in atherosclerotic lesions in the first forty years of life. *Eur Heart J* 1990;11(Suppl E):3–19.

11. Sangiorgi G, Rumberger JA, Severson A, et al. Arterial calcification and not lumen stenosis is highly correlated with atherosclerotic plaque burden in humans: a histologic study of 723 coronary artery segments using non-decalcifying methodology. *J Am Coll Cardiol* 1998;31:126–133.

12. Vanhoutte PM. Endothelial dysfunction and vascular disease. In: Panza JA, Cannon RO, eds. *Endothelium, Nitric Oxide and Atherosclerosis.* New York: Futura Publishing, 1999:79–96.

13. Celermajer D, Sorensen K, Gooch V, et al. Non-invasive detection of endothelial dysfunction in children and adults at risk of atherosclerosis. *Lancet* 1992;340:1111–1115.

14. Celermajer DS, Sorensen KE, Georgakopoulous D, et al. Cigarette smoking is associated with a dose dependent and potentially reversible impairment of endothelium-dependent dilatation in healthy young adults. *Circulation* 1993;88:2149–2155.

15. Rajagopalan S, Brook R, Rubenfire M, et al. Abnormal brachial artery flow-mediated vasodilation in young adults with major depression. *Am J Cardiol* 2001;88:196–198.

16. Stein JH, Keevil JG, Wiebe DA, et al. Purple grape juice improves endothelial function and reduces the susceptibility of LDL cholesterol to oxidation in patients with coronary artery disease. *Circulation* 1999;100:1050–1055.

17. Nissen S. Coronary angiography and intravascular ultrasound. *Am J Cardiol* 2001;87:15A–20A.

18. Glagov S, Weisenberg E, Zarins CK, et al. Compensatory enlargement of human atherosclerotic coronary arteries. *N Engl J Med* 1987;317:1371–1375.

19. Schoenhagen P, Ziada KM, Vince DG, et al. Arterial remodeling and coronary artery disease: the concept of "dilated" versus "obstructive" coronary atherosclerosis. *J Am Coll Cardiol* 2001;38:297–306.

20. Furberg CD, Hennekens CH, Hully SB, et al. Task Force 2. Clinical epidemiology: the conceptual basis for interpreting risk factors. *J Am Coll Cardiol* 1996;27:976–978.

21. Grundy SM, Bazzarre T, Cleeman J, et al. Prevention V. Beyond secondary prevention: identifying the high-risk patient for primary prevention. Medical office assessment. *Circulation* 2001;101:E3–E11.

22. Hautaunen A, Toivanen P, Manttari M, et al. Joint effects of a aldosterone synthase (CYP11B2) gene polymorphism and classic risk factors on risk of myocardial infarction. *Circulation* 1999;100:2213–2218.

23. Haffner SM, Lehto S, Ronnemaa T, et al. Mortality from coronary heart disease in subjects with type 2 diabetes and in non diabetic subjects with and without prior myocardial infarction. *N Engl J Med* 1998;339:229–234.

24. Lagrand WK, Visser CA, Hermens WT, et al. C-reactive protein as a cardiovascular risk factor: more than an epi phenomenon? *Circulation* 1999;100:96–102.

25. National Cholesterol Education Program. *Second Report on the Detection, Evaluation, and Treatment of High Blood Cholesterol in Adults (Adult Treatment Panel II).* Bethesda, MD: National Institutes of Health, National Heart Lung and Blood Institute, 1993; NIH Publication No. 93-3095.

26. The sixth report of the Joint National Committee on Prevention, Detection, Evaluation, and Treatment of High Blood Pressure. *Arch Intern Med* 1997;157:2413–2446.

27. Wilson PWF, D'Agostino RB, Levy D, et al. Prediction of coronary heart disease using risk factor categories. *Circulation* 1998;97:1837–1847.

28. Gordon T, Kannel WB. Multiple risk functions for predicting coronary heart disease: the concept, accuracy, and applications. *Am Heart J* 1982;103:1031–1039.

29. D'Agostino RB, Grundy S, Sullivan LM, et al. Validation of the Framingham coronary heart disease prediction scores. Results of a multiple ethnic groups investigation. *JAMA* 2001;286:180–187.

30. Lloyd-Jones DM, Larson MG, Beiser A, et al. Lifetime risk of developing coronary heart disease. *Lancet* 1999;353:89–92.

31. Grundy SM. Primary prevention of coronary heart disease. Integrating risk assessment with intervention. *Circulation* 1999;100:988–998.

32. Greenland P, Smith S, Grundy SM. Improving coronary heart disease risk assessment in asymptomatic people. Role of traditional risk factors and noninvasive cardiovascular tests. *Circulation* 2001;104:1863–1867.

33. Executive summary of the third report of the National Cholesterol Education Program (NCEP) Expert Panel on Detection, Evaluation, and Treatment of High Blood Cholesterol in Adults (Adult Treatment Panel III). *JAMA* 2001;285:2486–2497.

34. Lamarche B, Tchernof A, Mauriege P, et al. Fasting insulin, apolipoprotein B levels, and low-density lipoprotein particle size as risk factors for ischemic heart disease. *JAMA* 1998;279:1955–1961.

35. Superko HR. Beyond LDL cholesterol reduction. *Circulation* 1996;94:2351–2354.

36. Koenig W, Sund M, Frohlich M, et al. C-reactive protein, a sensitive marker of inflammation, predicts future risk of coronary heart disease in initially healthy middle aged men: results from the MONICA (Monitoring Trends and Determinants in Cardiovascular Disease) Augsburg Cohort Study, 1984 to 1992. *Circulation* 1999;99:237–242.

37. Ridker PM. Evaluating novel cardiovascular risk factors: can we better predict heart attacks? *Ann Intern Med* 1999;130:933–937.

38. Ridker PM, Rifai N, Clearfield M, et al. Measurement of C-reactive protein for the targeting of statin therapy in the primary prevention of acute coronary events. *N Engl J Med* 2001;344:1959–1965.

39. Ridker PM, Cushman M, Stampfer MJ, et al. Inflammation, aspirin, and the risk of cardiovascular disease in apparently healthy men. *N Engl J Med* 1997;336:973–979.

40. Smith SC, Amsterdam E, Balady GJ, et al. Prevention Conference V. Beyond secondary prevention: identifying the high-risk patient for primary prevention. Tests for silent and inducible ischemia. *Circulation* 2000;101:e12–e15.

41. Gibbons LW, Mitchell TL, Wei M, et al. Maximal exercise test as a predictor of risk for mortality from coronary heart disease in asymptomatic men. *Am J Cardiol* 2000;86:53–58.

42. O'Leary DH, Polak JF, Kronmal RA, et al. For the Cardiovascular Health Study Collaborative Research Group. Carotid artery intima and medial thickness as a risk factor for myocardial infarction and stroke in older adults. *N Engl J Med* 1999;340:14–22.

43. Hodis HN, Mack WJ, LaBree L, et al. The role of carotid intima-media thickness in predicting clinical coronary events. *Ann Intern Med* 1998;128:262–269.

44. Rubenfire M, Cao N, Smith DE, et al. Usefulness of brachial artery reactivity to isometric handgrip exercise in identifying patients at risk and with coronary artery disease. *Am J Cardiol* 2000;86:1161–1165.

45. Criqui MH, Langer RD, Fronek A, et al. Mortality over a period of 10 years in patients with peripheral arterial disease. *N Engl J Med* 1992;326:381–386.

46. Arad Y, Spadaro LA, Goodman K, et al. Prediction of coronary events with electron beam computed tomography. *J Am Coll Cardiol* 200;36:1253–1260.

47. Detrano R, Hsiai T, Wang S, et al. Prognostic value of coronary calcification and angiographic stenosis in patients undergoing coronary angiography. *J Am Coll Cardiol* 1996;27:285–290.

48. O'Rourke RA, Brundage BH, Froehlicher VF, et al. American College of Cardiology/American Heart Association expert consensus document on electron-beam computed tomography for the diagnosis and prognosis of coronary artery disease. *Circulation* 2000;102:126–140.

49. Rumberger JA, Brundage BH, Rader DJ, et al. Electron beam computed tomographic coronary calcium screening: a review and guidelines in asymptomatic persons. *Mayo Clin Proc* 1999;74:243–252.

50. He Z-X, Hedrick TD, Pratt CM, et al. Severity of coronary artery calcification by electron beam computed tomography predicts silent myocardial ischemia. *Circulation* 2000;101:244–251.

51. Glantz S, Parmley WW. Passive smoking and heart disease—mechanisms and risk. *JAMA* 1995;273:1047–1053.

52. Frick MH, Elo O, Happa K, et al. Helsinki Heart Study. Primary prevention with gemfibrozil in middle age men with dyslipidemia. *N Engl J Med* 1987;317:1235–1245.

53. Shepard J, Cobbe SM, Ford I, et al. Prevention of coronary heart disease with pravastatin in men with hypercholesterolemia. *N Engl J Med* 1995;333:1301–1307.

54. The Lipid Research Clinics Coronary Primary Prevention Trial results. I. Reduction in incidence of coronary heart disease. *JAMA* 1984;251:351–364.

55. West of Scotland Study Group. Influence of pravastatin and plasma lipids on clinical events in the West of Scotland Coronary Prevention Study (WOSCOPS). *Circulation* 1998;97:1440–1445.

56. Downs JR, Clearfield M, Weis S, et al., for the AFCAPS/TexCAPS Research Group. Primary prevention of acute coronary events with lovastatin in men and women with average cholesterol levels: results of AFCAPS/TexCAPS. *JAMA* 1998;279:1615–1622.

57. Robins SJ, Collins D, Witte JT, et al. Relation of gemfibrozil treatment and lipid levels with major coronary events: VA-HIT: a randomized controlled trial. *JAMA* 2001;285:1585–1591.

58. Julius S, Jamerson K, Mehia A, et al. The association of borderline hypertension with target organ change and high coronary risk. Tecumseh Blood Pressure Study. *JAMA* 1990;264:354–358.

59. Barrett-Connor E, Orchard T. Insulin-dependent diabetes mellitus and ischemic heart disease. *Diabetes Care* 1985;8:65–70.

60. Waller BF, Palumbo PJ, Lie JT, et al. Status of the coronary arteries at necropsy in diabetes mellitus with onset after age 30 years. Analysis of 229 diabetic patients with and without clinical evidence of coronary heart disease and comparison to 183 control subjects. *Am J Med* 1980;69:498–506.

61. Grundy SM. Multifactorial causation of obesity: implications for prevention. *Am J Clin Nutr* 1998;67:563S–572S.

62. Fletcher GF, Balady G, Blair SN, et al. Statement on exercise: benefits and recommendations for physical activity for all Americans. A statement for health professionals by the committee on exercise and cardiac rehabilitation of the council on clinical cardiology, American Heart Association. *Circulation* 1996;94:857–862.

63. Kiechl S, Egger G, Mayr M, et al. Chronic infections and the risk of carotid atherosclerosis: prospective results from large population study. *Circulation* 2001;103:1064–1070.

64. Epstein SE, Zhou YF, Zhu J. Infection and atherosclerosis: emerging mechanistic paradigms. *Circulation* 1999;100:e20–e28.

65. Sanmuganathan PS, Ghahramani P, Jackson PR, et al. Aspirin for primary prevention of coronary heart disease: safety and absolute benefit related to coronary risk derived from meta-analysis of randomised trials. *Heart* 2001;85:265–271.

66. Hayden M, Pignone M, Phillips C, et al. Aspirin for the primary prevention of cardiovascular events: a summary of evidence for the US preventive services task force. *Ann Intern Med* 2002:136:161–172.

67. Mosca L, Collins P, Herrington DM, et al. Hormone replacement therapy and cardiovascular disease: statement for healthcare professionals from the American Heart Association. *Circulation* 2001:104:499–503.

68. Low-dose aspirin and vitamin E in people at cardiovascular risk: a randomised trial in general practice. Collaborative Group of the Primary Prevention Project. *Lancet* 2001:357:89–95.

69. Dietary supplementation with n-3 polyunsaturated fatty acids and vitamin E after myocardial infarction; results of the GISSI-Prevenzzione Trial. Gruppo Italiano per lo Studio della Sopravvivenza nell'Infarto miocardico. *Lancet* 1999;354:447–455.

70. Boston AG, Silbershatz H, Rosenberg IH, et al. Nonfasting plasma total homocysteine levels and all-cause and cardiovascular disease mortality in elderly Framingham men and women. *Arch Intern Med* 1999;159:1077–1080.

8

Secondary Prevention of Coronary Artery Disease

Claire Duvernoy and Melvyn Rubenfire

The secondary prevention of coronary artery disease can be defined as a long-term management strategy for patients who have sustained an acute coronary syndrome or have chronic coronary heart disease. Goals of secondary prevention include (a) long-term survival, (b) enhanced quality of life by restoring and maintaining normal activities and psychosocial function, (c) prevention of recurrent coronary events, and (d) reduction of new lesion formation and rate of coronary disease progression.

The field of cardiology in the modern era is fortunate to contain a large number of well-designed randomized clinical trials that have addressed many of the issues surrounding coronary disease management and that can serve to guide rational therapy choices. This chapter is divided into segments covering each of the strategies and major therapeutic drug classes used in secondary prevention, with specific sections on preventive cardiology services, patient subgroups (the elderly, women), diabetes, and compliance. A summary of the evidence-based secondary prevention strategies, and their potential benefit, is provided in Table 8.1.

RATIONALE FOR SECONDARY CORONARY PREVENTION

The pathogenesis of atherosclerosis includes injury to the endothelium or vessel wall and the thrombotic and inflammatory responses to that injury. The degree of injury, the development of occlusive plaque, and the characteristics of the plaque are dependent on the interaction between lifestyle factors and genetic predisposition that are collectively the *coronary risk factors* listed

in Table 8.2. Each of the major risk factors and several new risk factors have been associated with abnormal endothelial function in the absence of occlusive coronary disease, and most are risk markers for future coronary events. That the majority of known risk factors associated with acute coronary events and rate of plaque progression are modifiable is the basis for the success of medical management of coronary artery disease (CAD) known as secondary prevention.

The sentinel observations by Dr. Michael Davies in England in the mid-1980s (1) and Dr. Peter Libby in the United States 10 years later (2) provided extraordinary clarity regarding the pathobiology of acute coronary syndromes. The concept of "rupture of the vulnerable plaque" and the characteristics of the vulnerable plaque initially observed in gross and microscopic pathologic studies have been supported by innumerable studies of ST segment elevation and non–ST segment elevation myocardial infarction (MI) and unstable angina with coronary angiography, intravascular ultrasonography, and intracoronary angioscopy. The preponderance of coronary events are caused by an occlusive or mural thrombus superimposed on plaque fissuring or rupture of coronary lesions with less than 75% stenosis (Fig. 8.1). The characteristics of the vulnerable plaque include a thin fibrous cap, a large lipid pool, decrease in the ratio of smooth muscle and collagen matrix to lipid pool, and a large number of inflammatory cells capable of secreting the matrix metalloproteinases that are considered a major source of plaque instability. Davies and Thomas (1) demonstrated that a significant number of persons dying of noncardiac causes have evidence of unstable and even

TABLE 8.1. *Evidence-based treatment targets for secondary coronary prevention*

Intervention	Target	Potential benefit
Antiplatelet therapy	Aspirin, 160–325 mg/d; can ↓ to 81 mg/d for intolerance, or use clopidogrel, 75 mg, if ASA allergic; clopidogrel, 75 mg and ASA after acute coronary syndromes; carry ASA and chew and swallow in possible acute event	25% reduction in all vascular events with ASA Additional 20% reduction with clopidogrel and ASA in acute coronary syndromes
Antithrombotic therapy	Oral anticoagulation with warfarin for 3–6 months for large anterior MI or significant LV dysfunction	Reduced mural thrombi and emboli, including strokes
Beta-adrenergic blockers	Continue beta-adrenergic blocker therapy for at least 1 year and indefinitely with impaired LV function and higher risk subsets; BP < 135/80 mm HG	Reduction of 20% for risk of death, 25% for reinfarction, and 30% for sudden death
ACEI	Use ACEI indefinitely in CAD, diabetes, and vascular disease and titrate to tolerance; BP < 135/80 mm HG	25%–30% reduction in coronary deaths, recurrent MI, sudden death, CABG
Lipid therapy	AHA Step II diet/exercise; initially target LDL-C to <100 mg/dL with a statin, then non–HDL-C to <130 mg/dL with statin combined with niacin or fibrates if necessary, and attempt to increase HDL-C to >45 mg/dL with niacin or fibrates	>25% reduction in mortality and other end points with statins when LDL-C > 100 mg/dL; 22% reduction in death or nonfatal MI with fibrates with HDL-C < 35 mg/dL
Diabetes	Near normal fasting blood glucose and HbA$_{1c}$ to <7% with diet and drug therapy; consider metformin and glitazones; BP < 130/80 mm HG	Decrease in microvascular and macrovascular complications
Folate	Folic acid supplementation (400 μg) for patients with homocysteine > 10 μmol/L; may require 2–10 mg	No evidence, but cost is minimal
Fish oil	Diet high in cold-water fish (twice per week) or up to 1,000 mg of omega-3 fatty acids	Over 20% reduction in mortality and sudden death
Calcium channel blockers	Consider diltiazem in non–ST elevation MI, diltiazem, or verapamil in hypertensives unable to tolerate beta-adrenergic blockers or those needing additional antianginal therapy	No survival benefit
Nitrates	Oral nitrate as adjunctive therapy for angina or CHF; all patients carry 0.4 mg sublingual nitrate for angina and possible acute coronary event	No evidence of survival benefit
Hormone replacement therapy	No current recommendations to initiate for coronary prevention	None
Smoking cessation	Emphasize stepped approach; prescribe nicotine replacement and/or buproprion if necessary	25%–50% reduction in coronary mortality within 1 to 2 years
Rehabilitation and stress management	Refer to cardiac rehabilitation program; exercise ≥20–30 minutes at least 3 days/week, upper body strength training, education, stress management	25% reduction in recurrent coronary events
Weight/dietary targets	Target to desirable BMI of 18.5–24.9 kg/m^2 with decrease in gut fat, AHA step II diet; limit salt to 5–6 g; consider Mediterranean diet; encourage nutrition consultation	Facilitated lipid and BP control, reduced progression of CAD, can reduce mortality up to 25%

ACEI, angiotensin converting enzyme inhibitor; AHA, American Heart Association; ASA, aspirin; BMI, body mass index; BP, blood pressure; CABG, coronary artery bypass graft; CAD, coronary artery disease; CVE, cardiovascular event; HbA$_{1c}$, hemoglobin A$_{1c}$; HDL-C, high-density lipoprotein cholesterol; LDL-C, low-density lipoprotein cholesterol; LV, left ventricular; MI, myocardial infarction.

TABLE 8.2. *Risk factors and risk markers for coronary and noncoronary atherosclerosis*

Classic risk factors	Novel and candidate risk factors/markers
Nonmodifiable	Apo B100
Age	Low apo A-1
Gender	Lipoprotein (a)
Family history of premature CAD	Small LDL particle size
	Insulin
Menopause	Insulin resistance
Low socioeconomic status	Triglycerides
Less educated	Homocysteine
Modifiable	Antioxidant status
Hypertension	Chronic infection
Diabetes	Dental hygiene
Total cholesterol	C-reactive protein
LDL cholesterol	PAI-1
IDL cholesterol	Activated factor VII
Low HDL cholesterol	Fibrinogen
ECG LVH	White blood cell count
Smoking	
Sedentary lifestyle	
Obesity	
Personality traits: hostility	
Stress, depression, anxiety	

CAD, coronary artery disease; ECG, electrocardiogram; HDL, high density lipoprotein; IDL, intermediate density lipoprotein; LDL, low density lipoprotein; LVH, left ventricular hypertrophy; PAI-1, plasminogen activator inhibitor-1.

ruptured plaque. The probability of a clinical event depends on the total plaque burden and the individual response to plaque instability. Each of the evidence-based secondary prevention strategies is designed to reduce thrombosis and en-

hance thrombolysis, decrease plaque growth, and increase plaque stability.

CLINICAL RISK STRATIFICATION

The risk factors associated with coronary disease (Table 8.2) are important predictors of long-term prognosis in established coronary disease. The major risks include increasing age, smoking, hypertension, diabetes, total cholesterol, low-density lipoprotein cholesterol (LDL-C), and high-density lipoprotein cholesterol (HDL-C). The 2-year risk of a major coronary event, stroke, or cardiovascular disease–related death in men and women with established CAD can be estimated from gender-specific tables developed by Califf et al. (3) (Table 8.3 for men, Table 8.4 for women). The average risk of a recurrent event in a 55-year-old man is about 6% annually but can be reduced to less than 2% through excellent control of modifiable risk factors. Although the exact score and probability of event by percentage should be used with caution, the information is of value when the cost benefit of each treatment is considered. In addition, the awareness of an estimate of overall risk, the risk attributable to each variable, and the knowledge that interventions are available for improving each variable (with the exception of age) can be used to motivate even the most recalcitrant patient in the office setting.

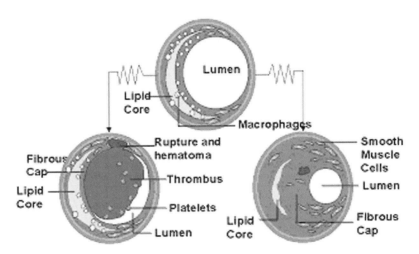

FIG. 8.1. Pathophysiology of plaque rupture.

TABLE 8.3. *Risk of recurrent event in patients with existing coronary artery disease: men*

Age (yr)	Points	Total cholesterol (mg/dL)	Points by HDL-C (mg/dL)									SBP (mm HG)	Points
			25	30	35	40	45	50	60	70	80		
35	0	160	6	5	4	4	3	2	1	1	0	100	0
40	1	170	6	5	5	4	3	3	2	1	0	110	1
45	1	180	7	6	5	4	4	3	2	1	1	120	1
50	2	190	7	6	5	4	4	3	2	2	1	130	2
55	2	200	7	6	5	5	4	4	3	2	1	140	2
60	3	210	7	6	6	5	4	4	3	2	1	150	3
65	3	220	8	7	6	5	5	4	3	2	2	160	3
70	4	230	8	7	6	5	5	4	3	3	2	170	4
75	4	240	8	7	6	6	5	4	4	3	2	180	4
		250	8	7	6	6	5	5	4	3	2	190	4
		260	8	7	7	6	5	5	4	3	2	200	5
		270	9	8	7	6	6	5	4	3	3	210	5
Other	Pts	280	9	8	7	6	6	5	4	4	3	220	5
Diabetes	1	290	9	8	7	7	6	5	4	4	3	230	6
		300	9	8	7	7	6	6	5	4	3	240	6
												250	6

Total points	2-yr Probability (%)	Average 2-yr risk in men with CVD	
		Age (yr)	Probability (%)
0	2	35–39	<1
2	2	40–44	8
4	3	45–49	10
6	5	50–54	11
8	7	55–59	12
10	10	60–64	12
12	14	65–69	14
14	20	70–74	14
16	28		
18	37		
20	49		
22	63		
24	77		

CVD, cerebrovascular disease; HDL-C, high-density lipoprotein cholesterol; SBP, systolic blood pressure.
From Antiplatelet Trialists Collaboration. Collaborative overview of randomised trials of antiplatelet therapy—1: prevention of death, myocardial infarction, and stroke by prolonged antiplatelet therapy in various categories of patients. *BMJ* 1994;308:81–106.

EVIDENCE-BASED SECONDARY PREVENTION STRATEGIES

Antiplatelet Agents

The risk of acute coronary syndromes is increased with increasing levels of fibrinogen, platelet count and aggregation, plasminogen activator inhibitor–1, and tissue plasminogen antigen and is inversely related to plasminogen activator activity. It is therefore not surprising that there is a strong, consistent reduction in MI and stroke risk with aspirin intake in CAD. Aspirin, a cyclooxygenase inhibitor, is irreversibly bound to platelets and blocks the formation of platelet thromboxane A_2, the potent stimulus for platelet aggregation. Aspirin also blocks vascular endothelium prostacyclin synthesis, but this effect is reversible. The use of low-dosage aspirin and its relatively short half-life tip the balance in favor of the vasodilating and antiplatelet properties of prostacyclin.

Among several risk categories of patients— including those with a history of acute MI or prior MI, stroke or transient ischemic attack, unstable angina, and chronic coronary disease—there was an approximate 25% risk reduction in "vascular events" (nonfatal MI, nonfatal stroke, or vascular death) in a review of trials comparing antiplatelet therapy with placebo (4). No significant increase

TABLE 8.4. *Risk of recurrent event in patients with existing coronary artery disease: women*

Age (yr)	Points	Total cholesterol (mg/dL)	Points by HDL-C (mg/dL)									SBP (mm HG)	Points
			25	30	35	40	45	50	60	70	80		
35	0	160	4	3	3	2	2	1	1	0	0	100	0
40	1	170	4	3	3	2	2	2	1	1	0	110	0
45	2	180	4	3	3	2	2	2	1	1	0	120	1
50	3	190	4	4	3	3	2	2	1	1	1	130	1
55	4	200	4	4	3	3	2	2	2	1	1	140	2
60	5	210	4	4	3	3	3	2	2	1	1	150	2
65	6	220	5	4	4	3	3	2	2	1	1	160	2
70	7	230	5	4	4	3	3	3	2	2	1	170	3
75	7	240	5	4	4	3	3	3	2	2	1	180	3
		250	5	4	4	4	3	3	2	2	1	190	3
		260	5	5	4	4	3	3	2	2	1	200	3
		270	5	5	4	4	3	3	2	2	2	210	4
Other	Pts	280	5	5	4	4	3	3	3	2	2	220	4
Diabetes	3	290	5	5	4	4	4	3	3	2	2	230	4
Smoking	3	300	6	5	4	4	4	3	3	2	2	240	4
												250	4

		Average 2-yr risk in women with CVD	
Total points	2-yr Probability (%)	Age (yr)	Probability (%)
0	0	35–39	<1
2	1	40–44	<1
4	1	45–49	<1
6	1	50–54	4
8	2	55–59	6
10	4	60–64	8
12	6	65–69	12
14	10	70–74	12
16	15		
18	23		
20	35		
22	51		
24	68		
26	85		

CVD, cerebrovascular disease; HDL-C, high-density lipoprotein cholesterol; SPB, systolic blood pressure.
From Antiplatelet Trialists Collaboration. Collaborative overview of randomised trials of antiplatelet therapy—1: prevention of death, myocardial infarction, and stroke by prolonged antiplatelet therapy in various categories of patients. *BMJ* 1994;308:81–106.

in benefit was shown for the combination of aspirin plus dipyridamole, when compared with aspirin alone (4).

Aspirin therapy is one of the most intensively studied and well-accepted strategies for the prevention of recurrent cardiovascular events. The usual recommendation for long-term aspirin therapy has been 160 to 325 mg daily. However, there is benefit for aspirin therapy in dosages as low as 75 mg daily. For long-term preventive use, low-dosage aspirin therapy (81 mg) is probably as effective as the standard dosages (160 and 325 mg). Enteric coating and lower dosages may reduce the risk of peptic symptoms, gastritis, peptic ulcers, and gastrointestinal bleeding. A valuable but often overlooked recommendation in the event of symptoms of MI is chewing a 325-mg aspirin tablet, which can be easily carried as four "baby" aspirin or one or two aspirin tablets in a packet.

An effective alternative to aspirin is clopidogrel, a thienopyridine derivative that binds to and blocks the adenosine diphosphate receptor on platelets. It is related to ticlopidine, another thienopyridine, which has a serious adverse effect—bone marrow suppression—that has limited its widespread use. Clopidogrel has gained widespread use because of its equivalent efficacy and more favorable side effect profile. The Clopidogrel versus Aspirin in Patients at Risk of Ischemic Events (CAPRIE) trial compared clopidogrel with aspirin in more than 19,000 patients with known vascular disease (cerebral, cardiovascular, or peripheral) and found an overall risk reduction of 8.7% in favor of clopidogrel in the reduction of the composite outcome stroke, MI, and vascular death. The major benefit occurred in patients with peripheral arterial disease, whereas patients with prior stroke and those with prior MI had negligible decreases in risk (5).

The Clopidogrel in Unstable Angina to Prevent Recurrent Events (CURE) trial showed additive benefit for clopidogrel with aspirin in over 12,500 patients with acute coronary syndromes, with a relative risk of 0.80 (range, 0.72 to 0.89) in comparison with placebo (6). Although the current American College of Cardiology/American Heart Association (ACC/AHA) guidelines (7,8) include no recommendations for antiplatelet therapy other than aspirin for long-term use, the data regarding the combination of aspirin and clopidogrel during the year after an acute coronary syndrome are compelling.

Anticoagulants

Long-term anticoagulation after acute MI is generally limited to a subset of patients at high risk for embolic events. Patients with atrial fibrillation after MI, whether paroxysmal or chronic, should be treated with warfarin to reduce the risk of embolic events. Patients with identifiable left ventricular (LV) thrombus or LV aneurysm after MI should receive oral anticoagulation for at least 3 to 6 months in order to prevent systemic embolization; treatment of other patients after MI remains controversial. Studies comparing anticoagulation with placebo have shown significant reductions in total mortality, reinfarction, and cerebrovascular events (9). One metaanalysis (10), performed to address the efficacy of combination anticoagulant/antiplatelet therapy, found no apparent benefit in the combination of low-intensity oral anticoagulation (target international normalized ratio, less than 1.5) with aspirin, whereas promise was shown by combination therapy involving moderate- and high-intensity anticoagulant therapy with aspirin. Large-scale studies

comparing anticoagulant with antiplatelet therapy have not yet been completed. To address this question, one such study, Warfarin and Antiplatelet Therapy in Chronic Heart Failure (WATCH), includes therapy with clopidogrel as one of three study arms (the others being aspirin and warfarin).

β-Adrenergic Blockers

There is strong evidence that treatment with beta-blocking agents after MI is beneficial in reducing rates of subsequent mortality, recurrent MI, and sudden death in all subsets. Treatment appears to be most efficacious in patients at highest risk (11), and benefits are similar in men and women. One of the first trials to systematically address the question was the Beta-blocker Heart Attack Trial (B-HAT), which compared the nonselective beta blocker propranolol to placebo after an acute MI. Significant risk reductions were seen in rates of total mortality, cardiovascular mortality, and sudden death (12). The majority of benefit was seen in smokers, those who had sustained an anterior MI, and those with impaired LV function. In years past, patients with significant LV dysfunction were generally excluded from receiving beta-blocker therapy because of concern that these agents would increase symptomatic heart failure. However, more recent trials have clearly demonstrated efficacy for several agents, including carvedilol, a nonselective beta blocker with some alpha$_1$ blocker effects, and metoprolol, a cardioselective beta blocker, in patients with both ischemic and nonischemic cardiomyopathy.

Beta-adrenergic blockade counteracts the adverse effects of neuroendocrine stimulation on the myocardium, reduces arrhythmic events, and improves LV function. Trials of beta-adrenergic blockers have consistently shown their benefit in patients with congestive heart failure (CHF) and LV dysfunction, which is additive to benefits seen with angiotensin-converting enzyme (ACE) inhibition.

Thus, long-term beta-adrenergic blockade is indicated for all patients after MI; the greatest benefit is seen in patients most at risk, including those with a history of CHF, decreased LV ejection fraction, hypertension, angina, and silent ischemia. In the Cooperative Cardiovascular

Project, a program designed to assess the benefits of beta blockers after MI in the Medicare population, use of beta blockers was associated with a 40% improvement in survival rates. The benefit did not vary with beta$_1$ selectivity or lipophilicity and was at least of equal value in patients with diabetes, chronic obstructive pulmonary disease, a history of CHF, and non–Q wave MI (13).

The benefit of prophylactic beta-blocker therapy in low-risk men and women (Table 8.1), particularly those without documented ischemia and hypertension, and after successful percutaneous or surgical coronary revascularization is not established. In consideration of the demonstrated benefits after MI, beta blockers should be used to manage symptomatic as well as silent ischemia (see later discussion), to control rhythm, and to control blood pressure.

Angiotensin-Converting Enzyme Inhibitors

Activation of the renin-angiotensin system clearly plays a role in increasing cardiovascular events in patients at risk. ACE inhibitors provide very effective therapy for hypertension and are the cornerstone of therapy for patients with CHF, in whom they have conclusively been shown to save lives, reduce the incidence of sudden death, and prevent the development of CHF in asymptomatic or mildly symptomatic persons with impaired LV systolic function (14, 15). ACE inhibitors act to interfere with LV remodeling and thereby limit LV cavity dilatation after MI. As in the beta blocker trials, some studies have suggested that the patients deriving the greatest benefit are those found to be at highest risk.

The use of ACE inhibitors in secondary prevention of cardiovascular events was limited to patients who had sustained a recent MI, those with CHF, and those with hypertension until the publication of the results of the Heart Outcomes Prevention Evaluation (HOPE) trial. This trial randomly assigned patients at high risk (those with known coronary, peripheral, or cerebral vascular disease and those with diabetes and one other cardiac risk factor) to receive ramipril or placebo; a significant reduction in cardiovascular as well as all-cause mortality, MI, CHF, and revascularization procedures was found with ramipril (16). These findings had

the dramatic implication that all patients with a history of cardiovascular disease could potentially benefit from ACE inhibition. Diabetic patients were found to derive additional benefit, because of a significant reduction in the incidence of nephropathy. Furthermore, there was a decrease in the development of type II diabetes with ramipril, which suggested an improvement in insulin sensitivity.

It is not clear that the benefits attributable to ramipril, an ACE inhibitor with high tissue selectivity titrated to 10 mg or tolerance in the HOPE trial, are a class effect of all ACE inhibitors. Tissue selectivity may be an advantage for ACE inhibitors, used specifically to reduce coronary events associated with plaque instability. As previously described, the vulnerable plaque contains a higher concentration of lymphocytes, macrophages, and proinflammatory cytokines. High dosages of non–tissue-selective ACE inhibitor can reduce proinflammatory cytokines, but until the effective and safe dosage for secondary prevention in atherosclerosis is identified in patients without hypertension and with normal LV function, it is reasonable to favor ramipril (17).

Although the benefit of ACE inhibition for treatment and prevention of CHF and LV systolic dysfunction is a class effect, dosage titration of these agents is important, inasmuch as all trials showing mortality benefit used moderate to high dosages of the drugs. This question was addressed specifically in a study comparing low-dosage (2.5 to 5 mg) with high-dosage (32.5 to 35 mg) lisinopril in patients with chronic CHF (18). The authors found significantly lower rates of mortality and hospitalizations for cardiovascular and other reasons in the high-dosage recipients and concluded that ACE inhibitor therapy should be pushed to the highest tolerated doses in most patients in whom it is initiated.

Blood Pressure Control

Hypertension in men and women with CAD is a major risk factor for death, MI, CHF, and stroke. Both CAD and hypertensive heart disease contribute to systolic and diastolic dysfunction and together markedly increase the risk of coronary events and CHF. Hypertension is associated with abnormal endothelial function, increased LV mass, and abnormal vasodilator reserve of intramyocardial resistance vessels. The twofold relative risk of death after MI in association with a blood pressure exceeding 160/95 mm HG approximates that of a cholesterol level of 200 versus 240 mg per deciliter (19). The risk of a coronary event increases by about 50% in men and women with CAD and a systolic blood pressure of 170 to 180 versus 110 to 120 mm HG (Tables 8.3 and 8.4).

The approach to hypertension in CAD, especially after MI, should follow the guidelines for post-MI management. Beta blockade and ACE inhibitor tolerance dosages are standard care in both nonhypertensive and hypertensive patients. The optimal blood pressure target is still not clear but is probably lower than the oft-quoted 140/90 mm HG, provided that renal function is adequate. The Hypertension Optimal Treatment (HOT) trial, designed to determine best blood pressure targets, included more than 3,000 men and women up to 80 years old with a previous MI or documented CAD. The maximal reduction in cardiovascular events occurred at 130 to 135 mm HG systolic and 80 to 85 mm HG diastolic pressures (20). Unfortunately, the study was not powered to determine whether there was an increased rate of mortality with lower blood pressure (J-shaped curve).

Lipid Management

The National Cholesterol Education Guidelines, the most recent being the Adult Treatment Panel III (ATP-III) published in 2001, emphasize the value of optimizing serum lipids (21) For established CAD, 3-hydroxy-3-methylglutaryl coenzyme A (HMG Co-A) reductase inhibitor (statin) therapy is one of the few long-term medical treatments that reduces the cost of each year of life saved. Through inhibition of HMG-CoA reductase, the rate-limiting enzyme of endogenous cholesterol synthesis, statins have the ability to reduce plasma LDL-C levels by 20% to 60%. That translates to a 25% to 50% reduction in coronary events and death. The Scandinavian Simvastatin Survival Study (4S), a comparison of simvastatin with placebo in 4,444 patients with angina or previous MI, conclusively demonstrated that treatment targeted to reduce total cholesterol levels to less than 200 mg per deciliter but greater than 116 mg per deciliter resulted in a 30% reduction ($p = 0.0003$) in all-cause mortality (22). Indeed, all cardiovascular events were favorably affected in the 5.4-year trial. In both the Cholesterol and Recurrent Events (CARE) study and the Long-term Intervention with Pravastatin in Ischemic Disease (LIPID) study, treatment with 40 mg of pravastatin per day was associated with impressive reductions in coronary heart disease events in men and women with heart disease and average LDL-C levels (23,24).

Statin therapy has other benefits in addition to lowering total cholesterol and LDL-C, which may help explain the strong and consistent reductions in mortality and MI. Improvement in endothelium-dependent coronary vasoreactivity has been documented and is postulated to lead to stabilization of the atherosclerotic plaque. Furthermore, statins have been shown to lower levels of C-reactive protein, an inflammatory marker that confers additive risk for cardiovascular events when levels are elevated.

Results from the Heart Protection Study (HPS) have helped to further delineate optimal treatment strategies for statin therapy. Significant benefit in favor of therapy with simvastatin was shown in this trial of more than 20,000 patients with stable atheroscerotic disease, regardless of baseline LDL-C level. Reductions were seen in all-cause mortality, cardiovascular events, and stroke (25). Substantial benefit was shown in the reduction of stroke and MI in diabetic patients without prior vascular disease. One inference from these findings is that "lower is better" (for LDL-C) and that all patients with coronary disease should be treated with high-dose statins to very low levels. Another consideration is that there is a major role for the non–lipid-lowering value of the statin class of drugs, and some researchers therefore argue for simply treating all patients with high-dose statins without necessarily treating to target level.

The majority of persons with CAD have a relatively normal LDL-C level. The most common lipid phenotype is a mild elevation of triglyceride level and low HDL-C level. The National Cholesterol Education Program ATP-III guidelines provides an expanded strategy for managing lipids in coronary and other vascular diseases that recognizes the importance of LDL-C, HDL-C, and the atherogenicity of triglyceride-rich very low density lipoprotein (VLDL) remnant particles (21). The first target or goal in CAD and other forms of atherosclerosis is to use a statin to reduce the LDL-C to less than 100 mg per deciliter. If the triglyceride levels exceed 200 mg per deciliter, the non-HDL cholesterol is targeted to be reduced to less than 130 mg per deciliter (non-HDL cholesterol = cholesterol − HDL-C). Because intermediate-density lipoprotein is negligible except in patients with the rare condition dysbetalipoproteinemia, non-HDL cholesterol is composed predominantly of LDL-C and VLDL-C. Figure 8.2 is a suggested algorithm for the management of lipids for secondary prevention.

Although therapy should always include dietary counseling to achieve an AHA Step 2 diet (less than 7% saturated fat, less than 200 mg of cholesterol intake per day), reality dictates that nearly all patients require pharmacologic lipid-lowering therapy. The effect of statins on plaque stability, as has been discussed, is not attributable solely to lipids. In the recent Myocardial Ischemia Reduction with Aggressive Cholesterol Lowering (MIRACL) study, atorvastatin given in the early phase of acute coronary syndromes reduced recurrent ischemic events by 25%, in comparison with placebo, in the first 16 weeks after discharge (26).

In patients with an LDL-C level less than 125 mg per deciliter who have a mild elevation of triglyceride level and/or low HDL-C level, there are several options: (a) Target the LDL-C to very low levels (60 to 80 mg per deciliter), as suggested by HPS; (b) if the triglyceride levels exceed 150 to 200 mg per deciliter and the non-HDL cholesterol level exceeds 130 mg per deciliter, treat with niacin, fibrates, or statins; and (c) if the HDL-C level is less than 35 to 40 mg per deciliter, treat with niacin or a fibrate. Many prevention enthusiasts (albeit without clinical trials) recommend optimizing each of the atherogenic plasma lipids with diet, exercise, and single or combination drug therapy as necessary: for example, LDL-C less than 70 mg per deciliter, triglyceride levels less than 100 mg per deciliter (converts to VLDL-C to less than 20 mg per deciliter), and HDL-C to more than 45 mg per deciliter.

The available drugs for treating lipids and the range of their effects are summarized in Table 8.5. The absorptive strategy for cholesterol lowering includes the bile resins, plant stanols, and synthetic absorbents, which reduce LDL-C by upregulating LDL receptor activity and can lower the total cholesterol and LDL-C in a dose-dependent manner by 5% to 15%. Each can be used as a supplement to statin therapy or as an alternative in the fewer than 1% of patients who are unable to tolerate the statins. Intensive lifestyle changes, including very low fat diets, as advocated by Dr. Dean Ornish, have shown benefit in reducing angina and even lead to modest plaque regression (27). Such interventions are extremely austere, however, and in general, only the most dedicated patients are able to adhere to such a strict regimen long term.

The evidence that raising an isolated low HDL-C level or lowering triglyceride levels with drug therapy is of benefit is limited in comparison with lowering LDL-C. A low HDL-C level does increase the risk of coronary events and mortality even in patients treated with statins. Furthermore, there is abundant evidence that the "atherogenic lipid phenotype"—the triad of small LDL particle size, low HDL-C, and increased triglyceride levels—is an important determinant of clinical events and disease progression. Both gemfibrozil and niacin, agents whose primary effects are to increase HDL-C and lower triglyceride levels, have been shown to reduce coronary event rates in CAD. Niacin was the first drug shown to reduce rates of coronary mortality in CAD, and, remarkably, the benefit persisted for 10 years after the study drug was discontinued (28). The reasons why it was not widely accepted in the United States are not entirely clear but include the annoying flush, potential for hepatic toxicity, and lack of industry support. With the introduction of new, safe, and well-tolerated sustained-release niacin products (Niaspan™, Slo-Niacin™), niacin alone and in combinations with statins Advicor™ is receiving much

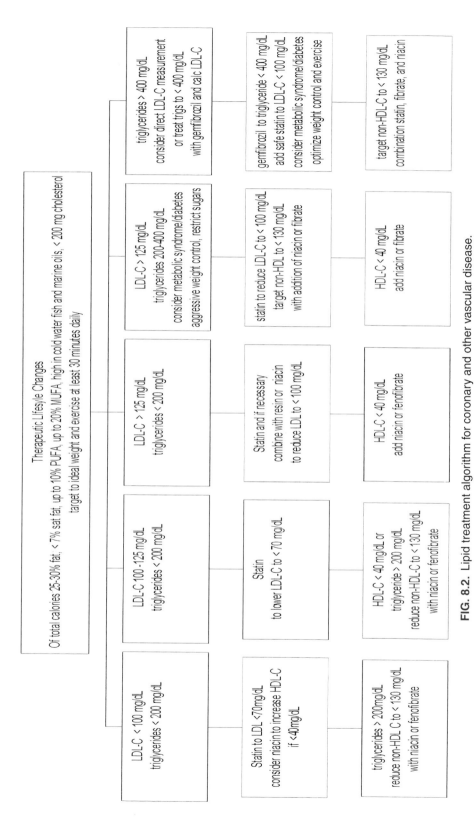

Therapeutic Lifestyle Changes
Of total calories 25-30% fat, < 7% sat fat, up to 10% PUFA, up to 20% MUFA, high in cold water fish and marine oils, < 200 mg cholesterol
target to ideal weight and exercise at least 30 minutes daily

LDL-C < 100 mg/dL
triglycerides < 200 mg/dL

Statin to LDL <70mg/dL
consider niacin to increase HDL-C
if <40mg/dL

triglycerides > 200mg/dL
reduce non-HDL C to < 130 mg/dL
with niacin or fenofibrate

LDL-C 100 - 125 mg/dL
triglycerides < 200 mg/dL

Statin
to lower LDL-C to < 70 mg/dL

HDL-C <40 mg/dL or
triglyceride > 200 mg/dL
reduce non-HDL-C to < 130 mg/dL
with niacin or fenofibrate

LDL-C > 125 mg/dL
triglycerides < 200 mg/dL

Statin and if necessary
combine with resin or niacin
to reduce LDL to < 100 mg/dL

HDL-C < 40 mg/dL
add niacin or fenofibrate

LDL-C > 125 mg/dL
triglycerides 200-400 mg/dL
consider metabolic syndrome/diabetes
aggressive weight control , restrict sugars

statin to reduce LDL-C to < 100 mg/dL
target non-HDL to < 130 mg/dL
with addition of niacin or fibrate

HDL-C < 40 mg/dL
add niacin or fibrate

triglycerides > 400 mg/dL
consider direct LDL-C measurement
or treat trigs to < 400 mg/dL
with gemfibrozil and calc LDL-C

gemfibrozil to triglyceride < 400 mg/dL
add safe statin to LDL-C < 100 mg/dL
consider metabolic syndrome/diabetes
optimize weight control and exercise

target non-HDL-C to < 130 mg/dL
combination statin, fibrate, and niacin

FIG. 8.2. Lipid treatment algorithm for coronary and other vascular disease.

TABLE 8.5. *Drugs affecting lipid metabolism*

Drug class agents, and daily doses	Lipid/lipoprotein effects	Safety and efficacy with combinations	Side effects	Contraindications
HMG-CoA reductase inhibitors (statins)[a]	LDL: ↓ 18%–55% HDL: ↑ 5%–15% TG: ↓ 7%–30%	Safe with resins and probably with nicotinic acid Do not use lovastatin or atorvastatin with fibrates	Myopathy; increased liver enzymes; monitor ALT 6–12 wk, then annually	*Absolute:* active or chronic liver disease *Relative:* with concomitant use of certain drugs,[b] reduce dose in renal disease
Bile acid sequestrants[c]	LDL: ↓15%–30% HDL: ↑ 3%–5% TG: No change or increase	Resins decrease absorption of other drugs, including warfarin and thyroid Take 1 hr before or 4 hr after; safe with nicotinic acid	Gastrointestinal distress; constipation; decreased absorption of fat-soluble vitamins	*Absolute:* dysbetalipoproteinemia; TG > 400 mg/dL *Relative:* TG > 200 mg/dL
Nicotinic acid[d]	LDL: ↓ 5%–25% HDL: ↑ 10%–35% TG: ↓ 10%–25%	Established safety with lovastatin and pravastatin Advicor: combination of niacin and lovastatin	Flushing; hyperglycemia; hyperuricemia (or gout); upper gastrointestinal distress; hepatotoxicity	*Absolute:* chronic liver disease; severe gout *Relative:* diabetes; hyperuricemia; peptic ulcer disease
Fibric acids[e]	HDL: ↑ 10%–20% TG: ↓20%–50% LDL: ↓5%–25% (may increase in patients with high TG)	Relatively safe with pravastatin and possibly simvastatin; screen with CK at 6 weeks or with any muscle ache; can be used with nicotinic acid	Dyspepsia; gallstones; myopathy; unexplained non-CHD deaths in WHO study	*Absolute:* severe renal disease; severe hepatic disease

ALT, alanine aminotransferase; CHD, coronary heart disease; CK, creatine kinase; HDL, high-density lipoprotein; HMG-CoA, 3-hydroxy-3-methylglutaryl coenzyme A; LDL, low-density lipoprotein; TG, triglycerides; WHO, World Health Organization.
[a]Lovastatin (20–80 mg), pravastatin (20–40 mg), fluvastatin (20–80 mg), atorvastatin (10–80 mg), simvastatin (10–80 mg).
[b]Cyclosporine, macrolide antibiotics, various antifungal agents, and other cytochrome P-450 inhibitors, including grapefruit juice. Pravastatin is relatively safe with other drugs as it is not metabolized via the P-450 system. Fibrates and niacin should be used with appropriate caution and monitoring of liver function.
[c]Cholestyramine (4–16 g), colestipol (5–20 g), and colesevelam (2.6–3.8 g). About 4% reduction in LDL cholesterol per initial dose equivalent.
[d]Immediate-release (crystalline) nicotinic acid (1.5–3 g), extended-release nicotinic acid (1–2 g), and sustained-release nicotinic acid (1–2 g).
[e]Gemfibrozil (600 mg twice daily), fenofibrate (160 mg daily), and clofibrate (1000 mg twice daily). Before using combinations of statins and fibrates, consider consultation with a lipid-specialist.

better acceptance. The combination of moderate doses of niacin (1,500 mg) and a statin is particularly attractive, because the combination may reduce the LDL-C by 30% to 50% and increase the HDL-C by 20% to 50%.

The recent Veterans Affairs High-Density Lipoprotein Cholesterol Intervention Trial (VA-HIT) demonstrated convincingly that treatment of an isolated low HDL-C level with gemfibrozil is effective in reducing coronary events in CAD. In VA-HIT, 2,531 men with established CAD, low HDL-C (mean, 32 mg per deciliter and all less than 40 mg per deciliter), and low LDL-C (mean, 111 mg per deciliter and all less than 140 mg per deciliter) were randomly assigned to receive gemfibrozil or placebo. By 5-year follow-up, there was a relative risk reduction of 22% in the primary endpoint of death or nonfatal MI with gemfibrozil (29). A second fibrate, fenofibrate, reduced angiographic progression of disease in type II diabetes (30). Although the study was not powered to assess clinical endpoints, there were fewer events with fenofibrate (30).

Practice guidelines for management of lipids are, by necessity, relatively simple, and parameters such as small LDL particle, apolipoprotein B, or lipoprotein (a) are not considered. Small LDL particle size is associated with an increased risk for CAD and disease progression by angiography, is commonly found in patients with diabetes and insulin resistance, and should be a direct or indirect target. The recommendation for targeting non-HDL cholesterol (to less than 130 mg per deciliter in established cardiovascular disease) when triglyceride levels exceed 200 mg per deciliter is in part derived from the recognition of the importance of LDL particle size. The LDL particle size is nearly uniformly small (phenotype B or high risk) when the triglyceride levels are over 175 mg per deciliter, when HDL-C level is less than 35 to 40 mg per deciliter, or both. Statins lower LDL-C by reducing the number of both large and small LDL particles but do not change the distribution. LDL particle distribution shifts to the less atherogenic large buoyant type as a result of therapeutic lifestyle measures, such as exercise, diet, and weight loss, that decrease triglyceride and VLDL-C levels. The benefit of exercise on lipids is frequently trivialized.

However, the combination of diet and exercise in patients with low levels of HDL-C, increased triglyceride levels, and elevated LDL-C levels is considerably more efficacious than either alone. Through treatment of the triglyceride, VLDL-C, and HDL-C levels to targets with lifestyle change and drugs such as niacin, fenofibrate, and gemfibrozil, there is a decrease in the number of small particles and a shift of overall LDL particle size to the larger and less atherogenic particles.

Antioxidants

Therapy with various antioxidants has been proposed for both primary and secondary prevention of cardiovascular events. Vitamin C, vitamin E, beta-carotene, and combinations of these have all been proposed as effective therapy to lower the rate of cardiovascular events, with benefit shown in observational studies for the vitamins (31). Randomized, placebo-controlled trials have been conducted with beta-carotene and vitamin E, with conflicting results. The Cambridge Heart Antioxidant Study (CHAOS) treated more than 2,000 patients with documented coronary atherosclerosis with vitamin E versus placebo and found a significant reduction in the incidence of nonfatal MI but no reduction in cardiovascular or all-cause mortality (32).

In contrast, in the more recent HOPE trial, there was no effect of vitamin E on survival or event rate in more than 20,000 men and women after MI or with other forms of atherosclerosis (33). The HPS, conducted in more than 20,000 patients, was also not able to demonstrate a reduction in cardiovascular events or death by treatment with a combination of vitamin E (600 mg), vitamin C (250 mg), and beta-carotene (20 mg) (25). It thus appears that, in spite of promising observational data and plausible mechanistic explanation for benefit, the antioxidant family cannot be recommended for secondary prevention of CAD.

Folic Acid

Homocysteine has been shown to be an independent risk factor for coronary and other atherosclerotic vascular diseases. The normal range (ninety-fifth percentile) is 5 to 15 μmol per liter. Although risk is continuous, a level above 10 μmol per liter is generally considered worth treating. Dietary supplementation with moderate doses of folic acid (400 μg, as available in multivitamins) lowers the homocysteine level by 3 to 4 μmol per liter, which is adequate for more than 90% of people. A combination of folic acid, pyridoxine, and oral vitamin B_{12} has been shown to improve endothelium-dependent vasodilation in human atherosclerotic disease (34). There exist no controlled studies documenting reduced clinical events through dietary supplementation with folate, but several authors have performed population analysis in order to argue for the potential to reduce cardiovascular events through dietary supplementation or through fortification of the food supply. Because supplemental intake of these vitamins is innocuous, it seems prudent to recommend this practice for secondary prevention.

Calcium Channel Blockers and Nitrates

Therapy with two additional types of medications, calcium channel blockers and oral nitrate preparations, is very widespread in the treatment of patients after MI and stable CAD despite lack of data to support any mortality benefit. Calcium channel blockers are excellent antihypertensives, and both agents are very effective as antianginal therapy in patients who remain symptomatic in spite of beta blockers. Their use should be limited to these indications, when drugs of known benefit are not adequate. In selected cases in which beta-blocking agents are not tolerated, calcium channel blockers with rate-slowing properties (e.g., verapamil and diltiazem) may be used for secondary prevention. Patients in whom such an alternative therapy is considered should have reasonable LV systolic function (35).

PREVENTIVE CARDIOLOGY SERVICES

Cardiac rehabilitation after MI, percutaneous coronary intervention, and coronary artery bypass graft is a routine component of care. Several studies have been performed to compare outcomes in patients randomly assigned to receive formal cardiac rehabilitation or usual care. Both all-cause and cardiovascular mortality rates have been reduced by cardiac rehabilitation (36). In addition to improving hard clinical endpoints, participation improves compliance with prescribed therapies, improves lipid and exercise performance, diminishes the emotional distress that often accompanies cardiac events, and improves overall quality of life. The benefits are seen in men and women of all ages, and studies have shown a particular benefit in the elderly.

All patients with coronary and other vascular disease can benefit from formal training in exercise and nutrition. Benefits can include improvement in weight, blood pressure, and glycemic control; a decrease in insulin resistance, triglyceride levels, and non-HDL cholesterol and an increase in HDL-C; reduced sympathetic tone and increased heart rate variability; and improved psychologic well-being. Exercise is associated with improved endothelial function, which promotes vasodilator reserve, and with a decrease in plasminogen activator inhibitor–1 level. Also increased is the level of tissue plasminogen activator, which promotes fibrinolysis and reduces thrombosis (37). Chronic participation in regular exercise may be the most important component of cardiac rehabilitation. In a controlled study, cardiopulmonary fitness or work capacity was the sole independent variable associated with a reduced progression of angiographic coronary disease at a 6-year follow-up. Unfortunately, there exist many barriers that lower participation of eligible patients in cardiac rehabilitation programs; only 10% to 15% of qualified patients participate, and rates for women are even lower. Physicians in the United States have traditionally been slow to refer patients to formal rehabilitation programs, and patients are unwilling or unable to participate for various reasons such as logistic or financial constraints, poor motivation, and lack of perceived benefit. Concerted efforts must be undertaken by physicians caring for post-MI patients to refer patients to these programs, facilitate enrollment and encourage compliance, and remove barriers to participation.

Cardiac rehabilitation historically encompassed a supervised exercise program and

TABLE 8.6. *Comprehensive cardiac rehabilitation or preventive cardiology services*

Standard cardiac rehabilitation: uniformly reimbursable
  Supervised exercise with ECG monitoring three times weekly for 2–12 weeks
  Series of five lectures on risk factors, diet, stress management, exercise, medication
  Prescription for home-based exercise program
  Follow-up varies from none to semiannual return visits: usually patient pays
Nutrition counseling or medical nutrition therapy: patients pay except those in managed care
  Individualized counseling for lipids, hypertension, weight control, diabetes
  Group sessions
  Interaction with behaviorist
Lipid management: consultation usually reimbursable
  Physician lipid specialist provides consultation, care, or both
  Nurse case management, short term, long term, or both
  Advanced laboratory testing
Stress management : reimbursed by some plans but not by managed care plans in general
  Psychological testing with SCL-90 or comparable measure
  Consultation and care by a psychosocial clinician
  Group therapy
  Weekly stress reduction seminars
Special programs: patients pay with the exception of those in a few managed care plans
  Yoga
  Tai chi
  Mindfulness meditation

ECG, electrocardiographic; SCL-90, Symptom Checklist-90.

education about coronary risk factors. Group exercise and education sessions have been an important component of the rehabilitation process. In many centers, cardiac rehabilitation has evolved into comprehensive Preventive Cardiology Services (Table 8.6). There is an increased emphasis on nutrition, psychosocial elements, and barriers to compliance with a long-term commitment to necessary lifestyle changes. Despite the recognized benefits 1 year after cardiac rehabilitation, participation in regular exercise and adherence to diet and stress reduction is seen in fewer than 50% of patients. For this reason, many centers have developed comprehensive medically based programs designed to assist cardiologists and primary care physicians by providing the facilities and staff to effect the necessary long-term commitment to lifestyle changes.

PSYCHOSOCIAL STATUS

Depression, anxiety, lack of social support, the general category of distress (referring to easily annoyed, feeling blue, fearful, self-conscious with others), and personality traits characterized by rage and hostility are associated with risk of fatal and nonfatal coronary disease and increasing mortality after MI. The inclusion of psychosocial interventions can provide an added benefit to what is generally referred to as cardiac rehabilitation. It is important that the cardiologist and primary care physicians are sensitive to and can identify features that are treatable by counseling or drug therapies. Also, they must value the possible contributions of psychosocial clinicians, who are capable of providing individual, group, and family counseling. Formal assessment of the psychologic profile with validated tools, and lectures on stress reduction and methods of relaxation have become part of post-MI care in many centers and are given the same consideration as diet and exercise.

MEDICAL NUTRITION

The ATP-III guidelines emphasize the importance of therapeutic life style changes, including diet, exercise, and maintenance of ideal weight (21). The AHA Step 2 diet is recommended for all forms of atherosclerotic vascular disease (21). This diet is restrictive in fat and enriched in soluble and nonsoluble carbohydrate fiber, fruits, and vegetables. The contents of the Step 2 diet and commonly accepted recommendations for other food substances are provided in Table 8.7. Considering the influence of diet on serum lipids, weight, hypertension, heart failure, and diabetes in coronary disease, *medical nutrition therapy* by qualified dietitians should be incorporated into the care paradigm.

The total number of calories should be targeted to achieving and maintaining a desirable weight; normal weight is defined as a body mass index between 18.5 and less than 25 kg per meter squared. Unfortunately, although fat intake in the United States is declining overall, total caloric intake is increasing, and obesity is currently

TABLE 8.7. *Dietary recommendations for coronary disease*

Nutrient	Sources of nutrients and effects	Practical hints
Carbohydrate (4 kcal/g)	55%–75% of total calories excluding alcohol; complex carbohydrates from fruits, whole grains, beans, reduced sugars and flours; micronutrient rich; high carbohydrates may increase triglycerides, decrease HDL-C, and worsen diabetes	25–30 g of viscous fiber from oats and beans; soluble and insoluble in fruits, vegetables; best are oat bran muffins and cereal (not wheat), multigrain breads, brown rice rather than white,
Fat Total fat (9 cal/g)	20%–30% of total calories; fats are high energy (calorie) per gram and need to be restricted for weight loss	Avoid frying, which saturates the food with fat regardless of source of oil; reduction in fat calories may decrease HDL-C
Saturated fat (SFA)	5%–7% of total calories Stearic acid from meats has less effect on LDL-C, but avoid palm and coconut oil	5–6 oz of lean meat per day; choose skim milk, yogurt, low-fat cheeses; avoid butter, cream, cheese, hydrogenated fats, cakes, cookies, crackers
Polyunsaturated fat (PUFA)	Up to 10% of total calories; lowers LDL-C if substituted for SFA but decreases HDL-C and increases LDL oxidation	
Linoleic (n-6)	Corn, safflower, soybean oils	Salad dressings, soft margarine, flaxseed, walnuts, margarine
Linolenic (n-3)	Flaxseed, canola and soybean oil, nuts	Salmon, sardines, mackerel, bluefish, tuna in water
Eicosapentanoic (n-3)	Cold-water fish; reduces platelet clumping and ventricular excitability; up to 15% of total calories	
Monounsaturated fats (MUFA)	Decrease LDL oxidation; sources are olive oil, peanut oil, canola oil, almonds, avocado	Substitute for calories from carbohydrates in diabetes and increased triglycerides; Use for salad dressing, pasta; substitute for spreads
Cholesterol	200 mg/day; all animal products	Reduce egg yolk, avoid organ meats
Protein (4 cal/g)	15%–20% of calories Meat, beans, dairy, yogurt	Chicken and fish contain about the same amount of fat; use skim milk
Alcohol (7 cal/g)	5%–7% of total calories; 4 oz of wine is equivalent in alcohol with 1.5 oz of spirits and 12 oz of beer, but calories differ. Women about $\frac{1}{2}$ the intake of men	All sources of alcohol in moderation (7–10 oz of spirits weekly) reduce CAD mortality, at least in part because of increase in HDL-C, and decrease clotting; red wines provide more antioxidants
Nuts	Almonds, walnuts, peanuts Decrease CAD risk in populations snacking on nuts	Liberal use in foods; snack on up to 1 oz daily, watching salt and calories; low-fat peanut butter
Allium	Garlic, onions, leeks; not cholesterol lowering but has antioxidant and possibly antithrombotic effects	Liberal use of garlic and onions is part of the Mediterranean diet
Phytosterols (plant sterols)	Plant sterols, beta sitosterol; have been incorporated into margarine	Sitostanol margarine (Benechol) with each meal can reduce the LDL-C by 10%–15%
Soy protein	Soy beans, soy milk, tofu with phytoestrogens and isoflavonoids (genistein); inhibits cell adhesion and proliferation	High intake of soy (25 g/day) can reduce LDL-C; good source of protein in comparison with beef
Fish oil and fish	Two or more fish servings a week (8 oz) decreases CAD mortality, particularly sudden death	Consider 1000 mg of fish oil (omega-3 PUFA) supplement if fish intake is low
Antioxidants from food sources	Food sources for antioxidants are high in MUFA, fruits and vegetables, and fortified cereals	Multivitamin with 400 μg of folic acid is fine Supplements may reduce absorption of dietary antioxidants and enhance disease progression

CAD, coronary artery disease; HDL-C, high-density lipoprotein cholesterol; LDL-C, low-density lipoprotein cholesterol.

epidemic; more than one third of American women are classified as overweight. Abdominal obesity, defined by waist circumferences exceeding 40 inches for men and 35 inches for women, is particularly ominous. Abdominal obesity confers an added cardiovascular risk, is associated with the metabolic syndrome (insulin resistance) and the emergence of diabetes, and has been linked to impaired endothelial function in the peripheral and coronary vasculature.

Although there is no direct evidence to link overall weight loss with a decrease in cardiovascular risk, there is evidence from several diet and lifestyle trials that show favorable outcomes. Ornish et al. (27) pioneered a very strict vegetarian diet, with less than 10% total calories from fat, in addition to smoking cessation, yoga, aerobic exercise, and counseling/stress reduction, and showed slowing of angiographic coronary disease as well as a reduction in clinical events at 5 years. An alternative, more appealing approach is the Mediterranean diet, which, in comparison with a Western diet, consists of fewer total calories, primarily because of fewer saturated and polyunsaturated fats. It favors higher intake of monounsaturated fats, fruits, and vegetables and increased consumption of alpha-linolenic acids (38). An impressive 72% risk reduction in the rate of cardiac death and nonfatal MI was obtained with the Mediterranean diet in the Lyon Diet Heart Study, in comparison with a prudent Western diet (38).

Other readily available food sources have potential benefit in coronary disease; these include cold-water fish, fish oil supplements, foods high in fiber, soy protein, and dietary antioxidants (Table 8.7). Several studies have documented the value of regular fish consumption and omega-3 fatty acids. A daily supplement of 850 mg of marine oil [eicosapentaenoic acid, a 3-omega polyunsaturated fatty acid (PUFA)] reduced the combined endpoint of death, nonfatal MI, and nonfatal stroke to a degree comparable with that of beta blockade and the statins. Because it will be difficult to get more convincing data, it is reasonable to suggest marine oil supplements in men and women with CAD who consume less than 8 to 10 oz of fish weekly. Flaxseed oil contains alpha-linolenic acid, which converts to omega-3

fatty acid and can be used as a supplement for people allergic to, or who for other reasons cannot eat, fish.

Recommendations for regular alcohol intake must be made with extreme caution because of the many toxic effects associated with alcohol excess, but it nonetheless appears that regular, moderate alcohol intake is associated with a reduction in the risk of cardiovascular events (39). Wine, especially red wine, appears to be particularly beneficial because of the special antioxidant properties associated with it; this may be an additional explanation for the benefits of the Mediterranean diet.

SMOKING CESSATION

Smoking cessation is the most important intervention in secondary prevention of CAD. Smoking has several direct effects on coronary risk factors and factors associated with acute events, including decreasing HDL-C; increasing blood pressure, fibrinogen, and C-reactive protein; and enhancing thrombosis and decreasing fibrinolysis. In young men and women, smoking a single cigarette induces abnormal endothelial function. Smoking can induce coronary vasospasm and significantly increases ischemic episodes and duration in patients with coronary heart disease (40). Unfortunately, smoking cessation is extremely difficult; relapse rates are 30% to 50% by 6 to 12 months (41). Table 8.8 provides a

TABLE 8.8. *Physician-assisted patient stepwise approach to smoking cessation*

1. Provide the rationale for and give an unequivocal message about quitting smoking
2. Determine whether the patient is willing to quit
3. Describe proven alternatives, and have patient choose his or her quitting method of choice
4. Describe the potential problems associated with withdrawal, and develop a plan for coping with each
5. Have the patient set a quit date and sign a contract in the medical record
6. Make sure that the patient can articulate how to cope with urges to smoke
7. Assure the patient of your support and that of your office staff
8. Follow up by telephone call or visit
9. Develop a plan for dealing with failure

stepped approach to help patients with the process of quitting.

Patients should be encouraged to participate in community-based programs with the local hospital or the American Lung Association. Use of adjunctive pharmacologic agents to aid in smoking cessation has been shown to be helpful in achieving higher quit rates, at least over the short term. Nicotine gum and patches, now available without prescription, are effective in minimizing symptoms of nicotine withdrawal. Clonidine may have some utility in selected populations (42). Short-term use of bupropion, the antidepressant, has been well studied and found to be safe and efficacious for smoking cessation. Bupropion is effective in a dose-dependent manner, can be accompanied by reduced weight gain, and has minimal side effects (43).

COMPLIANCE

The major barrier to successful coronary prevention is long-term compliance. The many negative and positive factors that affect compliance are listed in Table 8.9. The most important may be the focus of the physician and his or her explanation of coronary disease to the patient and spouse. If the patient is led to believe that coronary stenosis is the equivalent of blocked plumbing, the value of lifestyle changes and medication seems meager. In contrast, if told that with comprehensive treatment the patient can lower his or her rate of heart attack, stroke, and death, as well as the need for revascularization, the prevention message is heard.

SILENT ISCHEMIA

Despite indications that silent ischemia may be a marker of increased rates of events and mortality, there is no compelling evidence that either screening with ambulatory electrocardiographic monitoring (AmbECG) or exercise testing followed by aggressive treatment of silent ischemia is effective. The largest trial undertaken to assess the benefit of treating silent ischemia, the Asymptomatic Cardiac Ischemia Pilot (ACIP), was a National Heart, Lung, and Blood Institute–sponsored study to test the feasibility and efficacy

TABLE 8.9. *Factors affecting compliance with coronary prevention strategies*

Poor compliance
  Cost of medication and diet
  Lack of health insurance
  Lack of enthusiasm by primary care physician
  Lack of enthusiasm by cardiologist who is focused on coronary "anatomy"
  No or poorly conducted cardiac rehabilitation program
  Less than high school education
  Poor spousal or family relationships
  Poor employer support or nonunderstanding supervisor
  Depression, anxiety, distress, denial
  Unavailability of exercise equipment or community facilities
  Inability to quit smoking or other substance abuse
Good compliance
  Enthusiastic spousal support
  Regular follow-up with primary care physician and cardiologist with focus on risk factors and prevention
  Enthusiastic support of employer and or union
  Exercise facilities at work
  Some college education or more
  Previous interest in exercise
  Membership in local health clubs
  Spirituality and religiosity
  Type A personality
  Retirees
  Elderly

of three treatment strategies aimed at suppressing ischemia in patients with stable CAD (44). The strategies included (a) angina-guided drug therapy, (b) angina plus AmbECG ischemia-guided drug therapy, and (c) revascularization by either percutaneous transluminal coronary angioplasty or coronary artery bypass graft. Patients in the two medical therapy arms were treated either with atenolol plus nifedipine or with diltiazem plus isosorbide dinitrate. At 2 years, there was a nonsignificant trend toward decreased death and MI in the ischemia-guided therapy, in comparison with the angina-guided therapy. Patients randomly assigned to undergo revascularization did significantly better than patients in either medical therapy arm. In an earlier study of atenolol as monotherapy versus placebo, Pepine et al. (45) reported a significant decrease in aggravation of angina in patients treated with atenolol but no significant decrease in death, ventricular tachycardia/fibrillation, MI, or need for hospitalization. Thus, although silent ischemia as documented by

AmbECG monitoring and stress ECG appears to be a marker for worsened prognosis, the efficacy of therapy targeted specifically to eliminate or reduce silent ischemia to improve outcome remains unproven.

SECONDARY PREVENTION FOR WOMEN

Women tend to be older and to have more comorbid conditions when they present with a cardiovascular event. As a result, their prognosis after MI is worse than that for men. Proven therapies, including aspirin, beta blockers, ACE inhibitors, and lipid-lowering agents, should be aggressively utilized, just as they are for men. Effective therapy for diabetes is especially important because of the even graver prognosis that it confers on women than on men.

Hormone replacement therapy deserves special mention because of the increasing controversies surrounding its effectiveness. No benefit for secondary prevention has yet been demonstrated with hormone replacement therapy in postmenopausal women. Observational studies have consistently shown reduced rates of coronary heart disease in postmenopausal hormone users in comparison with nonusers (46).

Estrogen has multiple beneficial biologic effects in postmenopausal women, including reduction in LDL-C and increase in HDL-C levels. Estrogen restores endothelium-dependent vasodilation by increasing nitric oxide release and may also act to inhibit platelet aggregation and inflammatory cell adhesion. However, in spite of these findings, the first prospective, randomized, placebo-controlled trial to examine hormone therapy in women with preexisting CAD found a slight increase in risk for hormone-assigned study patients in the first year of the Heart and Estrogen/Progestin Replacement Study (HERS) (47). The early increase in risk was thought to result from estrogen-mediated activation in coagulation factors. At just over 4 years, there were no differences in outcomes between the treatment and placebo arms of the study. The results of HERS, as well as those of several other secondary prevention trials, led to the release of an AHA/ACC scientific statement advising against initiating hormone replacement

therapy in women with known CAD (48). Studies of estrogen alternatives such as raloxifene, a selective estrogen receptor modulator, are currently under way to determine whether these agents can modulate cardiovascular risk.

SECONDARY PREVENTION IN THE VERY ELDERLY

Only 5% of the U.S. population are octogenarians, but they account for 20% of hospital admissions and 30% of deaths due to MI (49). Nearly 50% have CAD, peripheral vascular disease, cerebral vascular disease, CHF, or other complications. There is a relative paucity of information regarding the effectiveness of standard therapies and clinical strategies, particularly in the middle-old (aged 75 to 85 years) and old-old (older than 85 years). In clinical trials that include patients up to age 75, age alone does not appear to reduce the benefit of specific therapies. However, older patients in clinical trials do not resemble those in clinical practice with regard to comorbidity. Furthermore, coronary prevention trials focus on mortality, morbidity, and cost and pay little attention to quality-of-life years of independence. Fibrocalcific lesions predominate in the elderly and are less likely to rupture, but, as in other age groups, most events result from rupture of mildly occlusive plaques. Until further studies are available, each of the secondary prevention strategies should be applied in elderly patients for whom the quality of life is satisfactory. It should be noted that compliance with smoking cessation, exercise, diet, and medication is comparable or better in the elderly if cost is not an important consideration.

SECONDARY PREVENTION IN DIABETES MELLITUS

Diabetes increases both the mortality and recurrent event rate in men and women with CAD. Each of the large secondary prevention clinical trials in CAD has had a cohort of diabetic patients. The value of cholesterol lowering with statins (22–24) and of raising HDL-C levels with fibrates (29,30), aspirin and clopidogrel (4,6), beta blockers (13), and ACE inhibitors in diabetic patients with and without LV dysfunction (16) is at least equal to or greater than that in nondiabetic patients. The added value of ACE inhibitors in diabetic patients is the reduction in the rate of progression and new onset of microscopic albuminuria, proteinuria, and renal failure.

The optimal blood pressure in diabetes with CAD is less than 130/80 mm Hg (20). ACE inhibitors and angiotensin receptor blockers effectively lower the pressure and are renal protective in diabetic patients (50). The decrease in strokes and coronary events attributable to the ACE inhibitor ramipril in the HOPE trial has not yet been shown in clinical trials of angiotensin receptor blockers. Tight blood pressure control in type II diabetes, best shown in the United Kingdom Prospective Diabetes Study (UKPDS), was less than 120 mm Hg systolic and was associated with a marked reduction in microvascular disease, strokes, and diabetes-related deaths (51). Similarly, good glycemic control is associated with a reduction in microvascular and possibly macrovascular complications (52). Although the relative value of various hypoglycemic agents is not clear, there is evidence that metformin (in comparison with insulin and sulfonylurea) may have a better effect on macrovascular disease and reduce the rate of coronary events alone and in combination with sulfonylureas (53).

The American Diabetes Association–suggested standards for metabolic parameters are as follows: fasting blood glucose level, 90 to 115 mg per deciliter; 2-hour postprandial and 4:00 to 6:00 p.m. blood glucose level, less than 140 mg per deciliter; hemoglobin A_{1c} level, less than 7%; HDL-C level, higher than 45 mg per deciliter; LDL-C level, lower than 100 mg per deciliter; and triglyceride level, lower than 200 mg per deciliter (54). The first priority in managing lipids in diabetic patients is diet and exercise to achieve ideal body weight and glycemic control to targets, followed by treatment with a relatively high-dose statin. After achieving LDL-C goal (by statin, resin, or fenofibrate), the second goal is to reduce the non-HDL cholesterol level to less than 130 mg per deciliter with the addition of niacin or gemfibrozil (not in combination with certain statins). Niacin is relatively safe and effective in lowering the triglyceride level and raising the HDL-C level in patients with type II diabetes and, contrary to previous reports, has little negative effect on glycemic control (54).

SUMMARY

The understanding of the pathobiology of coronary disease has led to many clinical trials that have helped establish an effective treatment paradigm. As with revascularization, the enthusiasm for prevention regimens must be tempered by rigorous clinical trials and cost analysis before widespread acceptance. Two examples involving such regimens are the demonstration of a lack of benefit from vitamin E and the remarkable finding that home-based nursing intervention monthly for post-MI patients was of no value in men and, in fact, had a significantly negative impact on women (55). A brief list of important questions that remain to be answered, many of which are being studied in ongoing trials, is presented in Table 8.10.

Secondary prevention in stable coronary disease and after acute coronary syndromes involves a multifaceted strategy comprising

TABLE 8.10. *Potential secondary prevention strategies requiring further study*

Combination of antioxidants, vitamin E, and vitamin C or coenzyme Q-10
Treatment of homocysteine, optimal target, and dose of B vitamins
Oral L-arginine supplement
Antibiotic therapy
Antibiotic for specific infection (*chlamydia* pneumonia)
Antiinflammatory drugs other than aspirin
Dental hygiene
Target for LDL-C (how low is low enough?)
Targeting triglycerides
Targeting VLDL-C
Targeting LDL particle size
Treating Lp (a)
Comparison of intensive medical therapy vs. revascularization in patients eligible for revascularization, for patients with AHA/ACC class II indications
Anxiolytics and antidepressants
Estrogen receptor blockers (SERMs) in postmenopausal women
Beta blockade vs. ACEI vs. combination in low-risk subsets
Optimal target blood pressure; is there a J-shaped curve?
Asian methods including yoga, tai chi, and meditation
Spirituality and religion

ACEI, angiotensin-converting enzyme inhibitors; AHA/ACC, American College of Cardiology/American Heart Association; LDL-C, low-density lipoprotein cholesterol; Lp(a), lipoprotein a; SERMs, selective estrogen receptor modulators; VLDL-C, very low density lipoprotein cholesterol.

pharmacologic therapy known to be of benefit, lifestyle and behavior modification, and continued interaction between patients and their physi- cians. Doctors must act as advocates as well as coaches for their patients in order to maintain adherence to therapeutic interventions.

PRACTICAL POINTS

- Goals of secondary coronary prevention are to increase long-term survival, improve quality of life, prevent recurrent coronary events, and reduce new lesion formation and rate of rupture.

- An understanding of the pathobiology of acute coronary syndromes forms the basis for developing treatment strategies, which can be effective for secondary prevention.

- Evidence-based strategies include pharmacologic therapy with aspirin, beta blockers, ACE inhibitors, a statin, a diet low in saturated fat and high in micronutrients, exercise, stress management, and smoking cessation.

- Treatment with a statin is a cornerstone of effective secondary prevention, because of both lipid and nonlipid effects. Lipid therapy must be individualized with targeting of HDL-C and triglyceride levels with single or carefully administered combination in selected persons.

- Preventive cardiology services, including exercise programs, psychosocial interventions, and nutrition counseling, have demonstrated benefit and are markedly underutilized in the United States.

- Smoking cessation through a stepped approach remains the most important intervention in secondary prevention of CAD.

- Hormone replacement therapy with estrogen and with or without progestins for secondary prevention in postmenopausal women is ineffective and should not be initiated for that purpose, and its discontinuation should be considered.

- Outcomes in the very elderly and in diabetic patients are worse than in the general population; for that reason, proven therapies should be implemented aggressively in these patients.

REFERENCES

1. Davies MJ, Thomas AC: Plaque fissuring the cause of acute myocardial infarction, sudden ischaemic death, and crescendo angina. *Br Heart J* 1985;53:363–373.
2. Libby P: Molecular bases of the acute coronary syndromes. *Circulation* 1995;91:2844–2850.
3. Califf RM, Armstrong PW, Carver JR, et al. 27th Bethesda Conference: matching the intensity of risk factor management with the hazard for coronary disease events. Task Force 5. Stratification of patients into high, medium and low risk subgroups for purposes of risk factor management. *J Am Coll Cardiol* 1996;27:1007–1019.
4. Antiplatelet Trialists Collaboration. Collaborative overview of randomised trials of antiplatelet therapy—I: prevention of death, myocardial infarction, and stroke by prolonged antiplatelet therapy in various categories of patients. *BMJ* 1994;308:81–106.
5. CAPRIE Steering Committee. A randomised, blinded trial of Clopidogrel versus Aspirin in Patients at Risk of Ischaemic Events (CAPRIE). *Lancet* 1996;348:1329–1339.
6. The Clopidogrel in Unstable Angina to Prevent Recurrent Events Trial Investigators. Effects of clopidogrel in addition to aspirin in patients with acute coronary syndromes without ST-segment elevation. *N Engl J Med* 2001;345:494–502.
7. Ryan TJ, Anderson JL, Antman EM, et al. ACC/AHA guidelines for the management of patients with acute myocardial infarction. A report of the American College of Cardiology/American Heart Association Task Force on Practice Guidelines (Committee on Management of Acute Myocardial Infarction). *J Am Coll Cardiol* 1996;28:1328–1428.
8. Ryan TJ, Antman EM, Brooks NH, et al. 1999 update: ACC/AHA guidelines for the management of patients with acute myocardial infarction: executive summary

and recommendations: a report of the American College of Cardiology/American Heart Association Task Force on Practice Guidelines (Committee on Management of Acute Myocardial Infarction). *Circulation* 1999;100:1016–1030.

9. Smith P, Arnesen H, Holme I. The effect of warfarin on mortality and reinfarction after myocardial infarction. *N Engl J Med* 1990;323:147–152.

10. Anand SS, Yusuf S. Oral anticoagulant therapy in patients with coronary artery disease: a meta-analysis. *JAMA* 1999;282:2058–2067.

11. Yusuf S, Peto R, Lewis J, et al. Beta blockade during and after myocardial infarction: an overview of the randomized trials. *Prog Cardiovasc Dis* 1985;27:335–371.

12. A randomized trial of propranolol in patients with acute myocardial infarction. I. Mortality results. *JAMA* 1982;247:1707–1714.

13. Gottlieb SS, McCarter RJ, Vogel RA. Effect of beta-blockade on mortality among high-risk and low-risk patients after myocardial infarction. *N Engl J Med* 1998;339:489–497.

14. The SOLVD Investigators. Effect of enalapril on mortality and the development of heart failure in asymptomatic patients with reduced left ventricular ejection fractions. *N Engl J Med* 1992;327:685–691.

15. Pfeffer MA, Braunwald E, Moye LA, et al. Effect of captopril on mortality and morbidity in patients with left ventricular dysfunction after myocardial infarction. Results of the Survival And Ventricular Enlargement trial. *N Engl J Med* 1992;327:669–677.

16. Yusuf S, Sleight P, Pogue J, et al. Effects of an angiotensin-converting-enzyme inhibitor, ramipril, on cardiovascular events in high-risk patients. *N Engl J Med* 2000;342:145–153.

17. Gullestad L, Aukrust P, Ueland T, et al. Effect of high-versus low-dose angiotensin converting enzyme inhibition on cytokine levels in chronic heart failure. *J Am Coll Cardiol* 1999;34:2061–2067.

18. Packer M, Poole-Wilson PA, Armstrong PW, et al. Comparative effects of low and high doses of the angiotensin-converting enzyme inhibitor, lisinopril, on morbidity and mortality in chronic heart failure. *Circulation* 1999;100:2312–2318.

19. Kannel WB, Sorlie P, Castelli WP, et al. Blood pressure and survival after myocardial infarction: the Framingham study. *Am.J Cardiol* 1980;45:326–330.

20. Hansson L, Zanchetti A, Carruthers SG, et al. Effects of intensive blood-pressure lowering and low-dose aspirin in patients with hypertension: principal results of the Hypertension Optimal Treatment (HOT) randomised trial. *Lancet* 1998;351:1755–1762.

21. Executive summary of the third report of the National Cholesterol Education Program (NCEP) expert panel on detection, evaluation, and treatment of high blood cholesterol in adults (Adult Treatment Panel III). *JAMA* 2001;285:2486–2497.

22. Randomised trial of cholesterol lowering in 4444 patients with coronary heart disease: the Scandinavian Simvastatin Survival Study (4S). *Lancet* 1994;344:1383–1389.

23. Sacks FM, Pfeffer MA, Moye LA, et al. The effect of pravastatin on coronary events after myocardial infarction in patients with average cholesterol levels. *N Engl J Med* 1996;335:1001–1009.

24. The Long-Term Intervention with Pravastatin in Is-

chaemic Disease (LIPID) Study Group. Prevention of cardiovascular events and death with pravastatin in patients with coronary heart disease and a broad range of initial cholesterol levels. *N Engl J Med* 1998;339:1349–1357.

25. Collins R. Heart Protection Study Collaborative Group: MRC/BHF Heart Protection Study of cholesterol lowering with simvastatin in 20,536 high-risk individuals: a randomized placebo controlled trial. *Lancet* 360(9326):7

26. Schwartz G, Olsson A, Ezekowitz M, et al. Effects of atorvastatin on early recurrent ischemic events in acute coronary syndromes. The MIRACL study. *JAMA* 2001;285:1711–1718.

27. Ornish D, Brown SE, Scherwitz LW, et al. Can lifestyle changes reverse coronary heart disease? The Lifestyle Heart Trial. *Lancet* 1990;336:129–133.

28. Canner PL, Berge KG, Wenger NK, et al. Fifteen year mortality in Coronary Drug Project patients: long-term benefit with niacin. *J Am Coll Cardiol* 1986;8:1245–1255.

29. Rubins HB, Robins SJ, Collins D, et al. Gemfibrozil for the secondary prevention of coronary heart disease in men with low levels of high-density lipoprotein cholesterol. *N Engl J Med* 1999;341:410–418.

30. Diabetes Atherosclerosis Intervention Study Investigators: Effect of fenofibrate on progression of coronary-artery disease in type 2 diabetes: the Diabetes Atherosclerosis Intervention Study, a randomised study. *Lancet* 2001;357:905–910.

31. Rimm EB, Stampfer MJ, Ascherio A, et al. Vitamin E consumption and the risk of coronary heart disease in men. *N Engl J Med* 1993;328:1450–1456.

32. Stephens NG, Parsons A, Schofield PM, et al. Randomised controlled trial of vitamin E in patients with coronary disease: Cambridge Heart Antioxidant Study (CHAOS). *Lancet* 1996;347:781–786.

33. Yusuf S, Dagenais G, Pogue J, et al. Vitamin E supplementation and cardiovascular events in high-risk patients. The Heart Outcomes Prevention Evaluation Study Investigators. *N Engl J Med* 2000;342:154–160.

34. Chambers J, Ueland P, Obeid O, et al. Improved vascular endothelial function after oral B vitamins: an effect mediated through reduced concentrations of free plasma homocysteine. *Circulation* 2000;102:2479–2483.

35. The Multicenter Diltiazem Postinfarction Trial Research Group. The effect of diltiazem on mortality and reinfarction after myocardial infarction. *N Engl J Med* 1988;319:385–392.

36. O'Connor GT, Buring JE, Yusuf S, et al. An overview of randomized trials of rehabilitation with exercise after myocardial infarction. *Circulation* 1989;80:234–244.

37. Hambrecht R, Wolf A, Gielen S, et al. Effect of exercise on coronary endothelial function in patients with coronary artery disease. *N Engl J Med* 2000;342:454–460.

38. de Lorgeril M, Salen P, Martin JL, et al. Mediterranean diet, traditional risk factors, and the rate of cardiovascular complications after myocardial infarction: final report of the Lyon Diet Heart Study. *Circulation* 1999;99:779–785.

39. Gaziano JM, Buring JE, Breslow JL, et al. Moderate alcohol intake, increased levels of high-density lipoprotein and its subfractions, and decreased risk of myocardial infarction. *N Engl J Med* 1993;329:1829–1834.

40. Barry J, Mead K, Nabel EG, et al. Effect of smoking

on the activity of ischemic heart disease. *JAMA* 1989;261:398–402.

41. Burling TA, Singleton EG, Bigelow GE, et al. Smoking following myocardial infarction: a critical review of the literature. *Health Psychol* 1984;3:83–96.

42. Covey LS, Glassman AH: A meta-analysis of double-blind placebo-controlled trials of clonidine for smoking cessation. *Br J Addict* 1991;86:991–998.

43. Hurt RD, Sachs DP, Glover ED, et al. A comparison of sustained-release bupropion and placebo for smoking cessation. *N Engl J Med* 1997;337:1195–1202.

44. Davies RF, Goldberg AD, Forman S, et al. Asymptomatic Cardiac Ischemia Pilot (ACIP) study two-year follow-up: outcomes of patients randomized to initial strategies of medical therapy versus revascularization. *Circulation* 1997;95:2037–2043.

45. Pepine CJ, Cohn PF, Deedwania PC, et al. Effects of treatment on outcome in mildly symptomatic patients with ischemia during daily life. The Atenolol Silent Ischemia Study (ASIST). *Circulation* 1994;90:762–768.

46. Barrett-Connor E, Grady D. Hormone replacement therapy, heart disease, and other considerations. *Annu Rev Public Health* 1998;19:55–72.

47. Hulley S, Grady D, Bush T, et al. Randomized trial of estrogen plus progestin for secondary prevention of coronary heart disease in postmenopausal women. *JAMA* 1998;280:605–613.

48. Mosca L, Collins P, Herrington DM, et al. Hormone replacement therapy and cardiovascular disease: a statement for healthcare professionals from the American Heart Association. *Circulation* 2001; 104:499–503.

49. Wenger NK. Preventive cardiology—its applicability at elderly age. *Am J Geriatr Cardiol* 2001;10:76.

50. Lewis EJ, Hunsicker LG, Clarke WR, et al. Renoprotective effect of the angiotensin-receptor antagonist irbesartan in patients with nephropathy due to type 2 diabetes. *N Engl J Med* 2001;345:851–860.

51. Adler AI, Stratton IM, Neil HA, et al. Association of systolic blood pressure with macrovascular and microvascular complications of type 2 diabetes (UKPDS 36): prospective observational study. *BMJ* 2000;321:412–419.

52. Stratton IM, Adler AI, Neil HA, et al. Association of glycaemia with macrovascular and microvascular complications of type 2 diabetes (UKPDS 35): prospective observational study. *BMJ* 2000;321:405–412.

53. Fisman EZ, Tenenbaum A, Boyko V, et al. Oral antidiabetic treatment in patients with coronary disease: time-related increased mortality on combined glyburide/metformin therapy over a 7.7-year follow-up. *Clin Cardiol* 2001;24:151–158.

54. American Diabetes Association. Clinical practice recommendations 2000. *Diabetes Care* 2000;23(Suppl 1):S1–S116.

55. Frasure-Smith N, Lesperance F, Prince RH, et al. Randomised trial of home-based psychosocial nursing intervention for patients recovering from myocardial infarction. *Lancet* 1997;350:473–479.

9

Stable Angina

Steven W. Werns

USUAL CAUSES

The most common cause of typical angina pectoris is atherosclerotic coronary artery disease (CAD). Other, less common causes include coronary spasm, Kawasaki's disease, microvascular angina, and aortic stenosis.

PRESENTING SYMPTOMS AND SIGNS

The definition of typical angina pectoris has three components: (a) substernal chest discomfort with a characteristic quality and duration that is (b) provoked by exertion or emotional stress and (c) relieved by rest or nitroglycerin (NTG). Atypical angina meets two of the three criteria, and noncardiac chest pain meets one or none of the criteria.

Typical angina pectoris is characterized as a feeling of constricting, squeezing, burning, or heaviness. The location of the discomfort may be substernal or interscapular, and it may radiate to the neck, jaw, shoulders, or arms. The typical duration of discomfort is 2 to 10 minutes. Discomfort that lasts less than 15 seconds is unlikely to be angina. Pain that lasts longer than 10 minutes may be indicative of unstable angina, myocardial infarction (MI), or noncardiac chest pain. Some patients may have dyspnea as an anginal equivalent. Typical angina may be provoked by physical exertion, emotional stress, cold weather, or meals. The Canadian Cardiovascular Society Classification System (CCS) is employed to grade angina pectoris (Table 9.1)(1).

The physical examination findings are usually normal in patients with stable angina caused by chronic CAD. Patients with angina due to aortic stenosis or hypertrophic cardiomyopathy have a characteristic systolic murmur. A systolic murmur also may be audible in patients with mitral regurgitation caused by papillary muscle dysfunction.

HELPFUL TESTS

American College of Cardiology/American Heart Association Guideline Classification:

The American College of Cardiology/American Heart Association (ACC/AHA) and the American College of Physicians–American Society of Internal Medicine (ACP-ASIM) jointly published guidelines for the management of patients with chronic stable angina in 1999 (1). Diagnostic and therapeutic recommendations are categorized as Class I, II, or III. In Class I conditions, there is evidence or general agreement that a given procedure or treatment is useful and effective. In Class II conditions, there is conflicting evidence or a divergence of opinion about the usefulness or efficacy of a procedure or treatment. For Class IIa, the weight of evidence or opinion is in favor of usefulness or efficacy, and for Class IIb, the usefulness or efficacy is less well established by evidence or opinion. In Class III conditions, there is evidence or general agreement, or both, that the procedure or treatment is not useful or effective and in some cases may be harmful.

The recommended indications for noninvasive testing and coronary angiography fall into two categories: to establish a diagnosis in patients with suspected angina and to risk-stratify patients with chronic stable angina. Left ventricular (LV) function, the presence of inducible ischemia (Table 9.2), and the anatomic extent and severity of CAD are key predictors of long-term survival of patients with chronic stable angina, and they influence decisions regarding revascularization. Left ventricular ejection fraction (LVEF) may be

TABLE 9.1. *Grading of angina pectoris by the Canadian Cardiovascular Society Classification system*

Class I
  Ordinary physical activity, such as walking or climbing stairs, does not cause angina
  Angina (occurs) with strenuous, rapid, or prolonged exertion at work or recreation
Class II
  Slight limitation of ordinary activity; angina occurs on walking or climbing stairs rapidly, walking uphill, walking or stair climbing after meals, in cold, in wind, under emotional stress, or only during the few hours after awakening;
  Angina occurs on walking more than two blocks on the level and climbing more than one flight of ordinary stairs at a normal pace and in normal condition
Class III
  Marked limitations of ordinary physical activity; angina occurs on walking one to two blocks on the level and climbing one flight of stairs in normal conditions and at a normal pace
Class IV
  Inability to carry on any physical activity without discomfort; anginal symptoms may be present at rest

assessed noninvasively by echocardiography or radionuclide techniques or by contrast-enhanced ventriculography during cardiac catheterization. Exercise testing provides additional prognostic information. For example, a low Duke treadmill score, which combines parameters reflecting exercise capacity and ischemia, is predictive of 4-year survival in 99% of patients tested (1). The guidelines recommend the inclusion of either an echocardiographic or radionuclide imaging technique in patients with resting ST segment depression, left bundle branch block, ventricular paced rhythm, or preexcitation and those receiv-

TABLE 9.2. *Noninvasive risk stratification*

High risk (>3% annual mortality)
  Resting or exercise LVEF <35%
  Duke treadmill score ≤−11
  Large or multiple stress-induced perfusion defects
  Stress-induced LV dilation or increased lung uptake of thallium 201
  Echocardiographic evidence of ischemia involving more than two segments at HR <120 or dobutamine infusion ≤10 μg/kg/min
Intermediate risk (1%–3% annual mortality)
  LVEF 35%–49%
  Duke treadmill score < 5 and > −11
  Moderate stress-induced perfusion defect without LV dilation or increased lung uptake of thallium 201
  Echocardiographic evidence of ischemia involving two or fewer segments at dobutamine infusion >10 μg/kg/min
Low risk (<1% annual mortality)
  Duke treadmill score ≥5
  No or small perfusion defect at rest or with stress
  No stress-induced wall motion abnormalities

HR, head rate; LV, left ventricular; LVEF, left ventricular ejection fraction.

ing digoxin therapy. Also, patients with physical limitations, such as severe lung disease, arthritis, or peripheral vascular disease, should undergo pharmacologic stress testing in combination with an imaging modality.

Electrocardiography

A resting 12-lead electrocardiogram (ECG) should be obtained in all patients with symptoms suggestive of angina pectoris. The resting ECG is normal in approximately 50% of patients with chronic stable angina. ST-T changes are usually nonspecific. Q waves may indicate previous MI. LV hypertrophy may be caused by hypertension, aortic stenosis, or hypertrophic cardiomyopathy.

Echocardiography

The resting echocardiogram (Table 9.3) is useful for evaluating global and regional LV function and for excluding aortic stenosis or hypertrophic cardiomyopathy from the diagnosis.

Electron Beam Computed Tomography

Electron beam computed tomography (EBCT) is a highly sensitive technique for detecting coronary artery calcification, an abnormality found in atherosclerotic arteries but not normal arteries. An ACC/AHA Expert Consensus Document concluded that (a) EBCT has a high sensitivity, a much lower specificity, and overall predictive accuracy of 70% in a typical CAD patient population; (b) the predictive accuracy of EBCT

TABLE 9.3. *Indications for echocardiography or radionuclide ventriculography to establish diagnosis and to stratify risk according to Canadian Cardiovascular Society Classification system*

Class I
  Resting echocardiogram in patients with a systolic murmur suggestive of mitral regurgitation, aortic stenosis, or hypertrophic cardiomyopathy
  Resting echocardiogram or radionuclide ventriculogram to assess LV function in patients with history of MI, Q waves, complex ventricular arrhythmias, or symptoms suggestive of congestive heart failure
Class IIb
  Resting echocardiogram to diagnose mitral valve prolapse in patients with a click and/or murmur
Class III
  Resting echocardiogram in patients with a normal ECG, no history of MI, and no symptoms or signs of heart failure, valvular heart disease, or hypertrophic cardiomyopathy

ECG, electrocardiogram; LV, left ventricular; MI, myocardial infarction.

is equivalent to alternative methods for diagnosing CAD; and (c) EBCT is not recommended for diagnosing CAD because of its low specificity (2).

Noninvasive Stress Testing

The predictive accuracy of noninvasive stress testing (Table 9.4) depends on the sensitivity and specificity of the test and the prevalence of the disease in the population studied—that is, the pretest probability of CAD. The exercise ECG is useful in patients with a normal resting ECG and an intermediate pretest probability of CAD, whereas it is less useful in patients with an abnormal resting ECG or either a low or high pretest probability of CAD. The inclusion of an imaging technique (i.e., echocardiography or myocardial

TABLE 9.4. *Selected indications for noninvasive stress testing to establish diagnosis and to stratify risk according to Canadian Cardiovascular Society Classification system*

Class I
Exercise ECG without imaging in patients with an intermediate pretest probability of CAD (see exceptions listed in Classes II and III)
Exercise myocardial perfusion imaging or echocardiography in patients who are able to exercise have an intermediate pretest probability of CAD, and one of the following baseline ECG abnormalities:
  Preexcitation (Wolff-Parkinson-White) syndrome
  >1-mm resting ST depression
Exercise myocardial perfusion imaging or echocardiography in patients with prior PCI or CABG
Adenosine or dipyridamole myocardial perfusion imaging in patients with an intermediate pretest probability of CAD and one of the following baseline
ECG abnormalities:
  Electronically paced ventricular rhythm
  Left bundle branch block (LBBB)
Stress myocardial perfusion imaging or echocardiography to identify the extent, severity, and location of ischemia in patients who do not have LBBB or electronically paced ventricular rhythm, or to assess the functional significance of coronary lesions in planning PCI
Class IIa
Patients with suspected vasospastic angina
Class IIb
Exercise ECG in patients with high or low pretest probability of CAD
Exercise ECG in patients taking digitalis or with left ventricular hypertrophy and <1-mm ST segment depression
Exercise or dobutamine echocardiography in patients with LBBB
Class III
Exercise ECG without imaging in patients with the following baseline ECG abnormalities:
  Preexcitation (Wolff-Parkinson-White) syndrome
  Electronically paced ventricular rhythm
  >1-mm resting ST depression
  Complete LBBB
Patients with severe comorbidity that is likely to limit life expectancy or prevent revascularization

CABG, coronary artery bypass graft; CAD, coronary artery disease; ECG, electrocardiogram; PCI, percutaneous coronary intervention.

perfusion imaging) increases the sensitivity and specificity of noninvasive stress testing. Pharmacologic stress testing (e.g., dobutamine echocardiography and adenosine or dipyridamole myocardial perfusion imaging) should be performed in patients who are unable to exercise adequately because of lung disease, peripheral vascular disease, or musculoskeletal disease.

Cardiac Catheterization and Coronary Angiography

Direct referral for diagnostic coronary angiography (Table 9.5) may be indicated in patients with chest pain and either a high pretest probability of severe CAD or a contraindication to noninvasive testing. Coronary angiography is usually accompanied by left-sided heart catheterization to rule out aortic stenosis and by contrast-enhanced ventriculography to assess regional and global LV function. Coronary angiography delineates the extent and severity of CAD and may reveal less common nonatherosclerotic causes of angina, such as coronary spasm, Kawasaki's dis-

ease, coronary artery dissection or anomalies, and radiation-induced vasculopathy. Intracoronary ultrasound studies have demonstrated that diffuse coronary atherosclerosis may be associated with a "false-negative" coronary angiogram. The hemodynamic significance of a coronary stenosis can be assessed with a Doppler wire or pressure-sensing wire to measure coronary flow reserve.

DIFFERENTIAL DIAGNOSIS

The differential diagnosis of chest pain includes numerous cardiac and noncardiac causes. Common cardiac causes of chest pain not attributable to myocardial ischemia are pericarditis and aortic dissection. Pulmonary causes include pulmonary embolus, pulmonary hypertension, pneumothorax, pneumonia, and pleuritis. Gastrointestinal causes are esophagitis, esophageal spasm or reflux, peptic ulcer disease, pancreatitis, and pathologic processes of the biliary tract. Musculoskeletal causes of chest pain are costochondritis, fibromyalgia, rib fractures, cervical

---

TABLE 9.5. *Selected indications for coronary angiography to establish diagnosis and to stratify risk according to Canadian Cardiovascular Society Classification system*

Class I
Patients with known or possible angina who have survived sudden death
Patients with CCS Class III or IV angina despite medical therapy
Patients with high-risk criteria shown on noninvasive testing regardless of anginal severity
Patients with angina and symptoms or signs of congestive heart failure
Class IIa
Patients with an uncertain diagnosis after noninvasive testing in whom the benefit of a more certain diagnosis
   outweighs the risk and cost
Patients who cannot undergo noninvasive testing because of disability, illness, or obesity
Patients with an occupation requirement for a definitive diagnosis
Patients with a high pretest probability of left main or three-vessel CAD
Patients with LVEF <45%, CCS Class I or II angina, and demonstrable ischemia but less than high-risk criteria
   shown on noninvasive testing
Class IIb
Patients with recurrent hospitalization for chest pain
Patients with greater than a low probability of CAD and an overriding desire for a definitive diagnosis
Patients with LVEF >45%, CCS Class I or II angina, and less than high-risk criteria shown on noninvasive
   testing
Class III
Patients with significant comorbidity in whom the risk outweighs the benefit
Patients with CCS Class I or II angina who respond to medical therapy and have no evidence of ischemia on
   noninvasive testing
Patients who prefer to avoid revascularization
Patients with a personal desire for a definitive diagnosis but a low probability of CAD

CAD, coronary artery disease; CCS, Canadian Cardiovascular Society; LVEF, left ventricular ejection fraction.

radiculopathy, and herpes zoster. Finally, chest pain may occur in patients with various psychiatric conditions, such as anxiety and affective disorders.

COMPLICATIONS

The complications of stable angina consist of the complications that may ensue from CAD, i.e. unstable angina, MI, ischemic cardiomyopathy, congestive heart failure, atrial and ventricular arrhythmias, and sudden death.

THERAPY

The goals of treatment are to relieve symptoms and to reduce the risk of morbidity (e.g., MI) and death (1). Ideally, successful treatment results in a functional capacity of CCS Class I. The initial treatment program consists of the following:

A: aspirin and antianginal therapy
B: beta blocker and blood pressure control
C: cigarette smoking cessation and cholesterol treatment
D: diet and diabetes therapy
E: education and exercise

Pharmacologic Therapy

Antianginal Agents

Nitrates

Parker and Parker (3) have published a detailed review of nitrate therapy (Table 9.6). Sublingual NTG tablets and spray are useful both for treating attacks of angina and for preventing episodes of exertional angina. Multiple long-acting nitrate preparations, including transdermal NTG, oral isosorbide dinitrate, and oral isosorbide mononitrate, have been shown to prolong the time to onset of ischemia during exercise testing. Tolerance, the major limitation of nitrate therapy, can be avoided by dosage regimens that provide a nitrate-free interval. Also, studies have suggested that antioxidant vitamins, such as vitamin C (4) and vitamin E (5), may counteract nitrate tolerance. There is no published evidence to suggest

TABLE 9.6. *Recommendations for pharmacotherapy according to Canadian Cardiovascular Society Classification system*

Class I
Aspirin
Beta-blockers in patients with prior myocardial infarction
Calcium antagonists or long-acting nitrates when beta blockers are contraindicated or cause unacceptable side effects
Sublingual NTG or NTG spray for immediate relief of angina
Lipid-lowering therapy to achieve LDL <100 mg/dL
Class IIa
Clopidogrel when aspirin is contraindicated
Long-acting nondihydropyridine calcium antagonists instead of beta blockers
Class IIb
Low-intensity anticoagulation with warfarin in addition to aspirin
Class III
Dipyridamole
Chelation therapy

LDL, low-density lipoprotein; NTG, nitroglycerin.

that nitrates change the incidence of death or MI in patients with chronic stable angina.

Beta Blockers

The Atenolol Silent Ischemia Study (ASIST) was a double-blind, placebo-controlled, randomized study of atenolol, 100 mg daily, versus placebo in 306 patients with Class I or II angina (6). The entry criteria included evidence of ischemia during both exercise testing and Holter monitoring. Treatment with atenolol reduced the number and average duration of ischemic episodes recorded during 48 hours of ambulatory ECG monitoring. Also, 1-year event-free survival rates were higher among the atenolol recipients than among the placebo recipients. Although ASIST was a relatively small trial, the results suggest that beta blockers may improve the prognosis of patients with chronic stable angina.

Calcium Channel Blockers

The largest published placebo-controlled trial of a calcium channel blocker in patients with CAD was the Prospective Randomized Evaluation of the Vascular Effects of Norvasc Trial

(PREVENT) (7). The trial was designed to determine whether amlodipine retards progression of atherosclerosis in patients with CAD. Coronary angiography and carotid ultrasonography were performed in 825 patients at baseline and after y 3 years. Of these patients, 69% had a history of stable angina. During the 3 years of follow-up, there were fewer hospitalizations for unstable angina and coronary revascularization among the amlodipine recipients. There were no differences in mortality or MI rates. Carotid artery atherosclerosis measured by ultrasonography progressed in the placebo recipients but not in the amlodipine recipients. There was no effect of amlodipine on progression of coronary atherosclerosis as measured by coronary angiography.

The Angina Prognosis Study in Stockholm (APSIS) was a long-term study of metoprolol or verapamil in 809 patients with stable angina (8). Patients were randomly assigned in a double-blind manner to receive either metoprolol, 200 mg daily, or verapamil, 240 mg twice daily. After a median follow-up period of 3.4 years, there were no differences in total mortality, cardiovascular mortality, nonfatal cardiovascular events, or combined cardiovascular events.

The Total Ischaemic Burden European Trial (TIBET) was a long-term study of atenolol, nifedipine, and their combination in 682 patients with chronic stable angina (9). Patients were randomly assigned to receive atenolol, 50 mg twice daily; nifedipine, 20 or 40 mg twice daily; or the combination. Exercise parameters improved and ambulatory ischemia decreased in each group, with no differences between the groups. Also, there were no significant differences in the frequency of clinical events.

Heidenreich et al. (10) performed a meta-analysis of trials that compared beta blockers, calcium channel blockers, and nitrates for stable angina. Trials that compared nitrates with either beta blockers or calcium channel blockers were too few to determine their relative efficacy. Although 72 studies that compared beta blockers with calcium channel blockers were identified, the APSIS and TIBET trials discussed previously were the only trials longer than 6 months, and

they accounted for 103 of the 116 cardiac events that occurred in all of the trials.

Antiplatelet Agents

Aspirin

Several clinical trials have demonstrated that aspirin improves outcome in patients with chronic stable angina. The Physicians' Health Study, a trial of aspirin (325 mg daily) among 22,071 male physicians, included 333 men with chronic stable angina at the time of enrollment (11). After an average follow-up of 60 months, the incidence of MI was 7 in 178 among patients who received aspirin, in comparison with 20 in 155 among patients who received placebo (relative risk, 0.30; confidence interval, 0.04 to 0.42; $p < 0.001$). The Swedish Angina Pectoris Trial (SAPAT) randomly assigned 2,035 patients with chronic stable angina to receive either aspirin, 75 mg daily, or placebo (12). All patients were treated with sotalol for control of symptoms. After a median-duration follow-up of 50 months, the aspirin recipients had a 34% lower incidence of sudden death and nonfatal MI ($p = 0.003$). There was no significant difference in major bleeding. The guidelines recommend that aspirin, 75 to 325 mg, should be prescribed to all patients with angina and no contraindications (1).

Clopidogrel

Although there are no placebo-controlled trials of clopidogrel in patients with chronic stable angina, clopidogrel was superior to aspirin in patients with CAD who were enrolled in the Clopidogrel versus Aspirin in Patients at Risk of Ischemic Events (CAPRIE) trial (13). Therefore, patients who are intolerant of or truly allergic to aspirin should be treated with clopidogrel.

Anticoagulant Therapy

The Thrombosis Prevention Trial demonstrated that low-intensity anticoagulation with warfarin [International Normalized Ratio (INR), 1.5] decreased the risk of coronary death and fatal and nonfatal MI in patients with risk factors for atherosclerosis but no symptoms of angina pectoris (14). A meta-analysis of 31 trials of oral anticoagulant therapy in patients with CAD has been published (15). In comparison with controls, high-intensity anticoagulation (INR, 2.8 to 4.8) was associated with a reduction in mortality and a sixfold increase in major bleeding. Moderate intensity anticoagulation (INR, 2 to 3) increased major bleeding to a similar extent (7.7- fold) and was associated with a 52% reduction in the rate of MI. Low-intensity anticoagulation (INR, less than 2.0) plus aspirin was not superior to aspirin alone. Thus, because of the increased bleeding rates associated with anticoagulation, aspirin and clopidogrel are safer treatment options.

Lipid-Lowering Agents

Statins

The Scandinavian Simvastatin Survival Study (4S) was a randomized trial of simvastatin in 4,444 patients with a history of angina pectoris or MI. Among the 21% of patients who had angina but no history of MI at the time of enrollment, there was a 26% reduction in the risk of major coronary events (coronary deaths, nonfatal MI, and resuscitated cardiac arrest), but analysis of this subgroup was not prespecified, and the difference did not achieve statistical significance ($p = 0.08$) (16). The Regression Growth Evaluation Statin Study (REGRESS) was a randomized trial of the effects of pravastatin on progression and regression of CAD (17). Enrollment included 768 male patients with stable angina, documented CAD, and serum cholesterol levels of 155 to 310 mg per deciliter. Forty-eight-hour ambulatory ECGs that were obtained before and after random assignment to receive pravastatin, 40 mg daily, or placebo demonstrated that pravastatin significantly decreased the frequency and duration of ischemic episodes.

Current guidelines recommend titration of statin therapy to achieve a serum low-density lipoprotein (LDL) level lower than 100 mg per deciliter in patients with CAD (1), but ongoing clinical trials may provide the rationale for even more aggressive lowering of LDL.

Fibrates

The Veterans Affairs High-Density Lipoprotein Cholesterol Intervention Trial (VA-HIT) demonstrated a 22% reduction in the relative risk of nonfatal MI or coronary death among patients with CAD and low levels of high-density lipoprotein (HDL) (less than 40 mg per deciliter) who received gemfibrozil (18). Patients with a serum LDL cholesterol level higher than 140 mg per deciliter were excluded. Thirty-nine percent of the patients did not have a history of MI before enrollment, but the effect of gemfibrozil on outcomes in this subgroup was not reported.

Angiotensin-Converting Enzyme Inhibitors

On the basis of the results of trials such as the Study of Survival and Ventricular Enlargement (SAVE) (19) and the Studies of Left Ventricular Dysfunction (SOLVD) (20), angiotensin-converting enzyme (ACE) inhibitors are indicated for patients with a history of CAD and either congestive heart failure or asymptomatic LV dysfunction. The Heart Outcomes Prevention Evaluation (HOPE) Study was a double-blind, randomized trial with a two-by-two factorial design (21). It evaluated the effects of an ACE inhibitor, ramipril, and vitamin E in 9,541 patients at high risk of cardiovascular events. Of the subjects, 80% had a history of CAD, and 56% had a history of stable angina pectoris. The primary endpoint was a composite of MI, stroke, and death from cardiovascular causes. A total of 651 patients in the ramipril group (14.0%) reached the primary endpoint, in comparison with 826 patients in the placebo group (17.8%) [relative risk (RR), 0.78; $p < 0.001$]. Treatment with ramipril reduced the rates of death from any cause (RR, 0.84; $p = 0.005$), death from cardiovascular causes (RR, 0.74; $p < 0.001$), MI (RR, 0.80; $p < 0.001$), stroke (RR, 0.68; $p < 0.001$), and revascularization procedures (RR, 0.85; $p = 0.002$). Among the 4,759 patients with documented normal LVEF, treatment with ramipril was associated with significant reductions in the primary endpoint and each of its components. Two ongoing trials, the Prevention of Events with Angiotensin Converting Enzyme Inhibition Trial (PEACE) and the European Trial for the Reduction of Cardiac Events with Perindopril in Stable Coronary Artery Disease (EUROPA), also are comparing ACE inhibitors (trandolapril and perindopril, respectively) with placebo in patients with CAD. If the results of PEACE and EUROPA are concordant with HOPE, treatment with an ACE inhibitor will be indicated in all patients with CAD, regardless of the LVEF.

Antioxidants

The HOPE trial randomly assigned 4,761 patients to receive vitamin E, 400 IU daily, and 4,780 patients to receive placebo (22). Treatment with vitamin E had no effect on cardiovascular events. Recently, Cheung et al. (23) reported the results of a small clinical study of patients with CAD and low levels of HDL. Lipoprotein changes over 12 months were studied in 153 patients who were randomly assigned to four treatment groups: antioxidants (vitamins E and C, beta-carotene, and selenium); simvastatin plus niacin; simvastatin, niacin, and antioxidants; or placebo. Simvastatin plus niacin increased HDL cholesterol and lipoprotein a-1, whereas the combination of antioxidant supplements blocked the HDL response to simvastatin plus niacin. In a preliminary report, the same study group wrote that the antioxidant combination also had deleterious effects on the progression of CAD as measured by quantitative coronary angiography (24). Thus, patients with CAD should probably abstain from antioxidant vitamins.

Revascularization

The LVEF is a critical determinant of whether myocardial revascularization improves long-term survival of a patient with CAD. The angiographic extent of CAD affects the decision of whether to recommend medical therapy alone, percutaneous coronary intervention (PCI), or surgical revascularization. The presence of more than 70% stenosis of the left main coronary artery, more than 70% stenosis of the proximal left anterior descending coronary artery, or three-vessel CAD each is an indication for revascularization to improve survival. Also, exercise testing provides additional prognostic information that influences the decision whether to recommend revascularization. The Class I, II, and III recommendations for revascularization are listed in Table 9.7.

Coronary Artery Bypass Surgery

Patients with chronic stable angina were randomly assigned to undergo coronary artery bypass graft (CABG) or medical therapy in three major clinical trials: The Veterans Administration (VA) Cooperative Study, the Coronary Artery Surgery Study (CASS), and the European Coronary Surgery Study (ECSS). The general conclusions were that CABG prolongs survival of patients with stable angina who have the following characteristics: stenosis of more than 50% of the left main coronary artery; three-vessel CAD with LVEF of less than 50%; or two-vessel CAD with stenosis of more than 75% of the proximal left anterior descending coronary artery (25). An overview of the 10-year results from all randomized trials of CABG versus medical therapy supported the conclusion that CABG prolongs survival in certain high-risk and medium-risk subgroups of patients with stable CAD but not in low-risk patients (26).

The survival benefit conferred by CABG in this era may be underestimated by the randomized clinical trials conducted in the 1970s because operative mortality has decreased and arterial revascularization was rarely performed. In comparison with placement of saphenous vein grafts as conduits, a single internal mammary artery (IMA) graft to the left anterior descending coronary was associated with lower operative mortality; greater graft patency; reduced frequency of MI, recurrent angina, and need for subsequent cardiac interventions; and increased long-term survival, among nonrandomized cohorts of patients (27). The advantages conferred by IMA grafts presumably result from their greater patency rates in comparison with vein grafts. One surgical series reported long-term

TABLE 9.7. *Recommendations for revascularization for chronic stable angina*

Class I
CABG for significant left main stenosis
CABG for three-vessel CAD
CABG for two-vessel CAD with significant proximal LAD stenosis and either LVEF <50% or inducible ischemia
PTCA for two- or three-vessel CAD with significant proximal LAD stenosis if suitable anatomy, normal LVEF, and no diabetes
PTCA or CABG for one- or two-vessel CAD without proximal LAD stenosis if large area of viable myocardium and high-risk noninvasive criteria
CABG for one- or two-vessel CAD without proximal LAD stenosis for sustained VT or survivor of sudden death
CABG or PTCA for restenosis after PTCA if large area of viable myocardium or high-risk noninvasive criteria
PTCA or CABG if medical therapy unsuccessful and risk of revascularization acceptable
Class IIa
Repeat CABG if multiple graft stenoses
PTCA or CABG for one- or two-vessel CAD without proximal LAD stenosis if moderate area of viable myocardium and inducible ischemia
PTCA or CABG for one-vessel CAD with significant proximal LAD stenosis
Class IIb
PTCA for two- or three-vessel CAD with significant proximal LAD stenosis and diabetes or abnormal LVEF
PTCA for significant left main coronary artery stenosis if patient is not candidate for CABG
PTCA for one- or two-vessel CAD without significant proximal LAD stenosis for sustained VT or survivor of sudden death
Class III
PTCA or CABG for one- or two-vessel CAD without proximal LAD stenosis if symptoms mild, or inadequate trial of medical therapy, and small area of viable myocardium or no inducible ischemia
PTCA or CABG for 50%–60% stenosis (other than left main coronary artery) and no inducible ischemia
PTCA or CABG for <50% stenosis
PTCA for patients who have significant left main stenosis and are candidates for CABG

CABG, coronary artery bypass graft; CAD, coronary artery disease; LAD, left anterior descending artery; LVEF, left ventricular ejection fraction; PTCA, percutaneous transluminal coronary angioplasty; VT, ventricular tachycardia.

patency rates of 96% for IMA grafts (27). In the CASS trial, 84% of the conduits were saphenous veins, and the cumulative graft patency rates 18 months and 5 years after CABG were only 85% and 82%, respectively (28). A metaanalysis of 10 clinical reports concluded that bilateral IMA grafting provides better survival than does a unilateral IMA graft, but none of the 10 studies analyzed was a randomized trial (29).

The randomized trials of CABG versus medical therapy were performed before the availability of statins to treat hyperlipidemia. More recent studies indicated that statins and other lipid-lowering agents improve the long-term patency of saphenous vein bypass grafts (30,31). The largest trial was the National Heart, Lung, and Blood Institute's Post Coronary Artery Bypass Graft Clinical Trial (31). The study enrolled 1,351 patients with a history of CABG, at least one patent vein graft, and LDL cholesterol levels of 130 to 175 mg per deciliter. The patients were randomly assigned to undergo "aggressive" lowering of LDL, with a goal of 60 to 85 mg per deciliter, or to undergo moderate lowering, with a goal of 130 to 140 mg per deciliter. Treatment consisted of lovastatin, plus cholestyramine if needed. The mean LDL cholesterol level during treatment ranged from 93 to 97 mg per deciliter in the aggressive-treatment group, in comparison with 132 to 136 mg per deciliter in the moderate-treatment group ($p < 0.001$). Angiography was performed before and an average of 4.3 years after randomization. The rates of new graft occlusion were 6% for the aggressive-group and 11% for the moderate-treatment group ($p < 0.001$). The rates of new lesion formation in grafts were 10% for the aggressive-treatment group and 21% for the moderate-treatment group. There was a 29% lower rate of revascularization procedures in the aggressive-treatment group than in the moderate-treatment group ($p = 0.03$). The results strongly support the recommendation to treat elevated LDL cholesterol aggressively in patients who have undergone CABG.

Regardless of its effect on survival, CABG is an excellent therapy for relief of angina. The early randomized trials comparing CABG with medical therapy demonstrated excellent relief of angina after CABG but declining benefit after 5 years because of attrition of vein grafts. It is presumed that patients who receive arterial bypass grafts experience more durable relief of angina because of superior graft patency. The Bypass Angioplasty Revascularization Investigation (BARI) was a large trial that randomly assigned 1,829 patients with stable angina to receive treatment with CABG or percutaneous transluminal coronary angioplasty (PTCA) (32). At least one IMA graft was used in 82% of patients who underwent CABG. Of the patients who underwent CABG, 84% were free of angina 5 years after surgery (33).

Percutaneous Coronary Intervention

Patients with chronic stable angina were randomly assigned to undergo PCI or medical therapy in several clinical trials (34). The largest completed study, the Second Randomized Intervention Treatment of Angina trial (RITA-2), randomly assigned 1,108 patients with single- or double-vessel CAD to undergo medical therapy or PTCA (35). PTCA increased exercise time and reduced the frequency of angina among patients with Class II angina or worse at baseline, at a cost of seven procedure-related MIs in the PTCA group. Thus, after a median follow-up of 2.7 years, there were 21 nonfatal MIs (4.2%) among the patients undergoing PTCA versus 10 (2.0%) among those undergoing medical therapy. There was no significant difference in mortality rates, however.

A small, randomized trial was performed in Switzerland to compare invasive versus medical therapy in patients 75 years or older with chronic angina (36). The inclusion criteria included at least CCS Class II angina despite at least two antianginal drugs. One hundred fifty patients were randomly assigned to receive "optimum medical" therapy, consisting of an increase in the number or dosage of antianginal drugs. One hundred fifty-five patients were randomly assigned to undergo invasive treatment. The 147 patients who underwent cardiac catheterization were treated with PTCA ($n = 79$), CABG ($n = 30$), or medications ($n = 34$). 4 patients who were

assigned PTCA or CABG did not undergo revascularization. The primary endpoints were quality of life after 6 months and major adverse cardiac events (death, nonfatal MI, or hospital admission for acute coronary syndrome). Angina severity decreased and quality of life increased in both treatment groups, but the improvements were significantly greater after revascularization. Major adverse events occurred in 72 (49%) patients who received medical therapy and 29 (19%) patients who underwent invasive treatment ($p < 0.0001$). A much larger ongoing trial, Clinical Outcomes Utilizing Revascularization and Aggressive Drug Evaluation (COURAGE), will randomly assign 3,260 patients with Classes I to III angina to undergo PCI or medical therapy. The results of COURAGE will be important because the Swiss study was very small, and neither stents nor platelet glycoprotein IIb/IIIa receptor inhibitors were employed in the RITA-2 trial.

Percutaneous Coronary Intervention versus Coronary Artery Bypass Graft

Patients with chronic stable angina have been enrolled in numerous randomized trials of PTCA versus CABG. Pocock et al. (37) published a metaanalysis of 3,371 patients who were enrolled in eight randomized trials. There were 73 deaths in the CABG group and 79 in the PTCA group (RR, 1.08; 95% confidence interval, 0.79 to 1.50). One year after randomization, the prevalence of angina was higher among patients treated with PTCA (RR, 1.56; 95% confidence interval, 1.30 to 1.88), but 3 years after randomization, the difference was smaller (RR, 1.22; 95% confidence interval, 0.99 to 1.54). Another group of investigators performed a metaanalysis that included only five of the randomized trials and arrived at similar conclusions: The combined rate of mortality and nonfatal MI was not significantly different after PTCA or CABG at 1 to 3 years of follow-up, but CABG provided better relief of angina and was followed by fewer repeat revascularization procedures (38).

Each of the metaanalyses (37,38) was performed before completion of the large randomized BARI study (32). The BARI trial investigators randomly assigned 914 patients to undergo

CABG and 915 patients to undergo PTCA. All patients had multivessel CAD; 41% had three-vessel disease. The mean LVEF was 57%. Of the patients who underwent CABG, 82% received at least one IMA graft. During the first 5 years of follow-up, 8% of the CABG patients underwent additional revascularization procedures, in comparison with 54% of the PTCA patients. The 5-year survival rates were 89.3% for CABG patients and 86.3% for PTCA patients ($p = 0.19$).

Percutaneous Coronary Intervention versus Coronary Artery Bypass Graft in Patients with Diabetes

Diabetic patients have higher rates of restenosis and target vessel revascularization procedures after both PTCA and coronary stent placement (39,40). Also, coronary artery occlusion and an associated decrease in LVEF are frequent manifestations of restenosis in diabetic patients, a possible explanation of the increased mortality rate after PTCA in diabetic patients (41). A post hoc analysis of the 641 diabetics who were enrolled in the BARI trial revealed that the 5-year survival rate was greater among subjects who underwent CABG than among subjects who underwent PTCA (80.6% vs. 65.5%; $p = 0.003$). Among diabetic patients, the 7-year survival rates were 76.4% for those who underwent CABG and 55.7% for those who underwent PTCA ($p=0.0011$) (33). CABG greatly reduced the risk of death after Q wave MI. The mortality rate was 17% among patients who underwent CABG and subsequently suffered a Q wave MI, in comparison with 80% among patients who underwent PTCA (42).

Interpretation of the BARI trial results is confounded by several concerns. Only 641 diabetic patients were enrolled in the BARI trial, and they did not constitute a prespecified subgroup. The survival advantage conferred by CABG among diabetic patients in the randomized component of the BARI trial was not observed among the diabetic patients who were eligible for BARI but declined random assignment and selected their mode of revascularization (43). Most important, enrollment in the BARI trial was completed before the advent of stents and glycoprotein IIb/IIIa inhibitors, which dramatically improve the short-term and long-term results of PCI, especially in diabetic patients (40,44). The Evaluation of Platelet IIb/IIIa Inhibitor for Stenting Trial (EPISTENT) study randomly assigned patients undergoing PCI to three groups: stent with placebo ($n = 809$), stent with the glycoprotein IIb/IIIa inhibitor abciximab ($n = 794$), or PTCA with abciximab ($n = 796$) (39). Among the 491 patients with diabetes, the 6-month target vessel revascularization rates were 8.1% after stent placement with abciximab, 16.6% after stent placement with placebo, and 18.4% after PTCA with abciximab ($p = 0.021$) (39,40). The EPISTENT trial also demonstrated that abciximab therapy, irrespective of revascularization strategy, resulted in a significant reduction in the 6-month rates of death or MI: 12.7% for stent with placebo, 7.8% for PTCA with abciximab, and 6.2% for stent with abciximab ($p = 0.029$). Pooling of the results of three randomized trials of abciximab versus placebo in patients undergoing PCI demonstrated that abciximab decreased 1-year mortality, especially among patients who underwent multivessel PCI (44). The mortality rate among diabetic patients who underwent multivessel PCI was reduced from 7.7% to 0.9% with abciximab therapy ($p = 0.018$).

The Arterial Revascularization Therapies Study (ARTS) randomly assigned 1,205 patients with multivessel CAD to undergo CABG or stent implantation (45). It included 112 diabetic patients who received stents and 96 diabetic patients who underwent CABG (46). IMA bypass grafts were placed in 99.7% of the nondiabetic and 89.3% of the diabetic patients who underwent CABG (46). Diabetic patients who underwent CABG had a higher 1-year event-free survival rate than did diabetic patients who underwent coronary stent placement (84.4% vs. 63.4%; $p<0.001$), primarily because of a 21.6% lower rate of repeat revascularization.

Further information regarding outcomes after PCI in diabetic patients will be generated by the second BARI trial.

Stent versus Coronary Artery Bypass Graft Trials

Several randomized trials have been performed to compare CABG with coronary stent placement

(45,47). In the Stenting versus Internal Mammary Artery (SIMA) study, 123 patients with isolated *de novo* stenosis of the proximal left anterior descending coronary artery were randomly assigned to undergo coronary stent placement ($n = 62$) or CABG with an IMA graft ($n = 59$) (47). One patient who received a stent experienced subacute stent thrombosis 4 days after the procedure and died of a massive cerebral hemorrhage after receiving a thrombolytic drug. One patient in the CABG group died of an anterior MI 10 days after CABG. After a mean follow-up period of 2.4 years, additional revascularization procedures were performed in 24% of the patients who underwent stent placement but in none of the patients who underwent CABG.

The Coronary Angioplasty with Stenting versus Coronary Bypass Surgery in Patients with Multiple-Vessel Disease (ERACI) II study randomly assigned 450 patients with multivessel CAD to undergo either PCI ($n = 225$) or CABG ($n = 225$) (48). Rates of mortality and freedom from MI were lower among patients randomized to PCI with stent placement than among patients randomized to CABG. The ERACI II study has numerous limitations: relatively short duration of follow-up (mean, 18.5 months), small sample size, high postoperative mortality rate after CABG (5.7%), low use of glycoprotein IIb/IIIa inhibitors (28%), and use of a suboptimal stent design (Gianturco Roubin II) that has been associated with relatively high restenosis rates. Also, only 38 patients had stable angina before randomization.

In the ARTS, 1,205 patients with multivessel CAD were randomly assigned to undergo CABG or stent implantation (45). Among the 600 patients who underwent stent implantation, 57% had stable angina and 19% had diabetes; the mean LVEF was 61%; and 30% had three-vessel CAD and 68% had two-vessel CAD. Among the 605 patients who underwent CABG, 60% had stable angina and 16% had diabetes; the mean LVEF was 60%; and 33% had three-vessel CAD and 67% had two-vessel CAD. Among the patients who underwent CABG, 93% received at least one arterial conduit. After the procedure, creatine kinase values more than five times the upper limit of normal were found in 6.2% of

TABLE 9.8. *Prognosis*

Extent of coronary artery disease	5-Year survival rate (%)
One-vessel disease, 75%	93
>One-vessel disease, 50%–74%	93
One-vessel disease, ≥95%	91
Two-vessel disease	88
Two-vessel disease, both ≥95%	86
One-vessel disease, ≥95% proximal LAD	83
Two-vessel disease, ≥95%	83
Two-vessel disease, ≥95% proximal LAD	79
Three-vessel disease	79
Three-vessel disease, ≥95% in at least one	73
Three-vessel disease, 75% proximal LAD	67
Three-vessel disease, ≥95% proximal LAD	59

LAD, left anterior descending (artery).

the patients who underwent PCI, in contrast to 12.6% of the patients who underwent CABG ($p<0.001$). After 1 year of follow-up, there was no significant difference between the two groups in the rates of death, stroke, or MI. Among patients who survived without a stroke or MI, repeat revascularization procedures were performed in 16.8% of the patients who underwent PCI, in contrast to 3.5% of those who underwent CABG. After 1 year, 90% of CABG patients were free of angina, in comparison with 79% of patients who underwent PCI. Glycoprotein IIb/IIIa inhibitors were not employed routinely in the ARTS trial.

The Stent or Surgery (SOS) trial randomly assigned 967 patients with multivessel CAD and

TABLE 9.9. *Questions to ask at each follow-up visit*

Has the patient decreased the level of physical activity since the last visit?
Have the patient's anginal symptoms increased in frequency and become more severe since the last visit?
How well is the patient tolerating therapy?
How successful has the patient been in reducing modifiable risk factors and improving knowledge about ischemic heart disease?
Has the patient developed any new comorbid illnesses, or has the severity or treatment of known comorbid illnesses worsened the patient's angina?

severe angina refractory to medical therapy to undergo CABG ($n = 487$) or PCI ($n = 480$). After follow-up for 1 year, the rates of death and additional PCI or CABG were higher among patients who underwent PCI than among patients who underwent CABG.

The rapid evolution of PCI makes it difficult to apply the results of the randomized PCI versus CABG trials to clinical decision making today. After the early trials were completed, restenosis rates after PCI decreased dramatically because of the introduction of coronary stents. For example, a comparison of coronary artery stent placement with angioplasty for isolated stenosis of the proximal left anterior descending coronary artery demonstrated restenosis rates of 19% after stent placement, in comparison with 40% after PTCA ($p = 0.02$) (49). The 1-year rates of event-free survival were 87% after stent placement and 70% after PTCA ($p = 0.04$).

Currently, a new generation of stents coated with antiproliferative agents (e.g., sirolimus, paclitaxel, actinomycin D) is under investigation. An intravascular ultrasound study showed that there was minimal intimal hyperplasia 4 months after implantation of sirolimus-coated stents (50). The first completed, randomized clinical trial of stents coated with sirolimus, Randomized Study with the Sirolimus Coated Stent (RAVEL), reported a restenosis rate of 0% 12 months after stent implantation (51). If these impressive results are reproduced in larger studies, the results of previous PCI versus CABG trials will be obsolete.

Refractory Myocardial Ischemia

Some patients with chronic stable angina are not candidates for PCI or CABG and continue to have severe angina despite maximal medical therapy.

TABLE 9.10. *Recommendations for noninvasive testing and coronary angiography during follow-up according to Canadian Cardiovascular Society Classification system*

Class I
Chest radiograph for patients with evidence of new or worsening congestive heart failure
Assessment of LVEF and segmental wall motion in patients with new or worsening congestive heart failure or evidence of intervening MI by history or ECG
Echocardiography for evidence of new or worsening valvular heart disease
Treadmill exercise test for patients without prior revascularization who have a significant change in clinical status, are able to exercise, and do not have any of the ECG abnormalities listed in the next recommendation
Stress imaging for patients without prior revascularization who have a significant change in clinical status and are unable to exercise or have one of the following ECG abnormalities:
Preexcitation (Wolff-Parkinson-White) syndrome
Electronically paced ventricular rhythm
>1-mm resting ST depression
Complete LBBB
Stress imaging for patients who have a significant change in clinical status and required a stress imaging procedure on their initial evaluation because of equivocal or intermediate-risk treadmill results
Stress imaging for patients with prior revascularization who have a significant change in clinical status
Coronary angiography in patients with Class III angina despite maximal medical therapy
Class IIb
Annual treadmill exercise testing in patients who have no change in clinical status, can exercise, have none of the ECG abnormalities listed in number 5 above, and have an estimated annual mortality >1%.
Class III
Echocardiography or radionuclide imaging to assess LV function in patients with a normal ECG, no history of MI, and no evidence of congestive heart failure.
Repeat treadmill exercise testing in <3 years in patients who have no change in clinical status and an estimated annual mortality <1% on their initial evaluation.
Stress imaging for patients who have no change in clinical status and a normal rest ECG, are not taking digoxin, are able to exercise, and did not require a stress imaging procedure on their initial evaluation because of equivocal or intermediate-risk treadmill results.
Repeat coronary angiography in patients with no change in clinical status, no change on repeat exercise testing or stress imaging, and insignificant CAD on initial evaluation.

CAD, coronary artery disease; ECG, electrocardiogram; LBBB, left bundle branch block; LV, left ventricular; LVEF, left ventricular ejection fraction; MI, myocardial infarction.

Various investigational approaches have been explored to alleviate angina in this population of patients. Transmyocardial laser revascularization was widely advocated but eventually abandoned. Enhanced external counterpulsation may reduce the frequency of anginal episodes in patients with angina pectoris. Myocardial angiogenesis with genes and growth factors is a fertile area of research.

PROGNOSIS AND FOLLOW-UP

The 5-year survival rate among patients receiving only medical treatment can be predicted from the extent of CAD (Table 9.8) (1). The ACC/AHA and ACP-ASIM guidelines for the management of patients with chronic stable angina recommend follow-up evaluation every 4 to 12 months

(1). The guidelines recommend follow-up evaluations every 4 to 6 months during the first year of therapy and annual evaluations thereafter if the patient is stable and reliable. The guidelines recommend asking five questions during each follow-up evaluation (Table 9.9). Aggressive risk factor control should be pursued (see Chapter 8). The Classes I, II, and III indications for echocardiography, treadmill exercise testing, stress imaging studies, and coronary angiography during follow-up are summarized in Table 9.10. An assessment of LV function is advisable in patients with new or worsening heart failure or intervening MI. Stress testing is indicated for patients who have a significant change in clinical status. Coronary angiography is indicated for patients who develop Class III angina despite maximal medical therapy.

PRACTICAL POINTS

- Sublingual NTG or NTG spray is indicated for immediate relief of angina.
- Aspirin is indicated for all patients who can tolerate aspirin.
- Beta blockers are indicated as initial therapy in all patients who can tolerate them.
- Calcium channel blockers, long-acting nitrates, or both are indicated when beta blockers are contraindicated, are unsuccessful, or cause unacceptable side effects.

- Lipid-lowering therapy is indicated in patients with LDL cholesterol levels higher than 130 mg per deciliter.
- Coronary angiography should be performed in selected patients with chronic stable angina.
- Coronary revascularization in patients with chronic stable angina offers symptomatic relief and reduces mortality risk in certain subsets.

REFERENCES

1. Gibbons RJ, Chatterjee K, Daley J, et al. ACC/AHA/ACP-ASIM Guidelines for the management of patients with chronic stable angina: a report of the American College of Cardiology/American Heart Association Task Force on Practice Guidelines (Committee on the Management of Patients with Chronic Stable Angina). *J Am Coll Cardiol* 1999;33:2092–2197.
2. O'Rourke RA, Brundage BH, Froelicher VF, et al. American College of Cardiology/American Heart Association Expert Consensus Document on electron-beam computed tomography for the diagnosis and prognosis of coronary artery disease. *Circulation* 2000;102:126–140.
3. Parker JD, Parker JO. Nitrate therapy for stable angina pectoris. *N Engl J Med* 1998;338:520–531.
4. Watanabe H, Kakihana M, Ohtsuka S, et al. Randomized, double-blind, placebo-controlled study of the preventive effect of supplemental oral vitamin C on attenuation of development of nitrate tolerance. *J Am Coll Cardiol* 1998;31:1323–1329.
5. Watanabe H, Kakihana M, Ohtsuka S, et al. Randomized, double-blind, placebo-controlled study of supplemental vitamin E on attenuation of the development of nitrate tolerance. *Circulation* 1997;96:2545–2550.
6. Pepine CJ, Cohn PF, Deedwania PC, et al. Effects of treatment on outcome in mildly symptomatic patients with ischemia during daily life. The Atenolol Silent Ischemia Study (ASIST). *Circulation* 1994;90:762–768.
7. Pitt B, Byington RP, Furberg CD, et al. Effect of amlodipine on the progression of atherosclerosis and the occurrence of clinical events. *Circulation* 2000;102:1503–1510.
8. Rehnqvist N, Hjemdahl P, Billing E, et al. Effects of metoprolol vs verapamil in patients with stable angina pectoris. *Eur Heart J* 1996;17:76–81.
9. Dargie HJ, Ford I, Fox KM. Total Ischaemic Burden

European Trial (TIBET). *Eur Heart J* 1996;17:104–112.

10. Heidenreich PA, McDonald KM, Hastie T, et al. Meta-analysis of trials comparing beta-blockers, calcium antagonists, and nitrates for stable angina. *JAMA* 1999;281:1927–1936.

11. Ridker PM, Manson JE, Gaziano JM, et al. Low-dose aspirin therapy for chronic stable angina. *Ann Intern Med* 1991;114:835–839.

12. Juul-Moller S, Edvardsson N, Jahnmatz B, et al. Double-blind trial of aspirin in primary prevention of myocardial infarction in patients with stable chronic angina pectoris. *Lancet* 1992;340:1421–1425.

13. CAPRIE Steering Committee. A randomised, blinded, trial of Clopidogrel versus Aspirin in Patients at Risk of Ischaemic Events (CAPRIE). *Lancet* 1996;348:1329–1339.

14. The Medical Research Council's General Practice Research Framework. Thrombosis Prevention Trial: randomised trial of low-intensity oral anticoagulation with warfarin and low-dose aspirin in the primary prevention of ischaemic heart disease in men at increased risk. *Lancet* 1998;351:233–241.

15. Anand SS, Yusuf S. Oral anticoagulant therapy in patients with coronary artery disease: a meta-analysis. *JAMA* 1999;282:2058–2067.

16. Kjekshus J, Pedersen TR. Reducing the risk of coronary events: evidence from the Scandinavian Simvastatin Survival Study (4S). *Am J Cardiol* 1995;76:64C–68C.

17. van Boven AJ, Jukema JW, Zwinderman AH, et al. Reduction of transient myocardial ischemia with pravastatin in addition to the conventional treatment in patients with angina pectoris. *Circulation* 1996;94:1503–1505.

18. Rubins HB, Robins SJ, Collins D, et al. Gemfibrozil for the secondary prevention of coronary heart disease in men with low levels of high-density lipoprotein cholesterol. *N Engl J Med* 1999;341:410–418.

19. Pfeffer MA, Braunwald E, Moye LA, et al. Effect of captopril on mortality and morbidity in patients with left ventricular dysfunction after myocardial infarction. *N Engl J Med* 1992;327:669–677.

20. The SOLVD Investigators. Effect of enalapril on mortality and development of heart failure in asymptomatic patients with reduced left ventricular ejection fractions. *N Engl J Med* 1992;327:685–691.

21. The Heart Outcomes Prevention Evaluation Study Investigators. Effects of an angiotensin-converting-enzyme inhibitor, ramipril, on cardiovascular events in high-risk patients. *N Engl J Med* 2000;342:145–153.

22. The Heart Outcomes Prevention Evaluation Study Investigators. Vitamin E supplementation and cardiovascular events in high-risk patients. *N Engl J Med* 2000;342:154–160.

23. Cheung MC, Zhao X-Q, Chait A, et al. Antioxidant supplements block the response of HDL to simvastatin-niacin therapy in patients with coronary artery disease and low HDL. *Arterioscler Thromb Vasc Biol* 2001;21:1320–1326.

24. Brown BG, Zhao X-Q, Chait A, et al. Niacin plus simvastatin, but not antioxidant vitamins, protect against atherosclerosis and clinical events in CAD patients with low HDLC. *Circulation* 2000;102(Suppl II):II-506(abst).

25. Solomon AJ, Gersh BJ. Management of chronic stable angina: medical therapy, percutaneous transluminal coronary angioplasty, and coronary artery bypass graft surgery. Lessons from the randomized trials. *Ann Intern Med* 1998;128:216–223.

26. Yusuf S, Zucker D, Peduzzi P, et al. Effect of coronary artery bypass graft surgery on survival: overview of 10-year results from randomised trials by the Coronary Artery Bypass Graft Surgery Trialists Collaboration. *Lancet* 1994;344:563–570.

27. Loop FD, Lytle BW, Cosgrove DM, et al. Influence of the internal-mammary-artery graft on 10-year survival and other cardiac events. *N Engl J Med* 1986;314:1–6.

28. Campeau L, Lesperance J, Conbara F, et al. Aorto-coronary saphenous vein bypass graft changes 5 to 7 years after surgery. *Circulation* 1978;58(Suppl I):I-170–I-175.

29. Taggart DP, D'Amico R, Altman DG. Effect of arterial revascularisation on survival: a systematic review of studies comparing bilateral and single internal mammary arteries. *Lancet* 2001;358:870–875.

30. Frick MH, Syvanne M, Nieminen M, et al. Prevention of the angiographic progression of coronary and vein-graft atherosclerosis by gemfibrozil after coronary bypass surgery in men with low levels of HDL cholesterol. *Circulation* 1997;96:2137–2143.

31. The Post Coronary Artery Bypass Graft Trial Investigators. The effect of aggressive lowering of low-density lipoprotein cholesterol levels and low-dose anticoagulation on obstructive changes in saphenous-vein coronary-artery bypass grafts. *N Engl J Med* 1997;336:153–162.

32. The Bypass Angioplasty Revascularization Investigation (BARI) Investigators. Comparison of coronary bypass surgery with angioplasty in patients with multivessel disease. *N Engl J Med* 1996;335:217–225.

33. The BARI Investigators. Seven-year outcome in the Bypass Angioplasty Revascularization Investigation (BARI) by treatment and diabetic status. *J Am Coll Cardiol* 2000;35:1122–1129.

34. Blumenthal RS, Cohn G, Schulman S. Medical therapy versus coronary angioplasty in stable coronary artery disease: a critical review of the literature. *J Am Coll Cardiol* 2000;36:668–673.

35. RITA-2 trial participants. Coronary angioplasty versus medical therapy for angina: the Second Randomized Intervention Treatment of Angina (RITA-2) trial. *Lancet* 1997;350:461–468.

36. The TIME Investigators. Trial of invasive versus medical therapy in elderly patients with chronic symptomatic coronary-artery disease (TIME): a randomised trial. *Lancet* 2001;358:951–957.

37. Pocock SJ, Henderson RA, Rickards AF, et al. Meta-analysis of randomised trials comparing coronary angioplasty with bypass surgery. *Lancet* 1995;346:1184–1189.

38. Sim K, Gupta M, McDonald K, et al. A meta-analysis of randomized trials comparing coronary artery bypass grafting with percutaneous transluminal coronary angioplasty in multivessel coronary artery disease. *Am J Cardiol* 1995;76:1025–1029.

39. Lincoff AM, Califf RM, Moliterno DJ, et al. Complementary clinical benefits of coronary-artery stenting and blockade of platelet glycoprotein IIb/IIIa receptors. *N Engl J Med* 1999;341:319–327.

40. Marso SP, Lincoff AM, Ellis SG, et al. Optimizing the percutaneous interventional outcomes for patients with

diabetes mellitus. Results of the EPISTENT (Evaluation of Platelet IIb/IIIa Inhibitor for Stenting Trial) Diabetic Substudy. *Circulation* 1999;100:2477–2484.

41. van Belle E, Ketelers R, Bauters C, et al. Patency of percutaneous transluminal coronary angioplasty sites at 6-month angiographic follow-up. A key determinant of survival in diabetics after coronary balloon angioplasty. *Circulation* 2001;103:1218–1224.

42. Detre KM, Lombardero MS, Brooks MM, et al. The effect of previous coronary-artery bypass surgery on the prognosis of patients with diabetes who have acute myocardial infarction. *N Engl J Med* 2000;342:989–997.

43. Detre KM, Guo P, Holubkov R, et al. Coronary revascularization in diabetic patients. A comparison of the randomized and observational components of the Bypass Angioplasty Revascularization Investigation (BARI). *Circulation* 1999;99:633–640.

44. Bhatt DL, Marso SP, Lincoff AM, et al. Abciximab reduces mortality in diabetics following percutaneous coronary intervention. *J Am Coll Cardiol* 2000;35:922–928.

45. Serruys PW, Unger F, Sousa JE, et al. Comparison of coronary-artery bypass surgery and stenting for the treatment of multivessel disease. *N Engl J Med* 2001;344:1117–1124.

46. Abizaid A, Costa MA, Centemero M, et al. Clinical and economic impact of diabetes mellitus on percutaneous and surgical treatment of multivessel coronary disease patients. Insights from the Arterial Revascularization Therapy Study (ARTS) trial. *Circulation* 2001;104:533–538.

47. Goy J-J, Kaufmann U, Goy-Eggenberger D, et al. A prospective randomized trial comparing stenting to internal mammary artery grafting for proximal, isolated *de novo* left anterior coronary artery stenosis: the SIMA trial. *Mayo Clin Proc* 2000;75:1116–1123.

48. Rodriguez A, Bernardi V, Navia J, et al. Argentine randomized study: Coronary Angioplasty with Stenting versus Coronary Bypass Surgery in Patients with Multiple-Vessel Disease (ERACI II): 30-day and one-year follow-up results. *J Am Coll Cardiol* 2001;37:51–58.

49. Versaci F, Gaspardone A, Tomai F, et al. A comparison of coronary-artery stenting with angioplasty for isolated stenosis of the proximal left anterior descending coronary artery. *N Engl J Med* 1997;336:817–822.

50. Sousa JE, Costa MA, Abizaid A, et al. Lack of neointimal proliferation after implantation of sirolimus-coated stents in human coronary arteries. A quantitative coronary angiography and three-dimensional intravascular ultrasound study. *Circulation* 2001;103:192–195.

51. Morice MC, Serruys PW, Sousa JE, Fajadet J, Hayashi EB, Perin M, Colombo A, Schuler G, Barragan P, Guagliumi G, Molnar F, Falotico R. A randomized comparison of a sirolimus-eluting stent with a standard stent for coronary revascularization. *N Engl J Med* 2002;346:1773–80.

10

Unstable Angina/Non–ST Elevation Myocardial Infarction

Stanley Chetcuti, Francis D. Pagani, and Eric R. Bates

USUAL CAUSES

Unstable angina (UA) and non–ST segment elevation myocardial infarction (NSTEMI) form part of the spectrum of acute coronary syndromes (ACS) that includes acute ST segment elevation myocardial infarction (MI) and sudden cardiac death. The two conditions are pathophysiologically and clinically related and may be indistinguishable at the time of presentation. Patients with biochemical marker evidence for myocardial necrosis are ultimately defined as having NSTEMI instead of UA. The causes of UA and NSTEMI may be classified under five different headings (Table 10.1).

The usual cause of UA/NSTEMI is disruption of an atherosclerotic plaque and formation of a nonocclusive thrombus. Plaques prone to rupture have a large lipid core, high macrophage and activated T-lymphocyte density, low smooth muscle cell density, and a thin fibrous cap characterized by disorganized collagen (1,2). The plaque shoulder, at its junction with the arterial wall, is mechanically the weakest point and the point where most ruptures occur, exposing the lipid core that is very potent in stimulating platelet-rich thrombus formation (3,4). In two thirds of vessels with plaque ruptures with thrombus, there is less than 50% diameter stenosis before plaque rupture, and 97% of these vessels have less than 70% diameter stenosis (5). Thrombus occurring on a ruptured or fissured plaque results from a complex series of interactions among the exposed lipid core, macrophages, smooth muscle cells, collagen, circulating blood products, and coagulation factors. Platelet surface receptors recognize the vascular matrix components (collagen, von

Willebrand factor, vitronectin, and fibronectin), stimulating platelet activation and adhesion. Activated platelets secrete mitogenic, chemotactic, and vasoactive substances and undergo conformational changes with the recruitment and activation of glycoprotein (GP) IIb/IIIa receptors. The activated GP IIb/IIIa receptors mediate platelet aggregation by fibrinogen cross-linkage, forming the white thrombus on the surface of the plaque (6). Tissue factor interacts with activated factor VII to initiate the coagulation cascade, which results in the generation of fibrin, which in turn traps red blood cells and forms the overlying red thrombus (7). Myocyte necrosis in NSTEMI is believed to be caused by temporary arterial occlusion or embolization of platelet-thrombus aggregates and plaque material into the microcirculation.

Less common causes include dynamic obstruction, progressive atherosclerosis or restenosis, and inflammation. Vasoconstrictor substances acting on a segment of epicardial coronary artery with dysfunctional endothelium may lead to vasoconstriction or focal spasm (8,9). Progressive atherosclerotic obstruction can occur in stable calcified lesions or after percutaneous coronary intervention (PCI). Sites of plaque disruption usually exhibit features of inflammation (10). It is not completely clear what role certain infectious agents play in inflammation, but it may be related to increased concentrations of activated macrophages and T lymphocytes at the plaque shoulder.

Noncardiac events can cause a mismatch in myocardial oxygen demand and supply, resulting in UA/NSTEMI. They may be caused by (a) increased myocardial oxygen demand (fever,

TABLE 10.1. *Causes of unstable angina and non–O wave myocardial infarction[a]*

Nonocclusive thrombus on preexisting plaque
Dynamic obstruction (coronary artery spasm or vasoconstriction)
Progressive mechanical obstruction
Inflammation and/or infection
Secondary unstable angina

[a]These causes are not mutually exclusive; some patients have two or more causes.
From Braunwald E. Unstable angina: an etiologic approach to management. *Circulation* 1998;98:2219–2222.

thyrotoxicosis), (b) reduced myocardial oxygen delivery (anemia, hypoxemia), or (c) reduced coronary blood flow (arrhythmia, hypotension). Although there may be coexisting coronary artery disease, it is usually stable, and care should be focused on the precipitating condition.

PRESENTING SYMPTOMS AND SIGNS

The main complaint of patients with UA and NSTEMI is worsening or new-onset angina. There are three principal presentations of UA (11) (Table 10.2). The character of the angina is the same as that encountered in chronic stable angina but is usually more severe and of longer duration, may occur at rest, or may be precipitated by less exertion than previously. Classically, the pain is described as a sensation of pressure in the chest that often radiates to the left arm and neck. Associated with the chest pain in varying frequencies are the symptoms of diaphoresis,

TABLE 10.2. *Three principal manifestations of unstable angina*

Rest angina	Angina occurring at rest and prolonged, usually >20 minutes
New-onset angina	New-onset angina of at least CCS Class III severity
Increasing angina	Previously diagnosed angina that has become distinctly more frequent, longer in duration, or lower in threshold (i.e., increased by ≥1 CCS classes to at least CCS Class III severity

CCS, Canadian Cardiac Society.
From Braunwald E. Unstable angina: a classification. *Circulation* 1989;80:410–414.

dyspnea, nausea, and vomiting. Occasionally, patients (especially elderly women) may have no discernible chest pain but may complain of varying components of arm pain, neck pain, and epigastric discomfort. There may also be a decrease in exercise threshold with worsening dyspnea on exertion. When these non–chest pain symptoms are clearly related to physical or emotional stress and are relieved by nitroglycerin, they should be considered anginal equivalents. Progression in frequency and intensity should warrant the same degree of concern as that for chest pain. A careful documentation of the patient's history may unmask features in the chest pain syndrome that point to noncardiac origins. Pain of extreme duration, lasting for many hours or days or, at the other end of the spectrum, a few seconds, is less likely to be ischemic in origin. Pain that is clearly pleuritic or positional or located with the tip of one finger is also unlikely to be cardiac in origin. The physician should document in the medical record whether there is a high, intermediate, or low likelihood of acute ischemia caused by coronary artery disease (Table 10.3).

The physical examination results are often unremarkable, with no abnormal findings of the pulse, blood pressure, chest, or cardiovascular system. It is very important that the examination be performed in a meticulous and structured manner, because it may elucidate noncardiac causes of chest pain (pleurisy, pneumothorax) and nonischemic causes of cardiac pain (valvular disease, pericarditis, and vascular emergencies). Serial examinations may uncover signs such as hypotension, bradycardia/tachycardia, pulmonary rales, a third heart sound, or a new or worsening murmur that are predictive of higher risk and mandate a more aggressive management (diagnostic and treatment) pathway (12).

HELPFUL TESTS

Electrocardiography

The electrocardiogram (ECG) is important for both diagnostic and risk stratification purposes. Specific characteristics and the magnitude of pattern abnormalities increase the likelihood of coronary artery disease. New or dynamic ST

TABLE 10.3. *Likelihood that signs and symptoms represent an acute coronary syndrome secondary to coronary artery disease*

Feature	High likelihood: any of the following	Intermediate likelihood: absence of high-likelihood features and presence of any of the following	Low likelihood: absence of high- or intermediate-likelihood features but may have
History	Chest or left arm pain or discomfort as chief symptom reproducing prior documented angina Known history of CAD, including MI	Chest or left arm pain or discomfort as chief symptom Age >70 years Male sex Diabetes mellitus	Probable ischemic symptoms in absence of any of the intermediate likelihood characteristics Recent cocaine use
Examination	Transient MR, hypotension, diaphoresis, pulmonary edema, or rales	Extracardiac vascular disease	Chest discomfort reproduced by palpation
ECG	New, or presumably new, transient ST segment deviation ($\geq$0.5 mm) or T wave inversion ($\geq$2 mm) with symptoms	Fixed Q waves Abnormal ST segments or T waves not documented to be new	T wave flattening or inversion in leads with dominant R waves Normal ECG
Cardiac markers	Elevated cardiac TnI, TnT, or CK-MB	Normal	Normal

CAD, coronary artery disease; CK-MB, creatine kinase and myocardial band fraction; ECG, electrocardiogram; MI, myocardial infarction; MR, mitral regurgitation; TnI, troponin I; TnT, troponin T.

From Braunwald E, Antman EM, Beasley JW, et al. ACC/AHA guidelines for the management of patients with unstable angina and non–ST-segment elevation myocardial infarction: a report of the American College of Cardiology/American Heart Association Task Force on Practice Guidelines (Committee on the Management of Patients with Unstable Angina). *J Am Coll Cardiol* 2000;36:970–1062.

segment depression (greater than 0.5 mm) is suggestive of acute ischemia with an associated prothrombotic state (13). Inverted T waves may also suggest ischemia or NSTEMI, although the risk is lower than that for ST segment depression. Nonspecific ST segment changes (less than 0.5 mm) and T wave changes (less than 2 mm) are much less helpful and may also be related to drugs (e.g., phenothiazines, digitalis), hyperventilation, or repolarization abnormalities in association with left ventricular hypertrophy or conduction disturbances. Conversely, the ECG may be normal in 1% to 6% of patients with NSTEMI and more than 4% of patients with UA (14).

In the Global Utilization of Streptokinase and Tissue Plasminogen Activator for Occluded Coronary Arteries (GUSTO) IIb trial, the 30-day incidence of death or MI was 5.5% in patients with T wave inversion, 9.4% in those with ST segment elevation, 10.5% in those with ST segment depression, and 12.4% in patients with ST elevation and depression (15). All these ECG findings may be transient phenomena, and this illustrates the importance of serial tracings. In fact, continu-ous ST segment monitoring may reveal episodes of otherwise undiagnosed ischemic episodes.

Biochemical Markers

Although many markers and assays that detect myocardial necrosis are available, the cardiac troponins T and I and the creatinine kinase and myocardial band fraction (CK-MB) isoform are the most commonly used; the troponins have gained acceptance as the markers of choice in ACS. They have achieved an important role in diagnostic, prognostic, and treatment pathways by virtue of their high degree of sensitivity and specificity and their relative ease of use and interpretation. According to the joint statement of the European Society of Cardiology and the American College of Cardiology, myonecrosis may be diagnosed when the maximal concentration of troponin T or I exceeds the decision limit (ninety-ninth percentile for a reference group) on at least one occasion in a 24-hour period (16). This new definition has increased the frequency of the NSTEMI diagnosis in patients with ACS by 30%. Troponin I yields more accurate findings with renal insufficiency. Both the troponins are detectable about 6 hours after myocardial injury and are measurable for up to 2 weeks. Mortality risk is directly proportional to troponin levels, and the prognostic information is independent of other clinical and electrocardiographic risk factors (17,18) (Fig. 10.1).

CK-MB is less specific, being also present in skeletal muscle and in low levels in the blood of healthy persons. Unlike troponins, it is useful in detected recurrent myocardial necrosis early after the initial event, inasmuch as levels tend to return to normal within 36 to 48 hours after initial release.

The role of increased inflammatory activity as an independent risk marker in ACS continues to elicit vigorous research interest. C-reactive protein levels in ACS appear to be related to long-term mortality in an independent and additive manner with troponin levels (19). The role of other inflammatory markers, such as amyloid A and interleukin-6, in the day-to-day management of patients with ACS is as yet undefined.

Elevated levels of fibrinogen, fibrinopeptide-A, and plasminogen activator inhibitor–1 have all been shown, albeit not consistently, to be related to an increased and independent risk of long-term events in patients with ACS (20–22). Again, these markers are not yet routinely used in clinical practice because their additive role is not yet defined.

Noninvasive Testing

Echocardiography allows for the rapid determination of left ventricular function. Stress testing to risk stratify (Table 10.4) should be performed in patients at low risk and intermediate risk who are free of complications and are not referred for coronary angiography (23). Choice of stress test is based on the resting ECG, ability to exercise, and local expertise. Treadmill testing is suitable for patients with good exercise tolerance in whom the ECG is free of ST segment abnormalities, bundle branch block, left ventricular hypertrophy, intraventricular conduction delay, paced rhythm, preexcitation, and digoxin

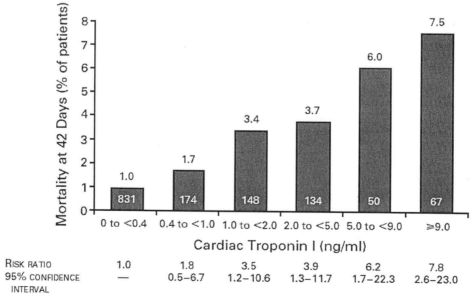

FIG. 10.1. Mortality rates at 42 days according to the level of cardiac troponin I measured at enrollment. (Adapted from Antman EM, Tanasijevic MJ, Thompson B, et al. Cardiac-specific troponin I levels to predict the risk of mortality in patients with acute coronary syndromes. *N Engl J Med* 1996;335:1342–1349.)

TABLE 10.4. *Noninvasive risk stratification*

High risk (>3% annual mortality rate)
1. Severe resting LV dysfunction (LVEF < 35%)
2. High-risk treadmill score (score ≤−11)
3. Severe exercise LV dysfunction (exercise LVEF < 35%)
4. Stress-induced large perfusion defect (particularly if anterior)
5. Stress-induced multiple perfusion defects of moderate size
6. Large, fixed perfusion defect with LV dilation or increased lung uptake (thallium 201)
7. Stress-induced moderate perfusion defect with LV dilation or increased lung uptake (thallium 201)
8. Echocardiographic wall motion abnormality (involving >2 segments) developing at a low dose of dobutamine ($\leq$10 mcg/kg^{-1}/min^{-1}) or at a low heart rate (<120 bpm)
9. Stress echocardiographic evidence of extensive ischemia

Intermediate risk (1%–3% annual mortality rate)
1. Mild/moderate resting LV dysfunction (LVEF 35%–49%)
2. Intermediate-risk treadmill score (−11 < score <5)
3. Stress-induced moderate perfusion defect without LV dilation or increased lung uptake (thallium 201)
4. Limited stress echocardiographic ischemia with a wall motion abnormality only at higher doses of dobutamine involving ≤2 segments

Low risk (<1% annual mortality rate)
1. Low-risk treadmill score (score ≥ 5)
2. Normal or small myocardial perfusion defect at rest or with stress
3. Normal stress echocardiographic wall motion or no change of limited resting wall motion abnormalities during stress

LV, left ventricular; LVEF, left ventricular ejection fraction.

From Braunwald E, Mark DB, Jones RH, et al. *Unstable angina: diagnosis and management*. Rockville, MD: Agency for Health Care Policy and Research and the National Heart, Lung, and Blood Institute, U.S. Public Health Service, U.S. Department of Health and Human Services, 1994:1; AHCPR Publication No 94-0602.

effect. Echocardiographic or nuclear stress imaging should be added for patients with ECG abnormalities that prevent accurate interpretation. Pharmacologic stress testing can be performed by patients who cannot achieve an adequate exercise stress on the treadmill.

Cardiac Catheterization

Cardiac catheterization defines regional and global left ventricular function, valvular function, and coronary artery anatomy. It is routinely performed 1 to 2 days after hospital admission in patients treated with the "early invasive strategy," which is directed toward immediate coronary revascularization. Alternatively, the "early conservative strategy" involves reserving cardiac catheterization for patients with recurrent angina who are receiving aggressive medical therapy or for those with ischemic stress test results. The test should not be performed in patients who are clearly not revascularization candidates, in those who do not want catheterization, or in those who are at low risk. Indications for cardiac catheterization are listed in Table 10.5 (24).

COMPLICATIONS

If left untreated, 5% to 10% of patients with UA die and 10% to 20% suffer nonfatal MI within 30 days. Of patients with NSTEMI, 25% develop Q wave MI; the remaining patients having non–Q wave MI. Arrhythmia, congestive heart failure, and cardiogenic shock are life-threatening complications. Recurrent ischemia may result in the need for urgent coronary artery revascularization. The Thrombolysis in Myocardial Infarction (TIMI) risk score (Fig. 10.2) (25) is one of a few prognostic tools (Table 10.6) (23) that has been shown to predict death, MI, and need for urgent revascularization.

DIFFERENTIAL DIAGNOSIS

Chest pain, the main manifestation of ACS, may be the manifestation of many nonischemic conditions. The rapid evaluation and treatment that is warranted for ACS should not be done at the expense of potentially missing an alternative condition that would warrant a significantly different approach and treatment.

Causes of nonischemic chest discomfort include: (a) musculoskeletal chest pain; (b) gastrointestinal discomfort (gastroesophageal reflux disease, peptic ulcer disease, biliary or pancreatic disease, or esophageal spasm); (c) cardiac nonischemic pain (valvular heart disease, hypertrophic cardiomyopathy, pulmonary hypertension, pericarditis); (d) pulmonary discomfort (pulmonary embolus, pneumothorax, pneumonia, exacerbation of chronic obstructive pulmonary disease); and (e) anxiety. This list is not meant to be exhaustive, but it demonstrates the spectrum of

TABLE 10.5. *American College of Cardiology/American Heart Association guidelines for invasive management of unstable angina non–ST segment elevation myocardial infarction*

Intervention	Class I	Class IIa	Class IIb	Class III
Cardiac catheterization	Recurrent angina at rest or with low activity Troponin positive New ST depression CHF High-risk stress test LVEF < 40% Hemodynamic instability Sustained VT PCI within 6 months Prior CABG In the absence of the above findings, either an invasive or a conservative strategy	Repeated ACS presentations without ischemia or high-risk features	—	Extensive comorbidities Low likelihood of ACS Unwilling to consent for revascularization
PCI	Two- to three-vessel CAD, normal LVEF, no DM One- to two-vessel CAD without proximal LAD, large area of viable myocardium	Focal SVG stenosis or poor candidate for repeat CABG One- to two-vessel CAD without proximal LAD, moderate area of viable myocardium One-vessel CAD, proximal LAD	Two- to three-vessel CAD, proximal LAD, DM or abnormal LVEF	One- to two-vessel CAD, no proximal LAD, no ischemia, mild or atypical symptoms Stenosis < 50%
CABG	Significant left main CAD Three-vessel CAD Two-vessel CAD with proximal LAD and LVEF < 50% or positive stress test One- to two-vessel CAD without proximal LAD, large area of viable myocardium One-vessel CAD, proximal LAD	Repeat CABG for multiple SVG stenoses Two- to three-vessel CAD, DM One- or two-vessel CAD without proximal LAD, moderate area of viable myocardium One-vessel CAD, proximal LAD	—	Left main, candidate for CABG One- to two-vessel CAD, no proximal LAD, no ischemia, mild or atypical symptoms Stenosis < 50%

ACS, acute coronary syndrome; CABG, coronary artery bypass graft surgery; CAD, coronary artery disease; CHF, congestive heart failure; DM, diabetes mellitus; LAD, left anterior descending artery; LVEF, left ventricular ejection fraction; PCI, percutaneous coronary intervention; SVG, saphenous vein graft; VT, ventricular tachycardia.

Adapted from Braunwald E, Antman EM, Beasley JW, et al. ACC/AHA guideline update for the management of patients with unstable angina and non–ST-segment elevation myocardial infarction. *J Am Coll Cardiol* 2002;40:1366.

Risk Factors

- Age $\geq$ 65y
- 3 CAD risk factors
- Stenosis $\geq$ 50%
- ST deviation
- Angina x3/24h
- ASA < 7 days
- Elevated Serum markers

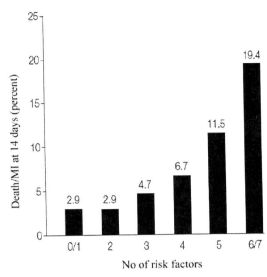

FIG. 10.2. Rates of all-cause mortality and myocardial infarction in the Thrombolysis in Myocardial Infarction (TIMI) 11B trial based on the TIMI risk score. (Adapted from Antman EM, Cohen M, Bernink PJLM, et al. The TIMI risk score for unstable angina/non-ST elevation MI. A method for prognostication and therapeutic decision making. *JAMA* 2000;284:835–842.)

conditions and underscores the importance of a rapid and accurate diagnosis (see Chapter 1).

THERAPY

UA results in more than 2 million hospital admissions per year, and NSTEMI accounts for more than 50% of all admissions for MI. The goals of an effective treatment strategy should be relief of ischemia and prevention of the serious adverse outcomes of MI or recurrent MI and death (Figs. 10.3, 10.4). These goals may be achieved by the initiation of appropriate therapy (Table 10.7), ongoing risk stratification, and selective coronary artery revascularization.

General Measures

Bed rest is strongly recommended in the presence of ongoing ischemia. When the patient is symptom free, mobility to a chair or bedside commode may be allowed. Supplemental oxygen, although widely used, appears to have no role when respiratory distress or hypoxemia (SaO_2 <90%) is absent and should be reserved for patients with cyanosis, respiratory distress, and high-risk fea-

tures. Continuous electrocardiographic monitoring for arrhythmias allows for the prompt detection and treatment of potentially fatal rhythm disorders. ST segment monitoring may have a role in detecting ongoing ischemia that may otherwise go undetected. Morphine sulfate has analgesic, anxiolytic, and hemodynamic effects that are beneficial in patients with persistent symptoms despite nitroglycerin.

Antiischemic Agents

Nitrates

Nitrates dilate venous capacitance vessels and peripheral arterioles, with a predominant decrease in preload and a lesser effect on afterload, thereby decreasing myocardial wall stress and oxygen demand. Nitrates also increase myocardial oxygen supply by dilating epicardial coronary arteries and increasing collateral flow. There are no placebo-controlled trials that address the effect of nitrates on symptom relief or reduction in cardiac events. In patients with signs and symptoms of ongoing ischemia after 3 sublingual nitroglycerin tablets in 10 minutes, intravenous

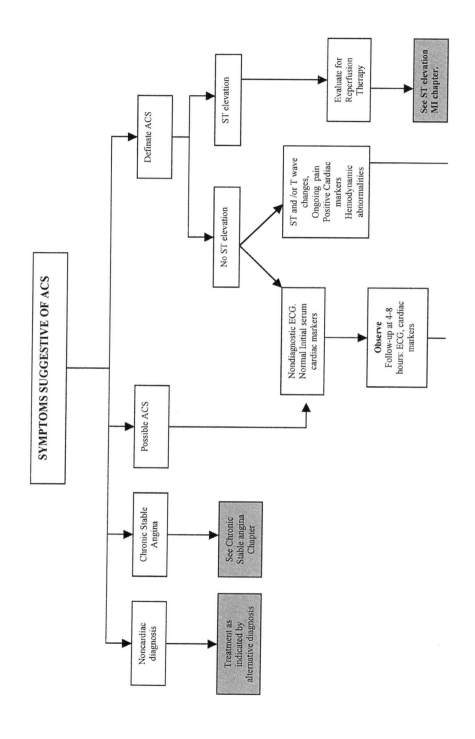

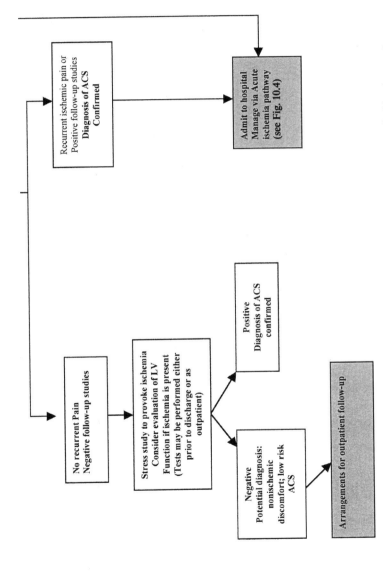

FIG. 10.3. Algorithm for the evaluation and management of patients suspected of having acute coronary syndrome. (Adapted from Braunwald E, Antman EM, Beasley JW, et al. ACC/AHA guideline update for the management of patients with unstable angina and non–ST-segment elevation myocardial infarction. *J Am Coll Cardiol* 2002;40:1366.)

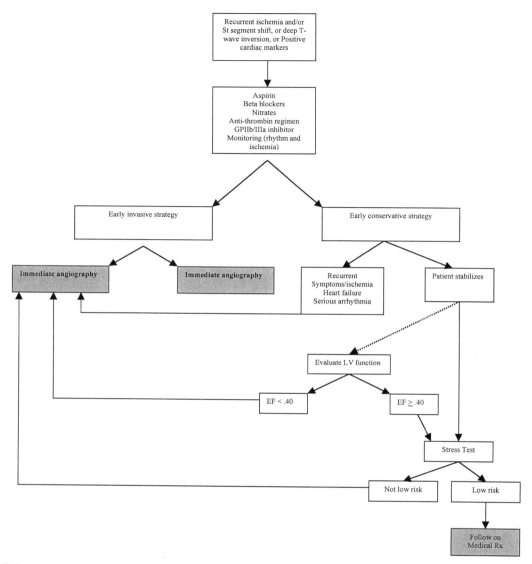

FIG. 10.4. Algorithm for the management of cardiac ischemia in patients admitted with acute coronary syndrome. (Adapted from Braunwald E, Antman EM, Beasley JW, et al. ACC/AHA guideline update for the management of patients with unstable angina and non-ST-segment elevation myocardial infarction. *J Am Coll Cardiol* 2002;40:1366.)

nitroglycerin should be started at $10\,\mu g$ per minute and increased every 3 to 5 minutes until ischemia is relieved or there is a significant drop in blood pressure (systolic blood pressure less than 110 mm Hg or more than a 25% decrease from starting) (Table 10.8). Because of the phenomenon of nitrate tolerance, the dose may have to be increased periodically. In patients without refractory symptoms, intravenous nitroglycerin should be converted to an oral or topical form within 24 hours, with nitrate-free periods to avoid tolerance. Use of sildenafil in the preceding 24-hour period represents a strong contraindication to the use of nitrates in any form.

TABLE 10.6. *Estimate of short-term risk of death or nonfatal myocardial infarction in patients with unstable angina*

Feature	High risk: At least one of the following features must be present	Intermediate risk: No high-risk feature but must have one of the following	Low risk: No high- or intermediate-risk feature but may have any of the following features
History	Accelerating tempo of ischemic symptoms in preceding 48 hr	Prior MI, peripheral or cerebrovascular disease, CABG, prior aspirin use	
Character of pain	Prolonged ongoing (>20 min) rest pain	Prolonged (>20 min) rest angina, now resolved, with moderate or high likelihood of CAD	New-onset CCS Class III or IV angina in the past 2 weeks without prolonged (>20 min) rest pain but with moderate or high likelihood of CAD
		Rest angina (<20 min) or relieved with rest or sublingual NTG	
Clinical findings	Pulmonary edema, most likely due to ischemia	Age >70 years	
	New or worsening MR murmur S_3, or new/worsening rales		
	Hypotension, bradycardia, tachycardia		
	Age >75 years		
ECG	Angina at rest with transient ST segment changes > 0.5 mm	T wave inversions > 2 mm Pathologic Q waves	Normal or unchanged ECG during an episode of chest discomfort
	Bundle branch block, new or presumed new		
	Sustained ventricular tachycardia		
Cardiac markers	Markedly elevated	Slightly elevated	Normal

CABG, coronary artery bypass graft; CAD, coronary artery disease; CCS, Canadian Cardiovascular Society; ECG, electrocardiogram; MI, myocardial infarction; MR, mitral regurgitation; NTG, nitroglycerin.
From Braunwald E, Antman EM, Beasley JM, et al. ACC/AHA guidelines for the management of patients with unstable angina and non–ST-segment elevation myocardial infarction: a report of the American College of Cardiology/American Heart Association Task Force on Practice Guidelines (Committee on the Management of Patients with Unstable Angina). *J Am Coll Cardiol* 2000;36:970–1062.

Beta Blockers

Beta blockers competitively inhibit beta₁ recep- tors, decreasing myocardial contractility, systolic blood pressure, sinus node rate, and atrioventric- ular node conduction velocity. This has the net effect of decreasing myocardial oxygen demand, shifting the oxygen supply-demand mismatch in favor of the ischemic myocardium. There are lim- ited clinical trial data on the use of beta blockers in UA and non–Q wave MI. A metaanalysis of three double-blind randomized trials suggested that beta blocker treatment was associated with a 13% relative reduction in the risk of progression to MI (26). There is no evidence of superior- ity for any member of this class over the others, although there is a general consensus that beta blockers with intrinsic sympathomimetic activ- ity should be avoided. In patients at high-risk, they are initially given intravenously and then orally. They are contraindicated in patients with asthma, severe conduction disturbances, conges- tive heart failure, bradycardia, or hypotension. When concern about patient tolerance is encoun- tered, short-acting intravenous esmolol should be used.

Calcium Channel Blockers

These agents variably produce vasodilation, a decrease in myocardial contractility, atrioven- tricular block, and sinus node slowing. Nifedip- ine, amlodipine, and felodipine have mostly

TABLE 10.7. *American College of Cardiology/American Heart Association guidelines for pharmacologic management of unstable angina/non–ST segment elevation myocardial infarction*

Therapy	Class I	Class IIA	Class IIB	Class III
Antiischemic	Bed rest Continuous ECG monitoring NTG for relief of symtoms O_2 for hypoxia MSO_4 for persistent pain, CHF, agitation Beta blocker Verapamil or diltiazem for recurrent pain if beta blocker contraindicated ACEI for CHF, HTN, DM	Long-acting Ca^{2+} blocker for recurrent pain after NTG/beta blocker ACEI IABP for recurrent angina on medical treatment	Verapamil or diltiazam instead of beta-blocker Nifedipine plus beta-blocker	NTG within 24 hours of sildenafil Nifedipine without beta blocker
Antiplatelet	ASA indefinitely Clopidogrel 1–9 months GP IIb/IIIa antagonists if PCI planned	Eptifibatide or tirofiban for persistent pain, (+) troponin, high risk if PCI not planned	Eptifibatide or tirofiban if no high risk features and PCI not planned	Fibrinolytic therapy Abciximab if PCI not planned
Anticoagulant	UFH or LMWH	Enoxaparin instead of UFH	—	—
Discharge	Sublingual NTG Drugs required in hospital to control symptoms if no revascularization ASA, 75–325 mg q.d. Clopidogrel, 75 mg orally q.d. for 9 mo Beta blocker Lipid-lowering drugs until LDL <100 mg/dL ACEI for CHF, LVEF < 40%	—	—	—

ACEI, angiotensin-converting enzyme inhibitor; ASA, aspirin; CHF, congestive heart failure; DM, diabetes mellitus; ECG, electrocardiogram; GP, glycoprotein; HTN, hypertension; IABP, intraaortic balloon pump; LDL, low-density lipoprotein; LMWH, low molecular weight heparin; LVEF, left ventricular ejection fraction; MSO_4, morphine sulphate; NTG, nitroglycerin; PCI, percutaneous coronary intervention; UFH, unfractionated heparin.
Adapted from Braunwald E, Antman EM, Beasley JW, et al. ACC/AHA guideline update for the management of patients with unstable angina and non–ST-segment elevation myocardial infarction. *J Am Coll Cardiol* 2002;40:1366.

vasodilatory properties, whereas verapamil and diltiazem have a greater effect on contractility and conduction. A metaanalysis of the use of this class in UA showed no effect on death and nonfatal MI (27). However, the mild benefit seen with diltiazem (28) and verapamil (29) was probably neutralized by the increased complications seen with short-acting nifedipine (30). Diltiazem and verapamil should not be used in patients with low ejection fractions or congestive heart failure, and nifedipine should not be used without a beta blocker. These agents may have added benefit in patients with coronary spasm, with recurrent ischemia during therapy with nitrates and beta blockers, with beta blocker intolerance, or with hypertension.

Antiplatelet Therapy

Aspirin

Aspirin, at doses ranging from 75 to 325 mg daily, irreversibly inhibits cyclooxygenase-1, blocking the formation of thromboxane A_2, thereby

TABLE 10.8. *Antiischemic agents*

Drug	Route	Dose
Nitrate		
Nitroglycerin	Sublingual tablets	0.3–0.6 mg up to 1.5 mg
	Spray	0.4 mg as needed
	Transdermal	0.2–0.8 mg/hr q12h
	Intravenous	10–200 mg/min
Isosorbide dinitrate	Oral	10–80 mg b.i.d. or t.i.d
Isosorbide mononitrate	Oral	30–240 mg q.d.
Beta blockers		
Propranolol	Oral	20–80 mg q.i.d.
Metoprolol	Intravenous	5 mg q5min three times
	Oral	50–200 mg b.i.d.
Atenolol	Intravenous	5 mg q5min two times
	Oral	50–200 mg q.d.
Esmolol	Intravenous	500 μg/kg over 1 min, repeated before each upward titration
		50 μg/kg infusion, increased by 50 μg/kg every 5 min up to 200 μg/kg/min
Calcium channel blockers		
Nifedipine-XL	Oral	30–180 mg
Amlodipine	Oral	5–10 mg q.d.
Diltiazem-CD	Oral	120–360 mg q.d.
Verapamil-SR	Oral	120–480 mg q.d.

reducing platelet aggregation (Table 10.9). When used in UA, it has repeatedly been shown to reduce the risk of cardiac death and nonfatal MI by approximately 50% (31–33). Consequently, aspirin is recommended for acute use in all patients with ACS and should be continued indefinitely, unless side effects are present. Contraindications to its use are allergy and active bleeding.

Thienopyridines

The thienopyridines, ticlopidine and clopidogrel, inhibit adenosine diphosphate–induced platelet aggregation. Ticlopidine used in the setting of UA decreased the rate of fatal and nonfatal MI by 46% in one study (34). The risk of neutropenia, thrombocytopenia, and gastrointestinal side effects has limited its use to short duration and

TABLE 10.9. *Antitrombotic agents*

Class	Drug	Route	Dose
Cyclooxygenase inhibitor	Aspirin	Oral	325 mg, then 81–325 mg q.d.
Thienopyridines	Clopidogrel	Oral	300 mg, then 75 mg q.d.
	Ticlopidine	Oral	500 mg, then 250 mg b.i.d.
Glycoprotein IIb/IIIa receptor antagonists	Abciximab	Intravenous	0.25 mg/kg bolus, then 0.125 μg/kg/min (max, 10 μg/min) for 12–24 hr
	Eptifibatide	Intravenous	180 μg/kg bolus, then 2 μg/kg/min up to 72 hr
	Tirofiban	Intravenous	0.4 μg/kg for 30 min, then 0.1 μg/kg/min up to 108 hr
Heparins	Heparin	Intravenous	60–70 U/kg (max, 5,000 U) bolus, then 12–15 U/kg/hr (max, 1,000 U/kg/hr) titrated to aPTT 1.5–2.5 times control
	Dalteparin	Subcutaneous	120 IU/kg (max, 10,000 IU) b.i.d.
	Enoxaparin	Subcutaneous	1 mg/kg b.i.d. (may start with 30-mg IV bolus)
Direct thrombin inhibitors	Bivalirudin	Intravenous	1 mg/kg bolus, then 2.5 mg/kg/hr for 4 hr, then 0.2 mg/kg/hr up to 20 hours if needed

aPTT, activated partial thromboplastin time; IV, intravenous.

to patients with aspirin intolerance. Clopidogrel has a faster onset of action and fewer side effects and has become the preferred thienopyridine. In the Clopidogrel in Unstable Angina to Prevent Ischemic Events (CURE) (35) trial, 12,562 patients with UA/NSTEMI were randomly assigned to receive aspirin alone or aspirin plus clopidogrel. There was a 20% reduction in the composite endpoint of cardiovascular death, MI, or stroke with only a slight increase in the risk of bleeding with combination antiplatelet therapy. Clopidogrel therapy is now recommended for 9 months after an ACS, in addition to aspirin (24).

Glycoprotein IIb/IIIa Inhibitors

The binding of fibrinogen to GP IIb/IIIa receptors on different platelets is the final event in platelet aggregation. GP IIb/IIIa antagonists occupy these receptors, preventing fibrinogen from cross-linking platelets and thereby prevent platelet aggregation. There are currently three intravenous agents approved for clinical use: abciximab, a monoclonal antibody; eptifibatide, a

cyclic heptapeptide; and tirofiban, a nonpeptide mimetic. These agents have been used both as medical therapy and as adjuncts to PCI. Three large studies using the different agents have each shown a significant early reduction in death and MI that was sustained at 30 days (36–38). According to a metaanalysis of the 12,296 patients enrolled in these studies, there was a 34% relative reduction in the rates of death or MI during a 24-hour period of medical management without revascularization (2.5% vs. 3.5%; $p = 0.001$) (39). This benefit is most pronounced in high-risk patients and is further amplified in such patients who underwent PCI as part of an early invasive strategy. In an overview of non–ST elevation ACS patients enrolled in PCI trials, the rates of death and MI at 30 days were reduced by 30% to 70% (Fig. 10.5). Tirofiban or eptifibatide should be administered, in addition to aspirin and heparin, to patients with continuing ischemia or high-risk features (Table 10.6) and to patients in whom PCI is planned. Abciximab is approved for patients with UA/NSTEMI in whom an early invasive strategy with PCI is planned within 12 hours (24).

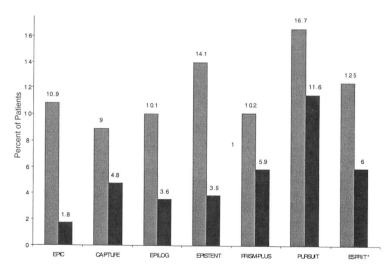

FIG. 10.5. Death and myocardial infarction at 30 days after percutaneous coronary intervention in patients with acute coronary syndrome: glycoprotein (GP) IIb/IIIa trials. ■, placebo; ■, GP IIb/IIIa inhibitor. (Adapted from Braunwald E, Antman EM, Beasley JW, et al. ACC/AHA guidelines for the management of patients with unstable angina and non–ST-segment elevation myocardial infarction: a report of the American College of Cardiology/American Heart Association Task Force on Practice Guidelines (Committee on the Management of Patients with Unstable Angina). *J Am Coll Cardiol* 2000;36:970–1062.)

Antithrombin Agents

Unfractionated Heparin

Heparin is a glycosaminoglycan made up of multiple different polysaccharide chain lengths with different anticoagulant activity. Antithrombin III, when bound to heparin, undergoes a conformational change that accelerates its inhibition of thrombin and factor Xa. Heparin also binds competitively to other plasma proteins (acute-phase reactants), blood cells, and endothelial cells that have varying concentrations, which thus affects its bioavailability. Another limitation of heparin is its lack of effect against clot-bound or platelet-rich thrombus and its degradation by platelet factor 4.

In a metaanalysis of six small trials in UA, the addition of unfractionated heparin to aspirin reduced risk by 33% in comparison with aspirin alone (40). Its beneficial effect does not appear to be sustained, which may be a result of reactivation of the disease process after its discontinuation.

Because of variable protein binding and bioavailability, patients receiving heparin therapy require frequent monitoring to ensure that a safe therapeutic range is maintained. The target activated partial thromboplastin time should be 1.5 to 2.5 times the control and should be checked every 6 hours after a dose change and every 24 hours after two consecutive therapeutic values. Serial platelet counts are also recommended to monitor for heparin-induced thrombocytopenia.

Low Molecular Weight Heparin

Low molecular weight heparin is prepared by depolymerization of the polysaccharide chains of heparin (41). The majority of chains contain fewer than 18 saccharide units and inactivate only factor Xa, in contrast to the longer chains, which inhibit both factor Xa and thrombin (factor IIa). This results in more potent inhibition of thrombin generation. In comparison with unfractionated heparin, low molecular weight heparin has lower plasma protein binding, greater bioavailability, more resistance to neutralization by platelet factor 4, greater release of tissue factor pathway in-

hibitor (TFPI), and a lower incidence of thrombocytopenia.

Dalteparin appears to be as effective as unfractionated heparin in UA/NSTEMI (42). Two trials with enoxaparin showed a 20% reduction in death or MI at 8, 14, and 43 days, in comparison with heparin (43). It is not clear whether the more favorable results with enoxaparin are attributable to different study populations, study design, dose regimens, drug properties, other unrecognized influences, or chance. The main advantages of these agents are the ease of subcutaneous administration and the absence of need for laboratory monitoring of activity.

Direct Thrombin Inhibitors

Direct thrombin inhibitors have the theoretical advantage over heparin of inhibiting clot-bound thrombin and not being inhibited by circulating plasma proteins and platelet factor 4 (44). The activated partial thromboplastin time can be used to monitor anticoagulation activity, but this is usually not necessary. Hirudin was shown in several trials to produce a small short-term reduction in death and MI, but bleeding was increased (45). Likewise, bivalirudin has shown efficacy, but, in contrast to hirudin, bleeding risk appears less than with unfractionated heparin. Bivalirudin is approved as a substitute for unfractionated heparin in patients with UA undergoing PCI. Hirudin or bivalirudin should be use in place of heparin in patients with heparin-induced thrombocytopenia.

Coronary Revascularization

Coronary artery revascularization is a treatment alternative to medical therapy in many patients (Table 10.5). Those with left main coronary artery disease or three-vessel disease, especially with left ventricular dysfunction, are often managed by coronary artery bypass graft (CABG) surgery, which has been shown to improve life expectancy and quality of life and to reduce readmissions (46). Despite improvements in surgical technique and myocardial preservation, morbidity and mortality rates are higher than with elective surgery; therefore, medical stabilization is strongly encouraged before proceeding to surgery. Technologic advances, high success rates, and low complication rates have increasingly made PCI a revascularization alternative, particularly in patients with preserved left ventricular function, one- or two-vessel disease, or contraindications for surgery (47). The decision to pursue an early conservative strategy versus an early invasive strategy aimed toward revascularization has been evaluated in six major trials (48–53). Although similar in scope, they differed in design and level of disease acuity. No difference in death or MI was seen in the first two studies (48,49). However, there was a large crossover rate from the conservative arms to the invasive arms, one study had an excessive CABG mortality rate, and GP IIb/IIIa antagonists and coronary stents were not utilized. Fragmin and Fast Revascularisation during InStability in Coronary artery disease (FRISC) II (50), TIMI-18 (51), VINO (52), and Randomized Intervention Treatment of Angina (RITA) III (53) represent more contemporary management of patients with UA/NSTEMI. In all four trials, an early invasive strategy was preceded by modern antiischemic and antithrombotic medications and was associated with a reduced risk of death, MI, and rehospitalization. The benefits were most significant in high-risk subsets (patients older than 65 years, those with positive findings of troponin, those with ST segment depression).

PROGNOSIS AND FOLLOW-UP

Newer treatments have improved the prognosis of these conditions, which were initially described as a predeath syndrome in the Ebers papyrus, around 2600 B.C. In patients with UA/NSTEMI, the greatest risk of progression to MI (or recurrent MI) and death is at the time of presentation and returns to the same level as in patients with stable angina at 2 months. Ongoing plaque instability and endothelial dysfunction persist for weeks as the healing process is taking place. There is also evidence of continued inflammation and a prothrombotic state. Many clinical and electrocardiographic features have been shown to increase the risk of death at 1 year, and they include persistent ST segment depression, congestive heart failure, advanced age, ST segment elevation, severe chronic obstructive pulmonary disease, positive troponin levels, prior CABG, renal insufficiency, and diabetes. In some studies, mental depression is also included as an independent risk factor for adverse events at 1 year.

Most patients are discharged on an antiischemic regimen that is similar to their inpatient regimen. The medications that are considered to have a Class I indication in the ACC/AHA guidelines for UA/NSTEMI are listed in Table 10.7.

After discharge, patients should be seen in the outpatient setting within 1 to 2 weeks. They should be reassessed for the need for cardiac catheterization and revascularization (54). Aggressive lifestyle and risk factor modification should be undertaken in all patients. The goals should be (a) tight glycemic control in diabetic patients (HbA$_{1c}$ less than 7.0); (b) hypertension control to a blood pressure of less than 130/85 mm Hg; (c) low-density lipoprotein cholesterol level less than 100 mg per deciliter; (d) smoking cessation; (e) initiation of a daily exercise program; (f) diet low in saturated fats; and (g) maintenance of optimal weight.

Patients with chronic coronary artery disease but no clinical events have a benign prognosis. Patients who develop UA/NSTEMI have sustained an important clinical event and need more aggressive long-term follow-up.

PRACTICAL POINTS

- The usual cause of UA/NSTEMI is atherosclerotic plaque disruption and nonocclusive thrombus formation.
- The history, physical examination, ECG, and troponin values provide critical information for early risk stratification.

- Initial pharmacotherapy should include aspirin, heparin or low molecular weight heparin, nitrates, and beta blockers. GP IIb/IIIa antagonists should be used in patients at high risk and those undergoing PCI.

(continued)

- An early invasive strategy should be followed in patients at high risk. Either an early conservative or an early invasive strategy can be followed for patients at intermediate or low risk.
- Coronary artery revascularization should be performed in appropriate candidates.
- Long-term pharmacotherapy should include aspirin, clopidogrel, beta blockers, lipid-lowering drugs if indicated, and an angiotensin-converting enzyme inhibitor if indicated.
- Aggressive risk factor control to goals should be pursued.

REFERENCES

1. Fuster V, Badimon JJ, Chesebro JH. The pathogenesis of coronary artery disease and the acute coronary syndromes. *N Engl J Med* 1992;326:242–250,310–318.
2. Fuster V, Lewis A. Conner Memorial Lecture. Mechanisms leading to myocardial infarction: insights from studies of vascular biology. *Circulation* 1994;90:2126–2146.
3. van der Wal AC, Becker AE, van der Loos CM, et al. Site of intimal plaque rupture or erosion of thrombosed coronary atherosclerotic plaques is characterized by an inflammatory process irrespective of the dominant plaque morphology. *Circulation* 1994;89:36–44.
4. Fernandez-Ortiz A, Badimon JJ, Falk E, et al. Characterization of the relative thrombogenicity of atherosclerotic plaque components: implications for consequences of plaque rupture. *J Am Coll Cardiol* 1994;23:1562–1569.
5. Little WC, Constantinescu M, Applegate RJ, et al. Can coronary angiography predict the site of a subsequent myocardial infarction in patients with mild-to-moderate coronary artery disease? *Circulation* 1988;78:1157–1166.
6. Coller BS. The role of platelets in arterial thrombosis and the rationale for the blockade of GPIIb/IIIa receptors as antithrombotic therapy. *Eur Heart J* 1995;16(Suppl L):11–15.
7. Moreno PR, Bernardi VH, Loez-Cuellar J, et al. Macrophages, smooth muscle cells, and tissue factor in unstable angina. Implications for cell-mediated thrombogenicity in acute coronary syndromes. *Circulation* 1996;94:3090–3097.
8. Ludmer PL, Selwyn AP, Shook TL, et al. Paradoxical vasoconstriction induced by acetylcholine in atherosclerotic coronary arteries. *N Engl J Med* 1986;315:1046–1051.
9. Willerson JT, Golino P, Eidt J, et al. Specific platelet mediators and unstable coronary artery lesions: experimental evidence and potential clinical implications. *Circulation* 1989;80:198–205.
10. Muller JE, Abela GS, Nesto RW, et al. Triggers, acute risk factors and vulnerable plaques: the lexicon of a new frontier. *J Am Coll Cardiol* 1994;23:809–813.
11. Braunwald E. Unstable angina: a classification. *Circulation* 1989;80:410–414.
12. Braunwald E, Mark DB, Jones RH, et al. *Unstable angina: diagnosis and management.* Rockville, MD: Agency for Health Care Policy and Research and the National Heart, Lung, and Blood Institute, U.S. Public Health Service, U.S. Department of Health and Human Services, 1994:1; AHCPR Publication No 94-0602.
13. Eisenberg PR, Kenzora JL, Sobel BE, et al. Relation between ST segment shifts during ischemia and thrombin activity in patients with unstable angina. *J Am Coll Cardiol* 1991;18:898–903.
14. Slater DK, Hlatky MA, Mark DB, et al. Outcome in suspected acute myocardial infarction with normal or minimally abnormal admission electrocardiographic findings. *Am J Cardiol* 1987;60:766–770.
15. Savonitto S, Ardissino D, Granger CB, et al. Prognostic value of the admission electrocardiogram in acute coronary syndromes. *JAMA* 1999;281:707–713.
16. The Joint European Society of Cardiology/American College of Cardiology Committee. Myocardial infarction redefined—a consensus statement of the Joint European Society of Cardiology/American College of Cardiology Committee for the redefinition of myocardial infarction. *J Am Coll Cardiol* 2000;36:959–969.
17. Lindahl B, Venge P, Wallentin L. Relation between troponin T and the risk of subsequent cardiac events in unstable coronary artery disease. *Circulation* 1993;96:1651–1657.
18. Antman EM, Tanasijevic MJ, Thompson B, et al. Cardiac-specific troponin I levels to predict the risk of mortality in patients with acute coronary syndromes. *N Engl J Med* 1996;335:1342–1349.
19. Morrow D, Rifai N, Antman E, et al. C-reactive protein is a potent predictor of mortality independently of and in combination with troponin T in acute coronary syndromes: a TIMI 11A substudy. *J Am Coll Cardiol* 1998;31:1460–1465.
20. Becker RC, Cannon CP, Bovill EG, et al. Prognostic value of plasma fibrinogen concentration in patients with unstable angina and non–Q-wave myocardial infarction (TIMI-IIIB Trial). *Am J Cardiol* 1996;78:142–147.
21. Ardissino D, Merlini PA, Gamba G, et al. Thrombin activity and early outcome in unstable angina pectoris. *Circulation* 1996;93:1634–1639.
22. Hamsten A, de Faire U, Walldius G. Plasminogen activator in plasma: risk factor for recurrent myocardial infarction. *Lancet* 1987;2:3–9.
23. Braunwald E, Antman EM, Beasley JW, et al. ACC/AHA guidelines for the management of patients with unstable angina and non–ST-segment elevation myocardial infarction: a report of the American College of Cardiology/American Heart Association Task Force on Practice Guidelines (Committee on the Management of Patients with Unstable Angina). *J Am Coll Cardiol* 2000;36:970–1062.
24. Braunwald E, Antman EM, Beasley JW, et al. ACC/AHA guideline update for the management of patients with unstable angina and non–ST-segment elevation

myocardial infarction. *J Am Coll Cardiol* 2002;40: 1366.

25. Antman EM, Cohen M, Bernink PJLM, et al. The TIMI risk score for unstable angina/non–ST elevation MI. A method for prognostication and therapeutic decision making. *JAMA* 2000;284:835–842.

26. Yusuf S, Wittes J, Friedman L. Overview of results of randomized clinical trials in heart disease: II. Unstable angina, heart failure, primary prevention with aspirin, and risk factor modification. *JAMA* 1988;260:2259–2263.

27. Held P, Yusuf S, Furberg CD. Calcium channel blockers in acute myocardial infarction and unstable angina: an overview. *BMJ* 1989;299:1187–1192.

28. Gibson RS, Boden WE, Theroux P, et al. Diltiazem and reinfarction in patients with non–Q-wave myocardial infarction: results of a double-blind, randomized, multicenter trial. *N Engl J Med* 1986;315:423–429.

29. Yusuf S, Held P, Furberg C. Update of effects of calcium antagonists in myocardial infarction or angina in light of the second Danish Verapamil Infarction Trial (DAVIT-II) and other recent studies. *Am J Cardiol* 1991;67:1295–1297.

30. The Holland Interuniversity Nifedipine/Metoprolol Trial (HINT) Research Group. Early treatment of unstable angina in the coronary care unit: a randomized, double blind, placebo controlled comparison of recurrent ischaemia in patients treated with nifedipine or metoprolol or both. *Br Heart J* 1986;56:400–413.

31. Lewis HD Jr, Davis JW, Archibald DG, et al. Protective effects of aspirin against acute myocardial infarction and death in men with unstable angina: results of a Veterans Administration Cooperative Study. *N Engl J Med* 1983;309:396–403.

32. Cairns JA, Gent M, Singer J, et al. Aspirin, sulfinpyrazone or both in unstable angina: results of a Canadian multicenter study. *N Engl J Med* 1985;313:1369–1375.

33. Theroux P, Ouimet H, McCans J, et al. Aspirin, heparin, or both to treat acute unstable angina. *N Engl J Med* 1988;319:1105–1111.

34. Balsano F, Rizzon P, Viola F, et al. Antiplatelet treatment with ticlopidine in unstable angina: a controlled multicenter clinical trial. The Studio della Ticlopidina nell'Angina Instabile Group. *Circulation* 1990;82:17–26.

35. Yusuf S, Zhao F, Mehta SR, et al. Effects of clopidogrel in addition to aspirin in patients with acute coronary syndromes without ST-segment elevation. *N Engl J Med* 2001;345:494–502.

36. The CAPTURE Investigators. Randomised placebo-controlled trial of abciximab before and during coronary intervention in refractory unstable angina: the CAPTURE Study. *Lancet* 1997;349:1429–1435.

37. Platelet Receptor Inhibition in Ischemic Syndromes Management in Patients Limited by Unstable Signs and Symptoms (PRISM-PLUS) Study Investigators. Inhibition of the platelet glycoprotein IIb/IIIa receptor with tirofiban in unstable angina and non–Q-wave myocardial infarction. *N Engl J Med* 1998;338:1488–1497.

38. The PURSUIT Trial Investigators. Inhibition of platelet glycoprotein IIb/IIIa with eptifibatide in patients with acute coronary syndromes. *N Engl J Med* 1998;339:436–443.

39. Boersma E, Akkerhuis KM, Theroux P, et al. Platelet glycoprotein IIb/IIIa receptor inhibition in non–ST-elevation acute coronary syndromes: early benefit during medical therapy only, with additional protection during percutaneous coronary intervention. *Circulation* 1999;100:2045–2048.

40. Oler A, Whooley MA, Oler J, et al. Adding heparin to aspirin reduces the incidence of myocardial infarction and death in patients with unstable angina. A meta-analysis. *JAMA* 1996;272:811–815.

41. Weitz JI. Low-molecular-weight heparins. *N Engl J Med* 1997;337:688–698.

42. Klein W, Buchwald A, Hillis SE, et al. Comparison of low-molecular weight heparin with unfractionated heparin acutely and with placebo for six weeks in the management of unstable coronary artery disease study. FRagmin In unstable Coronary artery disease study (FRIC). *Circulation* 1997;96:61–68.

43. Antman EM, Cohen M, Radley D, et al. Assessment of the treatment effect of enoxaparin for unstable angina/non–Q-wave myocardial infarction: TIMI-11B–ESSENCE meta-analysis. *Circulation* 1999;100:1602–1608.

44. Bates ER. Bivalirudin for percutaneous coronary intervention and in acute coronary syndromes. *Curr Cardiol Rep* 2001;3:348–354.

45. The Direct Thrombin Inhibitor Trialists' Collaborative Group. Direct thrombin inhibitors in acute coronary syndromes: principal results of a meta-analysis based on individual patients' data. *Lancet* 2002;359:294–302.

46. Yusuf S, Zucker D, Peduzzi P et al. Effects of coronary artery bypass graft surgery on survival: overview of 10-year results from randomized trials by the Coronary Artery Bypass Graft Surgery Trialists Collaboration. *Lancet* 1994;344:563–570.

47. Morisson DA, Sethi G, Sacks J, et al. Percutaneous coronary intervention versus coronary artery bypass graft surgery for patients with medically refractory myocardial ischemia and risk factors for adverse outcomes with bypass: a multicenter, randomized trial. *J Am Coll Cardiol* 2001;38:143–149.

48. The TIMI IIIB Investigators. Effects of tissue plasminogen activator and a comparison of early invasive and conservative strategies in unstable angina and non–Q-wave myocardial infarction. Results of the TIMI IIIB trial. *Circulation* 1994;89:1545–1556.

49. Boden WE, O'Rourke RA, Crawford MH, et al. Outcomes in patients with acute non–Q-wave myocardial infarction randomly assigned to an invasive as compared with a conservative management strategy. *New Engl J Med* 1998;338:1785–1792.

50. FRagmin and Fast Revascularisation during InStability in Coronary artery disease (FRISC II) Investigators. Invasive compared with non-invasive treatment in unstable coronary-artery disease: FRISC II prospective randomised multicentre study. *Lancet* 1999;354:708–715.

51. Cannon CP, Weintraub WS, Demopoulos L, et al. A comparison of early invasive versus conservative strategies in patients with unstable coronary syndromes treated with the glycoprotein IIb/IIIa inhibitor tirofiban. *N Engl J Med* 2001;344:1879–1887.

52. Spacek R, Widimsky P, Straka E, et al. Value of first

day angiography/angioplasty in evolving non–ST segment elevation myocardial infarction: an open multicentre randomized trial: the VINO study. *Eur Heart J* 2002;23:230–238.

53. Fox KAA, Poole-Wilson PA, Henderson RA, et al. Interventional versus conservative treatment for patients with unstable angina or non–ST-elevation myocardial infarction: the British Heart Foundation RITA 3 randomised trial. *Lancet* 2002;360:743–751.

54. Stone PH, Thompson B, Zaret BL, et al. Factors associated with failure of medical therapy in patients with unstable angina and non–Q wave myocardial infarction: a TIMI-IIIb database study. *Eur Heart J* 1999;20:1084–1093.

11

Acute ST Elevation Myocardial Infarction

Debabrata Mukherjee and Eric R. Bates

Acute myocardial infarction (AMI) remains a major public health issue and is the leading cause of death in the United States. The American Heart Association estimated that in the year 2001, 1,100,000 Americans would have a myocardial infarction (MI) (1). About 650,000 of these would be first attacks and 450,000 would be recurrent attacks.

USUAL CAUSES

Atherosclerotic coronary artery disease and plaque rupture with resultant thrombosis remains the most common cause of AMI (2). Other, less common causes include arteritis, trauma, embolization, congenital anomalies, hypercoagulable states, and substance abuse. Table 11.1 lists a number of pathologic processes other than atherosclerosis that may cause AMI (3).

PRESENTING SYMPTOMS AND SIGNS

History

A well-documented history is extremely important in establishing the diagnosis of AMI. The classic symptom is crushing retrosternal chest discomfort with radiation to the left arm (4). Some individuals may present with epigastric pain, which can lead to the misdiagnosis of heartburn or another abdominal disorder. Elderly individuals may not have any chest discomfort but may present with symptoms of left ventricular failure, marked weakness, or syncope (5). Postoperative patients and diabetic patients are other subgroups that may not experience classic symptoms with AMI. Patients may also present with neck, jaw, back, shoulder, or right arm pain as the sole manifestation. Other associated symptoms include diaphoresis, dysp-

nea, fatigue, weakness, dizziness, palpitations, acute confusion, nausea, or emesis. Nausea and emesis are seen more frequently with inferior wall MI.

Physical Examination

Physical examination is more important in excluding other diagnoses and in risk-stratifying patients rather than in establishing the diagnosis of AMI. Patients presenting with AMI often appear anxious and in distress. A fourth heart sound is almost universally present in patients who are in sinus rhythm. All patients should have a thorough cardiac examination as a baseline to monitor for mechanical complications that may develop. Systolic blood pressure, heart rate, rales, and a third heart sound are important prognostic determinants, besides age, in patients with AMI (6,7). A thorough baseline neurologic examination is also important.

HELPFUL TESTS

Electrocardiography

The electrocardiographic diagnosis of AMI requires at least 1 mm of acute ST segment elevation in two or more contiguous leads. The presence of prior left bundle branch block may confound the diagnosis of AMI, but striking ST segment deviation that cannot be explained merely by conduction abnormality is suggestive of AMI. Sgarbossa et al. (8) validated three electrocardiographic criteria with independent value in the diagnosis of AMI in patients with left bundle branch block: ST segment elevation of 1 mm or more that was concordant with (in the same direction as) the QRS complex; ST segment depression of 1 mm or more in lead V_1, V_2, or V_3;

TABLE 11.1. *Nonatherosclerotic causes of acute myocardial infarction*

Arteritis
  Takayasu's disease
  Polyarteritis nodosa
  Mucocutaneous lymph node (Kawasaki's) syndrome
  Systemic lupus erythematosus
  Rheumatoid arthritis
  Ankylosing spondylitis
Trauma to coronary arteries
Metabolic diseases with coronary artery involvement
  Mucopolysaccharidoses (Hurler's syndrome)
  Homocystinuria
  Fabry's disease
  Amyloidosis
Luminal narrowing by other mechanisms
  Spasm
  Dissection of the aorta extending into coronary
    artery
Emboli to coronary arteries
  Infective endocarditis
  Nonbacterial thrombotic endocarditis
  Prosthetic valve emboli
  Cardiac myxoma
  Paradoxical emboli
  Papillary fibroelastoma of the aortic valve
Congenital anomalies
  Anomalous origin of the left coronary from the pul-
    monary artery
  Left coronary from anterior sinus of Valsalva
Miscellaneous
  Carbon monoxide poisoning
  Polycythemia vera
  Thrombocytosis
  Cocaine abuse

Adapted from Cheitlin MD, McAllister HA, de Castro CM. Myocardial infarction without atherosclerosis. *JAMA* 1975;231:951–959.

TABLE 11.2. *Biochemical markers for detecting myocardial necrosis*

1. Any elevation of troponin T or I during the first 24 hr after the index clinical event
2. Any elevation of CK-MB in two sequential samples
3. CK-MB twice upper reference limit at any time
4. CK-MB should rise and fall, stable elevated values are never due to MI
5. CK twice upper reference limit (less satisfactory)

CK, creatine kinase, MB, muscle band; MI, myocardial infarction.

Adapted from Tunstall-Pedoe H, Kuulasmaa K, Amouyel P, et al. Myocardial infarction and coronary deaths in the World Health Organization MONICA Project. Registration procedures, event rates, and case-fatality rates in 38 populations from 21 countries in four continents. *Circulation* 1994;90:583–612.

and ST segment elevation of 5 mm or more that was discordant with (in the opposite direction from) the QRS complex. The electrocardiogram (ECG) also remains a valuable clinical tool for the localization of AMI (9).

Cardiac Markers

The World Health Organisation (WHO) criteria for the diagnosis of AMI requires at least two of the following three elements: (a) history of typical chest discomfort, (b) electrocardiographic changes consistent with AMI, and (c) rise and fall in serum cardiac markers (10). The serum cardiac markers that are used in the diagnosis of AMI include creatine kinase (CK), creatine kinase–myocardial band fraction isoenzyme

(CK-MB), cardiac-specific troponins, and myoglobin. The American College of Cardiology and the European Society of Cardiology redefined the diagnosis of MI to include any elevation of serum cardiac markers (Table 11.2) (11). Both CK-MB and troponin should be measured in all patients; the examiner should not rely solely on troponin, because it interferes with the ability to diagnose recurrent infarction.

Echocardiography

The portability of echocardiography makes this a valuable clinical tool in the assessment of patients with AMI. This technique can be useful for confirming or excluding the diagnosis of AMI (12) and to help with risk stratification (13). The echocardiogram is very useful in diagnosing the mechanical complications of AMI.

DIFFERENTIAL DIAGNOSIS

Pericarditis

Pericardial pain is usually aggravated by inspiration and lying supine. It is important to distinguish pericarditis from AMI because inadvertent fibrinolysis in patients with pericarditis may lead to hemopericardium. The ST changes in pericarditis are diffuse, with a concave upward slope. Other important diagnostic features include PR segment depression and absence of reciprocal ST segment depression.

Myocarditis

Symptoms and signs of myocarditis may closely mimic those of AMI. A thorough history may be helpful if it reveals a more gradual onset of symptoms and prior upper respiratory tract symptoms in a relatively young patient. Serum cardiac markers usually remain elevated rather than peaking and returning to baseline levels.

Aortic Dissection

The pain due to an acute aortic dissection is typically central, extremely severe, and often described by the patient as a tearing sensation. The pain is maximal at onset and persists for many hours. It is extremely important to diagnose this condition because fibrinolytic therapy usually results in death. Chest radiography often shows a widened mediastinum. A transthoracic echocardiogram may show an intimal flap in the proximal aorta. If the echocardiogram is nondiagnostic and dissection is still a clinical possibility, the patient should undergo more definitive testing in the form of computed tomography, magnetic resonance imaging, or transesophageal echocardiography.

Hypertrophic Cardiomyopathy

Patients with hypertrophic cardiomyopathy may present with chest discomfort similar to angina, related to increased myocardial oxygen demand. Transthoracic echocardiography is a useful test for diagnosing this condition. Use of nitroglycerin or dobutamine may precipitate hypotension and syncope in affected patients.

Pulmonary Embolism

Chest pain associated with severe shortness of breath without clinical or radiographic evidence of pulmonary edema should suggest pulmonary embolism. Echocardiography may be useful by demonstrating normal left ventricular wall motion and right ventricular dilatation and strain. Patients with pneumothorax and pleuritis may also present with substernal chest discomfort, but the character of the pain is different, and the pain is often worse with inspiration.

Cholecystitis

Patients with inferior AMI may present with epigastric or right upper quadrant pain that may mimic acute cholecystitis. Conversely, patients with acute cholecystitis may present with symptoms and occasionally ECG findings suggestive of an inferior AMI. The presence of fever, marked leukocytosis, and right upper quadrant tenderness favor the diagnosis of cholecystitis. Esophageal and other upper gastrointestinal symptoms may also mimic ischemic chest discomfort.

Costochondritis

Pain associated with costochondritis is usually associated with localized swelling and redness, and the character of the pain is usually sharp with marked focal tenderness.

Hyperventilation

Patients with panic attacks may present with chest discomfort that closely simulates angina. A thorough history is very useful for diagnosing this condition.

COMPLICATIONS

Sudden cardiac death before hospital admission is the most common cause of mortality in AMI. Inhospital mortality is primarily due to circulatory failure resulting from either severe left ventricular dysfunction or one of the mechanical complications. The complications of AMI may be broadly classified as mechanical, electrical, ischemic, embolic, and pericardial.

Mechanical

Cardiac Rupture

Ventricular septal rupture, papillary muscle rupture, and free wall rupture are serious, life-threatening mechanical complications of AMI. Reperfusion therapy has reduced the overall incidence of cardiac rupture and shifted its occurrence to earlier after AMI.

Ventricular septal rupture occurs in 0.5% to 2% of patients (14). The diagnosis should be suspected when a pansystolic murmur develops that was not present initially. Echocardiography with color flow imaging is the test of choice for diagnosing a ventricular septal rupture. Pulmonary artery catheterization with oximetry is also a useful diagnostic aid. This involves measuring oxygen saturations in the superior and inferior venae cavae, right atrium, right ventricle, and pulmonary artery under fluoroscopy. An intraaortic balloon pump (IABP) should be inserted as early as possible as a bridge to surgery, unless there is significant aortic regurgitation. This decreases systemic vascular resistance, decreases shunt fraction, increases coronary perfusion, and maintains blood pressure. After insertion of IABP, vasodilators can be used with close hemodynamic monitoring. Surgical closure is the treatment of choice.

Most mitral regurgitation associated with AMI is transient, asymptomatic, and benign. However, severe mitral regurgitation due to papillary muscle rupture is a life-threatening but treatable complication of AMI that contributes to 5% of the cases of mortality after AMI. The overall incidence of papillary muscle rupture is 1%. Papillary muscle rupture is more common with an inferior MI and involves the posteromedial papillary muscle because its blood supply is solely via the posterior descending artery. In contrast, the anterolateral papillary muscle is perfused by both the left anterior descending and the left circumflex arteries. Complete transection of the papillary muscles is rare and usually results in immediate shock and death. Patients with rupture of one or more papillary muscle heads typically present with sudden severe respiratory distress from development of pulmonary edema and may rapidly develop cardiogenic shock. A new pansystolic murmur is audible at the cardiac apex with radiation to the axilla or to the base of the heart. In posterior papillary muscle rupture, the murmur radiates up the left sternal border and may be confused with the murmur of ventricular septal rupture or aortic stenosis. Two-dimensional echocardiography, with Doppler and color flow imaging, is the diagnostic modality of choice. Hemodynamic monitoring with a pulmonary artery catheter may reveal large V waves in the pulmonary capillary wedge pressure (PCWP) tracing. Vasodilator

and IABP therapy are very important in patients with acute severe mitral regurgitation. IABP decreases left ventricular afterload, improves coronary perfusion, and increases forward cardiac output. Surgical therapy should be considered immediately in patients with papillary muscle rupture. The prognosis is very poor in patients treated medically, and even though perioperative mortality (20% to 25%) is higher than for elective surgery, surgical repair should be considered in every patient.

Cardiac free wall rupture occurs in 3% of patients and accounts for about 10% of cases of AMI mortality. Advanced age, female gender, hypertension, first AMI, and poor coronary collateral vessels are risk factors for free wall rupture. Free wall rupture constitutes part of the "early hazard" in patients treated with fibrinolytics (the mortality rate among patients who receive fibrinolytics is actually higher for the first 24 hours and is attributable partially to cardiac rupture). Emergency thoracotomy with surgical repair is the definitive therapy and may save a few patients who can be taken to surgery immediately. Pseudoaneurysm results from a contained rupture of the left ventricular free wall by the pericardium and mural thrombus. Pseudoaneurysms communicate with the body of the left ventricle through a narrow neck, the diameter of the neck being less than 50% of the diameter of the fundus. Spontaneous rupture occurs without warning in approximately one third of these patients; therefore, surgical resection is recommended for both symptomatic and asymptomatic patients, irrespective of the size of the aneurysm.

Left Ventricular Failure and Cardiogenic Shock

The severity of left ventricular dysfunction correlates with the extent of myocardial injury. Patients with a small AMI may have regional wall motion abnormalities but overall normal left ventricular function because of compensatory hyperkinesia of the nonaffected segments. Killip and Kimball (6) classified four subsets of patients on the basis of clinical presentation and physical findings at the onset of AMI (Table 11.3). More recently, in comparison with the 81% mortality in their original paper (6), the 30-day mortality rate

TABLE 11.3. *30-day mortality based on Killip class*

Killip class	Physical findings	Mortality (inhospital)
Class I	Clear lungs, no S3 gallop	6%
Class II	Basal rales and/or S3 gallop	17%
Class III	Pulmonary edema	38%
Class IV	Cardiogenic shock	81%

Adapted from Killip T 3rd, Kimball JT. Treatment of myocardial infarction in a coronary care unit. A two year experience with 250 patients. *Am J Cardiol* 1967;20:457–464.

was 58% among patients in the Global Utilization of Streptokinase and Tissue Plasminogen Activator for Occluded Coronary Arteries (GUSTO) I trial (15) who presented with cardiogenic shock and who were treated with fibrinolytics. An IABP should be inserted as soon as possible in a patient with cardiogenic shock. In the SHould we emergently revascularize Occluded Coronaries for cardiogenic shocK? (SHOCK) trial (16), patients with cardiogenic shock were randomly assigned to undergo emergency revascularization ($n = 152$) or initial medical stabilization ($n = 150$). The rates of overall mortality at 30 days did not differ significantly between the revascularization and medical therapy groups because of sample size (46.7% vs. 56.0%; difference, 9.3%; 95% confidence interval, 20.5% to 1.9%; $p = 0.11$). However, the 6-month mortality rate was significantly lower among the patients who underwent revascularization than in those receiving medical therapy (50.3% vs. 63.1%; $p = 0.027$). Therefore, emergency revascularization should be strongly considered for patients with AMI complicated by cardiogenic shock.

Right Ventricular Failure

Mild right ventricular dysfunction is common after inferior MI, but hemodynamically significant right ventricular impairment is seen in only 10% of patients. Right ventricular involvement depends on the location of the right coronary artery occlusion; significant dysfunction is noted only if occlusion is proximal to a large acute marginal branch. The triad of hypotension, jugular venous distention, and clear lungs is very specific but has poor sensitivity for right ventricular infarction. Patients with severe right ventricular failure have symptoms of low cardiac output. These include diaphoresis, clammy extremities, and altered mental status. Patients are often oliguric and hypotensive. The ECG usually shows an inferior MI. ST elevation in V4R in the setting of suspected right ventricular infarction has a positive predictive value of 80%. Hemodynamic monitoring with a pulmonary artery catheter usually reveals high right atrial (RA) pressures relative to the PCWP. Acute right ventricular failure results in underfilling of the left ventricle and a low cardiac output state. A RA pressure higher than 10 mm Hg and a RA/PCWP ratio of 0.8 or higher are strongly suggestive of right ventricular infarction (17). Treatment of right ventricular infarction involves volume loading, inotropic support with dobutamine, and maintenance of atrioventricular synchrony. Patients who undergo successful reperfusion of the right coronary artery and the right ventricular branches have improved right ventricular function and decreased 30-day mortality rates (18).

Left Ventricular Aneurysm

An acute aneurysm expands in systole, wasting contractile energy generated by the normal myocardium. Chronic true aneurysms develop in 10% of patients after AMI and are more commonly seen after anterior AMI. Chronic aneurysms are defined as those persisting more than 6 weeks after AMI. Patients with acute aneurysms may present with heart failure and even cardiogenic shock. Patients with chronic aneurysms may present with heart failure, ventricular arrhythmias, and systemic embolism, or they may be asymptomatic. Heart failure with acute aneurysms is treated with intravenous vasodilators and IABP. Anticoagulation with warfarin (Coumadin) is indicated for patients with mural thrombus. In patients with refractory heart failure or refractory ventricular arrhythmias, surgical resection of the aneurysm should be considered. Revascularization may be beneficial in patients with a large amount of viable myocardium in the aneurysmal segment.

Electrical Complications of Acute Myocardial Infarction

Arrhythmias are the most common complications after AMI, affecting approximately 90% of patients. Conduction abnormalities causing hypotension may necessitate temporary or permanent pacemaker therapy. These are briefly summarized in Table 11.4.

Ischemic Complications of Acute Myocardial Infarction

Infarct extension is a progressive increase in the amount of myocardial necrosis within the same arterial territory as the original AMI. This may manifest as a subendocardial AMI extending to a transmural AMI or as AMI that extends and involves the adjacent myocardium. Recurrent angina within a few hours to 30 days after an acute AMI is defined as postinfarction angina. The incidence is between 23% and 60%. The frequency of postinfarction angina is higher after non–Q wave MI and fibrinolytic therapy than after primary PCI. Patients with postinfarction angina have an increased incidence of sudden death, reinfarction, and acute cardiac events. Either percutaneous or surgical revascularization improves prognosis in these patients. Infarction in a separate territory may be difficult to diagnose in the first 24 to 48 hours after the initial event. It may be very difficult to differentiate ECG changes of reinfarction from the evolving ECG changes of the index MI. Recurrent elevations in CK-MB after normalization or to more than 50% of the prior value are diagnostic for reinfarction. Echocardiography may also be useful by revealing a wall motion abnormality in a new area.

Embolic Complications of Acute Myocardial Infarction

The incidence of clinically evident systemic embolism after AMI is approximately 2%; the incidence is higher in patients with anterior AMI. The overall incidence of mural thrombus after AMI is approximately 20%. Large anterior MIs may be accompanied by associated mural thrombus in 60% of patients. Patients with large anterior MI or mural thrombi should be treated with intravenous heparin for 3 to 4 days with a target partial thromboplastin time of 50 to 70 seconds. Oral therapy with warfarin should be continued for at least 3 months in patients with mural thrombi and in those with large akinetic areas detected by echocardiography.

Pericarditis

The incidence of early pericarditis after AMI is approximately 10%, and it usually develops within 24 to 96 hours (19). Patients complain of progressive, severe chest pain that lasts for hours. The pain is postural, worse with lying supine, alleviated if the patient sits up and leans forward, usually pleuritic in nature, and worsened with deep inspiration, coughing, and swallowing. Radiation to the trapezius ridge is nearly pathognomonic for acute pericarditis and is not seen in patients with ischemic pain. Postinfarction pericarditis is treated with aspirin in doses of 650 mg every 4 to 6 hours. Nonsteroidal anti-inflammatory agents and corticosteroids should not be administered to these patients because they may interfere with myocardial healing and contribute to infarct expansion (20). Colchicine may be beneficial in patients with recurrent pericarditis. Dressler's syndrome (post-MI syndrome) occurs in 1% and 3% of patients and is seen 1 to 8 weeks after AMI. Patients present with chest discomfort suggestive of pericarditis, fever, arthralgia, malaise, elevated leukocyte count, and elevated erythrocyte sedimentation rate. Treatment is similar to that for early postinfarction pericarditis.

THERAPY

A general treatment algorithm (21) is outlined in Fig. 11.1. Initial diagnostic and treatment measures are listed in Table 11.5. One of the most important goals is to quickly select appropriate patients for reperfusion therapy with either fibrinolytic therapy or coronary angioplasty. The National Heart Attack Alert Program Coordinating Committee (22) set a 30-minute target time within which diagnosis is to be completed and

TABLE 11.4. *Electrical complications of acute myocardial infarction and their management*

Category	Arrhythmia	Objective	Treatment
1. Electrical instability	Ventricular premature beats	Correction of electrolyte deficits and increased sympathetic tone	Potassium and magnesium replacement, beta blockers
	Ventricular tachycardia	Prophylaxis against ventricular fibrillation, restoration of hemodynamic stability	Antiarrhythmic agents; cardioversion
	Ventricular fibrillation	Urgent reversion to sinus rhythm	Defibrillation
	Accelerated idioventricular rhythm	Observation unless hemodynamic function is compromised	Increase sinus rate (atropine, atrial pacing); antiarrhythmic agents
	Nonparoxysmal atrioventricular junctional tachycardia	Search for precipitating causes (e.g., digitalis intoxication); suppress arrhythmia only if hemodynamic function is compromised	Atrial overdrive pacing; antiarrhythmic agents; cardioversion relatively contraindicated if digitalis intoxication present
2. Pump failure/excessive sympathetic stimulation	Sinus tachycardia	Reduce heart rate to diminish myocardial oxygen demands	Antipyretics; analgesics; consider beta blocker unless congestive heart failure present; treat latter with diuretics and afterload reduction
	Atrial fibrillation and/or atrial flutter	Control ventricular rate; restore sinus rhythm	Diltiazem, verapamil, digitalis; anticongestive measures (diuretics, afterload reduction); cardioversion; rapid atrial pacing (for atrial flutter)
	Paroxysmal supraventricular tachycardia	Reduce ventricular rate; restore sinus rhythm	Vagal maneuvers; verapamil, digitalis, beta-adrenergic blockers; cardioversion; rapid atrial pacing
3. Bradyarrhythmias and conduction disturbances	Sinus bradycardia	Acceleration of heart rate only if hemodynamic function is compromised	Atropine; atrial pacing
	Junctional escape rhythm	Acceleration of sinus rate only if loss of atrial "kick" causes hemodynamic compromise	Atropine; atrial pacing
	Atrioventricular block and intraventricular block	—	Ventricular pacing

Adapted from Ryan TJ, Anderson JL, Antman EM, et al. ACC/AHA guidelines for the management of patients with acute myocardial infarction: a report of the American College of Cardiology/American Heart Association Task Force on Practice Guidelines (Committee on Management of Acute Myocardial Infarction). *J Am Coll Cardiol* 1996;28:1328–1428.

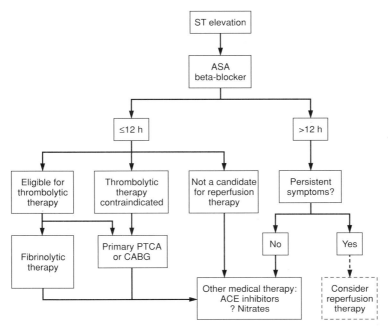

FIG. 11.1. General treatment algorithm. All patients with ST segment elevation on the electrocardiogram should receive aspirin, beta blockers, and heparin (unless receiving streptokinase). Eligible patients evaluated within 12 hours should be expeditiously treated with one of the currently available fibrinolytic agents [recombinant tissue plasminogen activator (rt-PA), recombinant plasminogen activator (rPA), tenecteplase–tissue plasminogen activator (TNK-tPA), streptokinase (SK)] or be considered for primary percutaneous coronary intervention (PCI). Primary PCI should also be considered when fibrinolytic therapy is absolutely contraindicated and in patients with cardiogenic shock. Individuals treated after 12 hours should receive medical therapy and, on an individual basis, may be considered for reperfusion therapy or angiotensin-converting enzyme inhibitors (particularly if left ventricular systolic function is impaired). (Adapted from Ryan TJ, Anderson JL, Antman EM, et al. ACC/AHA guidelines for the management of patients with acute myocardial infarction: a report of the American College of Cardiology/American Heart Association Task Force on Practice Guidelines (Committee on Management of Acute Myocardial Infarction). *J Am Coll Cardiol* 1996;28:1328–1428.)

suitable candidates are to be given fibrinolytic therapy. The committee divided the treatment delay period into four time points ("the four Ds"): arrival and triage in the emergency department (door), obtaining an ECG (data), deciding to administer fibrinolytic therapy (decision), and initiating the fibrinolytic infusion (drug). The target time for angioplasty is less than 90 minutes (23). A worksheet documenting the precise timing of these events should be completed and used as part of the continuous quality improvement program to improve efficiency.

Patients with more than 1-mm ST segment elevation in two or more contiguous leads or new left bundle branch block within 12 hours of symp-

tom onset should be administered one of the currently available fibrinolytic agents (Table 11.6) if they do not have a contraindication (Table 11.7) (21,23). Fibrinolytic therapy has been a major advance in the management of AMI (24). However, it continues to be underused or administered later than is optimal. Fibrinolysis works by dissolving infarct artery thrombus and restoring myocardial perfusion, thereby reducing infarct size, preserving left ventricular function, and improving survival. The most effective fibrinolytic regimens achieve epicardial infarct artery patency in 75% of patients within 90 minutes. Red blood cell transfusion is required in approximately 5% and hemorrhagic stroke occurs in approximately

TABLE 11.5. *Diagnostic and treatment measures in patients with ST segment elevation myocardial infarction*

Initial diagnostic measures
  Use continuous ECG; automated BP, HR monitoring
  Take targeted history (for AMI inclusions, fibrinolysis exclusions); check vital signs, perform focused examination
  Start IV administration, draw blood for serum cardiac markers, hematology, chemistry, lipid profile
  Obtain 12-lead ECG
  Obtain chest radiograph (preferably upright)
General treatment measures
  Aspirin, 160–325 mg (chew and swallow)
  Nitroglycerin, sublingual: test for Prinzmetal's angina, reversible spasm; antiischemic, antihypertensive effects
  Oxygen: sparse data; probably indicated, first 2–3 hr in all; continue if low arterial oxygen saturation (<90%)
  Adequate analgesia: small doses of morphine (2–4 mg) as needed
Specific treatment measures
  Reperfusion therapy: goals: door-to-needle time <30 min; door-to-balloon time <60 min
  Conjunctive antithrombotics: aspirin, heparin (especially with alteplase, reteplase, tenecteplase, angioplasty)
  Adjunctive therapies: beta-adrenoceptor blockade if eligible, intravenous nitroglycerin (for antiischemic or antihypertensive effects), ACE inhibitor [especially with large or anterior AMI, heart failure without hypotension (SBP >100 mm Hg), previous MI]

ACE, angiotensin converting enzyme; AMI, acute myocardial infarction; BP, blood pressure; ECG, electrocardiogram; HR, heart rate; IV, intravenous; SBP, systolic blood pressure.
  Adapted from Ryan TJ, Anderson JL, Antman EM, et al. ACC/AHA guidelines for the management of patients with acute myocardial infarction: a report of the American College of Cardiology/American Heart Association Task Force on Practice Guidelines (Committee on Management of Acute Myocardial Infarction). *J Am Coll Cardiol* 1996;28:1328–1428.

1% of patients, despite the fact that those at increased risk for bleeding are excluded from treatment.

Because of its widespread availability and proven ability to reduce mortality in several randomized trials, intravenous fibrinolytic therapy is the standard of care for patients with AMI; however, it has important limitations. Many patients are ineligible for treatment with fibrinolyt-ics. Of those given fibrinolytic therapy, 25% have persistent occlusion or reocclusion of the infarct-related artery. Consequently, primary percutaneous coronary intervention (PCI), with patency rates of more than 90% and few contraindications, is an attractive alternative reperfusion strategy. Weaver et al. (25) analyzed 10 trials, including data from 2,606 patients, comparing primary PCI with fibrinolytic therapy. PCI was

TABLE 11.6. *Comparison of approved fibrinolytic agents*

	Streptokinase	Anistreplase	Alteplase	Reteplase	Tenecteplase
Dose	1.5 MU in 30–60 min	30 mg in 5 min	100 mg in 90 min	10 U × 2 over 30 min	0.5 mg/kg once
Bolus administration	No	Yes	No	Yes	Yes
Antigenic	Yes	Yes	No	No	No
Allergic reactions (hypotension most common)	Yes	Yes	No	No	No
Systemic fibrinogen depletion	Marked	Marked	Mild	Moderate	Mild
90-min patency rates (%)	~50	~65	~75	~75	~75
TIMI grade 3 flow (%)	32	43	54	60	60
Cost per dose (US)	$294	$2,116	$2,196	$2,196	$2,196

TIMI, Thrombolysis in Myocardial Infarction.
  Adapted from Ryan TJ, Antman EM, Brooks NH, et al. 1999 update: ACC/AHA guidelines for the management of patients with acute myocardial infarction: a report of the American College of Cardiology/American Heart Association Task Force on Practice Guidelines (Committee on Management of Acute Myocardial Infarction). *J Am Coll Cardiol* 1999;34:890–911.

TABLE 11.7. *Absolute and relative contraindications for fibrinolytic therapy in acute myocardial infarction*

Contraindications
  Previous hemorrhagic stroke at any time; other strokes or cerebrovascular events within 1 year
  Known intracranial neoplasm
  Active internal bleeding (does not include menses)
  Suspected aortic dissection
Cautions/relative contraindications
  Severe uncontrolled hypertension on presentation (blood pressure >180/110 mm Hg)
  History of prior cerebrovascular accident or known intracerebral pathology not covered in contraindications
  Current use of anticoagulants in therapeutic doses (INR, 2.0–3.0); known bleeding diathesis
  Recent trauma (within 2–4 weeks), including head trauma or traumatic or prolonged (>10 min) CPR or major surgery (<3 wk)
  Noncompressible vascular punctures
  Recent (within 2–4 weeks) internal bleeding
  For streptokinase/anistreplase: prior exposure (especially within 5 d–2 yr) or prior allergic reaction
  Pregnancy
  Active peptic ulcer
  History of chronic severe hypertension

CPR, cardiopulmonary resuscitation; INR, International Normalized Ratio.
Adapted from Ryan TJ, Anderson JL, Antman EM, et al. ACC/AHA guidelines for the management of patients with acute myocardial infarction: a report of the American College of Cardiology/American Heart Association Task Force on Practice Guidelines (Committee on Management of Acute Myocardial Infarction). *J Am Coll Cardiol* 1996;28:1328–1428.

associated with a significant reduction in short-term mortality, reinfarction, and hemorrhagic stroke. Primary PCI may be the preferred reperfusion strategy when performed in a timely manner (balloon inflation in less than 2 hours) by individuals skilled in the procedure (performing more than 75 PCI procedures per year) and supported by experienced personnel in high-volume centers (more than 200 PCI procedures per year) (23,26). It is limited by the fact that fewer than 20% of U.S. hospitals have PCI capability and by the delay in time to treatment. It is the reperfusion strategy of choice in patients with cardiogenic shock. Patients with persistent ischemia refractory to medical therapy who are not candidates for primary PCI and patients in whom PCI fails should be considered for coronary bypass surgery. Coronary bypass surgery is also indicated in patients at the time of surgical repair of mechanical complications of AMI. Indications for the invasive management of AMI are summarized in Table 11.8.

Several interventions should quickly be undertaken while patients are being evaluated for reperfusion therapy (Tables 11.5, 11.9, and 11.10) (21,23). First, patients with overt pulmonary congestion and arterial oxygen desaturation (saturation less than 90%) should be given supplemental oxygen, as should all patients with AMI during the first 2 to 3 hours. Second, all patients should be given 160 to 325 mg of aspirin on presentation and continued it indefinitely. Clopidogrel is a reasonable alternative if a patient has a true allergy to aspirin. Third, heparin is indicated in all patients, except those receiving streptokinase. The recommended heparin regimen after fibrinolytic use is a bolus of 60 U per kilogram (maximum, 4,000 U) and a maintenance of 12 U per kilogram per hour (maximum, 1,000 U per hour) to maintain an activated partial thromboplastin time 1.5–2.0 times that of control times (i.e., 50 to 70 seconds) for 48 hours. Fourth, all patients should receive beta blockers unless they have bradycardia, atrioventricular heart block, hypotension, congestive heart failure, or bronchospasm. Fifth, intravenous nitroglycerin should be given for the first 24 to 48 hours in patients with congestive heart failure, large anterior infarction, persistent ischemia, or hypertension. It should be continued beyond 48 hours in patients with recurrent angina or persistent pulmonary congestion. Patients should be asked about recent use of sildenafil (Viagra) because administration of nitroglycerin within 24 hours of sildenafil ingestion may cause severe hypotension. Finally, angiotensin-converting enzyme (ACE) inhibitor therapy is recommended within the first 24 hours of AMI in patients with ST segment elevation in two or more anterior leads, with clinical heart failure in the absence of hypotension or known contraindications, and with left ventricular ejection fraction less than 40%. Other medications may be necessary to treat electrical complications or left ventricular failure (Table 11.11).

TABLE 11.8. *American College of Cardiology/American Heart Association guidelines for invasive management of acute myocardial infarction*

Interventions	Indications			
	Class I	Class IIA	Class IIB	Class III
Intraaortic balloon pump	Cardiogenic shock Acute MR or VSD Recurrent intractable ventricular arrhythmias Refractory post-MI angina	Hemodynamic instability Poor LV function, persistent ischemia, large area of myocardium at risk	Rescue PCI, three-vessel disease, and successful PCI Large area of myocardium at risk	—
Temporary pacing	Asystole Symptomatic bradycardia Bilateral/alternating BBB New trifascicular block Mobitz type II block	New bifascicular block First-degree AV block with RBBB LBBB new or indeterminate Overdrive pacing for incessant VT Recurrent sinus pauses >3 sec	Indeterminate-age bifascicular block New RBBB	First-degree AV block Mobitz type I block AIVR Old BBB or fascicular block
PA catheter	Severe or progressive CHF Progressive hypotension Cardiogenic shock VSD, acute MR, cardiac tamponade	Persistent hypotension without CHF	—	No cardiac or pulmonary complications
Arterial line	Systolic blood pressure <80 mm Hg Cardiogenic shock Use of IV vasopressors	Use of IV nitroprusside Other potent vasodilators	IV nitroglycerin IV inotrope use	Hemodynamically stable
Coronary angiography	Recurrent angina CHF, shock Persistent hypotension	EF <40% Prior revascularization Malignant arrhythmias Acute CHF, normal LVEF	Rescue PCI, anterior MI Risk stratification	Routine use after lytics Nonrevascularization candidates
PCI	As an alternative to fibrinolysis within 12 hours Cardiogenic shock within 36 hours of MI, age <75 years	Candidate for reperfusion with contraindication to fibrinolysis	No ST elevation but reduced flow of the infarct-related artery	Elective angioplasty of non–infarction-related artery 12 hours from symptom onset, no active ischemia No ischemia after fibrinolysis Alternative to fibrinolysis by a low-volume operator
CABG	Failed PCI and persistent ischemia Persistent symptoms and not candidate for PCI	Cardiogenic shock and suitable anatomy	Failed PCI, small MI, stable	Expected surgical mortality rate > medical mortality rate

AIVR, accelerated idioventricular arrhythmia; AV, atrioventricular; BBB, bundle branch block; CHF, congestive heart failure; EF, ejection fraction; IV, intravenous; LBBB, left bundle branch block; LV, left ventricular; LVEF, left ventricular ejection fraction; MI, myocardial infarction; MR, mitral regurgitation; PCI, percutaneous coronary intervention; RBBB, right bundle branch block; VSD, ventricular septal defect.

Adapted from Ryan TJ, Anderson JL, Antman EM, et al. ACC/AHA guidelines for the management of patients with acute myocardial infarction: a report of the American College of Cardiology/American Heart Association Task Force on Practice Guidelines (Committee on Management of Acute Myocardial Infarction). *J Am Coll Cardiol* 1996;28:1328–1428; and from Ryan TJ, Antman EM, Brooks NH, et al. 1999 update: ACC/AHA guidelines for the management of patients with acute myocardial infarction: a report of the American College of Cardiology/American Heart Association Task Force on Practice Guidelines (Committee on Management of Myocardial Infarction). *J Am Coll Cardiol* 1999;34:890–911.

TABLE 11.9. American College of Cardiology/American Heart Association guidelines for medical management of acute myocardial infarction

Interventions	Indications			
	Class I	Class IIa	Class IIb	Class III
Fibrinolysis	Ischemic symptoms, ST segment elevation or LBBB < 12 hr from symptom onset, age <75 years	Same as class I, age ≥ 75 years	Same as class I and IIa, > 12–24 hr from symptom onset, BP >180/110 mm Hg with high-risk MI	ST elevation, time to therapy > 24 hours, symptoms resolved
Aspirin	160–325 mg daily for all MI patients beginning on day 1	—	—	—
Heparin (unfractionated)	Patients undergoing primary PCI or bypass surgery	Patients receiving rtPA, rPA, TNK-tPA High risk for embolism: large MI, anterior MI, AF, prior emboli	Patients receiving streptokinase and not at high risk for emboli, 7,500–12,500 IU SC bid	Routine I.V. heparin in low-risk patients treated with streptokinase
Ticlopidine, clopidogrel	—	—	Alternative for aspirin-allergic patients	—
Beta blockers	Patients without contraindications within 12 hr of MI Continuing or recurrent ischemic pain Patients with tachyarrhythmias	—	Moderate LV failure or other relative contraindications to beta blockers	Severe heart failure second- or third-degree heart block Bronchospasm Hypotension Bradycardia
ACE inhibitors	Anterior MI within 24 hr Clinical heart failure Ejection fraction < 40%	All other MI patients within 24 hr without contraindications Ejection fraction 40%–50% and prior MI	Recent MI, no heart failure, normal or mildly decreased LV function	BP < 100 mm Hg
Nitrates	First 24–48 hr for large MI, heart failure, hypotension, persistent ischemia After 48 hr for ischemia, heart failure	—	First 24–48 hr in all MI patients After 48 hr in patients with large or complicated MI	Systolic BP < 90 mm Hg Heart rate < 50 bpm
Calcium channel blockers	—	Verapamil or diltiazem for ischemia or tachycardia in absence of heart failure or LV dysfunction if beta blockers are ineffective or contraindicated	—	Short acting dihydropyridines Diltiazem/verapamil in presence of heart failure/LV dysfunction

ACE, angiotensin-converting enzyme; AF, atrial fibrillation; BP, blood pressure; IV, intravenous; LBBB, left bundle branch block; LV, left ventricular; MI, myocardial infarction; PCI, percutaneous coronary intervention; rPA, reteplase; rtPA, alteplase; SC, subcutaneous; TNK-tPA, tenecteplase.

Adapted from Ryan TJ, Anderson JL, Antman EM, et al. ACC/AHA guidelines for the management of patients with acute myocardial infarction: a report of the American College of Cardiology/American Heart Association Task Force on Practice Guidelines (Committee on Management of Acute Myocardial Infarction). *J Am Coll Cardiol* 1996;28:1328–1428; and from Ryan TJ, Antman EM, Brooks NH, et al. 1999 update: ACC/AHA guidelines for the management of patients with acute myocardial infarction: a report of the American College of Cardiology/American Heart Association Task Force on Practice Guidelines (Committee on Management of Myocardial Infarction). *J Am Coll Cardiol* 1999;34:890–911.

TABLE 11.10. *Adjunctive pharmacologic management for acute myocardial infarction with doses*

Oxygen	2–4 L/min by nasal cannula
Sublingual nitroglycerin	0.4 mg every 2–5 min three times
Aspirin	160–325 mg every day
Morphine	2–5 mg every 5–30 min
Heparin	60 U/kg (max, 4,000 U), 12 U/kg/hr (max, 1,000/hr) adjusted to keep aPTT 50–70 sec × 48 hr
Beta blockers	
Metoprolol (Lopressor)	5 mg IV three times over 15 min; 50 mg orally 10 min later; then 100 mg orally twice daily
Atenolol (Tenormin)	5 mg IV twice over 10 min; 50 mg orally 10 min later; then 100 mg orally every day
Intravenous nitroglycerin	10–200 μg/min infusion
ACE inhibitors	
Captopril (Capoten)	6.25–50 mg orally t.i.d.
Enalapril (Vasotec)	2.5–20 mg orally b.i.d.
Lisinopril (Prinivil, Zestril)	2.5–20 mg orally daily
Ramipril (Altace)	2.5–20 mg orally daily
Warfarin (Coumadin)	2–10 mg orally adjusted to INR

ACE, angiotensin-converting enzyme; INR, International Normalized Ratio.

Evolving Therapy

There are several ways in which reperfusion rates and patient outcomes might be improved. Potential options include different dosing regimens of established agents; improved adjunctive therapy with direct thrombin inhibitors, low molecular weight heparin, or glycoprotein IIb/IIIa receptor antagonists; the development of novel fibrinolytic agents; and coronary stents. Bolus therapy with either reteplase (27) or tenecteplase (28) has been shown to be equivalent to therapy with alteplase and is easier to administer, potentially decreasing both time to treatment and dosing errors. The GUSTO V trial (29) compared the effect of full-dose reteplase with the combination of half-dose reteplase plus abciximab, a glycoprotein IIb/IIIa receptor antagonist. There was no significant difference in 30-day mortality rates between the treatment groups, but combination therapy led to a reduction in ischemic complications, including reinfarction, and may facilitate PCI. The Assessment of the Safety and Efficacy of a New Thrombolytic Regimen (ASSENT)–3 study (30) randomly assigned patients to one of three strategies: full-dose tenecteplase and enoxaparin; half-dose tenecteplase, weight-adjusted low-dose unfractionated heparin, and a 12-hour infusion of abciximab; or full-dose tenecteplase with weight-adjusted unfractionated heparin. There was a lower rate of death, reinfarction, and refractory ischemia among the enoxaparin and abciximab recipients than among the patients receiving unfractionated heparin; the ease of administration may make tenecteplase plus enoxaparin the more attractive option. Abciximab and coronary stent placement have improved patency rates and outcomes in patients undergoing PCI and are now routinely employed (31,32).

PROGNOSIS

The Thrombolysis in Myocardial Infarction (TIMI) risk score for ST segment elevation AMI is a simple tool for bedside risk assessment (33,34). This score has been validated in multiple clinical trials. The elements of the TIMI score are shown in Fig. 11.2 and include history, physical examination, and electrocardiographic findings on presentation. The actual score is a summed weighted integer score based on eight characteristics. Application of the TIMI risk score has revealed a significant, nearly linear, 30-fold graded increase in risk between patients with a score of 0 and those with a score of 8 or higher. The TIMI study group has expanded their TIMI risk calculator for handheld organizers, and the calculator can be downloaded from the TIMI study group web site (*http://www.timi.tv/*). Figure 11.2 shows the prediction of inhospital mortality with TIMI

TABLE 11.11. *Dosages of drugs commonly used in the management of complicated acute myocardial infarction*

Drug	Dose	Side effects
Bradycardia, atrioventricular block		
Atropine	0.5 mg IV q5min to maximum of 2.0 mg	Hallucinations, fever, VT/VF, urinary retention, acute angle glaucoma
Isoproterenol (Isuprel)	2–10 μg/min IV titrated to HR	Tachycardia, hypotension, increased O_2 demand
Aminophylline	300–400 mg IV over 15–30 minutes	Tachycardia, atrial arrhythmia, CNS toxicity
Supraventricular arrhythmias		
Esmolol (Brevibloc)	500 μg/kg IV over 1 min, repeated before each upward titration 50 μg/kg min infusion, increased by 50 μg/kg every 5 min up to 200 μg/kg/min	CHF, bronchospasm, hypotension, bradycardia, AV block
Propranolol (Inderal)	1 mg/min IV up to 0.1 mg/kg	Same as for esmolol
Metoprolol (Lopressor)	5 mg IV over 2 min; repeated q5min twice	Same as for esmolol
Atenolol (Tenormin)	5 mg IV over 2 min; repeated in 10 min	Same as for esmolol
Verapamil (Calan, Isoptin)	5 mg IV over 2 min; then 1–2 mg q2min up to 20 mg	CHF, hypotension, heart block, bradycardia
Diltiazem (Cardizem)	0.25 mg/kg IV over 2 min, then 5–15 mg/hr	Same as for verapamil
Digoxin (Lanoxin)	0.5 to 1 mg IV over 5 min, then 0.25 mg IV q4h to 1 mg	Ventricular dysrhythmias, heart block, increased infarction size
Procainamide (Pronestyl)	20–30 mg/min IV to 12–17 mg/kg, then 1–4 mg/min	Hypotension
Adenosine (Adenocard)	6 mg IV, then 12 mg IV if not effective	Flushing, chest pain, dyspnea, sinus pauses
Ventricular arrhythmias		
Lidocaine (Xylocaine)	1 mg/kg IV, 0.5 mg/kg IV q10min one to four times, followed by 2–4 mg/min infusion	Nausea, numbness, confusion, slurred speech, respiratory depression, tremors, seizures, sinus arrest
Amiodarone (Cordarone)	150 mg over 10 min, 1 mg/min × 6 hr, then 0.5 mg/min	Hypotension, myocardial depression, bradycardia, conduction block
Magnesium sulfate	2 g over 5 min, 8 g over 24 hours	Flushing, bradycardia
Heart failure, shock		
Nitroglycerin	50–200 μg/min as IV infusion	Hypotension
Nitroprusside (Nipride)	0.25–10 μg/kg/min IV infusion	Hypotension, thiocyanate toxicity
Enalaprilat (Vasotec)	0.625–1.25 mg IV q6h	Hypotension, azotemia
Labetalol (Normodyne)	20–80 mg IV q10min, then 2 mg/min IV infusion	Hypotension, bradycardia
Furosemide (Lasix)	20–160 mg IV	Hypokalemia, hypomagnesemia
Bumetanide (Bumex)	1–3 mg IV	Nausea, cramps
Dobutamine (Dobutrex)	5–20 μg/kg/min IV	Tolerance
Dopamine (Inotropin)	2–20 μg/kg/min IV	Increased oxygen demand
Norepinephrine (Levophed)	2–16 μg/min IV	Peripheral and visceral vasoconstriction
Milrinone (Primacor)	50 μg/kg over 10 min IV, then 0.375–0.75 μg/kg/min	Ventricular dysrhythmias

AV indicates atrioventricular; CHF, congestive heart failure; CNS, central nervous system; HR, heart rate; IV, intravenous; VF, ventricular fibrillation; VT, ventricular tachycardia.

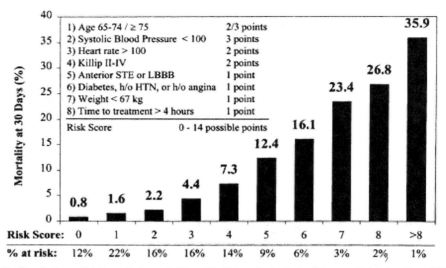

FIG. 11.2. Prediction of inhospital mortality with Thrombolysis In Myocardial Infarction (TIMI) risk score for ST-segment elevation myocardial infarction stratified by reperfusion therapy. NRMI, National Registry of Myocardial Infarction; InTIME II, Intravenous nPA for Treatment of Infarcting Myocardium Early. (Adapted from Morrow DA, Antman EM, Charlesworth A, et al. TIMI risk score for ST-elevation myocardial infarction: A convenient, bedside, clinical score for risk assessment at presentation: An Intravenous nPA for Treatment of Infarcting Myocardium Early II trial substudy. *Circulation* 2000;102:2031-2037.)

risk score for ST segment elevation MI, but the score has also been validated for outcomes at 30 days. Long-term prognosis is variable and depends on left ventricular function, ischemic burden, and revascularization status.

FOLLOW-UP

Figure 11.3 outlines the strategies for exercise testing for risk stratification after AMI (21). If patients are at high risk for ischemic events according to clinical criteria, they should undergo cardiac catheterization to determine whether they are candidates for coronary revascularization (strategy I). For patients initially deemed to be at low risk at the time of discharge after MI, one of two strategies for exercise testing can be used. One is a symptom-limited test at 14 to 21 days (strategy II). If the patient is taking digoxin, or if the baseline ECG precludes accurate interpretation of ST segment changes (e.g., baseline left bundle branch block, left ventricular hypertrophy), then an initial exercise imaging study is recommended. Results of exercise testing should

be stratified to determine need for additional invasive or exercise perfusion studies. A third strategy (strategy III) is to perform a submaximal exercise test 5 to 7 days after MI or just before hospital discharge. If the physician opts for strategy III and the exercise test result is negative, a second symptom-limited exercise test could be repeated at 3 to 6 weeks for patients engaging in vigorous activity. The ejection fraction should be estimated either with ventriculography during cardiac catheterization or by echocardiography in patients treated medically.

Secondary prevention is extremely important (see Chapter 8). All patients should be considered for a cardiac rehabilitation program and should follow diet and exercise prescriptions (35). All patients should be considered for long-term therapy with aspirin (36), beta blockers (37), statins (38), and ACE inhibitors (39). Individuals with a true allergy to aspirin should receive clopidogrel. Long-term anticoagulation is indicated for patients with persistent atrial fibrillation, for patients with left ventricular thrombus, and for secondary prevention in patients unable to take

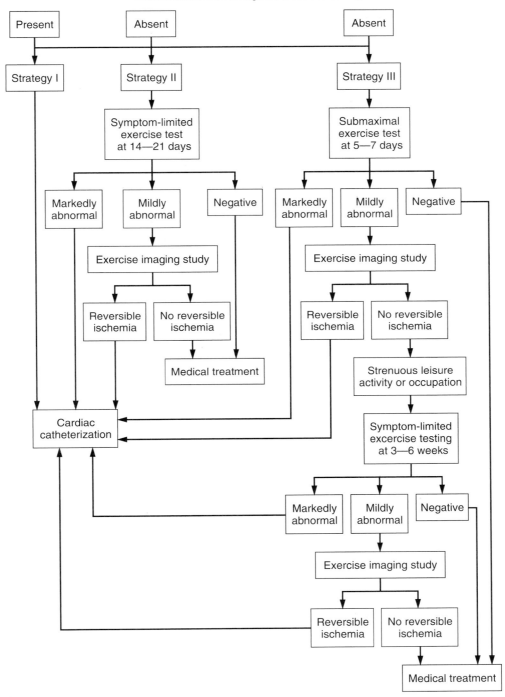

FIG. 11.3. Strategies for exercise testing for risk stratification after myocardial infarction. (Adapted from Ryan TJ, Anderson JL, Antman EM, et al. ACC/AHA guidelines for the management of patients with acute myocardial infarction: a report of the American College of Cardiology/American Heart Association Task Force on Practice Guidelines (Committee on Management of Acute Myocardial Infarction). *J Am Coll Cardiol* 1996;28:1328–1428.)

aspirin or clopidogrel. Smoking cessation and control of hypertension, dyslipidemia, diabetes, and weight to target values should be vigorously pursued.

PRACTICAL POINTS

- Age, blood pressure, heart rate, congestive heart failure, and ECG findings allow early risk stratification in the emergency department.

- Echocardiography should be performed in hemodynamically unstable patients to exclude mechanical complications.

- All patients should be given 160 to 325 mg of aspirin. Clopidogrel is an alternative if the patient has a true allergy to aspirin.

- Patients should receive heparin unless they are treated with streptokinase.

- Patients should receive beta blockers unless beta blockers are contraindicated.

- Expeditious reperfusion therapy should be the goal in all patients with AMI.

- Primary PCI may be superior to fibrinolytic therapy if performed in a timely manner (less than 2 hours) in an excellent interventional laboratory.

- ACE inhibitors are indicated in patients with large anterior AMI or left ventricular systolic dysfunction.

- Risk stratification should be performed to select high-risk patients for elective coronary artery revascularization.

- Aspirin, beta blockers, statins, and ACE inhibitors have each been shown to reduce long-term mortality.

- American Heart Association Step II diet, exercise, and complete smoking cessation are indicated. Control of hypertension, hyperlipidemia, diabetes, and weight to target values should be aggressively pursued.

REFERENCES

1. American Heart Association. *2001 Heart and Stroke Statistical Update.* Dallas: American Heart Association, 2000.
2. Horie T, Sekiguchi M, Hirosawa K. Coronary thrombosis in pathogenesis of acute myocardial infarction. Histopathological study of coronary arteries in 108 necropsied cases using serial section. *Br Heart J* 1978; 40:153–161.
3. Cheitlin MD, McAllister HA, de Castro CM. Myocardial infarction without atherosclerosis. *JAMA* 1975;231:951–959.
4. Willerson J, Cohen L, Maseri A. Coronary artery disease: pathophysiology and clinical recognition. In: Willerson J, Cohn J, eds. *Cardiovascular Medicine.* New York: Churchill Livingstone, 1995:333–357.
5. Muller RT, Gould LA, Betzu R, et al. Painless myocardial infarction in the elderly. *Am Heart J* 1990;119:202–204.
6. Killip T 3rd, Kimball JT. Treatment of myocardial infarction in a coronary care unit. A two year experience with 250 patients. *Am J Cardiol* 1967;20:457–464.
7. Lee KL, Woodlief LH, Topol EJ, et al. Predictors of 30-day mortality in the era of reperfusion for acute myocardial infarction: results from an international trial of 41,021 patients. *Circulation* 1995;91:1659–1668.
8. Sgarbossa EB, Pinski SL, Barbagelata A, et al. Electrocardiographic diagnosis of evolving acute myocardial infarction in the presence of left bundle-branch block. *N Engl J Med* 1996;334:481–487.
9. Murray C, Alpert JS. Diagnosis of acute myocardial infarction. *Curr Opin Cardiol* 1994;9:465–470.
10. Tunstall-Pedoe H, Kuulasmaa K, Amouyel P, et al. Myocardial infarction and coronary deaths in the World Health Organization MONICA Project. Registration procedures, event rates, and case-fatality rates in 38 populations from 21 countries in four continents. *Circulation* 1994;90:583–612.
11. Myocardial infarction redefined—a consensus document of the Joint European Society of Cardiology/American College of Cardiology Committee for the redefinition of myocardial infarction. *J Am Coll Cardiol* 2000;36:959–969.
12. Horowitz RS, Morganroth J, Parrotto C, et al. Immediate diagnosis of acute myocardial infarction by two-dimensional echocardiography. *Circulation* 1982;65:323–329.
13. Penco M, Sciomer S, Vizza CD, et al. Clinical impact of echocardiography in prognostic stratification after acute myocardial infarction. *Am J Cardiol* 1998;81:17G–20G.
14. Fox AC, Glassman E, Isom OW. Surgically remediable complications of myocardial infarction. *Prog Cardiovasc Dis* 1979;21:461–484.
15. Holmes DR, Jr., Bates ER, Kleiman NS, et al. Contemporary reperfusion therapy for cardiogenic shock: the GUSTO-I trial experience. *J Am Coll Cardiol* 1995;26:668–674.

16. Hochman JS, Sleeper LA, Webb JG, et al. Early revascularization in acute myocardial infarction complicated by cardiogenic shock. *N Engl J Med* 1999;341:625–634.

17. Dell'Italia LJ, Starling MR. Right ventricular infarction: an important clinical entity. *Curr Probl Cardiol* 1984;9:1–72.

18. Bowers TR, O'Neill WW, Grines C, et al. Effect of reperfusion on biventricular function and survival after right ventricular infarction. *N Engl J Med* 1998;338:933–940.

19. Lichstein E. The changing spectrum of post-myocardial infarction pericarditis. *Int J Cardiol* 1983;4:234–237.

20. Berman J, Haffajee CI, Alpert JS. Therapy of symptomatic pericarditis after myocardial infarction: retrospective and prospective studies of aspirin, indomethacin, prednisone, and spontaneous resolution. *Am Heart J* 1981;101:750–753.

21. Ryan TJ, Anderson JL, Antman EM, et al. ACC/AHA guidelines for the management of patients with acute myocardial infarction: a report of the American College of Cardiology/American Heart Association Task Force on Practice Guidelines (Committee on Management of Acute Myocardial Infarction). *J Am Coll Cardiol* 1996;28:1328–1428.

22. National Heart Attack Alert Program Coordinating Committee. Emergency department: rapid identification and treatment of patients with acute myocardial infarction. *Ann Emerg Med* 1994;23:311–329.

23. Ryan TJ, Antman EM, Brooks NH, et al. 1999 update: ACC/AHA guidelines for the management of patients with acute myocardial infarction: a report of the American College of Cardiology/American Heart Association Task Force on Practice Guidelines (Committee on Management of Acute Myocardial Infarction). *J Am Coll Cardiol* 1999;34:890–911.

24. White HD, Van de Werf FJ. Thrombolysis for acute myocardial infarction. *Circulation* 1998;97:1632–1646.

25. Weaver WD, Simes RJ, Betriu A, et al. Comparison of primary coronary angioplasty and intravenous thrombolytic therapy for acute myocardial infarction. *JAMA* 1997;278:2093–2098.

26. Cannon CP, Gibson CM, Lambrew CT, et al. Relationship of symptom-onset–to–balloon time and door-to-balloon time with mortality in patients undergoing angioplasty for acute myocardial infarction. *JAMA* 2000;283:2941–2947.

27. GUSTO-III Investigators. A comparison of reteplase with alteplase for acute myocardial infarction. *N Engl J Med* 1997;337:1118–1123.

28. ASSENT-2 Investigators. Single-bolus tenecteplase compared with front-loaded alteplase in acute myocardial infarction: the ASSENT-2 double-blind randomised trial. *Lancet* 1999;354:716–722.

29. The GUSTO V Investigators. Reperfusion therapy for acute myocardial infarction with fibrinolytic therapy or combination reduced fibrinolytic therapy and platelet glycoprotein IIb/IIIa inhibition: the GUSTO V randomised trial. *Lancet* 2001;357:1905–1914.

30. The ASSENT-3 Investigators. Efficacy and safety of tenecteplase in combination with enoxaparin, abciximab, or unfractionated heparin: the ASSENT-3 randomised trial in acute myocardial infarction. *Lancet* 2001;358:605–613.

31. Schomig A, Kastrati A, Dirschinger J, et al. Coronary stenting plus platelet glycoprotein IIb/IIIa blockade compared with tissue plasminogen activator in acute myocardial infarction. *N Engl J Med* 2000;343:385–391.

32. Montalescot G, Barragan, P, Wittenberg O, et al. Platelet glycoprotein IIb/IIIa inhibition with coronary stenting for acute myocardial infarction. *N Engl J Med* 2001;344:1895–1903.

33. Morrow DA, Antman EM, Charlesworth A, et al. TIMI risk score for ST-elevation myocardial infarction: A convenient, bedside, clinical score for risk assessment at presentation: an Intravenous nPA for Treatment of Infarcting Myocardium Early II trial substudy. *Circulation* 2000;102:2031–2037.

34. Morrow DA, Antman EM, Parsons L, et al. Application of the TIMI risk score for ST-elevation MI in the National Registry of Myocardial Infarction 3. *JAMA* 2001;286:1356–1359.

35. Balady GJ, Fletcher BJ, Froelicher ES, et al. Cardiac rehabilitation programs. A statement for healthcare professionals from the American Heart Association. *Circulation* 1994;90:1602–1610.

36. Antiplatelet Trialists' Collaboration. Collaborative meta-analysis of randomised trials of antiplatelet therapy for prevention of death, myocardial infarction, and stroke in high risk patients. *BMJ* 2002;324:71–86.

37. Yusuf S, Peto R, Lewis J, et al. Beta blockade during and after myocardial infarction: an overview of the randomized trials. *Prog Cardiovasc Dis* 1985;27:335–371.

38. Randomised trial of cholesterol lowering in 4444 patients with coronary heart disease: the Scandinavian Simvastatin Survival Study (4S). *Lancet* 1994;344:1383–1389.

39. Latini R, Maggioni AP, Flather M, et al. ACE-inhibitor use in patients with myocardial infarction: summary of evidence from clinical trials. *Circulation* 1995;92:3132–3137.

12

Primary Hypertension

Kenneth A. Jamerson

DEFINITION/DIFFERENTIAL DIAGNOSIS

Hypertension is a leading cause of mortality worldwide. Although the association between blood pressure and cardiovascular (CV) risk exists at every level of systolic and diastolic blood pressure, the diagnosis of hypertension is established by exceeding a blood pressure threshold of 140/90 mm Hg on two occasions (1). Repeat measures of blood pressure determine whether initial elevations persist and require immediate attention or whether they return to normal values and require only surveillance. The 140/90 mm Hg cut point is correlated with an acceleration in CV risk that has been established from natural history studies (the Framingham Heart Study) (2). However, the amount of CV risk that is acceptable in a population may vary from country to country. For example, Canada and Europe accept higher blood pressure cut points to confirm the diagnosis of hypertension (3). Over the decades, the United States has modified the threshold of elevated blood pressure that confers the diagnosis of hypertension, from 160/95 mm Hg to the current value of 140/90 mm Hg, thereby increasing the prevalence of hypertension from approximately 14.5% of the population to 23% (Table 12.1) (4).

The classification of blood pressure in the adult population is presented in Table 12.2. It is assumed that the blood pressure represent subjects who are not taking antihypertensive drugs and are not acutely ill. When systolic and diastolic blood pressures fall into different categories, the category with the higher value should be selected to classify the individual's blood pressure status. For example, 160/95 mm Hg should be classified as stage 2 hypertension, and 175/120 mm Hg

should be classified as stage 3 hypertension. Isolated systolic hypertension is defined as systolic blood pressure (SBP) of 140 mm Hg or higher and diastolic blood pressure (DBP) less than 90 mm Hg and is staged appropriately (e.g., 170/85 mm Hg is defined as stage 2 isolated systolic hypertension). In addition to classifying stages of hypertension on the basis of average blood pressure levels, clinicians should specify presence or absence of target organ disease and additional risk factors. This specificity is important for risk classification and treatment (see Table 12.3). For example, a patient with diabetes and a blood pressure of 142/94 mm Hg should be classified as having stage 1 hypertension with another major risk factor (diabetes). This patient's condition would be categorized as stage 1, risk group C, and immediate initiation of pharmacologic treatment would be recommended. Lifestyle modification should be relegated to adjunctive therapy for all patients recommended for pharmacologic therapy. Lifestyle modification is appropriate initial therapy for stage 1 uncomplicated hypertension.

Current national guidelines advocate even lower levels of blood pressure in the subpopulation of hypertensive patients at higher risk for cardiovascular disease (CVD) (diabetes and renal insufficiency), to targets below 130/85 mm Hg (5,6). However, the recommendations for aggressive targets for blood pressure control stem from epidemiologic studies and retrospective analyses of clinical trials. The studies are able to show an association between lower levels of blood pressure and lower CVD risk but do not prove that the intervention of lowering blood pressure to targets below 130/85 mm Hg is of any greater benefit than that seen with achieving more conventional targets of 140/90 mm Hg. Clinical trials

TABLE 12.1. *Age-adjusted and age-specific prevalence of hypertension.[a] U.S. population for 1991, aged 18–74 years*

Population group	NHANES III: prevalence of hypertension (%)
Aged 18–74 (all)	20.4
Men	22.8
Women	18.0
Black	30.2
Men	32.6
Women	28.1
White	19.2
Men	21.6
Women	16.7
Mexican American	19.9
Men	22.1
Women	17.4

NHANES, National Health and Nutrition Examination Survey.

[a]Hypertension is defined as systolic blood pressure ≥160 mm HG and/or diastolic blood pressure ≥95 mm HG and/or taking antihypertensive medication or as systolic blood pressure ≥140 mm HG and/or diastolic blood pressure ≥90 mm HG and/or currently taking antihypertensive medication. Values are percentages.

TABLE 12.2. *Classification of blood pressure for adults, aged 18 and older*

Category	Systolic (mm HG)		Diastolic (mm HG)
Optimal[a]	<120	and	<80
Normal	<130	and	<85
High-normal	130–139	or	85–89
Hypertension[b]			
Stage 1	140–159	or	90–99
Stage 2	160–179	or	100–109
Stage 3	≥180	or	≥110

[a]Optimal blood pressure with regard to cardiovascular risk is below 120/80 mm HG. However, unusually low readings should be evaluated for clinical significance.

[b]Based on the average of two or more readings taken at each of two or more visits after an initial screening.

Adapted from the sixth report of the Joint National Committee on Prevention, Detection, Evaluation, and Treatment of High Blood Pressure. *Arch Intern Med* 1997;157:2413–2446.

are needed to provide the evidence on which clinicians could make changes in patient management for more aggressive blood pressure targets. Clinical trials on aggressive blood pressure control are reviewed in this chapter (management of hypertension). There is a paucity of data demonstrating any clinical benefit of targeting a SBP much below 140 mm HG.

Natural history surveys indicate that both SPB and DBP confer risk for CVD; however, national guidelines before 1997 placed emphasis on the DBP for the purpose of defining hypertension (7). Current blood pressure guidelines define hypertension on the basis of either systolic or DBP levels. Moreover, SBP level may predict CV risk better than DBP (8). There is considerable evidence that pulse pressure (the difference between SBP and DBP) may provide even greater prognostic information on CV risk than either systolic or diastolic. In the Framingham Heart Study, middle-aged and elderly persons with SBP of 120 had increased CVD risk as the DBP decreased. This suggests that higher pulse pressure is an important component of risk. Ultimately, pulse pressure can be reduced or controlled only by targeting SBP (9). Thus, although all parameters of blood pressure are important for estimating CV risk, it is clinically prudent to focus special attention on lowering SBP for reducing CV risk.

TABLE 12.3. *Risk stratification and treatment*

BP Stages	Risk group		
	No risk factors	At least one risk factor	High risk, TOD/CCD, or diabetes
High normal (130–139/85–89)	Lifestyle modification	Lifestyle modification	Drug therapy
Stage 1 (140–150/85–89)	Lifestyle modification (up to 12 months)	Lifestyle modification (up to 6 months)	Drug therapy
Stage 2 and 3 (≥160/≥100)	Drug therapy	Drug therapy	Drug therapy

Adapted from the sixth report of the Joint National Committee on Prevention, Detection, Evaluation, and Treatment of High Blood Pressure. *Arch Intern Med* 1997;157:2413–2446.

Gender and ethnicity have a significant effect of the prevalence of hypertension in the United States. The estimated prevalence rate of hypertension is approximately 20% in the general population but as high as 30% among African Africans (Table 12.1). The epidemiology of hypertension may also help distinguish primary from secondary hypertension. Primary hypertension occurs most frequently in the fifth and sixth decades of life. African Americans have higher incident rates of hypertension occurring at earlier ages (10). Thus, the onset of hypertension in very young white women and in adults in during the seventh decade of life and beyond implies secondary hypertension more frequently than primary hypertension.

USUAL CAUSES OF HYPERTENSION

Subjects with hypertension can be subcategorized into two groups: those in whom the rise in blood pressure is secondary to another medical problem or ingestion of exogenous materials, or secondary hypertension, and those in whom the primary pathophysiologic process is elevated blood pressure, or primary (essential) hypertension. This chapter focuses only on essential hypertension. In essential hypertension, both hereditary and environmental factors contribute to elevated blood pressure.

Heredity

From epidemiologic surveys, it has been estimated that approximately 30% of the population variation in SPB can be accounted for by heritability or polygenetic factors (11). Evidence from twin studies and family cohorts provide heritability estimates as high as 70%. The differences in heritability estimates reflect the diversity of the population under study and the influence of obesity and other environmental factors that interact with genes in producing hypertension (12). Although the familial distribution of blood pressure is a plausible explanation for the aggregation of blood pressure in families, few studies have unequivocally confirmed that genetic relationships are more important than environmental components of family life (13). Advances in cellular and molecular biology have led to the identification of genes that influence blood pressure and have unmasked several candidate genes for hypertension; however, few of these genotypes explain more that 3% of the variance in blood pressure.

Environmental Factors

There are many environmental factors that might affect level of blood pressure. The following section briefly discusses the mutable factors that have been identified by the consensus of experts to have significant impact on the treatment of hypertension (1).

Obesity

Obesity is common in middle-aged Americans, especially in those who develop hypertension. In one follow-up study of the First National Health and Nutrition Examination Survey (NHANES I), adiposity as measured by body mass index was a strong predictor of hypertension; conversely, weight loss was associated with a decrease in blood pressure. In the Framingham Heart Study, nearly 70% of newly acquired hypertension was attributable to prior obesity (14). It is alleged that truncal obesity is more deleterious to the CV system than is generalized obesity (15). The mechanism whereby obesity is related to blood pressure is not well understood, but it remains a widely accepted risk factor for the development of hypertension. Of importance is that the risk of adiposity can be improved with weight loss of only a few kilograms (16).

Salt

There is significant data to suggest that dietary salt is linked to hypertension. In a small series of studies, it has been estimated that SBP is raised 1.2 mm HG per every 10-mmol increase in dietary sodium (17–19). There is considerable evidence, however, to contest the relationship between sodium intake and blood pressure within populations (19–23). Although there exists controversy in regard to a causal role for sodium in the genesis of hypertension, the impact of sodium restriction on lowering blood pressure has been clearly demonstrated. The Dietary Approach to Stop Hypertension (DASH) diet described a dose-related reduction in blood pressure in response to dietary sodium restriction. The reduction in sodium intake to levels below current recommendations of 100 mmol per day and the DASH diet led to reductions in blood pressure by 7.1 mm HG in normotensive participants and by 11.5 mm HG in hypertensive subjects (24).

Stress

Although perceived stress and experienced stress are associated with hypertension, there are few ways to quantify their impact on individuals. This technical lacuna has led to the use of maneuvers such as mental arithmetic and immersion of the arm into cold water as standard measures of stress. Although it is difficult to quantitate stress, it is becoming increasingly clear that stress reduction has important benefits for health (25,26). Transcendental meditation has resulted in significant reduction in blood pressure and regression in left ventricle hypertrophy. The effect of meditation in African Americans has led to blood pressure reductions (on average, 10.7 mm HG) that exceed those produced by most drug monotherapies (27).

Alcohol

A true direct relationship between regular alcohol use and hypertension remains unproven. In several series, researchers comparing periods of alcohol withdrawal (during hospitalization) have found a reduction in blood pressure during abstinence (28). The results of short-term intervention studies suggest a short-term pressor effect of drinking three to eight drinks per day (29). Although a cause-and-effect relationship has yet to be established, it remains prudent to restrict alcohol intake to 1 to 2 ounces per day, as suggested by the American Heart Association.

HELPFUL TESTS/PRESENTING SYMPTOMS AND SIGNS

When a patient's blood pressure has been documented at higher than 140/90 mm HG on more than two occasions, the diagnosis of hypertension is confirmed. The initial evaluation includes three components that all converge to estimated the amount of target organ damage that currently exists and to estimate the risk for future target organ damage.

The first component is a patient interview that includes a family history, a review of organ systems with particular attention to the CV system, and the identification of lifestyle factors that impart excess CV risk.

The second component includes a physical examination with careful attention to eye grounds, the neck, the heart, the lungs, the abdomen, and the peripheral vasculature. Abbreviated examinations of other organ system may be appropriate for the initial examination. Hemorrhages and exudates found on funduscopic examination, specific valvular murmurs, abdominal bruits, and polycystic kidneys are key findings that either characterize severity of hypertension or indicate the etiology of elevated blood pressure.

The third component includes laboratory assessment. The initial laboratory panel is a basic screening chemistry profile to measure electrolytes (Table 12.4). Electrolytes provide screening information of renal function, and serum potassium is the recommended screening test for primary hyperaldosteronemia. A urinalysis provides addition information on renal function and possible renal causes of hypertension. Electrocardiography is the recommended screening test for hypertension-induced changes in the heart. A complete blood cell count and measurement of uric acid level provide less information on target organ damage but do uncover the frequent association of gout and low hematocrit as risk factors for arteriosclerosis. A fasting glucose and lipid profile similarly

TABLE 12.4. *Initial laboratory evaluation*

Test	Implications
Urine examination	Helpful in ruling out renal disease
Urea nitrogen or serum creatinine determination	Can rule out kidney failure; provides an index of baseline kidney function
Serum potassium;	Hypokalemia (<3.5 mEq/L) in patients not taking medication suggests a search for primary hyperaldosteronism
Serum glucose elevation[a]	Assists in diagnosis of diabetes mellitus
Uric acid measurements[a]	Provides baseline; may be predictor of future gout
Serum cholesterol with HDL, LDL, and triglycerides if indicated[a]	Provides information about another risk factor for heart disease
Calcium level[a]	Excludes hypercalcemia as a primary cause of hypertension
Electrocardiogram	Helpful in determining the presence of LVH, ischemia, heart block, and other conditions

HDL, high-density lipoprotein; LDL, low-density lipoprotein; LVH, left ventricular hypertrophy.
[a]An automated bood chemistry may be less expensive than individual determinations.

uncovers increased CV risk from diabetes mellitus and dyslipidemia.

CLINICAL MANAGEMENT

There are two fundamental questions that guide hypertension management: (a) whether specific antihypertensive medications able to provide CV benefits beyond lowering blood pressure and (b) whether there is an ideal blood pressure target that confers maximal CV protection. In November 1997, when the Sixth Joint National Committee on Prevention, Detection, Evaluation, and Treatment of High Blood Pressure issued its recommendations, there was a paucity of data suggesting that antihypertensive agents other than diuretics and beta blockers could provide such benefits (1). However, clinical trials involving hundreds of thousands of subjects that have been conducted since that report have yielded new data. This review summarizes those data.

Ultimately, the findings suggest that targeting blood pressure reduction below the conventional goal of 140/90 (approximately 138/85) mm HG is advantageous, particularly for hypertensive diabetic patients. There appears to be no additional benefit of achieving more aggressive targets. No specific drug class has demonstrated superiority in modifying CV outcomes; however, blocking the renin-angiotensin system has proven superiority for retarding progression to dialysis in subjects with impaired renal function. A modified treatment algorithm is provided in Figure 12.1.

Trials Assessing the Impact of Aggressive Blood Pressure Control

Four clinical trials have assessed the impact of aggressive blood pressure control in CV risk in various patient populations: the Hypertension Optimal Treatment (HOT) study (30) in a general hypertensive population; the United Kingdom Prospective Diabetes Study (UKPDS) (31) in hypertensive diabetic patients; the Appropriate Blood Pressure Control in Diabetes (ABCD) trial (32–34) in normotensive and hypertensive diabetics; and the African American Study of Kidney Disease and Hypertension (AASK) (35) in hypertensive African American patients with renal insufficiency.

The investigators in the HOT study sought to determine the optimal DBP target in a cohort of 18,790 hypertensive patients, by measuring the incidence of CV events that occurred when DBP was lowered to each of three target levels: less than 90, less than 85, and less than 80 mm HG. The study participants were aged 50 to 80 years (mean age, 61.5 years) with DBP between 100 to 115 mm HG. Within this population, 8.0% had diabetes, 6.0% had coronary heart disease, and 1.2% had suffered a stroke. Felodipine was given to all patients, with additional therapy and dosage increases permitted to achieve target DBP. After almost 46 months of follow-up, the incidences of CV events were similar among the three target-level groups. Among the diabetic subpopulation, however, the incidence of CV events in the patients with lower than 80 mm HG group was half

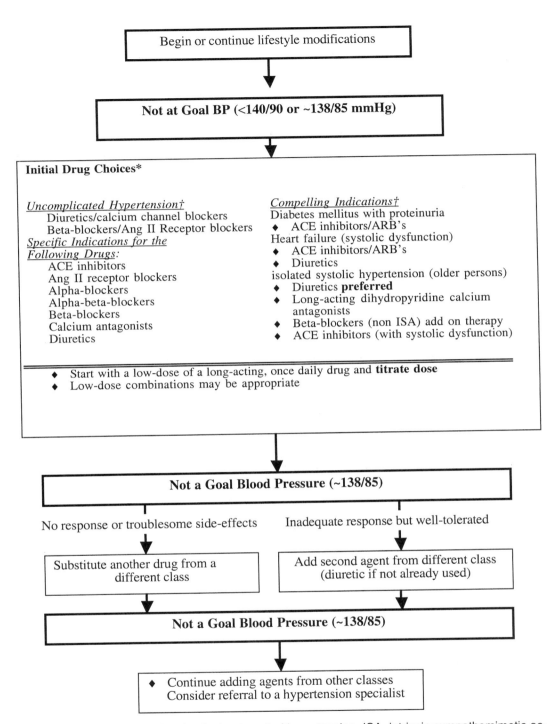

FIG. 12.1. Modified algorithm for the treatment of hypertension. ISA, intrinsic sympathomimetic activity. *Unless contraindicated. †Based on randomized controlled trials. (Adapted from Joint National Committee. The sixth report of the Joint National Committee on the Prevention, Detection, Evaluation, and Treatment of High Blood Pressure [JNC-VI]. *Arch Intern Med* 1997;157:2413–2446.)

that of the patients with lower than 90 mm HG (22 vs. 45; p for trend = 0.005). These results suggest a benefit of aggressive blood pressure control in diabetic patients, but only in a secondary analysis.

The UKPDS study examined whether the relatively more tight control of blood pressure would prevent microvascular and microvascular sequelae in 1,148 hypertensive patients with type 2 diabetes. The participants in this study, aged 25 to 65 years (mean age, 56.4 years), had a mean blood pressure of 160/94 mm HG. Participants were randomly assigned to undergo tight control (lower than 150/85 mm HG) or less tight control (lower than 180/105 mm HG). The data demonstrated a prominent reduction in CV risk, death, and complications from diabetes among the patients who underwent tight control (30). Blood pressure control was more important than glycemic control in this cohort. The study was not, however, able to recommend aggressive blood pressure targets below 140/90 mm HG.

The ABCD trial compared the effects of an intensive blood pressure control (goal DBP of 75 mm HG) with those of a moderate control (goal DBP of 80 to 89 mm HG) in 480 normotensive patients and 470 hypertensive patients with type 2 diabetes. The patients in this study were aged 40 to 74 years. Among patients without gross albuminuria, there was no difference between the intensive and moderate control in the progression of microvascular disease (32,33). The incidence of all-cause mortality was lower in patients who received intensive blood pressure control than in those who received moderate control.

The AASK study examined the effect of aggressive blood pressure control on progression to renal failure in 1,094 African Americans aged 18 to 70 years with hypertension and renal impairment (glomerular filtration rate of 25 to 65 mL per minute per 1.73 m^2 at baseline). The investigators compared a mean arterial blood pressure of less than 92 mm HG (SBP of 128 and DBP of 79 mm HG) with a one of 102 to 107 (SBP of 140 and DBP of 90 mm HG). In this trial, there was no advantage to achieving the more aggressive blood pressure target. (Abstract presented at American Heart Association Meetings, 2001.)

Is there an optimal target for blood pressure control? Only 29% of individuals with hypertension achieve control to 140/90 mm HG (10). There is a continuous trend toward recommending even more aggressive blood pressure targets for subjects with hypertension and higher risk for CV complications, including individuals with diabetes mellitus and renal insufficiency. It is estimated that only 11% of treated hypertensive patients currently achieve control to the more aggressive blood pressure target of less than 130/85 mm Hg. Moreover, achieving the aggressive targets has not been shown to provide any more CV protection than that obtained with targeting 140/90 mm HG; this lack of clinical evidence (from four prospective trials with more than 20,000 participants) detracts from the recommendation of the aggressive strategy. Instead, the primary goal for therapy in most hypertensive subjects, is to achieve control to less than 140/90 mm Hg (approximately 138/85 mm Hg).

Trials Assessing Cardiovascular Benefits of Specific Antihypertensive Regimens

The completion of several large clinical trials: the Captopril Prevention Project (CAPPP) (36), the Intervention as a Goal in Hypertension Treatment (INSIGHT) (35), the Nordic Diltiazem (NORDIL) study (37), the Swedish Trial in Old Patients with Hypertension–2 (STOP-2) (38), the UKPDS, the Reduction of Endpoints in NIDDM with the AII Antagonist Losartan (RENAAL), the Irbesartan Diabetic Nephrathy Trial (IDNT), and the AASK have provided important information on the selection of specific antihypertensive drug classes. The most robust of the prospective trials for assessing the cardioprotective benefits of specific drug classes is the Antihypertensive and Lipid Lowering Treatment to Prevent Heart Attack Trial (ALLHAT) and is currently ongoing. The findings of the recently completed and ongoing trials are summarized as follows.

The CAPPP trial examined the incidence of CV events in 10,985 patients randomly assigned to receive an angiotensin-converting enzyme inhibitor (ACEI), captopril, or conventional treatment with beta blockers or diuretics. The results demonstrated that captopril did not significantly reduce the number of CV-related deaths in comparison with conventional treatment (76 vs. 95; $p = 0.092$; relative risk $= 0.77$). The rates of fatal and nonfatal myocardial infarction (MI) did not differ according to therapy; however, the rate of fatal and nonfatal stroke was greater with captopril than with conventional treatment (189 vs. 148; $p = 0.044$; relative risk $= 1.25$) (36).

In the INSIGHT trial, the investigators compared the effects of nifedipine with that of a combination of diuretics in 6,321 white high-risk hypertensive patients, aged 55 to 80 years. The average blood pressure at entry was 150/90 mm HG. The primary outcomes were CV-related death, nonfatal stroke, MI, and heart failure. The results showed no difference between the two study regimens in preventing overall CV outcomes (39).

In the NORDIL study, a total of 10,881 patients were randomly assigned to receive diltiazem, diuretics and beta blockers, or both. The patients were aged 50 to 74 years and had an average DBP of 100 mm HG. The primary outcomes were fatal and nonfatal stroke, MI, and other CV-related death. The primary endpoints of the two regimens were identical (preventing stroke, MI, and other CV-related death) (37). In a secondary analysis of a few hundred participants, diltiazem was slightly more effective than diuretic and beta blocker therapy in preventing stroke (159 vs. 196; $p = 0.04$; relative risk $= 0.80$).

In the STOP-2 study, 6,614 patients aged 70 to 84 years, with an average SBP of 180 mm HG, DBP of 105 mm HG, were randomly assigned to receive treatment with newer antihypertensive agents (enalapril, lisinopril, felodipine, isradipine) or conventional antihypertensive agents (atenolol, metoprolol, pindolol, hydrochlorothiazide, amiloride). The results showed similar decreases in blood pressure among all the treatment groups; the newer and conventional antihypertensive agents were equally effective in preventing CV-related morbidity and mortality (38).

The UKPDS was designed to evaluate the impact of aggressive blood pressure control with either an ACEI or a beta blocker. Ultimately, the UKPDS demonstrated that in patients with concomitant type 2 diabetes, treatment with an ACEI was no more beneficial than that with a beta blocker (40).

The RENAAL trial examined the effects of a blood pressure regimen that contained an angiotensin receptor blocker to an equally effective blood pressure strategy that did not (placebo). The RENAAL endpoints focused on renal events, including doubling of serum creatinine level, dialysis, transplantation, and death. The IDNT trial selected a similar population as the RENAAL (hypertensive diabetic patients with a creatinine level of 2 mg per deciliter and significant proteinuria), but added a third comparator, amlodipine, to the angiotensin receptor blocker and placebo arms. In both trials, there was a clear advantage for blocking the renin-angiotensin system in comparison to regimens that did not contain this drug class. The AASK study confirmed that the renal protective effect of blocking the renin-angiotensin system extended to nondiabetic African Americans with hypertension.

The ALLHAT is evaluating 40,389 high-risk patients with hypertension, aged 55 years or older. The study is comparing chlorthalidone, a diuretic; amlodipine, a calcium channel blocker; and lisinopril, an ACEI. The primary outcome is a composite of fatal coronary heart disease and nonfatal MI. The trial initially included doxazosin, an alpha-adrenergic blocker, but that arm was discontinued because patients demonstrated a 25% increase in CV events, driven primarily by a twofold greater hospitalization rate for heart failure, in comparison with the participants receiving diuretics (41,42).

SUMMARY

As is evident from the completed and ongoing clinical trials mentioned here, investigators are still trying to determine whether there are distinctions among antihypertensive drug classes in conferring CV protection. In the meantime, key findings from these trials indicate that certain therapies are preferred and others should be avoided, or at least deferred to second-line status or used as add-on therapy.

Many of the large-scale trials have shown that blood pressure control is critical for the general hypertensive population. This is particularly true for subjects with hypertension and at higher risk for CV complications, such as those with concomitant diabetes or renal insufficiency. However, it appears that control of SPB to 138 mm HG is as effective in preventing CV events, as is achieving the more aggressive targets of SBP of 130 mm HG or less. These observations in prospective trials are in contrast to the recommendations of consensus panels that used retrospective studies to arrive at the recommendation for aggressive blood pressure control for diabetic patients and patients with renal insufficiency. It is expected that updated guidelines will reflect strict blood pressure control to less than 140 mm

HG for SPB and will be much less cavalier in advocating for more aggressive targets.

At this time, there appears to be no reason to recommend specific drug classes in the management of hypertension in a general population. An exception concerns blocking the renin-angiotensin system in hypertensive patients with diabetic nephropathy. The ALLHAT study continues, but its investigators have already determined that alpha blockers do not decrease CV risk as well as diuretics do and, accordingly, are relegated to second-line or add-on therapy status.

As the inquiry into the "best" antihypertensive drug class continues, it appears that diuretics, ACEIs, beta blockers, angiotensin receptor blockers, and calcium channel blockers (excluding their use in patients with impaired renal function) are still contenders. It is likely that multiple drugs are necessary to control blood pressure to a target of SBP less than 140 mm HG.

PRACTICAL POINTS

- Hypertension is diagnosed on the basis of persistent elevation in blood pressure above 140/90 mm HG.

- The treatment target for blood pressure control is to less than 140/90 mm HG (approximately 138/85).

- Diuretics, calcium channel blockers, and ACEIs are recommended selections for initial drug therapy.

- Combinations of classes may be necessary to achieve optimal control of blood pressure.

REFERENCES

1. Joint National Committee on Prevention, Disease, Detection, Evaluation, and Treatment of High Blood Pressure. The sixth report of the Joint National Committee on Prevention, Detection, Evaluation, and Treatment of High Blood Pressure. *Arch Intern Med* 1997;157:2413–2446.
2. Sytkowski PA, D'Agostino RB, Belanger AJ, et al. Secular trends in long-term sustained hypertension, long-term treatment, and cardiovascular mortality: the Framingham Heart Study, 1950 to 1990. *Circulation* 1996;93:697–703.
3. Guidelines Subcommittee of the World Health Organization–Internal Society of Hypertension (WHO-ISH) Mild Hypertension Liaison Committee. 1999 World Health Organization–International Society of Hypertension guidelines for the management of hypertension. *J Hypertens* 1999;17:151–183.
4. Kannel W, Wolf P, Garrison R. *The Framingham Study,*

Section 35. Survival following initial cardiovascular events. Bethesda, MD: National Institutes of Health 5, 1998.
5. American Diabetes Association. Clinical practice recommendations 2001 [Guideline. Practice Guideline]. *Diabetes Care* 2001;24(Suppl 1):S1–S133.
6. Bakris GL, Williams M, Dworkin L, et al., for the National Kidney Foundation Hypertension and Diabetes Executive Committee Working Group. Preserving renal function in adults with hypertension and diabetes: a consensus approach. *Am J Kidney Dis* 2000;36:646–661.
7. Joint National Committee on Prevention, Detection, Evaluation, and Treatment of High Blood Pressure. The fifth report of the Joint National Committee on Detection, Evaluation, and Treatment of High Blood Pressure. *Arch Intern Med* 1993;153:154–183.
8. Kannel WB, Gordon T, Schwartz MJ. Systolic versus

diastolic blood pressure and the risk of coronary heart disease. *Am J Cardiol* 1971;27:335–346.

9. Franklin SS, Khan SA, Wong ND, et al. Is pulse pressure useful in predicting risk for coronary heart disease: the Framingham Heart Study. *Circulation* 1999;100:354–360.

10. Burt VL, Cutler JA, Higgins M, et al. Trends in the prevalence, awareness, treatment, and control of hypertension in the adult US population. data from the Health Examination Surveys, 1960 to 1991. *Hypertension* 1995;26:60–69.

11. Ward RB, Chin PG, Prior IAM. Genetic epidemiology of blood pressure in migrating isolate: prospectus. In: Sing CF, Skolnick MII, eds. *Genetic analysis of common diseases.* New York: Alan R. Liss, 1979:675–709.

12. Thiel B, Weder AB. Genes for essential hypertension: hype, help or hope? *J Clin Hypertens* 2000;2(3):187–193.

13. Sing CF, Boerwinkle E, Turner ST. Genetic of primary hypertension. *Clin Exp Hypertens A* 1986;8:623–651.

14. Kannel WB, Brand N, Skinner JJ Jr, et al. The relation of adiposity to blood pressure and development of hypertension: the Framingham study. *Ann Intern Med* 1967;67:48–59.

15. Reaven GM, Lithell H, Landberg L. Hypertension and associated metabolic abnormalities: the role of insulin resistance and the sympathoadrenal system. *N Engl J Med* 1996;334:374–381.

16. Reisin E, Abel R, Modan M, et al. Effect of weight loss without salt restriction on the reduction of blood pressure in overweight hypertensive patients. *New Engl J Med* 1978;298:1–6.

17. Cutler JA, Follman D, Allender PS. Randomized trials of sodium reduction: an overview. *Am J Clin Nutr* 1997;65:643S–651S.

18. Law MR, Frost CD, Wald NJ. By how much does dietary salt reduction lower blood pressure? III. Analysis of data from trials of salt reduction. *BMJ* 1991;302:819–824. [Erratum, *BMJ* 1991;302:939.]

19. National High Blood Pressure Education Program Working Group. Report on primary prevention of hypertension. *Arch Intern Med* 1993;153:186–208.

20. Intersalt Cooperative Research Group. An international study of electrolyte excretion and blood pressure: results for 24 hour urinary sodium and potassium excretion. *BMJ* 1988;297:319–328.

21. Miller JZ, Weinberg MH, Daughtery SA, et al. Heterogeneity of blood pressure response to dietary sodium restriction in normotensive adults. *J Chronic Dis* 1987;40:245–250.

22. Longworth DL, Drayer JIM, Weber MA, et al. Divergent blood pressure responses during short-term sodium restriction in hypertension. *Clin Pharmacol Ther* 1980;27:544–546.

23. MacGregor GA. The importance of the response of the renin-angiotensin system in determining blood pressure changes with sodium restriction. *Br J Clin Pharmacol* 1987;23:21S–26S.

24. Sacks FM, Svetkey LP, Vollmer WM, et al., for the DASH-Sodium Collaborative Research Group. Effects on blood pressure of reduced dietary sodium and the Dietary Approaches to Stop Hypertension (DASH) diet. *New Engl J Med* 2001;344:3–10.

25. Schneider RH, Nidich SI, Salerno JW. The Transcendental Meditation program: reducing the risk of heart disease and mortality and improving quality of life in African Americans. *Ethn Dis* 2001;11:159–160.

26. Zarnarra JW, Schneider RH, Besseglini T, et al. Usefulness of the transcendental meditation program in the treat of patients with coronary artery disease. *Am J Cardiol* 1996;77:867–870.

27. Schneider RH, Staggers F, Alexander CN, et al. A randomized controlled trial of stress reduction for hypertension in older African Americans. *Hypertension* 1995;26:820–927.

28. Wallace RB, Lynch CF, Pomrehn PR, et al. Alcohol and hypertension: epidemiological and experimental considerations. *Circulation* 1981;64(Suppl III):41–47.

29. Friedman GD, Klatsky AL, Siegelaub AB. Alcohol intake and hypertension. *Ann Intern Med* 1983;98:846–849.

30. Hansson L, Zanchetti A, Carruthers SG, et al., for the HOT Study Group. Effects of intensive blood-pressure lowering and low-dose aspirin in patients with hypertension: principal results of the Hypertension Optimal Treatment (HOT) randomised trial. *Lancet* 1998;351:1755–1762.

31. UK Prospective Diabetes Study Group. Tight blood pressure control and risk of macrovascular and microvascular complications in type 2 diabetes: UKPDS 38. *BMJ* 1998;317:703–713.

32. Estacio RO, Schrier RW. Antihypertensive therapy in type 2 diabetes: implications of the Appropriate Blood Pressure Control in Diabetes (ABCD) trial. *Am J Cardiol* 1998;82:9R–14R.

33. Estacio RO, Jeffers BW, Hiatt WR, et al. The effect of nisoldipine as compared with enalapril on cardiovascular outcomes in patients with non–insulin-dependent diabetes and hypertension. *New Engl J Med* 1998;338:645–952.

34. Estacio RO, Jeffers BW, Gifford N, et al. Effect of blood pressure control on diabetic microvascular complications in patients with hypertension and type 2 diabetes. *Diabetes Care* 2000;23(Suppl 2):B54–B64.

35. The African American Study of Kidney Disease and Hypertension (AASK) Study Group. Effect of ramipril vs amlodipine on renal outcomes in hypertensive nephrosclerosis: a randomized controlled trial. *JAMA* 2001;285:2719–2727.

36. Hansson L, Lindholm LH, Niskanen L, et al., for the Captopril Prevention Project (CAPPP) Study Group. Effect of angiotensin-converting enzyme inhibition compared with conventional therapy on cardiovascular morbidity and mortality in hypertension: the Captopril Prevention Project (CAPPP) randomized trial. *Lancet* 1999;353:611–616.

37. Hansson L, Hedner TM, Lund-Johansen P, et al., for the NORDIL Study Group. Randomised trial effects of calcium antagonists compared with diuretics and β-blockers on cardiovascular morbidity and mortality in hypertension: the Nordic Diltiazem (NORDIL) study. *Lancet* 2000;356:359–365.

38. Hansson L, Lindholm LH, Ekbom T, et al., for the STOP–Hypertension-2 study Group. Randomised trial of old and new antihypertensive drugs in elderly patients: cardiovascular mortality and morbidity, the Swedish Trial in Old Patients with Hypertension-2 study. *Lancet* 1999;354:1751–1756.

39. Brown MJ, Palmer CR, Castaigne A, et al. Morbidity

and mortality in patients randomised to double-blind treatment with a long-acting calcium-channel blocker or diuretic in the International Nifedipine GITS study: Intervention as a Goal in Hypertension Treatment (INSIGHT). *Lancet* 2000;356:366–372.

40. UK Prospective Diabetes Study Group. Efficacy of atenolol and captopril in reducing risk of macrovascular and microvascular complications in type 2 diabetes: UKPDS 39. *BMJ* 1998;317:713–720.

41. Davis BR, Cutler JA, Gordon DJ, et al., for the ALLHAT Research Group. Rationale and design for the Antihypertensive and Lipid Lowering Treatment to Prevent Heart Attack Trial (ALLHAT). *Am J Hypertens* 1999;9:342–360.

42. The ALLHAT Officers and Coordinators for the ALLHAT Collaborative Research Group. Major cardiovascular events in patients randomized to doxazosin vs. chlorthalidone: the Antihypertensive and Lipid-Lowering Treatment to Prevent Heart Attack Trial (ALLHAT). *JAMA* 2000;283:1967–1975.

13

Approach to Secondary Hypertension

John D. Bisognano

Approximately 90% to 95% of people with hypertension have primary (essential) hypertension (1). This elevation of blood pressure is multifactorial in origin and probably represents a complex interaction of multiple genetic traits with lifestyle factors such as weight, sodium intake and excretion, and stress (2). In contrast, patients with secondary hypertension have a specific identifiable cause of the blood pressure elevation and may benefit by correction of the underlying defect. This chapter describes the most common causes of secondary hypertension, with particular focus on issues relating to patient management. It is important to remember that many people have secondary hypertension *in addition* to primary hypertension and that addressing the secondary issues can lead to reduction, but not necessarily elimination, of a patient's need for other blood pressure–lowering therapy.

The Sixth Report of the Joint National Commission on the Evaluation and Treatment of High Blood Pressure recommends considering secondary causes of hypertension if blood pressure cannot be controlled by a combination of three drugs (3). This three-drug guideline alone, although generally reasonable, is likely to yield a high proportion of negative workups for secondary hypertension and may well be a relic of previous days when triple-drug treatment of hypertension was fraught with side effects and was viewed as maximum medical treatment. It also does not acknowledge the additional difficulty in reaching lower target blood pressure levels for diabetic patients (130/80 mm Hg) and for patients with severe renal insufficiency (125/75 mm Hg), which almost always require numerous medications (4). In addition, evaluation for secondary hypertension may be appropriate, regardless of blood pressure level or intensity of treatment, for specific groups such as the young, those with specific symptoms suggesting a secondary origin, and those with a history of hypertensive emergencies or severe target organ damage.

CLINICAL APPROACH

Before instituting an extensive evaluation for secondary causes of hypertension, the clinician must be certain that the blood pressure readings obtained are indicative of the patient's true blood pressure during the majority of the day. Although blood pressures measured in the physician's office serve this purpose for most patients, a sizable subset of patients have significant hypertension in the physician's office ("white-coat" hypertension). Labile hypertension carries an increased risk of cardiovascular events (5) and generally warrants some treatment, and the use of home blood pressure readings or 24-hour ambulatory monitoring can be important in distinguishing a patient with severe hypertension from one who simply has a controlled hypertension that is significantly augmented in the physician's office. A workup for secondary causes in a patient with near-normal home blood pressure readings is likely to be unrevealing, and the cost of home blood pressure monitoring is low in comparison with most secondary evaluations. Moreover, home blood pressure readings can prevent overtreatment in patients with labile blood pressure, decrease drug side effects and increase the patient's ability to adhere to prescribed medical regimens.

In elderly patients, evaluation of pseudohypertension (6) is also important because measurement in the calcified and noncompressible brachial arteries of these patients can lead to falsely elevated cuff readings and to subsequent overtreatment of the elevated numbers. In these patients, alternative blood pressure–measuring devices such as wrist and finger monitors, or even arterial lines, can be useful when a calcified brachial artery is palpated.

The physician must also assess a patient's compliance before embarking on an extensive workup for secondary causes of hypertension. Moderate to severe hypertension is often treated with multiple drugs that are expensive and have adverse side effect profiles. Because of their power in lowering blood pressure, drugs such as clonidine, hydralazine, and minoxidil are often prescribed without regard for the patient's ability to tolerate their combined side effects. In short, patients are often not eager to spend money each month in order to feel miserable, particularly when they generally seem well despite their elevated blood pressure. Assessing medical compliance for treatment of an asymptomatic disease such as hypertension is absolutely essential for successful treatment.

Finally, all of the numerical and physical data from a patient should be consistent before a secondary evaluation is considered. A patient with years of extremely elevated blood pressure but no evidence of any target organ damage (microalbuminuria, left ventricular hypertrophy, retinal abnormalities) is unlikely to have sustained levels of blood pressure elevation out of the

physician's office and would be a poor candidate for a workup for secondary hypertension. Similarly, a patient with modestly elevated readings in the physician's office but evidence of target organ damage should be evaluated more aggressively.

Once the accuracy of the blood pressure measurements and pattern is confirmed and the patient's history of medical compliance is reasonably documented, an evaluation for secondary causes of hypertension can proceed. In this chapter, the evaluation and treatment of the more common secondary causes of hypertension— specifically, exogenous drug use (including oral contraceptives), renal parenchymal disease, renal artery disease, adrenal disease (hyperaldosteronism, pheochromocytoma, and Cushing's syndrome), thyroid and parathyroid abnormality, obstructive sleep apnea, and aortic coarctation—are discussed (Table 13.1).

EXOGENOUS DRUG USE

Evaluation for exogenous drug use is an important step in the evaluation of secondary (potentially reversible) causes of hypertension. Some of the more common drugs used by hypertensive patients include oral contraceptives and other estrogen-containing compounds, sympathomimetic drugs for weight loss and sinusitis, alcohol and cocaine, immunosuppressive drugs,

TABLE 13.1. *Overall approach to secondary hypertension*

Possible cause of secondary hypertension	Initial diagnostic approach
Labile (white coat) hypertension	Home or 24-hr ambulatory monitor
Medical noncompliance	Focused history, including drug cost and side effects
Pseudohypertension	Wrist, finger, or arterial blood pressure measurement
Exogenous drug use	Focused history, including over-the-counter drugs
Renal parenchymal disease	General chemistry, urinalysis, urine for microalbumin
Renal artery stenosis	Renal artery imaging, including MRI, ultrasonography, angiography
Primary aldosteronism	Serum potassium, aldosterone/renin ratio
Pheochromocytoma	Urine VMA, catecholamines, metanephrines or serum metanephrines
Cushing's syndrome	24-hr urine for free cortisol
Thyroid disease	TSH or free thyroxine
Parathyroid disease	Serum calcium and ionized calcium level
Obstructive sleep apnea	Sleep study
Aortic coarctation	Chest radiograph or CT

CT, computed tomography; MRI, magnetic resonance imaging; TSH, thyroid-stimulating hormone; VMA, vanillylmandelic acid.

anabolic steroids, and nonsteroidal antiinflammatory drugs.

A relatively large proportion of young women use oral contraceptive medications. Although these medications produce only small increases of blood pressure in most patients, a subset of patients experiences significant increases in systolic blood pressure, sometimes as great as 22 mm Hg. In one study, degree of hypertension was associated with increased age (older than 35 years), duration of antiovulatory therapy, and alcohol intake. The hypertensive effect of the medication reversed in 50% of the patients 3 to 6 months after discontinuation, leaving a residual elevation in blood pressure that was probably attributable to underlying primary hypertension. Estrogen replacement therapy does not appear to have a similar hypertensive effect (7). Because the population of women who are at highest risk for renal artery fibromuscular dysplasia also includes a high relative percentage who use of oral contraceptives, it may be worthwhile to consider a trial of discontinuation of oral contraceptives before embarking on an extensive evaluation (discussed later) for renal artery fibromuscular dysplasia.

Numerous sympathomimetic drugs can be purchased over the counter and at health food stores for the treatment of sinusitis (pseudoephedrine) or obesity (phenylpropanolamine and others) (8). These drugs can produce profound increases in blood pressure through peripheral vasoconstriction and tachycardia. Because many hypertensive patients are also overweight, it is useful to ask patients specifically whether they use over-the-counter weight-loss drugs during evaluation for secondary causes of hypertension. Inquiry should also be made about food supplements because sympathomimetics may be included and because some products from overseas may not be labeled in English.

Recreational use of cocaine can cause transient spikes in blood pressure but results in no chronic elevation of blood pressure. The transient spikes can also lead to significant myocardial ischemia and coronary spasm (9). Alcohol intake of more than 2 oz per day can be associated with severe hypertension resistant to medical therapy, and patients whose condition appears refractory to the effects of medical therapy should be questioned about alcohol intake. In such patients, the issue of compliance with the medical regimen should also be definitively evaluated before they embark on an extensive workup for other secondary causes of hypertension.

More patients are receiving solid organ transplants each year, and a greater proportion of these patients are surviving longer. The immunosuppressive medications cyclosporine and tacrolimus produce nephrotoxicity and hypertension in the majority of patients. The virtually unavoidable side effects are necessary to permit adequate immunosuppression while minimizing use of steroid drugs (which can also cause hypertension through volume increase). The mechanism of the hypertension caused by cyclosporine and tacrolimus is unclear but may be related to activation of the sympathetic nervous system (10). Because most patients' survival depends on adequate dosing with these drugs, blood pressure must simply be treated (often to low target levels dictated by the underlying renal insufficiency) with the usual armamentarium of antihypertensive drugs. Isradipine is frequently the favored calcium channel blocker because of its lack of effect on cyclosporine metabolism.

Exogenous intake of anabolic steroid medications, primary for bodybuilding, can lead to mild increases in blood pressure as a result of sodium retention. It may be important to counsel hypertensive patients who engage in bodybuilding to avoid exogenous steroid usage and also to inform them that that bodybuilding itself can exacerbate hypertension.

Finally, the increasing use of nonsteroidal antiinflammatory drugs can cause hypertension both acutely and chronically by causing an analgesic nephropathy. This class of drugs generally produces small, if any, elevation in blood pressure in most patients (11), but certain patients have a marked increase in blood pressure. It is important to consider nonsteroidal drugs as a cause of increased blood pressure, particularly in the elderly patients, who often use these drugs at high doses. Simply withholding these medications for a few weeks may result in normalization of blood pressure and eliminate the need to pursue a workup for other secondary causes of high blood pressure.

RENAL PARENCHYMAL DISEASE

Disease of the renal parenchyma can be responsible for acute and chronic hypertension. When a patient presents with a hypertensive crisis, it is mandatory to evaluate renal function through a general chemistry profile and a urinalysis. Although abnormalities may be the result of the hypertension itself, evaluation for acute renal processes such as acute glomerulonephritis, bilateral renal artery embolism, and bilateral ureteral obstruction should be considered (12). Other processes such as vasculitis and high-dose nonsteroidal drug ingestion can also lead to acute renal failure and hypertension, and prompt consultation with a nephrologist or, if indicated, a vascular surgeon or urologist should be made in these cases.

More commonly, chronic hypertension can be caused by chronic renal insufficiency (and vice versa). Long-standing diabetic nephropathy and chronic pyelonephritis, for example, can result in decreases in glomerular filtration rate and sodium retention and can worsen chronic hypertension (13). Much evidence now available suggests that angiotensin-converting enzyme inhibition or angiotensin receptor blockade (14) can result in decreased blood pressure as well as preservation of renal function. Patients who are likely to proceed to dialysis or renal transplantation should receive prompt referral to a nephrologist. Aggressive cardiovascular risk modification is also warranted in these patients with end-stage renal disease, in whom the primary cause of death is cardiovascular in origin (15).

RENAL ARTERY STENOSIS

Renal artery disease can result from either of two entirely separate entities: atherosclerotic renal artery stenosis and renal artery fibromuscular dysplasia (16). Both of these entities can cause hypertension but can also exist in many patients without significant elevations in blood pressure. Great strides have been made since 1990 in percutaneous revascularization, including renal

artery stent placement. The greatest challenge, however, remains in selecting the patients most likely to benefit from these procedures.

Atherosclerotic renal artery stenosis is primarily a disease of the renal artery ostium and the proximal one third of the renal artery (17). Because atherosclerosis is a systemic disease, renal artery stenosis occurs in patients with other cardiovascular risk factors, and a high proportion of patients with atherosclerotic renal artery disease also have coronary disease (18), an important consideration when renal revascularization is contemplated. Noninvasive imaging with renal magnetic resonance angiography, Doppler ultrasonography, or computed tomography (CT) can be helpful in screening patients for invasive angiography and revascularization. Other tests such as selective renal vein renins and captopril renograms can further guide the decision of whether to perform revascularization, and there is some evidence that renal artery resistive indices may be useful in predicting responsiveness to renal artery revascularization (19). There is wide variability in the sensitivity, specificity, and availability of these modalities among institutions, and it is most important for the clinician to explore a particular institution's area of expertise when ordering renal artery imaging. Invasive arteriography remains the gold standard for determining the degree of stenosis and also enables the operator to measure gradients to evaluate the hemodynamic significance of a lesion (20). Patients who experience onset of severe hypertension at a late age or rapid deterioration of hypertension control should be considered for renal artery evaluation, particularly if they have other atherogenic risk factors. Selection of patients most likely to benefit from renal artery revascularization remains an area of controversy.

In contrast to atherosclerotic renal artery disease, renal artery fibromuscular dysplasia responds exceeding well to balloon angioplasty (21). Affected patients generally have abnormalities in the arterial media, leading to weblike stenoses in the distal two thirds of the renal artery. The disease occurs in both sexes and at all ages, but young women are the most frequently affected by this disease. Most noninvasive imaging studies do not provide an adequate assessment of the distal two thirds of the renal arteries; it is often necessary to perform arteriography in patients in whom medial fibromuscular dysplasia is suspected. This disease is worth finding in afflicted patients because a significant improvement in hypertension can be accomplished in 60% to 70% of patients with simple balloon angioplasty, without stent placement.

ADRENAL DISEASE

Adrenal hormonal excesses are responsible for a variety of causes of secondary hypertensions. This section describes the evaluation and treatment of the three most common causes.

Hyperaldosteronism

Primary aldosteronism, or oversecretion of aldosterone unregulated by angiotensin II, is classically thought to manifest with low serum potassium or an exaggerated potassium loss with small doses of diuretic. In the modern era, many cases of aldosteronism are uncovered through routine screening of aldosterone and plasma renin activity. Patients with suspected primary aldosteronism can be further evaluated with a ratio of plasma aldosterone to renin activity; a ratio of greater than 10 is abnormal, and a ratio exceeding 20 is highly suggestive of hyperaldosteronism. Once a screening has identified a patient as having aldosteronism, the next step is to determine whether the aldosterone level can be suppressed by either saline infusion or captopril (22). This testing often requires referral to an endocrinologist or a hypertension specialist. Most antihypertensive medications have an effect either on plasma renin or on serum aldosterone levels, but the option of taking a patient off all drugs before testing may increase the risk of cardiovascular complications, particularly in patients with severe elevations of their blood pressure. One report suggested that increasing the threshold for a positive aldosterone/renin ratio permits its use in treated patients (23). Once primary aldosteronism is confirmed with biochemical testing, the key diagnostic decision is whether a patient with primary aldosteronism is suffering from a benign solitary adenoma, an adrenal adenocarci-

noma, or bilateral adrenal hyperplasia. Adrenal CT or magnetic resonance imaging (MRI) can suggest this diagnosis, and solitary lesions can be further characterized with NP-59 scintigraphy after dexamethasone suppression. Benign lesions take up the isotope, adenomas unilaterally and hyperplasia bilaterally, whereas malignant ones generally do not. Lesions thought to be malignant, on the basis of either NP-59 scans or size (larger than 4 cm suggests malignancy) should be resected. Smaller, presumably benign lesions can be monitored expectantly, but improvement in blood pressure is expected in many patients after resection of solitary adrenal adenomas. With the development of laparoscopic techniques, adrenalectomy is an increasingly attractive alternative. Patients with bilateral adrenal hyperplasia are treated with spironolactone but can also be treated effectively with other antihypertensive medications (24).

Pheochromocytoma

The diagnosis of pheochromocytoma can be made primarily from the patient's history, but the symptoms of pheochromocytoma overlap considerably with those of numerous other diseases, including panic attacks, atrial tachyarrhythmias, alcohol withdrawal, and perimenopausal hot flashes, as well as with those caused by intermittent compliance with hypertensive medications. The classic patient with a pheochromocytoma has wide, unprovoked fluctuations in blood pressure accompanied by tachycardia, pallor, sweating, headaches, and sometimes cardiac failure caused by progressive catecholamine-induced left ventricular failure.

In patients with an appropriate history, the most widely used screening test is a 24-hour urine collection for metanephrine, normetanephrine, and vanillylmandelic acid. Labetalol can interfere with older fluorometric assays, but the now more commonly used high performance liquid chromatography determination is not similarly affected. Another screening test is the determination of plasma metanephrine; a random sample has a 99% sensitivity for diagnosis (25).

Once there is biochemical evidence for a pheochromocytoma, the next step is to localize the tumor for resection. Eighty-five percent of pheochromocytomas are in the adrenal glands and can be demonstrated by CT or MRI (26). In patients without obvious adrenal masses, metaiodobenzylguanidine (MIBG) scanning with I 131–labeled benzylguanidine can localize the tumor, which is usually found along the sympathetic chain or in the bladder.

Once localized, pheochromocytomas should be resected with careful perioperative blood pressure control, usually with phenoxybenzamine and other medications. Beta blockers should be used cautiously until alpha blockade is established, to prevent further increases in blood pressure. Malignant pheochromocytomas can be treated with various agents such as metyrosine (27) and streptozocin (28).

Cushing's Syndrome

Cushing's syndrome, an unusual secondary hypertension, is caused by excess glucocorticoid secretion. The hypertension can be severe (29) and is associated with a lack of a normal nocturnal decline in blood pressure. This syndrome should be suspected in patients with depression, as well as in those with the physical features of Cushing's syndrome, such as central obesity and purple striae. In patients in whom Cushing's syndrome is suspected, a 24-hour urine collection for free cortisol yields nearly 100% sensitivity (30). Additional evaluation would include a dexamethasone suppression test and, if the result is positive, radiologic studies for isolation of the lesion. If hypercortisolism is independent of adrenocorticotropic hormone (ACTH), the adrenal glands should be imaged by CT or MRI (31). If the hormonal tests suggest that the disease is ACTH dependent, then the pituitary gland is the likely location of the tumor. Hypertensive patients with hypercortisolism are likely to benefit from referral to an endocrinologist for full evaluation, including evaluation for more unusual causes of cortisol excess.

THYROID AND PARATHYROID ABNORMALITIES

Patients with symptoms of hyperthyroidism or hypothyroidism should be screened by thyroid-stimulating hormone (TSH) measurement. Patients with hypothyroidism often have a depressed cardiac output with a markedly increased peripheral vascular resistance, which results in hypertension. Similarly, patients with hyperthyroidism have tachycardia and increased inotropism and can be hypertensive for those reasons. Elderly patients often have atypical manifestations of thyroid dysfunction, and it is prudent to screen all elderly hypertensive patients for hypothyroidism or hyperthyroidism. Treatment of these patients can yield improvement in blood pressure, both systolic and diastolic (32).

Hyperparathyroidism can lead to left ventricular hypertrophy (33) and hypertension. These conditions may be caused by increased vascular reactivity to catecholamines (34) or long-term calcium deposition in the kidneys, which lead to renal parenchymal disease. Hyperparathyroidism should be considered in hypertensive patients with elevated serum calcium levels.

OBSTRUCTIVE SLEEP APNEA

Obstructive sleep apnea may occur in as many of 30% of hypertensive patients (35), although some investigators have noted no daytime hypertension among patients with obstructive sleep apnea (36). Observational studies have shown that systemic and pulmonary pressures rise during apneic episodes (37), which have also been associated with increased sympathetic activity (38). Screening patients with clinical signs of obstructive sleep apnea may yield a secondary cause of hypertension that can be easily reversed with weight loss and continuous positive airway pressure ventilation.

AORTIC COARCTATION

Significant aortic coarctation is generally diagnosed in childhood and is often amenable to balloon dilatation (39). However, patients with less severe coarctation often survive into adulthood and develop hypertension as a result of a postobstructive vasoconstriction. These patients often have activation of the renin-angiotensin system and excessive catecholamine increases during exercise (40). Adult patients with aortic coarctation often present with heart failure, aortic rupture, bacterial endocarditis, and intracranial hemorrhage (41). The diagnosis can sometimes be made by evaluating the aortic contour on plain chest radiography, but it is more definitively made by CT, MRI, or transesophageal echocardiography. The prevalence of hypertension among adults with coarctation approaches 33% (42). Evaluation of young patients with hypertension should include consideration of aortic coarctation, not only because repair of the coarctation can improve the hypertension but also, more important, so that the sequelae of the coarctation itself can be minimized or prevented.

CONCLUSIONS

In considering an evaluation for secondary causes of hypertension, it is important to realize that the overwhelming majority of patients with hypertension, even severe hypertension, have primary (essential) hypertension. It is important to take a close look at a patient's medical regimen with a special focus on its cost and the pa-tient's ability to adhere to the regimen before labeling a patient's hypertension as "refractory to treatment." In addition, it is essential to look for exogenous causes of a patient's blood pressure elevation, because attention to these causes can result in reversal of much of a patient's hypertension and, in many ways, these causes are among the most treatable "secondary" causes of hypertension. Once it has been established that a patient's hypertension is truly refractory to treatment or has characteristics (either laboratory or clinical) suggestive of other secondary causes, prompt and complete evaluation can lead to marked improvement or even complete resolution of hypertension. Most important, an evaluation for hypertension is not simply a reason for the physician to treat the elevated numbers; it is also an opportunity—perhaps one that will not occur again in a decade—for examination of the patient's overall cardiovascular risk profile and for action to be taken to decrease cardiovascular risk.

PRACTICAL POINTS

- Approximately 90% to 95% of people with hypertension have primary (essential) hypertension.
- Before instigating an extensive evaluation for secondary causes of hypertension, the clinician must be certain that the blood pressure readings obtained are indicative of the patient's true blood pressures during the majority of the day.
- In elderly patients, evaluation of pseudohypertension is important, because measurement in noncompressible brachial arteries can lead to falsely elevated cuff readings.
- The physician must also assess a patient's adherence to a medical regimen before embarking on an extensive workup for secondary hypertension.
- Renal parenchymal disease and renovascular hypertension are the most common causes of secondary hypertension.
- Primary aldosteronism, Cushing's syndrome, hyperthyroidism and hypothyroidism, and pheochromocytoma are endocrine causes of secondary hypertension.
- The role of renal artery revascularization in renovascular hypertension remains controversial.
- Although primary hypertension is the most common cause of elevated blood pressure in adolescents, secondary causes of hypertension are more prevalent in the young hypertensive population.

REFERENCES

1. Rudnick KV, Sackett DL, Hirst S, et al. Hypertension in family practice. *Can Med Assoc J* 1977;117:492.
2. Harrap SB. An appraisal of the genetic approaches to high blood pressure. *J Hypertens* 1996:15(Suppl 5): S111–S115.
3. The Sixth Report of the Joint National Committee on

Prevention, Detection, Evaluation and Treatment of High Blood Pressure. *Arch Intern Med* 1997;157:2413.

4. Pontremoli R, Robaudo C, Gaiter A. Long term minoxidil treatment in refractory hypertension and renal failure,. *Clin Nephrol* 1991;35:39–43.

5. Vasan RS, Larson MG, Leip EP, et al. Impact of high-normal blood pressure on the risk of cardiovascular disease. *N Engl J Med* 2001;345:1291–1297.

6. Zweifler AJ, Shahab ST. Pseudohypertension: a new assessment. *J Hypertens* 1993;11:1–6.

7. Royal College of General Practitioners. Hypertension. In: *Oral Contraceptives and Health*. London: Pitman Medical, 1974.

8. Lake CR, Gallant S, Masson E, et al. Adverse drug effects attributed to phenylpropanolamine: a review of 142 case reports. *Am J Med* 1990;89:195–208.

9. Om A, Ellahham S, DiSciascio G. Management of cocaine-induced cardiovascular complications. *Am Heart J* 1993;125:471–475.

10. Singer DR, Jenkins GH. Hypertension in transplant recipients. *J Hum Hypertens* 1996;10:395–402.

11. Brook RD, Blaxall BC, Kramer M, et al. Nonsteroidal anti-inflammatory drugs and hypertension. *J Clin Hypertens* 2000;(5):319–323.

12. Ghose RR, Harinda V. Unrecognized high pressure chronic retention of urine presenting with systemic arterial hypertension. *BMJ* 1989;297:1626.

13. Gaede P, Vedel P, Parving H, et al. Intensified multifactorial intervention in patients with type 2 diabetes mellitus and microalbuminuria, *Lancet* 1999;353:617.

14. Jafar TH, Schmid CH, Landa M, et al. Angiotensin-converting enzyme inhibitors and progression of non-diabetic renal disease: a meta-analysis of patient-level data. *Ann Intern Med* 2001;135:73–87.

15. Pfeffer MA, Sacks FM, Moye LA. Cholesterol and recurrent events: a secondary prevention trial for normolipidemic patients. CARE Investigators. *Am J Cardiol* 1995;76:73C–106C.

16. Mann SJ, Pickering TG. Detection of renovascular hypertension: state of the art 1992. *Ann Intern Med* 1992;227:845.

17. Bookstein JJ. Segmental renal artery stenosis in renovascular hypertension. *Radiology* 1968;90:973.

18. NCEP III. Cholesterol treatment guidelines. *JAMA* 2001;285:2508.

19. Radermacher J, Chavan A, Bleck J, et al. Use of Doppler ultrasonography to predict the outcome of therapy for renal-artery Stenosis. *N Engl J Med* 2001;344:410–417.

20. van de Ven PH, Kaatee R, Beutler JJ. Arterial stenting and balloon angioplasty in ostial atherosclerotic renovascular disease, a randomized trial. *Lancet* 1999;353:282.

21. Aurell M, Jensen G, Treatment of renovascular hypertension. *Nephron* 1997;75:373.

22. Holland OB, Brown H, Huhnert L. Further evaluation of saline infusion for the diagnosis of primary aldosteronism. *Hypertension* 1984;6:717–723.

23. Gallay BJ, Ahmad S, Xu L, et al. Screening for primary aldosteronism without discontinuing hypertensive medications: plasma aldosterone-renin ratio. *Am J Kidney Dis* 2001;37:699–705.

24. Mantero F, Opocher G, Rocco S. Long term treat-

ment of mineralocorticoid excess syndromes. *Steroids* 1995;60:81–86.

25. Lenders JWM, Keiser HR, Goldstein DS, et al. Plasma metanephrines in the diagnosis of pheochromocytoma. *Ann Intern Med* 1995;123:101–109.

26. Freitas JE. Adrenal cortical and medullary imaging. *Semin Nucl Med* 1995;25:235–250.

27. Serri O, Comtois R, Bettez P. Reduction in the size of a pheochromocytoma pulmonary metastasis by metyrosine therapy. *N Engl J Med* 1984;310:1264–1265.

28. Feldman JM. Treatment of metastatic pheochromocytoma with streptozocin. *Arch Intern Med* 1983; 143:1799–1800.

29. Fallo F, Paoletta A, Tona F. Response of hypertension to conventional antihypertensive treatment and/or steroidogenesis inhibitors in Cushing's syndrome. *J Intern Med* 1993;234:595–598.

30. Mengden T, Hubmann P, Muller J. Urinary free cortisol versus 17-hydrosycorticosteroids: a comparative study of their diagnostic value in Cushing's syndrome. *Clin Invest* 1992;70:545–548

31. Doppman J. The dilemma of bilateral adrenocortical nodularity in Conn's and Cushing's syndromes. *Radiol Clin North Am* 1993;31:1039–1050.

32. Streeten DHP, Anderson GH, Howland T. Effects of thyroid function on blood pressure. Recognition of hypothyroid hypertension. *Hypertension* 1988;11:78–83.

33. Stefenelli T, Abela C, Frank H. Cardiac abnormalities in patients with primary hyperparathyroidism: implications for follow-up. *J Clin Endocrinol Metab* 1997;82:106–112

34. Gennari C, Nami R, Gonnelli S. Hypertension and primary hyperparathyroidism: the role of adrenergic and renin-angiotensin-aldosterone system. *Miner Electrolyte Metab* 1995;21:77–81.

35. Young T, Palta M, Dempsey J. The occurrence of sleep-disorder breathing among middle-aged adults. *N Engl J Med* 1993;328:1230–1235.

36. Davies RJO, Drosby J, Prothero A, et al. Ambulatory blood pressure and left ventricular hypertrophy in subjects with untreated obstructive sleep apnea and snoring and their response to treatment. *Clin Sci* 1984;86:417–424.

37. Mateika J, Mateika S, Slutsky A, et al. The effect of snoring on mean arterial blood pressure during non-REM sleep, *Am Rev Respir Dis* 1992;145:141–146.

38. Somers F, Dyken M, Clary M, et al. Sympathetic neural mechanisms in obstructive sleep apnea. *J Clin Invest* 1995;96:1897–1904.

39. Huggon I, Qureshi S, Baker E, et al. Effect of introducing balloon dilation of native aortic coarctation on overall outcome in infants and children. *Am J Cardiol* 1994;73:799–801.

40. Ross RD, Clapp SK, Gunther S. Augmented norepinephrine and renin output in response to maximal exercise in hypertensive coarctectomy patients. *Am Heart J* 1992;123:1293–1298.

41. Campbell M. Natural history of coarctation of the aorta. *Br Heart J* 1970;32:633–640.

42. Cohen M, Fuster V, Steele P. Coarctation of the aorta. Long-term follow-up and prediction of outcome after surgical correction. *Circulation* 1989;80:840–845.

14

Heart Failure Due to Left Ventricular Systolic Dysfunction

Todd M. Koelling and Robert J. Cody

Heart failure is a clinical syndrome that occurs when any disease causes impairment of the heart's ability to pump blood. According to this definition, heart failure can be caused by any process that inhibits heart chamber filling or reduces myocardial contractile function. Patients with impaired cardiac pumping function experience symptoms related to abnormal perfusion and retention of vascular fluid volume. The cardinal symptoms of heart failure include fatigue, dyspnea, and edema, although other related symptoms may also occur. Heart failure may be caused by disorders of the pericardium, myocardium, heart valves, or great vessels, but most patients manifest the syndrome through abnormalities in systolic function. Reduction in myocardial contractility is more commonly referred to as *systolic dysfunction* and may also coexist with chamber filling abnormalities, also referred to as *diastolic dysfunction.*

The term *heart failure* is now preferred to *congestive heart failure,* inasmuch as not all patients with heart failure are "congested," and experts believe that the latter description has limited diagnostic accuracy. Heart failure occurs commonly in clinical practice and represents the most common Diagnosis-Related Group discharge diagnosis in the Medicare (elderly) population. Nearly 4,700,000 patients (2,300,000 men and 2,400,000 women) in the United States suffer from heart failure, and approximately 550,000 new cases of heart failure are diagnosed each year. Of Americans older than age 65, approximately 6% to 10% have experienced heart failure. Although heart failure can occur at any age, most patients with heart failure are older than 65 years, and 78% of men and 85% of women hospitalized because of heart failure belong to this older age group.

Heart failure is a common cause of mortality in the population; nearly 300,0000 patients die of heart failure each year. Over the period 1979 to 1998, deaths from heart failure increased by 135%, and hospitalizations for heart failure as a primary diagnosis rose by 159% (377,000 in 1979 to 978,000 in 1998) (Table 14.1). The annual estimated rate of new and recurrent heart failure events for nonblack men aged 65 to 74 is 21.5 per 1,000 population; for those aged 75 to 84, it is 43.3; and for those aged 85 and older, it is 73.1. For black men, the rates are 21.1, 52.0, and 66.7, respectively. For nonblack women in the same age groups, the rates are 11.2, 26.3 and 64.9, respectively, and for black women, the rates are 18.9, 33.5, and 48.4, respectively. Because heart failure necessitates frequent hospitalizations in the population, the costs of caring for this syndrome are considerable. The total inpatient and outpatient costs for heart failure in 1991 were $38.1 billion, about 5.4% of the health care budget at that time.

USUAL CAUSES

It has been well recognized that the myocardium undergoes structural changes in response to cardiovascular disease states. Irrespective of the initial cause, myocardial damage results in reduced power output of the heart, which occurs in a varying time frame, depending on the severity of disease and the cause of myocardial damage. Myocardial ischemia is usually manifested initially by regional impairment of myocardial function. Nonischemic dilated cardiomyopathies

TABLE 14.1. *Causes of systolic heart failure*

Primary myocardial diseases
Inherited cardiomyopathic disorders
    Dilated cardiomyopathy
    Late remodeling stage of hypertrophic
       cardiomyopathy
Muscular dystrophies
Secondary myocardial diseases
Energy supply deficit
    Coronary atherosclerosis
    Coronary dissection
    Coronary embolus
Excess ventricular afterload
    Hypertension
    Aortic stenosis
    Aortic coarctation
Excess ventricular preload
    Mitral regurgitation
    Aortic insufficiency
Tachycardia mediated
    Atrial fibrillation/flutter
    Supraventricular tachycardia
Infectious
    Viral myocarditis
    Septicemia
    Human immunodeficiency virus
Endocrine
    Hypothyroidism
    Hyperthyroidism
Connective tissue diseases
    Systemic lupus erythematosus
    Sarcoidosis
Infiltrative diseases
    Amyloidosis
    Hemochromatosis
    Wilson's disease
Toxins
    Alcohol
    Anthracycline
       Doxorubicin
       Daunarubicin
       Epirubicin
       Paclitaxel
    Trastuzumab (Herceptin)
    Cyclophosphamide
    Interferon
    Interleukin-2
    Chloroquine
    Zidovudine
Congenital heart disease
Peripartum
Idiopathic

caused by such insults as viral infections, exogenous toxins, regurgitant valvular lesions, and hereditary factors normally manifest with global left ventricular dysfunction. Abnormalities that begin by causing elevated myocardial strain include hypertension, aortic stenosis, and hypertrophic cardiomyopathy. Most patients with these abnormalities present with myocardial hypertrophy, either concentric (hypertension, aortic stenosis) or focal (hypertrophic cardiomyopathy). Although the types of insults that occur may be very different in the initial appearance of the myocardium, the chronic adaptations that occur in the body as a response to myocardial dysfunction reach a common pathway, as it is understood today (Fig. 14.1).

COMMON MECHANISMS

Occurrence of the primary disorder leads first to myocyte injury or increased myocyte strain, or both (Fig. 14.2); second, to myocardial remodeling in structure and function; and, third, to loss of systolic or diastolic function, which in turn leads to decreased cardiac output and elevated filling pressures. Structural changes in the myocardium and vasculature are important contributors to the progression of left ventricular dysfunction. Myocardial fibroblasts and vascular smooth muscle cells may hypertrophy or proliferate, or both, in response to a variety of stimuli. These structural effects lead to changes in the compliance of arteries that augment the left ventricular load and to increases in the volume, mass, or both of the left ventricle (1). The role of such ventricular remodeling in heart failure has been further described in patients who have had myocardial infarctions.

Many of the adaptive and maladaptive responses in congestive heart failure occur at sites distal to the initial myocardial damage. Decrements in cardiac output and elevations in central venous pressure result in reduced organ perfusion (Fig. 14.2). Underperfusion of the kidney and underfilling of the arterial vasculature results in a cascade of adaptations that lead to neurohormonal alterations that have been found to have direct myocardial toxicity through myocyte hypertrophy, myocardial fibrosis, and/or apoptosis (2). Nonetheless, these distal abnormalities are integrally related to reduction of systolic function. Because cardiac myocytes cannot replicate at a rate sufficient to contribute to repair a direct injury, the response to injury is limited primarily to hypertrophy and increased interstitial tissue alterations.

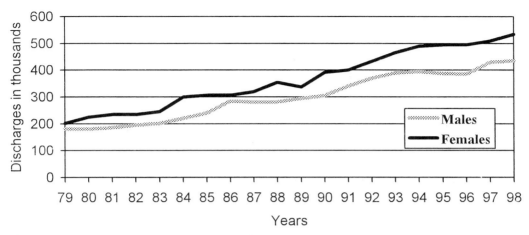

FIG. 14.1. Hospital discharges in the United States by sex from 1979 to 1998. (From Centers for Disease Control and Prevention/National Center for Health Statistics and the American Heart Association.)

The mechanisms that lead to progression of disease in heart failure include neural and hormonal factors that increase the load on the left ventricle, stimulate growth of myocytes, and may have direct toxic effects on the myocardium. The concentrations of several neurohormones and cytokines, including plasma norepinephrine, plasma renin activity, atrial natriuretic peptide (ANP), and tumor necrosis factor, have been shown to be increased in plasma in patients with congestive heart failure. The elevation in the levels of these compounds becomes more marked as clinical symptoms of heart failure advance and is associated with increased mortality rates. There also exists evidence that elevations of these compounds may be a more sensitive method of monitoring disease progression, as Benedict et al. (3) showed in the Studies of Left Ventricular Dysfunction (SOLVD) prevention trial that plasma norepinephrine levels continued to be predictive of mortality and development of clinical events related to the onset of heart failure despite the patients' being asymptomatic or minimally symptomatic.

Renin-Angiotensin-Aldosterone System

Activation of the renin-angiotensin-aldosterone system is one of the predominant abnormalities of heart failure. The degree of increase in plasma renin activity provides an indicator for prognosis in patients with heart failure (4). Studies in mild and asymptomatic heart failure demonstrate relatively less activation, but even these values are increased in comparison to normal. The degree of renin activity is intensified in the presence of diuretic therapy. Angiotensin II causes constriction of the systemic vasculature and vasoconstriction of both the afferent and efferent renal arterioles. In some patients with severe heart failure, treatment with angiotensin-converting enzyme (ACE) inhibitors may cause a deterioration of renal function. This may be related to fixed renal artery disease or, alternatively, to selective blocking of the constrictor action of angiotensin II on the efferent arteriole (5). Renin system components have been identified in the myocardium and vasculature, where they adversely affect fibrosis and remodeling, as well as cellular dysfunction. These findings suggest that the renin-angiotensin-aldosterone system has effects on cardiac function beyond altering sodium excretion and cardiac afterload. Not only is angiotensin II a potent vasoconstrictor, but it also causes a direct effect on hypertrophy of myocytes and may lead to energy supply mismatch as the capillary bed perfuses a larger bed.

In addition to vasoconstriction, angiotensin II stimulates aldosterone secretion by the adrenal gland, producing sodium retention and

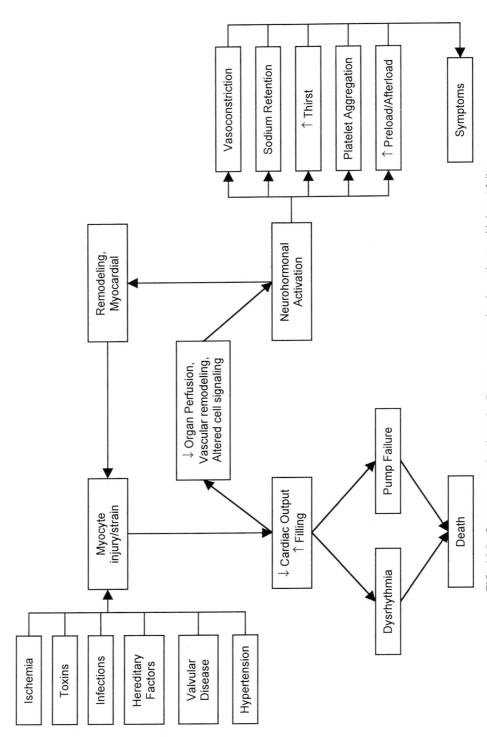

FIG. 14.2. Common mechanisms in disease progression in patients with heart failure.

potassium excretion at the distal nephron. Elevations in the activity of aldosterone leads to a sodium-retentive state found in patients with heart failure. Although adrenergic stimulation and angiotensin II increase sodium transport in the proximal tubule of the kidney, patients with increased activity from aldosterone overcome this effect, and sodium delivery to the distal tubules is attenuated, leading to the edematous state. It has been shown previously that although ACE inhibition continues to suppress angiotensin II levels over the course of 1 year, levels of aldosterone are initially suppressed during the first 1 to 3 months of therapy but fail to be suppressed beyond 6 months of therapy (6). This is thought to occur because stimuli in the form of glucocorticoids, hyperkalemia, hypermagnesemia, melanocyte-stimulating hormone, and endothelin continue to increase aldosterone secretion, although angiotensin II levels are low. Analysis of the Cooperative North Scandinavian Enalapril Survival Study (CONSENSUS) revealed that elevated levels of aldosterone were associated with the lowest rates of survival, and a reduction in plasma aldosterone during the course of therapy was associated with a favorable impact on survival (7). Although elevated aldosterone levels may track the clinical state of patients with congestive heart failure, they may also be responsible in part for progression of myocardial dysfunction through mechanisms that lead to abnormal accumulation of collagen, which surrounds and encases myocytes, resulting in diastolic and systolic ventricular dysfunction. Such deposition of collagen may lead to pathologic hypertrophy of the myocardium and has been shown to be prevented by spironolactone in a rat model of arterial hypertension (8). Spironolactone at doses of 25 to 50 mg per day can be used safely in conjunction with ACE inhibitors, diuretics, and digitalis. In a minority of patients, however, hyperkalemia may occur, leading to discontinuation of the drug. Findings of the Randomized Aldactone Evaluation Study (RALES) revealed that doses of spironolactone as low as 12.5 mg per day significantly reduce atrial natriuretic factor levels in patients with Classes II to IV heart failure without a significant effect on serum potassium levels (9). Moreover, the RALES investigators also found that treatment groups had lower levels of aldosterone, norepinephrine, and plasma renin activity.

Sympathetic Nervous System

The baroreceptor-mediated increase in sympathetic tone that occurs with ventricular dysfunction has several consequences, including increased myocardial contractility, tachycardia, arterial vasoconstriction and thus increased cardiac afterload, and venoconstriction with increased cardiac preload. Beta-adrenergic receptors in the heart either are downregulated (beta$_1$-adrenegic receptors) or have abnormalities in signal-transduction activity that effectively uncouple them from effector mechanisms (beta$_1$- and beta$_2$-adrenergic receptors) (5). Increased local and circulating concentrations of norepinephrine may contribute to myocyte hypertrophy, either directly through stimulation of alpha$_1$- and beta-adrenergic receptors or secondarily by activating the renin-angiotensin-aldosterone system. Norepinephrine is directly toxic to myocardial cells, an effect mediated through calcium overload, the induction of apoptosis, or both. Norepinephrine-induced death of myocytes can be prevented by concomitant nonselective beta-adrenergic blockade. Patients with plasma norepinephrine concentrations greater than 800 pg per milliliter (4.7 nmol per liter) have a 1-year survival rate of less than 40% (10). Through renal vasoconstriction, stimulation of the renin-angiotensin-aldosterone system, and direct effects on the proximal convoluted tubule, increased renal adrenergic activity contributes to the avid renal sodium and water retention that occurs in patients with heart failure.

Substantiating the importance of the sympathetic nervous system in the heart failure syndrome, multiple randomized controlled trials have demonstrated the benefits of beta-adrenergic blockade on clinical outcomes in patients with heart failure (11–13). In the past, beta-adrenergic blockade was thought to be contraindicated in patients with heart failure. However, if patients can tolerate short-term beta-adrenergic blockade, ventricular function subsequently improves.

Natriuretic Peptides

The roles of ANP and brain natriuretic peptide (BNP) in congestive heart failure and mitral regurgitation are not well understood. Investigators have shown that these compounds are produced by cardiac myocytes and their levels correlate inversely with left ventricular ejection fraction, directly with left atrial pressure, and directly with New York Heart Association (NYHA) class and mortality (14). Administration of exogenous ANP, 0.10 μg per kilogram per minute to normal subjects was found to increase sodium (450%) and free water (100%) excretion, while decreasing plasma renin (33%) and aldosterone (40%). Similar administration of ANP to patients with congestive heart failure had no effect on sodium or free water excretion, although significant decreases in pulmonary capillary wedge pressure (19%), systemic vascular resistance (13%), and plasma aldosterone (51%) and increases of cardiac index (17%) were noted. More recently, use of intravenous BNP has been shown to improve symptoms and reduce elevated filling pressures in patients treated for heart failure in the emergency department (15). BNP has also been shown to be an independent prognostic indicator in patients with cardiac disease (16). Omland et al. (16) favored the assessment of BNP over ANP because of its enhanced *in vitro* stability and relative simplicity of analysis.

Endothelin

Endothelin (ET) is a family of potent vasoconstrictor peptides of vascular endothelial origin. Although it has been proposed that the vasoconstrictor effects of ET are produced at the local vascular level, increased plasma concentration of ET has been identified in cardiovascular disorders (17). ET levels have been demonstrated to be nearly threefold higher in patients with congestive heart failure than in normal controls. ET was used a decade ago as a potent vasoconstrictor. The peptides were originally identified from rodent sources (ET-3) as well as human and porcine sources (ET-1). ET-1, ET-2, and ET-3 all have potent vasoconstrictor properties. ET-1 levels have a close association with pulmonary pressures, as well as the resistance ratio (pulmonary vascular resistance/systemic vascular resistance). Preliminary studies of ET antagonists have suggested that ET may provide relative selectivity for pulmonary vasculature vasoconstriction. Whether ET-1 is a regional mediator of pulmonary hypertension or a marker for its occurrence is unknown.

According to current data, the increase of plasma ET represents a biologic marker for vascular damage, and ET probably contributes to the pathophysiologic processes of vasoconstrictive disorders. To resolve the issue of the pathophysiologic contribution of ET to heart failure, specific inhibitors of ET are required. There are several ET antagonists in varying stages of development. They vary to the extent of ET_A and ET_B receptor activity. The vasoconstrictor effects of ET at the ET_A receptor suggest that this should be the site of blockade. However, some authorities have argued that blockade of both receptors would be important for improved endothelial cell function. This issue has not been settled. It is too early to comment on the potential clinical role of ET antagonists for the patient with heart failure.

Arginine Vasopressin

Arginine vasopressin (AVP) has affinity for two receptor subsets, V1 and V2, that govern free water clearance by the kidney and vasoconstriction, respectively. AVP production is increased in heart failure (18), as a result of angiotensin II stimulation and the indirect effect of thirst. Under resting conditions, AVP level is increased in patients with heart failure, in comparison with normal subjects and hypertensive patients. During the postural adjustment of head-up tilt, little additional modulation could be identified. Additional physiologic studies have demonstrated that AVP exhibits the spectrum of abnormalities observed with other major hormonal pathways, while still maintaining a responsiveness to adjustment of free water and other known physiologic changes. Preliminary clinical studies with AVP receptor antagonists has been performed. Design and outcomes of these studies have been determined by the receptor subtype against which the compound has physiologic activity. The spectrum of current compounds under experimental or clinical evaluation include primary V1, primary V2, and compounds with combined receptor activity. The latter class of pharmacologic probes, although the most desirable, are the most difficult to develop, and for this reason, clinical studies documenting the clinical role of AVP and its inhibition lag behind those for other hormonal compounds.

Specific Etiologies

The term *cardiomyopathy* is an ill-described, general category for a large group of unrelated disease processes that share only the clinical characteristic of substantially reduced cardiac pumping function and power output. Practical and graphic descriptions have been used to describe cardiomyopathy, and this classification is firmly anchored in the pathologic description of the heart. Thus, *dilated cardiomyopathy, hypertrophic cardiomyopathy,* and *infiltrative cardiomyopathy* are descriptive pathologic terms. Alternatively, cardiomyopathy is characterized by the specific clinical or disease process with which it is associated. Thus, terms such as *peripartum cardiomyopathy, diabetic cardiomyopathy,* and *toxic cardiomyopathy* are used. In clinical practice, the etiology of left ventricular systolic dysfunction can be identified in patients with coronary artery ischemia or infarction, infectious vectors, toxins, hereditary conditions, and conditions for which no cause can be identified (idiopathic) (Table 14.1). These disorders, in aggregate, account for the majority of cases of heart failure resulting from myocardial disease.

Ischemia

In patients with coronary artery disease, a cardiomyopathy can develop as the result of one extensive myocardial infarction, multiple smaller myocardial infarctions, ongoing ischemia from severe triple-vessel disease, or coronary artery disease associated with significant mitral regurgitation. Myocardial dysfunction may also develop after coronary artery bypass surgery, even in the setting of otherwise technically adequate graft placement. Early identification of myocar-

dial dysfunction associated with coronary artery disease is important, in view of the potential for reversal of dysfunction with effective management. When overt angina is not apparent, because of limited exercise capacity, subclinical myocardial ischemia may nonetheless produce abnormal systolic and diastolic ventricular dysfunction. Additional subclinical loss of viable myocardium may also occur.

When ischemia-related myocardial dysfunction prevents identification of reversible disease during exercise, viable hibernating myocardium may be identified by nuclear imaging studies. The predictive value of ^{201}Tl and ^{99m}Tc scintigraphy for detecting hibernating myocardium has been enhanced by newer redistribution and reinjection protocols, and these techniques are more readily available than positron emission testing at most institutions. Once identified, reversible ischemia caused by hibernation can be managed by interventional or surgical techniques, to prevent further deterioration of myocardial function.

Infections

A long list of infectious agents can be identified as vectors for this subgroup of myocardial disease. Myocardial dysfunction develops from a nonspecific immune or inflammatory response, or both, or from structural damage to cardiac myocytes. "Viral" myocarditis is frequently suspected among the patients who are otherwise classified as having idiopathic cardiomyopathy. Myocarditis can be diagnosed by endomyocardial biopsy and has been shown to be present in 12% of patients presenting with dilated cardiomyopathy in the absence of coronary artery disease within 6 months of their original diagnosis (19). With the exception of a few welldescribed viral causes that can be inferred from serial immune titers, isolation of a specific viral vector remains difficult. Molecular biologic techniques permit enhancement of viral messenger ribonucleic acid. However, in evaluations of myocardial tissue by histologic techniques, the occurrence of viral particles is equally distributed between patients with active myocarditis and those with nonspecific cardiomyopathy. Etiologic origin is therefore difficult to assign.

Diagnosing and treating active myocarditis remains a challenge. In general, the diagnosis can be confirmed only on myocardial biopsy, and the occurrence may be sporadic and related to fluctuation in Coxsackie virus prevalence. Endomyocardial biopsy can also be utilized for histologic documentation when there is a strong clinical suspicion of myocarditis. Endomyocardial biopsy evidence of myocarditis on the whole carries a prognosis similar to that for heart failure of idiopathic origin.

Among patients with history of a flu-like syndrome and there is clinical suspicion of myocarditis, biopsy evidence of inflammatory infiltrates is seen in approximately 25%, and yet almost half of these patients may have other concurrent disorders. Investigators have shown that the shorter the duration of illness, the greater the likelihood of a biopsy sample positive for inflammation; the likelihood reaches almost 90% in patients presenting within 4 weeks of their initial symptoms (20). Seasonal and yearly variations exist in the clinical presentation. The Myocarditis Treatment Trial demonstrated better-than-expected prognosis in patients with myocarditis (21). Specific immunosuppression did not alter outcome. Additional analyses are in progress to determine immunologic markers that identify patients who may benefit from immunosuppressive therapy.

Myocarditis may be present in cases in which the biopsy result is negative. One possible explanation is that the transvenous technique does not sample enough myocardial sites to detect each case of a disease that may have a focal or multifocal distribution. Acute myocarditis may occur as a regional process and can mimic acute myocardial infarction, with striking electrocardiographic changes. The regional nature of this disorder is evident with invasive and noninvasive assessment of ventricular performance. Depending on clinical presentation, this disorder may necessitate cardiac catheterization, which is the only means of definitively excluding epicardial coronary artery disease.

Myocardial dysfunction due to Chagas' disease remains the most common worldwide cause of cardiomyopathy (22). Infection in humans is caused by a bite from the reduviid insect, which harbors the protozoa *Trypanosoma cruzi* in its gastrointestinal tract. *T. cruzi* is the infectious etiology of Chagas' disease and gains entry into a human host by fecal deposition after a bite from the reduviid. After initial infection, acute trypanosomiasis occurs, followed by a long latent period; chronic Chagas' disease appears up to 20 years later. Myocardial dysfunction and congestive heart failure develop during this time. *T. cruzi* parasites within a cellular infiltrate may be present during the acute phase, but cardiac manifestations occur during the chronic phase. There is no correlation between the severity of disease and parasitemia. T lymphocytes may destroy normal myocardial cells, and antibody-mediated responses to specific myocyte components, such as the sarcoplasmic reticulum, have been identified.

In the Western Hemisphere, the greatest concentration of this disorder is in Central and South America, where 20 million people may be infected with the parasite (22). However, with increasing migration from these regions to the United States, consideration must be given to this diagnosis in patients of Latin American or South American origin from endemic regions. The concern regarding Chagas' disease as an etiology of myocardial dysfunction is not limited to the endemic populations. Currently, donor blood products are not routinely screened for *T. cruzi*. Thus, blood donation is conceivably a means by which *T. cruzi* may be spread by a nonvector pathway. An acceptable method to routinely screen blood products for *T. cruzi* has not been established. This has not proved to be a significant problem at the current time, but as much as 10 to 15 years may separate acute parasitemia and overt myocardial dysfunction.

Toxins

Several exogenous toxins are well known to cause left ventricular systolic dysfunction and subsequent heart failure. The most common of these is alcohol, represented in 3.4% of cases of systolic heart failure in the absence of coronary artery disease. Myocardial toxicity due to anthracyclines (e.g., doxorubicin) is a common cause of systolic heart failure in patients with a prior history of receiving chemotherapy for the treatment of cancer (23). Other exogenous toxins known to lead to systolic heart failure include cocaine, other chemotherapeutic agents (cyclophosphamide, and trastuzumab), interferon, interleukin-2, and chloroquine. In the mid-1960s, a clustering of cases of acute-onset cardiomyopathy developing in patients with heavy beer consumption led to the discovery that cobalt represented a myocardial toxin. When the practice of adding cobalt to beer was stopped, no further cases occurred.

Alcoholic Cardiomyopathy

Alcohol may be associated with heart failure in several different ways. Alcohol causes an acute depressant effect on myocardial contractility that can result in measurable dysfunction with binge drinking. Evidence suggests that the fundamental mechanism of injury induced by ethanol is structural and chemical disorganization of membranes, interference with ion transport, and derangement of various biochemical functions that possibly allow calcium to accumulate in the cell (24). Heavy alcohol consumption may also cause atrial tachyarrhythmias, termed *holiday heart,* which may contribute to the development of systolic dysfunction. The amount of alcohol necessary to cause this is unknown, because the testimony of alcoholic patients regarding intake cannot be validated. Studies have shown that ejection fraction correlates inversely with reported alcohol intake in alcoholic patients, and women may be more sensitive to the myocardial toxicity of alcohol than are men.

The pathologic and physiologic characteristics of alcoholic cardiomyopathy are similar to those of idiopathic dilated cardiomyopathy in gross appearance. The morphometric evaluation of endomyocardial biopsy does not provide adjunctive prognostic information in these patients. As many as one fourth of patients with systolic failure due to alcohol may present with elevated cardiac output, caused by concomitant liver disease and development of arteriovenous fistulae. Patients with alcoholic cardiomyopathy may have a favorable prognosis in comparison with those with idiopathic cardiomyopathy; approximately 50% of alcoholic patients experience improved left ventricular function once abstinence is established.

Athracycline-Induced Cardiomyopathy

Doxorubicin and daunorubicin are anthracycline analogues that are widely employed as chemotherapeutic agents. One important side effect caused by anthracyclines is cardiotoxicity. Cardiotoxicity due to anthracycline derivatives has been shown to be dependent on the cumulative dose (23). Measurable left ventricular systolic dysfunction is rare in patients receiving less than 350 mg per square meter of doxorubicin but may be seen in as much as 30% of patients receiving more than 600 mg per square meter (25). The peak levels of the drug may be a determinant for developing the disorder: Some evidence suggests that giving the same total dose weekly rather than every 3 weeks or administering the drug by slow continuous infusion rather than by bolus may reduce the incidence of cardiotoxicity. The risk factors for development of doxorubicin-induced cardiomyopathy include age older than 70, use in combination with other chemotherapeutic agents, concomitant or prior mediastinal radiotherapy, prior cardiac diseases, hypertension, liver disease, and whole body hyperthermia. Most authors on this topic have recommended monitoring patients serially with radionuclide ventriculography as patients are treated with anthracyclines (23). The diagnostic test with the greatest specificity and sensitivity for doxorubicin-induced cardiomyopathy is endomyocardial biopsy (26). Endomyocardial tissue from the right ventricle shows typical histopathologic changes, including loss of myofibrils, distention of the sarcoplasmic reticulum, and vacuolization of the cytoplasm and may appear before measurable changes in left ventricular systolic function occur. A biopsy scoring system has been described to show that patients in whom more than 25% of cells exhibit histopathologic changes will probably develop substantial changes in the ejection fraction, which suggests that treatment should be terminated (26). However, it is still possible that patients with lower biopsy grades will develop cardiomyopathy 4 to 20 years later.

Hereditary Influences

Studies have shed light on the role of the genetic background in the onset and the development of heart failure due to diastolic dysfunction (hypertrophic disease) and systolic dysfunction. Familial forms of dilated cardiomyopathy are common and have been described in as many as 30% of patients with nonischemic cardiomyopathy. Various modes of inheritance and phenotypes have been reported, and this condition appears genetically highly heterogeneous. Genetic abnormalities found to be associated with familial dilated cardiomyopathy include mutations in protein kinase A and protein kinase C (27) and the lamin A/C gene (28), among others. It has been postulated that the molecular defect involved in hereditary forms of heart disease causing left ventricular systolic dysfunction is an abnormality in the transmission of contractile force. Polymorphisms in the Ile164 $beta_2$-adrenergic receptor have been shown to be associated with poor prognosis in patients with dilated cardiomyopathy (29). In a study of 259 patients with dilated cardiomyopathy and NYHA Classes II to IV symptoms, patients with the Ile164 polymorphism displayed a striking difference in survival rates, with a relative risk of death or need for cardiac transplantation of 4.81. Further studies of the genetic determinants of dilated cardiomyopathy should allow better understanding of the underlying mechanisms that promote the progression of the disease, to identify subjects at risk of the disease who would benefit from early medical management and promote the development of pharmacogenetics.

Idiopathic Causes

Idiopathic remains the designation for many forms of dilated cardiomyopathy, when coronary artery disease and specific causes such as those listed earlier have been excluded. With the exception of primary causes, which are clinically identified, there are limited screening procedures that can identify a specific cause. Of these, per-

haps the most fruitful is the screen test for thyroid disease, which may be particularly important in the evaluation of the elderly patient. Both hyperthyroidism and hypothyroidism may produce left ventricular dysfunction. Abnormalities of trace substances such as selenium have been suggested, but deficiencies do not routinely occur in Western diets. Patients may also present with left ventricular systolic dysfunction due to chronic tachycardia conditions, such as atrial fibrillation with rapid ventricular response. Rate control with beta blockers, digitalis, or both has been shown to lead to improvements in left ventricular function on follow-up testing.

PRESENTING SYMPTOMS AND SIGNS

The cardinal manifestations of heart failure are dyspnea, fatigue, and fluid retention. Both dyspnea and fatigue may limit exercise tolerance, and fluid retention may be demonstrated by peripheral edema, abdominal ascites, or pulmonary edema. All of these symptoms can impair the functional capacity and quality of life of affected individuals; however, these are not all necessarily present in patients with heart failure. Many patients with advanced heart failure do not show physical signs of pulmonary congestion, because of the chronic changes that occur in the pulmonary vasculature. These patients may have only symptoms of dyspnea and fatigue. Other patients may have overt signs of volume overload, with lower extremity edema and jugulovenous distention, but have no problem with dyspnea. In these patients, the impairment of exercise tolerance may occur so gradually that it may not be noted unless the patient is questioned carefully and specifically about a change in activities of daily living.

New York Heart Association Classification

Functional status of patients has been standardized according to the NYHA classification system, a system that allows physicians to compare functional strata within the population of patients with heart failure (Table 14.2.) This approach assigns patients to one of four functional classes,

TABLE 14.2. *New York Heart Association classification*

Class I: Symptoms only at levels of activity that would produce symptoms in normal individuals; ordinary physical activity does not cause undue dyspnea or fatigue
Class II: Symptoms on ordinary exertion, resulting in mild limitation of physical activity
Class III: Symptoms on less than ordinary exertion, resulting in marked limitation of physical activity
Class IV: Symptoms at rest or minimal exertion, resulting in inability to carry on any physical activity without discomfort

depending on the degree of effort that brings on either fatigue or dyspnea. NYHA Class I represents patients without symptoms with any activity, except those that would bring on symptoms in normal individuals. NYHA Class II represents patients who develop fatigue or dyspnea on ordinary exertion (e.g., with one or more flights of stairs or with walking one or more blocks on a flat surface). NYHA Class III represents patients who develop symptoms at less than ordinary exertion (e.g., with less than one flight of stairs or with less than one block of walking on a flat surface). NYHA Class IV represents patients who experience symptoms at rest (e.g., sitting in a chair, lying in bed) or with minimal activity (e.g., eating, dressing, showering). Although much effort is made to assign a NYHA classification to patients, the functional status of a given patient need not be static. Patients may present in NYHA Class IV and, after appropriate medical therapy, change to being asymptomatic, or NYHA Class I. Nevertheless, assignment of a functional classification is important in the care of patients with heart failure, because current therapies indicated for treatment may have been tested only in patient populations selected on the basis of distinct NYHA classifications.

Exercise tolerance and functional status are not determined by resting left ventricular function; instead, they correlate better with exercise cardiac reserve. Patients with very low ejection fraction may be entirely asymptomatic, whereas others with mild to moderate dysfunction are symptomatic at rest or with mild exertion. Many factors contribute to exercise tolerance, including skeletal muscle function, respiratory function, peripheral vascular function, and psychologic factors.

American College of Cardiology/American Heart Association Stages of Heart Failure

Because NYHA classification is a designation in flux, the American College of Cardiology and American Heart Association (ACC/AHA) Task Force on Practice Guidelines, in the ACC/AHA Guidelines for the Evaluation and Management of Chronic Heart Failure in the Adult, published in 2001 (29a), established a staging system to act as a complement to the NYHA classification. The ACC/AHA stages represent the evolution and the progression of heart failure (Table 14.3). Stage A represents patients who are at high risk for developing a structural disorder of the heart but have not yet done so. This stage includes patients with hypertension, coronary artery disease risk factors, or a family history of cardiomyopathy. Stage B represents patients with a structural disorder of the heart but without symptoms. These patients are analogous to those represented by NYHA Class I. Stage C represents patients with a structural disease of the heart and with symptoms of heart failure. This stage includes patients represented by NYHA Classes II to IV. Stage D represents patients in the terminal phase of the disease who require repeated and prolonged hospitalizations or specialized treatment strategies such as mechanical circulatory support, continuous inotropic infusions, cardiac transplantation, or

TABLE 14.3. *American College of Cardiology/American Heart Association stages of heart failure*

Stage A: Patients at risk for developing a structural disorder of the heart
Stage B: Patients with a structural disorder of the heart but without symptoms
Stage C: Patients with a structural disorder of the heart and with symptoms of heart failure (New York Heart Association Classes II–IV)
Stage D: Patients in the end stage of chronic heart failure who require repeated or prolonged hospitalizations or specialized treatment strategies such as mechanical circulatory support, continuous inotropic infusions, cardiac transplantation, or hospice care

hospice care. These patients have marked symptoms of heart failure at rest despite maximal medical therapy and may require specialized interventions. The classification scheme recognized that heart failure has established risk factors; that the evolution of heart failure has asymptomatic and symptomatic phases, and that interventions may be necessary at every stage to help prevent the progression of the disease and to help relieve the suffering of the patient.

CLINICAL FEATURES AND LABORATORY TESTS

Cardiac History

The usual reason the patient seeks medical attention is breathlessness or fatigue that limits exercise tolerance. Sometimes the first recognized manifestation of heart failure is orthopnea or paroxysmal nocturnal dyspnea; in other patients, pedal edema may be the first recognized abnormality. Thus, the secondary manifestations of heart failure (such as circulatory congestion) bring the patient to medical attention, rather than the primary cardiac contractile abnormality. A complete history and review of systems are crucial for understanding the cause of heart failure. Direct inquiry may reveal prior evidence of myocardial ischemia, infarction, or both; valvular disease; or a family history of heart ailments.

When documenting a history from the patient with heart failure, the examiner should begin by identifying the dominant symptom of the patient, whether it is fatigue, dyspnea, chest discomfort, palpitations, syncope or near syncope, edema, cough, or wheezing. Clarifying the conditions in which the symptom occurs is critical: whether they occur at rest, with recumbency, or with mild, moderate, or heavy exertion; how long the episodes have been occurring; how frequently the episodes last; how severe the symptoms are; and what relieves the symptoms. Establishing the activity level of the patient is important, because many patients will report no symptoms and yet they have assumed a sedentary lifestyle to avoid experiencing the effects of their heart condition. Patients with modest limitations of activity should be asked about their participation in sports or their ability to carry out strenuous exercise, whereas patients with substantial limitations of activity should be asked about their ability to get dressed without stopping, take a shower, climb stairs, or carry out specific routine household chores. Documenting a dietary history is helpful, particularly for the patient with edema, because some patients may be consuming large amount of sodium and free water that may override attempts to establish euvolemia. Patients should be asked about a history of hypertension, diabetes, hypercholesterolemia, coronary disease, valvular disease, peripheral vascular disease, rheumatic fever, chest irradiation, and exposure to cardiotoxic agents. Patients should be questioned carefully regarding illicit drug use, alcohol consumption, tobacco use, and exposure to sexually transmitted diseases. A travel history may be helpful in identifying patients exposed to trypanosomes, which lead to Chagas' disease. The history should also include questions related to noncardiac diseases such as collagen vascular diseases, infections, and thyroid excess or deficiency.

Physical Examination

General Appearance

Asymptomatic patients may not have distinguishing characteristics on general appearance. Patients with chronic heart failure have features of chronic disease, such as pallor and general weakness. In more advanced stages of the disease, wasting of limb-girdle and facial muscles is common, and there may be the appearance of overall cachexia. The abdomen may be distended from hepatomegaly and ascites. Long-standing peripheral edema is accompanied by darkened skin as a result of chronic hemosiderin deposition and scarring from chronic skin lesions. Body weight may be misleading in documentation of heart failure. Accumulation of edema may be insidious and balanced by loss of lean body mass, thereby masking fluid retention. Virtually any weight abnormality may be present, and the presence of obesity certainly will completely obscure any attempt to characterize weight in relation to the severity of heart failure.

Pulse and Blood Pressure

Tachycardia, in the absence of other known causes, represents chronotropic compensation for the reduced cardiac output of pump failure. A two-to-one ratio of apical to radial pulse may reflect pulses alternans, secondary to the severity of heart failure. Alternatively, very slow peripheral pulses may represent sinus node dysfunction (structural or secondary to medications) or heart block. An irregular pulse most typically reflects atrial fibrillation. A narrow pulse pressure is consistent with a low stroke volume or inadequate diastolic filling time. Assessment of the carotid arteries and pulses therefore provides information regarding ventricular contraction and the overall circulatory status.

The measurement of systolic and diastolic blood pressure provides important clues to the origin of heart failure. If blood pressure exceeds 140/90 mm HG on repeated measurements, lowering the blood pressure is mandatory in patients with heart failure. In contrast, many patients with long-standing heart failure have hypotension, which is accentuated with upright posture ("orthostatic hypotension"). When documented, this should be correlated with symptoms of dizziness and fatigue. In general, most therapies for heart failure produce low blood pressure and may require adjustment in the setting of symptomatic orthostatic hypotension.

Venous System

The magnitude of jugular venous distention provides an estimate of cardiac filling pressure and circulatory volume status. It is most convenient to use the right atrium as the reference point for this measurement by measuring at the midaxillary point at the nipple level. The simplest stress test is the hepatojugular reflux test, performed by exerting constant firm pressure over the right upper quadrant of the abdomen. A positive result of the hepatojugular reflux test may be interpreted as evidence for impaired right ventricular response to volume load, a dilated heart that can be compressed by a rising diaphragm, and a volume overload state. An alternative approach to stressing the circulation is leg raising or exercise.

In evaluating the peripheral venous system, the examiner should look for varicose veins or prior surgical scars, which may increase the tendency for edema, particularly in an asymmetric manner. Peripheral pitting edema secondary to heart failure should be distinguished from the heavy ankles of lipedema. The pitting quality of edema distinguishes it from lymphedema.

Lungs

Tachypnea is a typical finding of heart failure and may be present under resting conditions during the physical examination. Dyspnea in the course of a patient interview is a finding of inadequate cardiac compensation. The most characteristic finding on pulmonary examination is the presence of rales, indicative of increased pulmonary capillary pressure and transudation of fluid into the alveolar airspace. In general, rales provide an estimate of the severity of left ventricular decompensation, inasmuch as the height of the rales in the lung fields is proportionate to the severity of the decompensation. Rales are obscured by the presence of pleural effusion, which is more often a marker of chronic decompensation.

Cardiac Findings

Precordial palpation provides valuable information in heart failure, indicating the extent of cardiac enlargement and providing information regarding the degree of contractile impairment and valvular function. Displacement of the apical impulse away from the midsternal line is typical of heart failure. A diffuse apical impulse is characteristic of ventricular enlargement, and a heaving quality may indicate ventricular dyskinesis or underlying left atrial lift. The palpation of thrills may provide a clue to the presence of valvular disease. Auscultation of the heart should confirm the abnormalities already identified by observation and palpation. In particular, the examiner should check for the presence of murmurs or diastolic filling sounds. Mitral regurgitation is common in patients with heart failure and may result in an apical murmur that radiates toward the axilla. Tricuspid regurgitation may also be present on auscultation. An accentuated pulmonic closure sound (P_2) suggests pulmonary hypertension, a fourth heart sound (S4) indicates abnormal atrial-ventricular filling characteristics, and a third heart sound (S3) indicates ventricular dysfunction or decompensation.

Echocardiography and Radionuclide Ventriculography

Ventricular function can be quantitated by imaging techniques, either echocardiography or radionuclide ventriculography. A left ventricular ejection fraction of less than 45% at rest is considered abnormal. Echocardiography provides information about valve function and regional wall motion as well as quantitative assessment of the dimensions, geometry, and thickness of the left ventricle. Qualitative information about right ventricular size and function is available from echocardiography. Doppler flow measurements also identify the functional significance of observed stenotic and regurgitant valve lesions, which provides a better global assessment of the impact of heart failure on cardiac function, as well as etiologic information. The comprehensive evaluation offered by echocardiography is helpful in assessing the patient with heart failure, inasmuch as it is not uncommon for patients to have more than one abnormality contributing to the heart failure syndrome. Radionuclide ventriculography offers enhanced precision in measuring left ventricular ejection fraction in comparison with echocardiography and may be more useful when monitoring ventricular function serially is important in the care of the patient (i.e., monitoring patients treated with anthracyclines).

Electrocardiography

Prior or acute myocardial infarction can be identified by Q waves on the electrocardiogram. Myocardial hypertrophy almost invariably accompanies heart failure, and so increased voltage or conduction abnormalities are often present. Left ventricular hypertrophy and cardiomyopathy may manifest with what appears to be localized loss of electrical forces that may be mistaken for a prior myocardial infarction. Evidence of

atrial conduction delay–related prolongation of the PR interval, QRS duration, and QT interval are common in patients with heart failure. These changes may predispose patients to cardiac arrhythmias. Both atrial and ventricular dysrhythmias are common manifestations of heart failure, and evidence for their existence may be detected on a random electrocardiogram. Monitoring for longer periods, especially 24-hour Holter monitoring, is likely to detect these arrhythmias.

Chest Radiograph

The chest radiograph provides an estimate of ventricular chamber size, but it often serves as a screening technique to identify the presence of heart disease. The cardiothoracic ratio measured on a standard posteroanterior chest film provides an estimate of overall heart enlargement. The degree of left ventricular enlargement is better assessed by lateral or oblique views. In the presence of a high pulmonary capillary pressure secondary to left ventricular failure, pulmonary blood volume often is redistributed to the upper lobes in an upright film, producing the cephalization characteristic of left-sided heart failure. Pulmonary infiltrates and fibrosis occasionally masquerade as heart failure.

Stress Testing

Exercise testing can be conducted safely in the patient with heart failure, and the information obtained from this test is important in diagnostic and therapeutic efforts. An exercise test can be performed either informally in the examining room, by having the patient perform a 6-minute walk test, or formally with the use of a cardiopulmonary exercise test with either a bicycle ergometer or a treadmill, simultaneously with respiratory gas analysis. The cardiopulmonary exercise test provides more detailed information regarding the cause of the exercise limitation. Monitoring the electrocardiogram during exercise provides additional information that can give a clue to the presence of ischemic heart disease. Performing the stress test while monitoring gas exchange allows more precise assessment of the exercise burden at the point when the patient reaches his or her anaerobic threshold and the peak oxygen consumption that he or she can achieve. Its added value is in distinguishing among cardiac, pulmonary, deconditioning, and nonmotivational disability.

Coronary Arteriography

Coronary angiography is often necessary to clarify the origin of left ventricular dysfunction. Coronary artery disease is responsible for 50% to 60% of cases of heart failure due to left ventricular systolic dysfunction. It may be useful to define the presence, anatomic characteristics, and function significance of coronary artery disease in patients with heart failure. This may be particularly useful in three types of patients: (a) those with known coronary artery disease and angina; (b) those with known coronary artery disease without angina; and (c) those in whom the possibility of coronary artery disease has not been evaluated. Identification of high-grade coronary artery disease should prompt analysis for revascularization in patients with angina, because ongoing ischemia is a prominent cause of left ventricular dysfunction and heart failure. For patients without angina, functional testing with nuclear imaging or stress echocardiography may be able to identify viable myocardium or ischemic myocardium that may respond favorably with revascularization. In patients with left ventricular systolic dysfunction and unknown coronary anatomy, cardiac catheterization may be able to identify lesions amenable for revascularization that could change the course of the disease. This applies in particular to patients with regional dysfunction, episodic heart failure symptoms, and chest discomfort or anginal equivalent. Although there are no clear guidelines for coronary arteriography in patients with heart failure due to left ventricular systolic dysfunction and no anginal equivalent, many of these patients would benefit by knowing the coronary anatomy, inasmuch as the sensitivity of noninvasive functional studies is limited and many patients with ischemic disease have clinically silent events. In patients in whom coronary artery disease has previously been excluded as the cause

for left ventricular dysfunction, repeated invasive or noninvasive assessment for ischemia is generally not indicated.

Right-Sided Heart Catheterization

The role of invasive hemodynamic measurements in the management of heart failure remains uncertain. Most drugs used for the treatment of heart failure are prescribed on the basis of the symptoms, rather than hemodynamic measurements, of the individual patient. Nevertheless, invasive hemodynamic measurements may assist in the determination of volume status and in distinguishing heart failure from other disorders (pulmonary disease and sepsis). Right-sided heart catheterization is important when moderate to severe pulmonary hypertension has been suggested by physical examination or noninvasive studies. This procedure can be valuable in the management of complex heart failure. With quality echocardiography and Doppler studies, right-sided heart catheterization is not required in all patients. Although hemodynamic measurements can be estimated with the use of noninvasive methods such as transthoracic bioimpedance, routine use of those techniques cannot be recommended until they have been shown to be valid in the population of patients with heart failure.

Endomyocardial Biopsy

The usefulness of endomyocardial biopsy is not well established. Most patients with nonischemic cardiomyopathy show nonspecific changes on biopsy (hypertrophy, cell loss or apoptosis, and fibrosis). Biopsy specimens showing lymphocytic infiltration consistent with myocarditis are of diagnostic but, at present, not of therapeutic value. Many patients with myocarditis improve on their own, and directed immunosuppression has not been shown to be helpful in these patients. Biopsy specimens showing giant-cell myocarditis are of prognostic utility, because this disease has been shown to have a virulent course. Nonetheless, therapies for giant cell myocarditis are, at present, anecdotal. The biopsy findings can be used to make a diagnosis of sarcoidosis, amyloidosis, hemochromatosis, eosinophilic myocarditis, Loeffler's syndrome, and endocardial fibroelastosis. However, evidence that biopsy results lead to successful therapies in these conditions is lacking. There is no evidence that outcomes would be improved by performing biopsies to screen for these diseases. Although the risk of serious complication is less than 1%, endomyocardial biopsy is not indicated in the routine evaluation of cardiomyopathy and should be performed only when there is a strong reason to believe that the results will have a meaningful impact on subsequent therapeutic decisions.

Laboratory Testing

The most important blood studies in the patient with heart failure are the serum electrolyte and renal function measurements. A low serum sodium concentration indicates a stimulated renin-angiotensin system as well as increased vasopressin levels and is observed in patients requiring large doses of loop diuretics. A low serum potassium level and contraction alkalosis may also be observed in patients receiving diuretic therapy. An elevated blood urea nitrogen or serum creatinine level suggests either organic or functional renal impairment, caused by vasoconstriction, and decreased cardiac output. Liver function abnormalities may suggest hepatic congestion. Thyroid-stimulating hormone should be measured at the initial evaluation, because both hypothyroidism and hyperthyroidism can be a primary contributor to the cause of heart failure. In the setting of an acute presentation of heart failure, measurement of creatine phosphokinase and isoenzymes, as well as troponin I or troponin T may indicate the presence of active inflammation or ischemic injury to the heart. Serum ferritin and transferrin saturation measurements may be useful for detecting hemochromatosis, although they are of limited yield in the absence of other manifestations of hemochromatosis such as diabetes, liver disease, and skin changes. Screening for human immunodeficiency virus is recommended for patients with high-risk exposures or history of sexually transmitted diseases, with manifestations of infection with the virus such as lymphopenia, anemia, cachexia, or history of opportunistic infections.

Interest has been developing in using the measurement of BNP to diagnose heart failure in the setting of unexplained dyspnea and to monitor patients with chronic heart failure. In the past, measurement of BNP has required a complex radioimmune assay, and in many hospitals, this meant that the test needed to be sent to a referral center for analysis. More recently, results of studies of the use of a portable apparatus capable of rapid analysis of blood samples have shown the utility of measuring samples on site in the emergency department (30). Natriuretic peptide levels have been shown to distinguish heart failure from pulmonary causes of dyspnea and to enable examiners to correctly classify the severity of heart failure (Fig. 14.3) (14). Whether measurement of BNP offers additional information over that of a history and physical examination is not known.

DIFFERENTIAL DIAGNOSIS

Determination of the underlying cause of systolic heart failure may provide additional avenues for therapies that can lead to improvement of the condition of the patient. Because of the prevalence of atherosclerosis in the population, the first diagnosis that must be considered is ischemia or infarction (Fig. 14.4). Because coronary artery disease is the causal factor in more than half the cases of systolic heart failure, measures taken to distinguish the remaining causes are less likely to produce a diagnosis. During the initial evaluation of the patient, the clinician should be able to identify patients with primary valve disorders (such as aortic stenosis, aortic insufficiency, and mitral regurgitation) causing heart failure. For patients with aortic stenosis, and in many cases of aortic insufficiency, valve surgery can result in a vast improvement of the heart failure syndrome. Although prior reports advised against mitral replacement in the setting of mitral regurgitation and systolic heart failure, repair of the mitral valve (sparing the papillary muscle function and ventricular geometry) has been shown to improve symptoms in these patients in uncontrolled series (31). Patients with uncontrolled hypertension should be treated with maximally titrated doses of ACE inhibitors, beta blockers, and, if necessary, amlodipine and other antihypertensives.

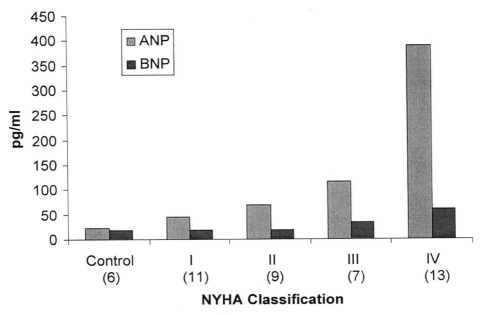

FIG. 14.3. Relationship between serum atrial natriuretic peptide and brain natriuretic peptide levels and New York Heart Association classification. (Modified from Wei CM, Heublein DM, Perrella MA, et al. Natriuretic peptide system in human heart failure. *Circulation* 1993;88:1004–1009.)

Evaluation of the patient should uncover exposure to cardiac toxins, such as alcohol or cocaine. Detoxification from alcohol and prolonged abstinence may allow for recovery of cardiac function. Patients with tachyarrhythmias such as atrial fibrillation with rapid ventricular response should be treated with cardioversion or rate control, because ventricular function may improve once the tachycardia ceases. Both hypothyroidism and hyperthyroidism may result in systolic heart failure, which merits a check of thyroid-stimulating hormone on initial presentation. It is well documented that treatment of these disorders leads to clinical improvement. Initial assessment of the laboratories of patients with systolic heart failure may reveal evidence of hypocalcemia or uremia, both documented causes of dilated cardiomyopathy capable of improvement with correction of the abnormality. Other nutritional (selenium) and metabolic (carnitine) deficiencies have been described as leading to dilated cardiomyopathy. These deficiencies, when corrected, may lead to improvements in cardiac function.

Endomyocardial biopsy is not recommended in the routine evaluation of patients with sys-

tolic heart failure. However, treatment of patients presenting with signs and symptoms highly suggestive of diagnoses that may be made through biopsy (particularly if the diagnosis has a proven therapy) may benefit by endomyocardial biopsy and the directed therapy that ensues. Patients presenting with fever, myalgias, or pleuritic chest pain may be suffering from myocarditis or myopericarditis. Findings on electrocardiography may also be suggestive of myocarditis or myopericarditis. At the time of this writing, however, no effective therapies for myocarditis beyond supportive therapy and medical therapy for heart failure have been identified. Patients with a history of extracardiac sarcoid or signs of atrioventricular block may be suffering from cardiac sarcoid. Reports of improvements in these patients have been made with the use of corticosteroids. Patients with concomitant liver disease, especially in the setting of diabetes and skin bronzing, may have systolic heart failure as a result of hemochromatosis, a diagnosis that can be made by endomyocardial biopsy. Investigators have also shown utility of magnetic resonance imaging in the diagnosis of cardiac

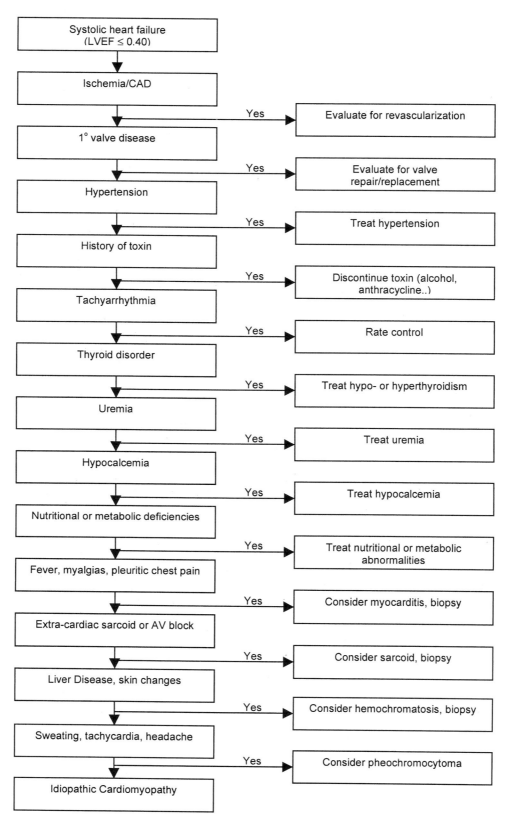

FIG. 14.4. Decision tree for determining the cause of systolic heart failure.

hemochromatosis. Some patients with pheochromocytoma have dilated cardiomyopathy, which is reversible in at least some cases with operative removal of the tumor. Patients presenting with symptoms of sweating, tachycardia (also common in other forms of cardiomyopathy), or headaches may benefit from measurement of plasma and urinary catecholamines and their metabolites and from imaging of the abdomen with computed tomography.

In the absence of identifiable causes of systolic heart failure, patients are assigned a diagnosis of "idiopathic" dilated cardiomyopathy. In series of 1,230 patients presenting with nonischemic dilated cardiomyopathy, 50% were assigned a diagnosis of idiopathic dilated cardiomyopathy (32). Because no etiologic agent can be identified with these patients, no specific therapy is available beyond medical therapies proved to benefit patients with systolic heart failure as a group, which are outlined later in this chapter.

COMPLICATIONS

Morbidity and mortality are, unfortunately, common complications in patients suffering from systolic heart failure. One of the most common complications in heart failure is the need for hospitalization for the treatment of worsening heart failure. These hospitalizations result from acute worsening of the chronic condition or from gradual worsening that is refractory to outpatient management. The rate of hospitalization varies, depending on the severity of the illness. Of ambulatory patients (largely in NYHA Classes II to III) enrolled into the placebo arm of the U.S. Carvedilol trials, 19.6% were hospitalized over a mean follow-up period of 6.5 months, in comparison with 14.1% of the patients receiving carvedilol (11). Patients in the RALES study who were in NYHA Class IV at the time of enrollment or in NYHA Class III but had been in NYHA Class IV within the previous 6 months were more likely to be hospitalized; 40% of the placebo group required hospitalization over the 24-month follow-up period, and 31.6% of the patients received spironolactone.

Patients with heart failure may suffer from heart rhythm disturbances. More than 10% of patients with heart failure and systolic dysfunction suffer from concomitant atrial fibrillation. Ventricular tachyarrhythmias are also common, inasmuch as approximately 10% of patients with advanced heart failure experience syncope or high-grade ventricular ectopy that necessitates the placement of an implantable cardiac defibrillator. Lower grades of ventricular ectopy, such as nonsustained ventricular tachycardia, are seen more commonly; approximately one third of patients show at least three beats of ventricular tachycardia on ambulatory electrocardiographic monitoring.

Patients with heart failure may also experience stroke, because of either atrial fibrillation or a low-flow state. The incidence of stroke may be reduced with the use of warfarin. Low cardiac output in advanced heart failure may lead to complications resulting from poor organ perfusion, which leads to renal insufficiency, hepatic insufficiency, and central nervous system dysfunction. These complications can compound the problem of heart failure in that they can exacerbate fluid retention, lead to metabolic derangements, and interfere with compliance with medical and dietary therapies. Quality of life and prognosis take a progressive decline when heart failure is joined by multisystem failure. Palliation with intravenous inotropic medications in this setting may improve the clinical status of the patient temporarily.

THERAPY FOR HEART FAILURE DUE TO LEFT VENTRICULAR SYSTOLIC DYSFUNCTION

The goals of treatment for congestive heart failure include identification of correctable causes and cofactors, prevention of disease progression, maintenance of physical activity, reversal of sodium retention, and reduction of the risk of mortality. Of course, some of these factors can be achieved or optimized only through medical therapy for heart failure, particularly as the disorder reaches advanced stages. ACE inhibitors are recommended for all stages of heart failure, not only for treatment but also to prevent progression of ventricular dysfunction. Spironolactone, an aldosterone antagonist, has been shown to significantly reduce mortality rates when added to standard therapy. Diuretic therapy is used for the symptomatic and clinical relief of edema, but there are no data that identify a primary role in prevention of disease progression. Most clinicians believe that digoxin is safe and effective in reducing the risk of hospitalization. More recently, beta-adrenergic blockade has emerged as important therapy for heart failure, dispelling previous misconceptions regarding lack of benefit, or even additive risk.

Diet and Lifestyle Issues

The effective therapy of heart failure requires compliance with dietary limitations and other lifestyle issues. In all patients with heart failure, dietary sodium intake should be limited to 2 to 3 g per day, and a fluid restriction should be established in a range of 48 to 64 oz per day. In the absence of dietary restrictions, patients consuming liberal amounts of sodium and water can overcome the even the most potent diuretic regimens. Cessation of smoking is required of all patients with heart failure, particularly those with underlying ischemic disease. In patients with heart failure in whom the cause is coronary artery disease and the lipid profile is abnormal, dietary and pharmacologic reduction of cholesterol and triglyceride levels is recommended. Normal or near normal body weight should also be achieved. Obesity can be a major confounding factor in the successful management of heart failure, in view of the direct effects of obesity on ventricular geometry and function.

Exercise

Historically, bed rest was recommended for the management of acute heart failure, particularly when the cause was myocarditis. This is no longer recommended beyond the initial first days of management of acute decompensation. Current studies indicate that cardiac rehabilitation and a supervised exercise prescription are important for the maintenance of overall circulatory conditioning and skeletal muscle function. Development of a cardiac rehabilitation program should be considered for all patients, as part of the long-term management of heart failure.

Specific Drug Classes

Since the mid-1980s, there has been a radical shift in the accepted endpoints for safety and efficacy of drug therapy for heart failure. Although acute and chronic hemodynamic endpoints are important for characterizing the pharmacologic response to a new drug, more desirable long-term endpoints include reduction of symptoms (improved quality of life), improved exercise or exertional capacity, reversal of abnormal neurohormonal profile, and reduction of mortality. The studies in heart failure that dominated the later 1980s and the early 1990s were large, multicenter clinical trials. These trials were powered to detect the effect of pharmacologic therapy on mortality, efficacy endpoints, and meaningful side effect profiles. Ancillary data derived from these studies included the influence of therapy on subclasses of patients, changes in ventricular arrhythmias, quality of life, symptoms, and concomitant drug usage. Frequently, these studies did not provide information regarding mechanism of pharmacologic action, specific details of pathophysiologic processes, or clear explanations for drug failure when they occurred. General guidelines for the treatment of systolic heart failure according to ACC/AHA stage are given in Tables 14.4 to 14.8.

Diuretics

Diuretics are evaluated with the efficacy endpoint of weight reduction and reversal of edema and pulmonary vascular congestion and are a traditional therapy for the edema of heart failure. Although there have been no long-term randomized controlled studies showing the effects of diuretic therapy on morbidity and mortality in heart failure, shorter term studies have shown that diuretics improve symptoms and exercise tolerance in patients with volume overload. Diuretic choices include loop diuretics (e.g., furosemide, bumetanide, and torsemide), thiazide diuretics [e.g., HydroDIURIL (hydrochlorothiazide) and

TABLE 14.4. *Recommendations for patients at high risk of developing heart failure (Stage A)*

Class I
1. Control of systolic or diastolic hypertension, in accordance with recommended guidelines
2. Treatment of lipid disorders, in accordance with recommended guidelines
3. Avoidance of patient behaviors that may increase the risk of developing heart failure (smoking, alcohol, cocaine)
4. ACE inhibitor for patients at high risk for occurrence of a cardiovascular event (history of atherosclerotic vascular disease, diabetes, hypertension, hyperlipidemia, smoking)
5. Periodic evaluation for signs and symptoms of heart failure

Class IIa
1. Control of ventricular rate in patients with rapid supraventricular tachyarrhythmias
2. Weight loss in patients with obesity

Class IIb
1. Noninvasive evaluation of LV function in patients with a strong family history of cardiomyopathy

Class III
1. Routine exercise to maintain cardiovascular conditioning
2. Reduction of dietary salt in patients without hypertension or fluid retention
3. Routine testing to detect left ventricular dysfunction in patients without signs or symptoms of heart failure or a history of structural heart disease

ACE, angiotensin-converting enzyme; LV, left ventricular.
From Hunt SA, Baker DW, Chin MH, et al. ACC/AHA guidelines for the evaluation and management of chronic heart failure in the adult. *J Am Coll Cardiol* 2001; 104:2996–3007.

TABLE 14.5. *Recommendations for patients with asymptomatic systolic left ventricular dysfunction (Stage B).*

Class I
1. Beta blockade in patients with a recent myocardial infarction, regardless of ejection fraction
2. Beta blockade in patients with a reduced ejection fraction, whethre or not they have experienced a myocardial infarction
3. ACE inhibition in patients with a recent or remote history of myocardial infarction, regardless of ejection fraction
4. ACE inhibition in patients with a reduced ejection fraction, whether or not they have experienced a myocardial infarction
5. Treatment of heart failure risk factors (hypertension, and hyperlipidemia), in accordance with recommended guidelines
6. Periodic evaluation for signs and symptoms of heart failure

Class IIa
1. Exercise to maintain cardiovascular conditioning

Class IIb
1. Routine use of anticoagulants and antiplatelet agents in patient with asymptomatic LV dysfunction without prior myocardial infarction
2. Reduction of dietary salt in patients without hypertension or fluid retention

Class III
1. Antiarrhythmic drug treatment for asymptomatic ventricular arrhythmias
2. Treatment with digitalis glycosides in patients in sinus rhythm

ACE, angiotensin-converting enzyme; LV, left ventricular.
From Hunt SA, Baker DW, Chin MH, et al. ACC/AHA guidelines for the evaluation and management of chronic heart failure in the adult. *J Am Coll Cardiol* 2001; 104:2996–3007.

metolazone], and potassium-sparing diuretics (e.g., spironolactone, triamterene, and amiloride). Loop diuretics act in the proximal tubule and maintain their efficacy unless renal function is severely impaired. Thiazide diuretics tend to be less potent when used alone and are not effective in patients with moderately impaired renal function. Because patients with chronic heart failure tend to have at least mild abnormalities of renal function, loop diuretics generally tend to be the diuretic of first choice in view of mild renal impairment in this population. However, this does not exclude use of thiazide-type diuretics in milder heart failure. In more severe heart failure, loop diuretics are much more efficacious when combined with a thiazide-type diuretic, as they block different sites in the nephron and have an additive effect. The goal is optimization of diure-

sis, prevention of hypokalemia, and assessment of the risk of hyperkalemia. In the absence of signs or symptoms of volume overload, diuretics are not necessary.

When diuretic therapy is initiated in a stable but volume-overloaded patient with heart failure, furosemide, 20 to 40 mg daily, is preferred. Baseline chemistry profiles should be drawn and rechecked 5 to 7 days after initiation of the drug, to assess for signs of hypokalemia and volume contraction. If the baseline serum potassium level is in the lower range of normal, then supplemental potassium chloride is added along with the diuretic. The patient should be advised to weigh himself or herself every morning after voiding and record the result. The goal weight change should rarely be in excess of 0.5 to 1.0 kg per

TABLE 14.6. *Recommendations for treatment of symptomatic left ventricular systolic dysfunction (Stage C)*

Class I
1. Diuretics in patients who have evidence for or a prior history of fluid retention
2. ACE inhibition in all patients, unless contraindicated
3. Beta-adrenergic blockade in all stable patients, unless the patient has fluid retention on physical examination or has recently received treatment with a positive inotropic agent
4. Digitalis in all patients, unless contraindicated
5. Withdrawal of drugs known to adversely affect the clinical status of patients (NSAIDs, antiarrhythmic drugs other than amiodarone, and calcium channel–blocking drugs other than amlodipine)

Class IIa
1. Spironolactone in patients with recent or current Class IV symptoms, preserved renal function, and normal potassium concentrations, who can be closely monitored for changes in serum potassium concentration and renal function
2. Exercise training as an adjunctive approach to improve clinical status in stable ambulatory patients
3. Angiotensin receptor blockade or a combination of hydralazine and a nitrate in patients who are receiving treatment with digitalis, diuretics, and a beta blocker and who cannot receive an ACE inhibitor; the hydralazine-nitrate combination is preferred if the reason for not taking an ACE inhibitor is hypotension or renal insufficiency

Class IIb
1. Addition of an angiotensin receptor blocker to an ACE inhibitor in patients who are also receiving digitalis, diuretics, and a beta blocker
2. Addition of a nitrate (alone or in combination with hydralazine) to an ACE inhibitor in patients who are also receiving digitalis, diuretics, and a beta blocker

Class III
1. Long-term intermittent use of an infusion of positive inotropic drug
2. Use of an angiotensin receptor blocker instead of an ACE inhibitor in patients with HF who have not received or can tolerate an ACE inhibitor
3. Use of a calcium channel–blocking drug as a treatment for heart failure
4. Routine use of nutritional supplements (coenzyme Q10, carnitine, taurine, and antioxidants) or hormonal therapies (growth hormone or thyroid hormone) for the treatment of heart failure

ACE, angiotensin-converting enzyme; HF, heart failure; NSAID, nonsteroidal antiinflammatory drug.
From Hunt SA, Baker DW, Chin MH, et al. ACC/AHA guidelines for the evaluation and management of chronic heart failure in the adult. *J Am Coll Cardiol* 2001;104:2996–3007.

TABLE 14.7. *Recommendations for patients with refractory heart failure (Stage D)*

Class I
1. Meticulous evaluation and management of fluid status
2. Referral for cardiac transplantation in eligible patients

Class IIa
1. Referral to a heart failure program with expertise in the management of refractory heart failure, if available
2. Continuous intravenous infusion of a positive inotropic agent for palliation of symptoms

Class IIb
1. Pulmonary artery catheter placement to guide therapy in patients with persistently severe symptoms
2. Mitral valve repair or replacement for secondary mitral regurgitation

Class III
1. Left ventriculectomy
2. Routine intermittent infusions of positive inotropic agents

From Hunt SA, Baker DW, Chin MH, et al. ACC/AHA guidelines for the evaluation and management of chronic heart failure in the adult. *J Am Coll Cardiol* 2001;

day. The patient should be contacted within a week of starting the initial diuretic dose to determine whether further upward titration is necessary. Dosages are normally titrated upward by doubling the baseline dose until an adequate diuretic response is achieved; this usually results in urination within 30 to 60 minutes of taking a dose, and increased urination is noted 3 to 6 hours after the dose is taken. If euvolemia is achieved, then dosages need not be increased, and attention should be paid to signs and symptoms of dehydration. If the patient remains volume overloaded despite an adequate diuretic response, then the regimen can be increased to twice a day. If twice-a-day loop diuretic does not result in euvolemia, then addition of a thiazide diuretic should be considered (e.g., hydrochlorothiazide, 25 to 50 mg daily). Intermittent doses of high-dose diuretics (metolazone) are not recommended, because these result in large volume shifts and in

TABLE 14.8. *Dosages of medications used in heart failure*

Medication	Starting dose	Peak dose
Diuretics		
Loop diuretics		
Furosemide	20 mg daily	200 mg twice daily
Bumetanide	0.5 mg daily	4 mg twice daily
Torsemide	5 mg daily	100 mg twice daily
Thiazide diuretics		
Hydrochlorothiazide	25 mg daily	50 mg daily
Chlorthalodone	50 mg daily	100 mg daily
Metolazone	2.5 mg daily	10 mg twice daily
K^+-sparing diuretics		
Spironolactone	25 mg daily	100 mg daily
Amiloride	5 mg daily	10 mg daily
Triamterene	50 mg daily	100 mg twice daily
Angiotensin-converting enzyme inhibitors		
Captopril	6.25 mg t.i.d.	50 mg t.i.d.
Enalapril	2.5 mg q.d.	10 mg b.i.d.
Lisinopril	2.5 mg q.d.	10 mg q.d.
Fosinopril	2.5 mg q.d.	10 mg q.d.
Ramipril	2.5 mg q.d.	5 mg b.i.d.
Quinapril	5 mg b.i.d.	20 mg b.i.d.
Beta blockers		
Metoprolol Succinate	12.5 mg q.d.	150 mg q.d.
Bisoprolol	1.25 mg q.d.	10 mg q.d.
Carvedilol	3.125 mg b.i.d.	25 mg b.i.d. (50 if weight > 85 kg)
Digitalis		
Digoxin	0.125 mg q.d.	0.125 – 0.25 mg q.d.

episodes of hypokalemia that can precipitate ventricular dysrhythmias.

Patients may become resistant to diuretics as a result of intestinal edema, hypoperfusion, or renal mechanisms. In general, patients with diuretic resistance respond better to higher doses of drug or addition of a thiazide diuretic, or both. Because the bioavailability of furosemide may be affected by changes in intestinal edema, bumetanide and torsemide may be more reliably absorbed in these patients. Patients with inadequate response to all oral diuretics should be treated with intravenous diuretics. Diuretic responsiveness may be restored after alleviation of the edematous state.

Spironolactone

Although therapy with ACE inhibitors may initially lead to reductions in elevated aldosterone levels in heart failure patients, some patients may develop "aldosterone escape" after a period of months. Serum aldosterone levels have been shown to correlate with NYHA class. Elevated levels of aldosterone have been shown to correlate with myocyte hypertrophy and fibrosis in animal models of heart failure (33).

The addition of spironolactone (aldosterone inhibitor) to the combination of digoxin, loop diuretic, and ACE inhibitor in patients with severe heart failure (those in NYHA Class IV and those in NYHA Class III who have had symptoms at rest within the previous 6 months) has been evaluated in the RALES trial (34). The addition of low doses of spironolactone (12.5 to 50 mg daily) reduced the risk of death by 30% in these patients. The role of spironolactone in patients with mild heart failure (NYHA Classes I and II) has not been defined, and, as result, the drug is not included in the treatment guideline for these patients.

The most common reported adverse reactions to spironolactone are hyperkalemia and gynecomastia. Because spironolactone causes the potassium level to rise by an average of 0.2 mmol per liter, attention should be paid to concomitant doses of supplemental potassium. Serum potassium levels should be checked at baseline and again 5 to 7 days after spironolactone therapy is initiated. Patients with serum potassium levels greater than 5.0 mmol per liter and serum creatinine levels greater than 2.5 mg per deciliter should have these abnormalities corrected before initiating spironolactone therapy. If the serum potassium level rises between 5.0 and 6.0 mmol per liter after therapy begins, then the dosage should be reduced by half and the laboratory measurements should be checked in 5 to 7 days. If the serum potassium level rises above 6.0 mmol per liter, then the drug should be discontinued until the abnormality resolves before a lower dosage is attempted.

Direct Vasodilators

Despite conventional wisdom that "vasodilators" are a mainstay of chronic heart failure therapy, only the combination of hydralazine and isosorbide dinitrate has a favorable efficacy and mortality benefit in heart failure. By older classifications, hydralazine was considered a direct arterial vasodilator, and nitrate preparations such as isosorbide dinitrate were considered venodilators. Such arbitrary classification of vasodilators does not withstand current scrutiny. Hydralazine does exert an effect on vascular smooth muscle cells that is direct. The marked increases of cardiac output and heart rate produced by hydralazine may suggest a direct inotropic effect, although confirmatory studies are needed. Although nitrates are venodilators, it is clear that they are also arterial vasodilators, inasmuch as they mimic endothelium-dependent nitric oxide vasodilation. This combination of therapy is effective in all forms of congestive heart failure. A Veterans Administration Cooperative Study, the Vasodilator–Heart Failure Trial (V-HeFT) in moderate heart failure, was the first trial to demonstrate a favorable effect on mortality when the combination of hydralazine and isosorbide dinitrate was compared with placebo (35). The V-HeFT II trial compared the combination of hydralazine and isosorbide dinitrate with enalapril in patients with moderate congestive heart failure, without a placebo arm (36). Mortality in the hydralazine-isosorbide dinitrate group was virtually superimposed with the hydralazine-isosorbide dinitrate group in the V-HeFT I trial.

Although the enalapril treatment produced a greater reduction of mortality, the hydralazine–isosorbide dinitrate treatment in a greater improvement in exercise tolerance and a significant increase of ejection fraction.

The alpha-antagonist prazosin, with potent vasodilator properties, has been tested extensively in patients with heart failure. The V-HeFT study demonstrated that the prazosin treatment did not confer a mortality benefit, in comparison with placebo. Activation of the renin system and adverse stimulation from "unopposed beta"–adrenergic effects have been implicated. As a class of drugs, alpha antagonists are not currently used in chronic therapy for heart failure. Other types of vasodilators such as epoprostenol prostaglandin (Flolan), minoxidil, moxonidine, and nifedipine have all shown detrimental effects in patients with systolic heart failure. The disappointing results of trials with these drugs that provide potent vasodilatory effects have shown that a treatment strategy to provide vasodilation to patients with systolic heart failure has a weak foundation. Medications that have been shown to be successful in reducing deaths and hospitalizations in patients with systolic heart failure have demonstrated significant effects on the neurohormonal adaptations that occur in the disease, rather than pure hemodynamic effects.

Renin-Angiotensin System Suppression

(ACE inhibitors, in contrast to direct-acting vasodilators, have been highly successful in all stages of congestive heart failure. Although ACE inhibitors have vasodilator properties, their mechanism of action extends to other effects of suppressing angiotensin II and modulation of additional vasoactive substances. ACE serves to catalyze the conversion of angiotensin I to angiotensin II, a potent vasoconstrictor and stimulant for aldosterone release. ACE also acts as a kininase, and inhibition of this enzyme leads to decreased breakdown of bradykinin. It is the kininase activity that may explain the advantage of ACE inhibitors over angiotensin receptor blockers.

Many studies have identified the clinical and mortality benefit of ACE inhibitors for all stages of heart failure. The CONSENSUS trial investigators reported in 1987 that the addition of enalapril in patients with NYHA Class IV symptoms led to a 31% reduction in mortality. A significant improvement in NYHA classification was observed in the enalapril recipients, together with a reduction in heart size and a reduced requirement for other medications for heart failure. The effects of ACE inhibitors on patients with asymptomatic heart failure (NYHA Class I) and mild to moderate (NYHA Classes II and III) were demonstrated in the SOLVD trial, which also evaluated the ACE inhibitor enalapril. The treatment substudy evaluated the efficacy of enalapril versus placebo for the treatment of established heart failure (37). In this group, enalapril was associated with a reduction of overall mortality (16% reduction), although rates of mortality attributed to sudden death were not substantially altered. In a separate prevention substudy in patients with asymptomatic left ventricular dysfunction, enalapril prevented progression of congestive heart failure (38). Overall mortality rates were not improved in comparison with those for placebo. Enalapril recipients also experienced a lesser incidence of subsequent clinically evident myocardial infarction, in comparison with those receiving placebo. Subsequent studies of ACE inhibitors used in patients with systolic heart failure have demonstrated that the benefits provided are not restricted to any particular compound, but instead represent a "class effect."

In addition to studies that have documented the benefit of ACE inhibitors in mild or asymptomatic heart failure, studies have demonstrated the benefit of ACE inhibitors in patients who have experienced an acute myocardial infarction. The Survival and Ventricular Enlargement (SAVE) study assessed the effects of captopril in an asymptomatic post-infarction population with ejection fractions of less than 40% (39). This study also demonstrated reduction of recurrent myocardial infarction with captopril. Subsequent studies of ramipril in a symptomatic postinfarction population showed reduction in mortality with the addition of an ACE inhibitor (40). More recently, ramipril has been shown to reduce the risk of cardiovascular events (HOPE trial), including a 23% reduction in the risk of developing heart failure, in a population without preexisting heart disease but with cardiovascular

risk factors (41). It is overly simplistic to label these drugs vasodilators, because patients in this study had an average systolic/diastolic pressure drop of only 3/2 mm HG with the active drugs. The drugs appear to have effects on the vasculature, heart, and kidneys that go far beyond their rather small blood pressure–lowering effects. Inhibition of the renin-angiotensin-aldosterone system at the tissue level allows the vasculature, heart, and kidneys to escape some of the ravages of long-term activity of angiotensin II and aldosterone, including growth, hypertrophy, proliferation, deposition of collagen, and tissue remodeling.

The choice of ACE inhibitor dosage should be based on individual patient characteristics, such as baseline blood pressure and serum creatinine and serum sodium levels (+8). Development of mild hypotension (e.g., systolic blood pressure of 80 to 90 mm HG) and azotemia (serum creatinine concentration of 2.0 to 2.5 mg per deciliter) may be encountered during drug titration and should be tolerated in the absence of symptoms to attain the benefits offered by the drug. Symptomatic hypotension, progressive azotemia, or an intolerable cough, however, occasionally forces the discontinuation of the ACE inhibitor. Other side effects, including rash and angioedema, are rare. The optimal dosage of an ACE inhibitor and the treatment target (blood pressure vs. trial goal doses) has not been established. Evidence suggests that aspirin and nonsteroidal antiinflammatory drugs can block the favorable effects and increase the likelihood for renal insufficiency of ACE inhibitors. Whether other ACE inhibitors will afford the same benefits provided by ramipril in the HOPE Trial is unknown at the time of this writing. There are differences between the relative blockade provided by individual ACE inhibitors at the level of the kidney and at that of other tissues (myocyte, vascular endothelium).

Beta-Adrenergic Blockade

The sympathetic nervous system is activated in patients with advanced heart failure. Evidence for this change rests in observations that norepinephrine levels correlate with mortality in heart failure, and low-frequency heart rate responses by heart rate spectral analysis are augmented in patients with severe heart failure. In view of failed trials of dobutamine and other positive inotropic agents on clinical outcomes, relatively small studies performed in Europe initially hinted at the beneficial effects of beta blockade in heart failure (42). The Metoprolol in Dilated Cardiomyopathy (MDC) trial evaluated progressive increase of metoprolol dosage in patients with moderate to severe dilated cardiomyopathy; patients with coronary artery disease were excluded. Metoprolol improved functional status and was associated with a reduction of combined endpoints (combined mortality or listing for cardiac transplantation) in comparison with placebo. Despite these results, skepticism regarding the use of beta blockers in the treatment of heart failure prevailed until the U.S. Carvedilol trials demonstrated a 65% reduction in mortality with carvedilol, a nonselective beta blocker with additional alpha-blocking properties, in patients with largely NYHA Classes II and III symptoms (11). After this, trials using selective beta₁ blockade (metoprolol) and nonselective beta blockade in the absence of alpha blockade (bisoprolol) have demonstrated that the benefits of beta blockade in heart failure are largely a class effect (12,13). Only the Beta blocker Efficacy and Survival Trial (BEST) failed to demonstrate a benefit of a beta blocker (bucindolol) over placebo in heart failure. Most recently, the Cardivol Prospective Randomized Cumulative Survival (COPERNICUS) trial showed that beta blockade with carvedilol reduces mortality in patients with severe heart failure (rest symptoms without signs of volume overload).

As a class, beta blockers produce the greatest increase in ejection fraction during therapy in comparison with other forms of therapy. Reduction of heart rate and improved diastolic filling time may contribute to this benefit. Beta blockers directly suppress renin release and thereby interrupt the renin system at its origin. The antioxidant properties of carvedilol may also contribute to its efficacy in heart failure, either by direct chemical redox effects or by indirect effects as a consequence of decreased oxygen consumption or oxidative stress.

Patients with NYHA Class II and III symptoms and patients with rest symptoms who do not have signs of volume overload should be treated with beta blockade unless a contraindication exists. During the initiation of beta blockers, and with each dose titration, patients may experience a temporary reduction in functional status and worsening of fluid retention. This period generally lasts for 2 to 4 weeks and is usually tolerated without additional diuretics. Beta blockers should not be started by patients who are hospitalized for the treatment of volume overload. Patients with heart rate less than 60 beats per minute should receive beta blockers with caution. Patients with low systolic blood pressure generally tolerate beta blockade; trials have generally shown little to no blood pressure reduction in patients with low to normal blood pressure at baseline. Patients with significant bronchospastic disease may not tolerate beta blockade, although patients with heart failure and wheezing as a manifestation of pulmonary congestion should be considered candidates if the wheezing resolves with diuresis.

Treatment with carvedilol should be initiated at 3.125 to 6.25 mg twice daily, and metoprolol succinate should be initiated at 12.5 to 25 mg daily. The dose of beta blocker may be titrated upward by doubling the dose every 2 to 4 weeks as tolerated. Patients should report symptoms of weight gain, breathlessness, or hypotension that might delay upward titration. Carvedilol should be titrated upward to the maximally tolerated dose with a goal of achieving 25 mg twice daily or, for patients weighing more than 85 kg, 50 mg twice daily. However, doses as low as 6.25 mg twice daily have demonstrated mortality benefit in comparison with placebo. Patients treated with metoprolol should be targeted to receive a daily dose of 150 mg. Patients admitted to the hospital for the treatment of volume overload during treatment with beta blockade should receive intravenous diuretics. If diuresis is not adequate with intravenous diuretics, the physician may try to reduce the dose of beta blocker, rather than discontinue the beta blocker abruptly.

Calcium Channel Antagonists

Calcium channel antagonists have not been successful in the treatment of congestive heart failure, and largely do not have a role in therapy of heart failure patients except in patients with coexistent hypertension or active myocardial ischemia. Hypotheses for the lack of efficacy in congestive heart failure include a direct negative inotropic effect and activation of adverse neurohormonal pathways. This class of compounds is pharmacologically diverse. Verapamil and diltiazem do not increase heart rate, whereas the dihydropyridines increase both resting and peak exercise heart rate. Plasma catecholamines are also increased in response to many of the dihydropyridines. Newer dihydropyridines may not produce these adverse effects. Both felodipine and amlodipine have been shown to be safe but not efficacious in patients with heart failure (43).

Digoxin

Although forms of digitalis glycosides have been used by physicians to treat edematous states for more than 200 years, its efficacy has been a point of dispute until much more recently. Digitalis exerts its effect through the inhibition of Na^+-K^- adenosine triphosphatase (ATPase). Inhibition of this enzyme leads to augmentation of the myocardial contractility but also blocks vagal afferent nerve function, thereby leading to sensitization of cardiac baroreceptors. Baroreceptor responses to physiologic maneuvers are normalized in many patients. By slowing the ventricular response in atrial fibrillation, digoxin improves ventricular filling, coronary perfusion time, and myocardial oxygen consumption. Inhibition of Na^+-K^- ATPase in the kidney reduces the renal tubular reabsorption of sodium, thereby leading to natriuresis. Digitalis therapy administration decreases plasma renin activity and plasma aldosterone. Acutely, catecholamines are also reduced with digitalis.

Two studies evaluated the effect of digoxin withdrawal on clinical and exercise parameters. These were the Randomized Digoxin and Inhibitor of Angiotensin Converting Enzyme (RADIANCE) and the Prospective Randomized Study of Ventricular Failure and the Efficacy of Digoxin (PROVED) trials (44). In both trials, patients randomly assigned to undergo withdrawal of digoxin experienced reduction of exercise performance and clinical deterioration. Deterioration was evident within 4 to 8 weeks, consisting of subjective clinical deterioration, requirement for medication change, and increase of outpatient and inpatient medical management. More recently, the Digitalis Investigation Group (DIG), a long-term trial of 7,500 patients randomly assigned to receive digoxin or placebo, showed no mortality benefit with digoxin. However, the risk of hospitalization was reduced by 8% in these patients (45).

Patients with heart failure who are at risk for hospitalization (NYHA Classes II to IV) should be considered for treatment with digoxin. Therapy with beta blockers should not be withheld to facilitate the initiation of digoxin, however. Therapy with digoxin is initiated and maintained at a dose of 0.125 to 0.25 mg per day. Lower doses (0.125 mg every other day) may be given to elderly patients or patients with impaired renal function. Previously, the therapeutic range of digoxin was thought to be up to a serum level of 2.0 ng per milliliter. Analysis of data from the DIG trial, however, has shown that patients achieving these levels are more likely to experience adverse effects.

Inotropic Therapy

Several randomized trials comparing the effects of inotropic therapies (dobutamine, milrinone, vesnarinone, pimobendan, ibopamine, enoximone, and others) to standard therapy for heart failure have shown that these agents increase the likelihood of death. The presumed mechanism for the added risk is through increased ventricular dysrhythmias, but these agents may also hasten the progression of heart failure by creating a mismatch between myocardial energy supply and demand and through neurohormonal mechanisms. These positive inotropic drugs should be avoided in patients with heart failure if at all possible. Patients with advanced heart failure, who require frequent hospitalizations despite adherence to dietary restrictions, treatment with medical therapies known to improve clinical outcomes, and optimization of volume status, may be candidates for continuous intravenous inotropic support for palliative purposes only. The goal of such therapy should be to increase systemic blood flow to improve organ perfusion, improve appetite, and enhance the likelihood that volume status can be maintained so that these patients can enjoy their remaining days outside the hospital. There is no role for intermittent administration of positive inotropic medications to patients with heart failure.

Implantable Cardiac Defibrillators

Many patients with heart failure due to left ventricular systolic dysfunction die unexpectedly from sudden cardiac death (in the setting of ventricular fibrillation, pulseless ventricular tachycardia, or severe bradycardia). Implantable cardiac defibrillators have the capacity to continuously monitor the cardiac electrogram and deliver therapy (cardioversion or backup cardiac pacing) on the basis of the program algorithm. Two primary prevention trials have demonstrated that patients with ischemic heart disease, left ventricular systolic dysfunction, and nonsustained ventricular tachycardia benefit from implantable defibrillators if malignant ventricular arrhythmias can be induced during electrophysiologic testing (46,47). Ambulatory electrocardiographic monitoring is a useful tool for risk-stratifying patients with cardiomyopathy and coronary artery disease. Even without inducible arrhythmias, the risk of sudden cardiac death is substantial with nonsustained ventricular tachycardia in patients with ischemic cardiomyopathy (46). Less is known about the utility of ambulatory electrocardiographic monitoring in the nonischemic population. The Sudden Cardiac Death in Heart Failure Trial (SCD-HeFT) is in progress and has been designed to determine whether amiodarone or the implantable cardiac defibrillator will decrease overall mortality rates among patients with coronary artery disease or nonischemic cardiomyopathy who are in NYHA Class II or III heart failure and have a left ventricular ejection fraction of less than 35%. The use of the implantable cardiac defibrillator in patients with heart failure may be understood better when the results of this study is available.

Biventricular Pacemaker Therapy

Many patients with systolic heart failure have right ventricular dyssynchrony that is caused by an intraventricular conduction delay or bundle branch block. Left ventricular pacing can be offered through specially designed pacemakers and combination defibrillator/pacemakers that allow for the placement of a lead into the coronary sinus, terminating in the anterior interventricular vein or the middle cardiac vein. Studies have shown that left ventricular or biventricular pacing can improve this dyssynchrony in patients with left bundle branch block and can lead to higher cardiac output, higher blood pressure, and improved exercise tolerance. The long-term benefits of biventricular pacing on mortality and hospitalizations attributable to heart failure are not known at this time.

Mechanical Assist Devices

Patients waiting for a donor heart to become available may be considered for mechanical assist therapy if it is thought that they are unlikely to survive to the time of transplantation. Intraaortic balloon counterpulsation (IABP), originally developed for short-term augmentation of cardiac output and coronary blood flow, has been used for this purpose to a limited degree. Use of IABP longer than a few days carries the risk of infection (groin access), limb ischemia, and sacral decubitus ulcer. Patients require continuous systemic anticoagulation and must be immobilized for IABP treatment. Since the early 1990s, left ventricular assist devices (LVADs) have become available for the purpose of "bridging" to transplantation. These devices provide full cardiac support (device output, more than 5 L per minute) and in some cases are implanted into the body with only a power supply cannula exiting the skin. Newer devices that are totally implanted into the body, including the power supply, are in development. These LVADs allow for improved organ blood flow and clinical improvement before the time of transplantation. Patients may be ambulatory with these devices in place and, in some cases, leave the hospital to live at home while they are waiting for transplantation. The Randomized Evaluation of Mechanical Assistance for the Treatment of Congestive Heart Failure (REMATCH) trial has shown that placement of the HeartMate LVAD reduces the risk of death by 48% in carefully selected patients with advanced heart failure. The mortality rate in the LVAD group at 2 years was 77%, however, and significant improvements are required before this device can be used for long-term myocardial replacement therapy.

PROGNOSIS

The prognosis of patients suffering from congestive heart failure has improved significantly since the mid-1980s. Patients with NYHA Class IV heart failure symptoms enrolled in the placebo arm of the CONSENSUS trial had a 44% rate of mortality at 6 months of follow-up (48). The patients treated with enalapril in this study had a 40% reduction in mortality at 6 months. The RALES trial showed in 1999 that the addition of spironolactone to the medication regimen of patients with severe heart failure reduced the risk of death by 30%. Most of the patients in the RALES trial were taking ACE inhibitors at baseline. More recently, the COPERNICUS trial demonstrated that carvedilol reduces the risk of all-cause mortality by approximately 35%. Although most patients in the COPERNICUS trial were receiving ACE inhibitors at baseline, only a minority of the patients was receiving spironolactone. However, if the effects of these three classes of drugs are assumed to be additive, the expected mortality of patients with NYHA Class IV symptoms would be reduced by 72% (12% rate of 6-month mortality) in comparison with the group enrolled in the CONSENSUS trial.

Although statistics can be gleaned from clinical trials in regard to the expected survival of populations of patients with systolic heart failure, predicting the prognosis of an individual patient is difficult. Predictions regarding how many months a patient has to live should be avoided, because they are invariably wrong. Nonetheless, patients with heart failure benefit from understanding their general prognosis, as it helps them understand the need to prepare for end-of-life events.

Perhaps the best-documented predictor of prognosis is functional status, usually with the NYHA classification. Asymptomatic patients with heart failure enrolled in the SOLVD Prevention Trial had a 15% rate of mortality over an average of 37 months of follow-up (38). Patients with NYHA Classes II and III symptoms enrolled in the treatment arm of the Metoprolol CR/XL Randomised Intervention Trial in Congestive Heart Failure (MERIT-HF) had a 7.2% rate of mortality at 12 months of follow-up (13). In contrast, patients with NYHA Class IV symptoms enrolled in the COPERNICUS trial had an 18% mortality rate over 12 months of follow-up. Ejection fraction has also been shown to be a potent predictor of mortality in a heterogeneous population of patients with heart failure, but it is less helpful when groups of patients with severe left ventricular systolic dysfunction are compared (49). Several additional predictors of prognosis have been identified, including peak exercise oxygen consumption, cardiothoracic ratio as measured by chest radiograph, left ventricular end-diastolic volume, QRS interval, heart rate, mean arterial blood pressure, presence of coronary artery disease, presence of mitral regurgitation, ventricular arrhythmias as identified by Holter monitoring, pulmonary capillary wedge pressure, serum sodium, and levels of plasma norepinephrine as well as other neurohormones/cytokine levels (e.g., BNP, ET, tumor necrosis factor). Statistical models have been derived and validated for the purposes of predicting prognosis in patients referred for evaluation for transplantation. Generalizing these models to patients with less severe heart failure is not possible.

RECOMMENDATIONS FOR END-OF-LIFE PLANNING

Education of patients with heart failure and their families regarding prognosis should be done at the time of initial evaluation and at subsequent times of follow-up care when conditions have changed so the parties can have a chance to plan for end-of-life events. Advanced planning should include treatment preferences such as implantable cardiac defibrillator placement, intravenous inotropic administration, surgical interventions, and transplantation. Because patients with systolic heart failure may experience sudden death, attention should be paid to living wills and advanced directives early in the treatment course. Patients with severe heart failure symptoms refractory to maximal medical therapy and who are ineligible for surgical interventions should be approached regarding preferences for resuscitation. Hospice services may be helpful for patients in the process of dying from severe heart failure.

FOLLOW-UP

Care of patients with systolic heart failure requires close follow-up and attention to detail to prevent decompensation, need for hospitalization, and death. Outpatient visits are necessary for monitoring subtle changes in signs and symptoms and for titrating medications to achieve the optimal medical regimen. Laboratory testing to monitor renal function and serum potassium level should be performed within 1 week of medication changes, because changes in renal perfusion and electrolyte excretion may lead to unwanted side effects. Because care of the patient with systolic heart failure patient requires significant time and resources to provide sufficient education and planning for follow-up laboratory testing, specialized multidisciplinary disease management programs designed to care for patients with heart failure may provide a distinct advantage over management by a single practitioner. Trials designed to study the benefits of multidisciplinary care delivery to elderly patients with heart failure have clearly been shown to improve clinical patient outcomes, as well as to lead to reduction in cost of care (50).

PRACTICAL POINTS

- In all patients with symptoms of heart failure, their left ventricular systolic function should be assessed.
- Coronary angiography should be performed in patients with heart failure and symptoms of angina or with risk factors for atherosclerosis.
- Patients with heart failure and a left ventricular ejection fraction less than 40% should be treated with an ACE inhibitor unless it is contraindicated.
- Patients with heart failure and a left ventricular ejection fraction less than 40% should be treated with a beta blocker, unless they are intolerant of this medication or unless rest symptoms and signs of volume overload are present.
- Patients with current or recent NYHA Class IV symptoms should be treated with spironolactone.

- All patients with heart failure should be advised to weigh themselves daily and report significant weight changes (more than 3 to 5 pounds) to their physicians.
- Patients requiring diuretic therapy or who have a history of volume overload should be instructed to limit daily dietary sodium intake to 2–3 g and limit daily dietary fluid intake to 48–64 oz.
- Patients with refractory heart failure symptoms require frequent office visits and meticulous management of medical therapy.
- Eligible patients with NYHA Class III or IV symptoms despite optimal medical care should be referred for cardiac transplantation evaluation.
- Patients with heart failure should understand how their disease influences their prognosis and should be advised to consider end-of-life issues.

REFERENCES

1. Cohn JN. The management of chronic heart failure. *N Engl J Med* 1996;335:490–498.
2. Weber KT. Extracellular matrix remodeling in heart failure: a role for *de novo* angiotensin II generation. *Circulation.* 1997;96:4065–4082.
3. Benedict CR, Shelton B, Johnstone DE, et al. Prognostic significance of plasma norepinephrine in patients with asymptomatic left ventricular dysfunction. SOLVD Investigators. *Circulation* 1996;94:690–697.
4. Francis GS, Cohn JN, Johnson G, et al. Plasma

norepinephrine, plasma renin activity, and congestive heart failure. Relations to survival and the effects of therapy in V-HeFT II. The V-HeFT VA Cooperative Studies Group. *Circulation* 1993;87:VI40–VI48.

5. Schrier RW, Abraham WT. Hormones and hemodynamics in heart failure. *N Engl J Med* 1999;341:577–585.

6. Staessen J, Lijnen P, Fagard R, et al. Rise in plasma concentration of aldosterone during long-term angiotensin II suppression. *J Endocrinol* 1981;91:457–465.

7. Swedberg K, Eneroth P, Kjekshus J, et al. Hormones regulating cardiovascular function in patients with severe congestive heart failure and their relation to mortality. CONSENSUS Trial Study Group. *Circulation* 1990;82:1730–1736.

8. Brilla C, Matsubara L, Weber K. Antifibrotic effects of spironolactone in preventing myocardial fibrosis in systemic arterial hypertension. *Am J Cardiol* 1993; 71:12A–16A.

9. Pitt B. RALES Investigators. The Randomized Aldactone Evaluation Study (RALES): parallel dose finding trial. *J Am Coll Cardiol* 1995;25:45A(abst).

10. Cohn JN, Levine TB, Olivari MT, et al. Plasma norepinephrine as a guide to prognosis in patients with chronic congestive heart failure. *N Engl J Med* 1984; 311:819–823.

11. Packer M, Colucci WS, Sackner-Bernstein JD, et al. Double-blind, placebo-controlled study of the effects of carvedilol in patients with moderate to severe heart failure. The PRECISE Trial. Prospective Randomized Evaluation of Carvedilol on Symptoms and Exercise. *Circulation* 1996;94:2793–2799.

12. The Cardiac Insufficiency Bisoprolol Study II (CIBIS-II): a randomised trial. *Lancet* 1999;353:9–13.

13. Effect of metoprolol CR/XL in chronic heart failure: Metoprolol CR/XL Randomised Intervention Trial in Congestive Heart Failure (MERIT-HF). *Lancet* 1999;353:2001–2007.

14. Wei CM, Heublein DM, Perrella MA, et al. Natriuretic peptide system in human heart failure. *Circulation* 1993;88:1004–1009.

15. Colucci WS, Elkayam U, Horton DP, et al. Intravenous nesiritide, a natriuretic peptide, in the treatment of decompensated congestive heart failure. Nesiritide study group. *N Engl J Med* 2000;343:246–253.

16. Omland T, Aakvaag A, Bonarjee VV, et al. Plasma brain natriuretic peptide as an indicator of left ventricular systolic function and long-term survival after acute myocardial infarction. Comparison with plasma atrial natriuretic peptide and N-terminal proatrial natriuretic peptide. *Circulation* 1996;93:1963–1969.

17. Cody RJ, Haas GJ, Binkley PF, et al. Plasma endothelin correlates with the extent of pulmonary hypertension in patients with chronic congestive heart failure. *Circulation* 1992;85:504–509.

18. Preibisz JJ, Sealey JE, Laragh JH, et al. Plasma and platelet vasopressin in essential hypertension and congestive heart failure. *Hypertension* 1983;5(Suppl I):I129–I138.

19. Kasper E, Agema W, Hutchins G, et al. The causes of dilated cardiomyopathy: a clinicopathologic review of 673 consecutive patients. *J Am Coll Cardiol* 1994; 23:586–590.

20. Dec GW Jr, Palacios IF, Fallon JT, et al. Active myocarditis in the spectrum of acute dilated cardiomyopathies. Clinical features, histologic correlates, and clinical outcome. *N Engl J Med* 1985;312:885–890.

21. Mason JW, O'Connell JB, Herskowitz A, et al. A clinical trial of immunosuppressive therapy for myocarditis. The Myocarditis Treatment Trial Investigators. *N Engl J Med* 1995;333:269–275.

22. Morris SA, Tanowitz HB, Wittner M, et al. Pathophysiological insights into the cardiomyopathy of Chagas' disease. *Circulation* 1990;82:1900–1909.

23. Alexander J, Dainiak N, Berger HJ, et al. Serial assessment of doxorubicin cardiotoxicity with quantitative radionuclide angiocardiography. *N Engl J Med* 1979;300:278–283.

24. Knochel JP. Cardiovascular effects of alcohol. *Ann Intern Med* 1983;98:849–854.

25. Henderson I, Frei E. Adriamycin and the heart. *N Engl J Med* 1979;300:310.

26. Bristow MR, Mason JW, Billingham ME, et al. Dose-effect and structure-function relationships in doxorubicin cardiomyopathy. *Am Heart J* 1981;102:709–718.

27. Wang J, Liu X, Arneja AS, et al. Alterations in protein kinase A and protein kinase C levels in heart failure due to genetic cardiomyopathy. *Can J Cardiol* 1999;15:683–690.

28. Gruver EJ, Fatkin D, Dodds GA, et al. Familial hypertrophic cardiomyopathy and atrial fibrillation caused by Arg663His beta-cardiac myosin heavy chain mutation. *Am J Cardiol* 1999;83:13H–18H.

29. Liggett SB, Wagoner LE, Craft LL, et al. The Ile164 beta$_2$-adrenergic receptor polymorphism adversely affects the outcome of congestive heart failure. *J Clin Invest* 1998;102:1534–1539.

29a. Hunt SA, Baker DW, Chin MH, et al. ACC/AHA guidelines for the evaluation and management of chronic heart failure in the adult: executive summary. A report of the American College of Cardiology and American Heart Association Task Force on Practice Guidelines (Committee to revise the 1995 Guidelines for the Evaluation and Management of Heart Failure). *J Am Coll Cardiol* 2001;38:2101–2113.

30. Dao Q, Krishnaswamy P, Kazanegra R, et al. Utility of B-type natriuretic peptide in the diagnosis of congestive heart failure in an urgent-care setting. *J Am Coll Cardiol* 2001;37:379–385.

31. Bolling SF, Pagani FD, Deeb GM, et al. Intermediate-term outcome of mitral reconstruction in cardiomyopathy. *J Thorac Cardiovasc Surg* 1998;115:381–386.

32. Felker GM, Thompson RE, Hare JM, et al. Underlying causes and long-term survival in patients with initially unexplained cardiomyopathy. *N Engl J Med* 2000;342:1077–1084.

33. Weber K, Brilla C. Pathological hypertrophy and cardiac interstitium: fibrosis and renin-angiotensin-aldosterone system. *Circulation* 1991;83:1849–1865.

34. Pitt B, Zannad F, Remme WJ, et al. The effect of spironolactone on morbidity and mortality in patients with severe heart failure. Randomized Aldactone Evaluation Study Investigators. *N Engl J Med* 1999;341:709–717.

35. Cohn JN, Archibald DG, Ziesche S, et al. Effect of vasodilator therapy on mortality in chronic congestive heart failure. Results of a Veterans Administration Cooperative Study. *N Engl J Med* 1986;314:1547–1552.

36. Cohn J, Johnson G, Ziesche S. A comparison of enalapril with hydralazine–isosorbide dinitrate in the treatment of chronic congestive heart failure. *N Engl J Med* 1991;325:303–310.

37. Effect of enalapril on survival in patients with reduced left ventricular ejection fractions and congestive heart failure. The SOLVD Investigators. *N Engl J Med* 1991;325:293–302.

38. Effect of enalapril on mortality and the development of heart failure in asymptomatic patients with reduced left ventricular ejection fractions. The SOLVD Investigators. *N Engl J Med* 1992;327:685–691.

39. Pfeffer MA, Braunwald E, Moye LA, et al. Effect of captopril on mortality and morbidity in patients with left ventricular dysfunction after myocardial infarction. Results of the Survival And Ventricular Enlargement trial. The SAVE investigators. *N Engl J Med* 1992;327:669–677.

40. Effect of ramipril on mortality and morbidity of survivors of acute myocardial infarction with clinical evidence of heart failure. The Acute Infarction Ramipril Efficacy (AIRE) Study Investigators. *Lancet* 1993;342:821–828.

41. Yusuf S, Sleight P, Pogue J, et al. Effects of an angiotensin-converting-enzyme inhibitor, ramipril, on cardiovascular events in high-risk patients. The Heart Outcomes Prevention Evaluation Study Investigators. *N Engl J Med* 2000;342:145–153.

42. Waagstein F, Bristow M, Swedberg K. Beneficial effects of metoprolol in idiopathic dilated cardiomyopathy. *Lancet* 1993;342:1441–1446.

43. Cohn JN, Ziesche S, Smith R, et al. Effect of the calcium antagonist felodipine as supplementary vasodilator therapy in patients with chronic heart failure treated with enalapril: V-HeFT III. Vasodilator-Heart Failure Trial (V-HeFT) Study Group. *Circulation* 1997;96:856–863.

44. Packer M, Gheorghiade M, Young JB, et al. Withdrawal of digoxin from patients with chronic heart failure treated with angiotensin-converting-enzyme inhibitors. RADIANCE Study. *N Engl J Med* 1993;329:1–7.

45. The effect of digoxin on mortality and morbidity in patients with heart failure. The Digitalis Investigation Group. *N Engl J Med* 1997;336:525–533.

46. Buxton A, Lee K, Fisher J, et al. A randomized study of the prevention of sudden death in patients with coronary artery disease. Multicenter Unsustained Tachycardia Trial Investigators. *N Engl J Med* 1999;341:1882–1890.

47. Moss AJ, Hall WJ, Cannom DS, et al. Improved survival with an implanted defibrillator in patients with coronary disease at high risk for ventricular arrhythmia. Multicenter Automatic Defibrillator Implantation Trial Investigators. *N Engl J Med* 1996;335:1933–1940.

48. Effects of enalapril on mortality in severe congestive heart failure. Results of the Cooperative North Scandinavian Enalapril Survival Study (CONSENSUS). The CONSENSUS Trial Study Group. *N Engl J Med* 1987;316:1429–1435.

49. Cohn JN, Johnson GR, Shabetai R, et al. Ejection fraction, peak exercise oxygen consumption, cardiothoracic ratio, ventricular arrhythmias, and plasma norepinephrine as determinants of prognosis in heart failure. The V-HeFT VA Cooperative Studies Group. *Circulation* 1993;87:VI5–VI16.

50. Rich MW, Beckham V, Wittenberg C, et al. A multidisciplinary intervention to prevent the readmission of elderly patients with congestive heart failure. *N Engl J Med* 1995;333:1190–1195.

15

Congestive Heart Failure with Preserved Systolic Function

Ragavendra R. Baliga, Mauro Moscucci, and Robert J. Cody

GENERAL ASPECTS

Definition

Diastolic heart failure is present when elevated filling pressure is necessary to achieve normal ventricular filling (1). Because it is logistically difficult to establish the diagnosis of diastolic heart failure, a working definition of this entity has been congestive heart failure with preserved systolic function (CHF-PSF). Clearly, not all patients with this diagnosis have diastolic left ventricular dysfunction, such as mitral stenosis or constrictive pericarditis. In an attempt to better define diastolic heart failure for both clinical and epidemiologic purposes, the Vasan-Levy criteria are used to classify this condition into three diagnostic categories: definite, probable, and possible (Table 15.1).

These diagnostic criteria are limited by the facts that they do not have exclusionary clauses for constrictive pericarditis and mitral stenosis and that they lump together several pathologic entities with varying prognoses, such as amyloidosis, hypertrophic cardiomyopathy, intermittent myocardial ischemia, and diffuse myocardial fibrosis (2).

Burden

Several hospital-based and community-based studies have suggested that diastolic heart failure is more common than acknowledged (3–7). Both epidemiologic and case studies based in the community suggest that as high as 40% to 50% percent of the patients with a diagnosis of congestive heart failure have normal systolic function (4–7). Exacerbations of heart failure due to diastolic dysfunction carry the same high hospital readmission rate as those of heart failure due to systolic dysfunction (8), and it has been estimated that diastolic heart failure is responsible for at least 25% of the total economic burden imposed by congestive heart failure (9). The incidence of diastolic dysfunction increases as an individual ages, and the incidence of congestive heart failure due to diastolic dysfunction dramatically rises with age (7,10–13). It has been suggested that diastolic heart failure may be more common in women (3,14) and black persons (15), and it has been proposed that this is due to gender and racial variation in responses to left ventricular remodeling that occurs in response to pressure overload (16).

Usual Causes

The classical causes of diastolic heart failure include nonobstructive hypertrophic cardiomyopathy, infiltrative cardiomyopathies, and restrictive cardiomyopathies (Table 15.2). However, most of the patients with CHF-PSF do not have an intrinsic myocardial disorder. Common causes include hypertension, ischemic heart disease (17), age, and valvular heart disease (particularly aortic stenosis). The typical CHF-PSF patient is an elderly hypertensive woman (14) with a small body surface area. The changes in the cardiovascular system that naturally accompany aging tend to affect the diastolic function of the left ventricle rather than the systolic function (18). Other causes of CHF-PSF, including hypertension, aortic sclerosis, coronary artery disease, and atrial fibrillation, are also more common in the elderly. Aging is also associated with myocardial fibrosis (and, consequently, the "stiff" heart) and impaired peripheral vasodilatory properties, and

TABLE 15.1. *Vasan-Levy criteria for diagnosis of diastolic dysfunction*

Probability of diastolic dysfunction	Definitive evidence of CHF[a]	Evidence of normal LV systolic function within 72 hours of heart failure[b]	Objective evidence of diastolic dysfunction[c]
Define	+	+	+
Probable	+	+	−
Possible	+	−(but present outside the 72-hr window)	−

CHF, congestive heart failure; LV, left ventricular.
[a]Clinical symptoms, signs, supporting tests such as chest radiograph, typical clinical response to treatment with diuretics, with or without documentation of elevated left ventricular filling pressure or a low cardiac index.
[b]Left ventricular ejection fraction of $\geq$50%.
[c]Abnormal LV relaxation/filling/distensibility indices on cardiac catheterization or echocardiography.

all these factors contribute to the increased occurrence of CHF-PSF in the elderly. Elderly women are more prone to CHF-PSF because of gender-dependent variation in cardiac remodeling in response to hypertension or diabetes (19). Diabetic patients have diastolic dysfunction in the absence of diabetic complications, hypertension, or coronary artery disease (20).

Presenting Symptoms and Signs

Symptoms and signs of congestive heart failure are indistinguishable from those of left ventricular systolic function (see Chapter 14). Diastolic dysfunction should be suspected in

TABLE 15.2. *Usual causes*

Physiologic adaptation
Hypertension
Ischemic heart disease (Dodek et al., 1972[17])
Aging
Diabetes mellitus
Intrinsic anatomic abnormalities
Valvular heart disease
Hypertrophic cardiomyopathy
Restrictive cardiomyopathy (abnormally rigid ventricles that are not necessarily thickened but with impaired diastolic filling and usually normal systolic function)
  Myocardial
    Noninfiltrative: idiopathic, scleroderma
    Infiltrative: amyloidosis, sarcoidosis
    Storage disorders: hemochromatosis, glycogen storage disorders
  Endomyocardial
    Endomyocardial fibrosis
    Hypereosinophilic syndromes
    Radiation therapy
    Metastatic tumors

the following circumstances (Table 15.3): when systolic blood pressure exceeds 160 mm HG or diastolic blood pressure exceeds 100 mg HG during the acute exacerbation of heart failure (21), when patients develop heart failure with infusion of small amounts of intravenous fluids, in elderly patients (particularly women) with long histories of hypertension and repeated admissions for heart failure, and when there is echocardiographic evidence of left ventricular hypertrophy without systolic dysfunction or without wall motion abnormalities.

Helpful Tests

- *Chest radiography* is used to confirm the presence of pulmonary edema and to monitor response to diuretic therapy (Fig. 15.1).
- The *electrocardiogram* (ECG) is used to look for evidence of left ventricular hypertrophy and atrial fibrillation. The presence of tachyarrhythmia or atrial fibrillation results in the

TABLE 15.3. *Suspect diastolic heart failure in the following circumstances*

When systolic blood pressure >160 mm HG or diastolic blood pressure >100 mg HG during the acute exacerbation of heart failure (Badgett et al., 1997[21])
Patient develops heart failure with infusion of small amounts of intravenous fluids
Elderly patients (particularly women) with long history of hypertension with repeated admissions for heart failure
Echocardiographic evidence of left ventricular hypertrophy without systolic dysfunction or without wall motion abnormalities

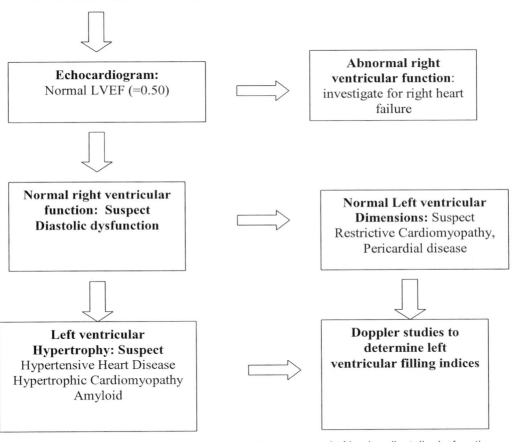

FIG. 15.1. Flow chart for investigation of a patient suspected of having diastolic dysfunction.

loss "atrial kick" during the episode of congestive heart failure.

- The *echocardiogram* is used to determine systolic function, chamber size, and diastolic filling characteristics (22). Two-dimensional Doppler echocardiography is a reliable and reproducible method for diagnosis and longitudinal follow-up of left ventricular diastolic dysfunction (23). The *Nishimura-Tajik grading* (Fig. 15.2) of diastolic dysfunction is based on clinical and echocardiographic criteria (23):

Grade 0: Normal (mitral inflow velocity curve with an E/A ratio greater than 1.0 and a deceleration time of approximately 200 milliseconds).

Grade I: Abnormal relaxation pattern on Doppler echocardiogram; patient develops symptoms on moderate exertion or with onset of atrial fibrillation.

Grade II: Pseudonormalization pattern of the mitral flow velocity and increased filling pressure at rest, producing symptoms at mild to moderate exertion.

Grade III: Restrictive filling pattern on mitral flow velocity curves and severe increase in filling pressures and symptoms at rest or on minimal exertion. Patients respond to diuretic therapy, and their condition improves to grade I or II.

Grade IV: Irreversible grade III changes; patients maintain a severe restrictive pattern despite aggressive diuretic therapy; poor prognosis.

- *Myocardial biopsy* is useful for demonstrating deposits of amyloid or iron, caseating granulomas, eosinophilic or lymphocytic infiltrates, or any interstitial inflammatory change.
- *Right- and left-sided heart catheterization* is the standard method for direct measurement

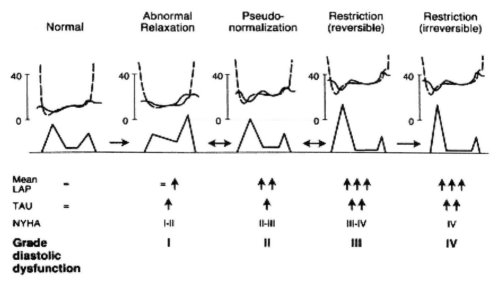

FIG. 15.2. Diagram of a proposed grading system for diastolic dysfunction, based on the progression of disease patterns in patients with cardiac disease. Below the high fidelity left atrial and left ventricular pressure curves is a schematic representation of the mitral flow velocity curve. Below this is the mean left atrial pressure (LAP), time constant of relaxation (TAU), and New York Heart Association (NYHA) class associated with the various mitral flow velocity curves. The natural progression is from the normal pattern to the abnormal relaxation pattern, to the pseudonormalization pattern, to a reversible restriction pattern, and finally to an irreversible restriction pattern. The grade of diastolic dysfunction on a scale of I to IV is shown. (From Nishimura RA, Tajik J. Evaluation of Doppler filling of left ventricle in health and disease: Doppler echocardiography is the clinician's Rosetta stone. *J Am Coll Cardiol* 1997;30:8–18.)

of left ventricular filling pressure and the rate of left ventricular relaxation but is not practical for routine use. Typically, the left ventricular end-diastolic filling pressure is elevated in the presence of normal or reduced left ventricular end-diastolic volume (24,25). Cardiac catheterization is also useful in differentiating from constrictive pericarditis and in confirming left ventricular diastolic dysfunction.

- *Magnetic resonance imaging* is used to exclude pericardial disease.

Differential Diagnosis

The differential diagnosis includes all causes of left ventricular systolic dysfunction (see Chapter 14), including episodic dysfunction (e.g., supraventricular tachycardia, hypertension, ischemia, alcohol), mitral stenosis, pericardial constriction or effusion, right ventricular systolic dysfunction, high-output cardiac failure, and inaccurate measurement of left ventricular systolic function.

Therapy

Currently, there have been no randomized clinical trials of CHF-PSF. Therefore, treatments for which the weight of evidence and expert opinion favor their usefulness and efficacy in this condition are discussed (Table 15.4) (26,27). The results of two ongoing randomized, controlled studies examining the treatment of patients with heart failure who have normal left ventricular ejection fraction are awaited: the Candesartan in Heart Failure—Assessment of Reduction in Mortality and Morbidity (CHARM) trial (28) and Perindopril for Elderly People with Chronic Heart Failure (PEP-CHF) study (29).

Treatment of Underlying Cause

Elevated blood pressure is associated with transient left ventricular dysfunction and pulmonary edema. In pulmonary edema due to hypertension, a normal ejection fraction after treatment suggests that edema was caused by exacerbation of diastolic dysfunction (and not by transient mitral regurgitation or transient systolic dysfunc-

TABLE 15.4. *Treatment of diastolic heart failure*

Treatment	Comments
Treat underlying cause	Hypertension, coronary artery disease, diabetes mellitus
Achieve euvolemia and avoid extremes of volume status	Cautious diuresis and preload-reducing agents when congested (avoid fluid depletion)
	Careful fluid replacement (avoid fluid overload)
Treat atrial fibrillation	Restoration of sinus rhythm to restore "atrial kick" (see page ***)
Facilitate adequate diastolic filling of left ventricles	Slow heart rate: beta blockers
	Avoid chronotropic or inotropic agents such as theophylline, ephedrine, caffeine, or digoxin
Reverse left ventricular hypertrophy and myocardial stiffness	ACE inhibitors, afterload reducing agents, spironolactone (see page ***)

ACE, angiotensin-converting enzyme.
Adapted from Cody RJ. The treatment of diastolic heart failure. *Cardiol Clin* 2000;18:589–596.

tion) (30). When the blood pressure is lowered, there is an improvement in pulmonary congestion (30,31). Management includes not only optimal control of blood pressure but also the recognition of secondary forms of hypertension. Even small increases in fluid status can result in flash pulmonary edema in these patients. This is because small increases in left-ventricular end-diastolic volume are associated with a marked elevation of diastolic pressure, resulting from reduced distensibility of the left ventricle.

Coronary artery disease can cause a "stiff" heart without cardiomegaly, resulting in pulmonary edema. Revascularization either percutaneously or surgically is the most definitive approach to reversing myocardial ischemia in these patients. However, coronary revascularization by itself may not be adequate to prevent flash pulmonary edema, and the control of hypertension is also important (32). Antianginal medications, nitrates, beta blockers, angiotensin-converting enzyme inhibitors, should be used in patients not eligible for revascularization and as adjunctive treatment in those who undergo this procedure. These approaches often reduce the incidence of transient episodes of left ventricular dysfunction and resulting pulmonary edema.

In the elderly, the heart is stiff because of the aging process (15,33–35), and there is no specific therapy to ameliorate this condition. Diuretic therapy is often useful in symptomatic patients (36). Verapamil has been shown to ameliorate age-related impairment in left ventricular diastolic filling (37). However, verapamil can produce considerable constipation in the elderly. Elderly patients with hypertension often have underlying renovascular disease. Angiotensin-converting enzyme inhibitors must be used cautiously because they can exacerbate renovascular disease. More recently, it has been suggested that aldosterone-receptor blockers such as spironolactone may reduce fibrosis associated with aging and retard the progression of diastolic dysfunction in the elderly (38).

Valvular heart disease is associated with complex remodeling of the left ventricle in response to a variable extent of cardiac fibrosis. Treatment of diastolic dysfunction includes repair or replacement of the affected valve. In aortic stenosis, typically there is initially left ventricular hypertrophy that is often associated with diastolic dysfunction. The diastolic dysfunction may persist for a considerable period of time after valve replacement. Improvement of diastolic function depends on the characteristics of the prosthetic valve.

In diabetic heart disease, patients have both coronary microvascular disease and epicardial disease. Diastolic dysfunction has not been extensively documented in this cohort of patients (20). Their symptoms have a more insidious onset because the patients typically have silent ischemia. These patients have insulin resistance and potentially may benefit from drugs that may ameliorate insulin resistance.

Treatment of Atrial Fibrillation

The loss of atrial kick in atrial fibrillation can result in rapid increases in pulmonary venous congestion and pulmonary edema in patients with diastolic dysfunction. Restoration of sinus rhythm often ameliorates symptoms and improves left ventricular hemodynamics in these patients. Return of the atrial transport mechanism may take several months after restoration of sinus rhythm. Patients in whom atrial fibrillation is refractory to cardioversion may benefit from rate control. Many such patients may require atrioventricular nodal ablation and a permanent pacemaker to control ventricular rate.

Achieving Euvolemia and Avoiding Extremes of Volume Status

In CHF-PSF, patients may be euvolemic for prolonged periods of time that may be punctuated by periods of flash pulmonary edema. Diuretics should be used to reduce volume overload and must not be used as the sole therapeutic agent for reducing left ventricular end-diastolic pressure (36). Patients should be advised to avoid excessive dietary sodium intake. Aggressive treatment of pulmonary edema in these patients may result in volume depletion, and diuretics should therefore be used cautiously in these patients. Volume depletion results in tachycardia and decreased diastolic filling, which in turn exacerbates left ventricular filling pressures. Also, volume depletion can result in collapse of the right ventricle and trigger vasodepressor syncope. Replacement of fluid should be done cautiously because these patients develop pulmonary edema with infusion of small amounts of intravenous fluids.

Lifestyle Modification

Dietary sodium intake should be limited to 3 g per day. Cessation of smoking and correction of an abnormal lipid profile is recommended in all patients with coronary artery disease. Because obesity is associated with abnormal left ventricular geometry and function, all obese patients should be encouraged to achieve an optimal body mass index.

Facilitating Adequate Diastolic Filling of Left Ventricle

Impaired relaxation of the left ventricle in these patients means that the time for filling of the ventricle is not optimal. Slowing the heart rate increases the time for ventricular filling; therefore, agents that slow the heart rate, such as beta blockers, should be beneficial in these patients. Although digoxin slows heart rate, it is also a positive inotropic agent, and hence its beneficial effects are negated by its inotropic action. Drugs that induce tachycardia or promote inotropism, such as ephedrine, theophylline, and over-the-counter decongestants should be avoided by these patients.

Reversing Left Ventricular Hypertrophy and Myocardial Stiffness

Reversal of left ventricular hypertrophy is an important goal because it is associated with decreased myocardial stiffness and improved diastolic filling, which in turn improves stroke volume. Substantial increases in afterload delay myocardial relaxation to such an extent that it causes an upward shift of the end-diastolic pressure-volume curve even in normal hearts, and the resulting diastolic dysfunction occurs because there is insufficient time for the ventricle to relax completely (39). Therefore, agents that reduce left ventricular afterload, such as angiotensin-converting enzyme inhibitors, should be beneficial in these patients. Hydralazine, another afterload-reducing agent, is not recommended because it causes reflex tachycardia and impairs diastolic filling.

Prognosis and Follow-up

Earlier reports suggested that patients with diastolic heart failure due to coronary artery disease, hypertension, or aging has a much better prognosis (3) than do those with systolic dysfunction, and it is therefore important to distinguish it from systolic heart failure. Although CHF-PSF carries a lower mortality risk than do cases with systolic dysfunction, there is a fourfold mortality risk in comparison to control subjects who are free of heart failure (4). However, a more recent 3-year follow-up study from the Mayo Clinic suggests that diastolic heart failure carries the same prognosis as systolic heart failure (Table 15.3) (7).

HYPERTROPHIC CARDIOMYOPATHY

Definition

Hypertrophic cardiomyopathy (HCM) is an intrinsic cardiac muscle disorder characterized by left ventricular hypertrophy, vigorous systolic function with or without left ventricular outflow obstruction, and impaired diastolic function. In the past it was referred to as idiopathic hypertropic subaortic stenosis or hypertrophic obstructive cardiomyopathy. Affected patients typically have left ventricular hypertrophy in the absence of hypertension or aortic stenosis; septal thickening; and impaired ventricular relaxation with high end-diastolic pressures (Figs. 15.3, 15.4). These patients are at risk for premature death. There are different anatomic and hemodynamic types of HCM (Table 15.5, Fig. 15.4). Histologic features include extensive myocardial hypertrophy, disarray of myocyte bundles, and interstitial replacement fibrosis (Fig. 15.6).

Etiology

Research estimates suggest that the incidence of this condition is as high as 1 per 500 individuals (40). It affects both men and women of all ages. The condition can be sporadic or familial. Of the familial cases, 70% are due to mutations of the sarcomeric protein genes, including beta-myosin heavy chain, cardiac troponin T, and beta-tropomyosin (Fig 15.7).

Presenting Symptoms and Signs

The manifestations are influenced by age, duration of the disease, genetic origin, and cardiovascular hemodynamics (41). The onset is in late adolescence and early adulthood, typically in the mid-twenties. Onset in early childhood is rare. Patients usually present with exertional dyspnea, angina, palpitations, orthostatic hypotension, syncope, and sometimes sudden death. Sudden death can also occur in well-established disease. The signs and symptoms of heart failure are usually due to progressive diastolic dysfunction and occasionally necessitate orthotopic heart transplantation despite preserved systolic function. About 10% to 20% of patients

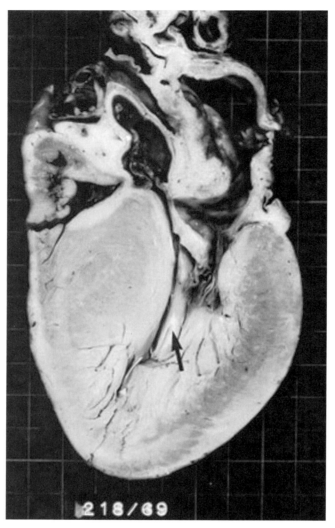

FIG. 15.3. Ventricular septal hypertrophy. Longitudinal section of the heart in a patient with subaortic obstructive hypertrophic cardiomyopathy who died suddenly while receiving propranolol therapy. Hemodynamic investigation had confirmed the presence of subaortic obstruction, as well as mitral regurgitation that was partially due to an abnormal mitral valve [insertion of an anomalous papillary muscle (*arrow*) onto the ventricular surface of the anterior mitral leaflet]. Note the asymmetric hypertrophy with a grossly thickened ventricular septum and a narrowed outflow tract between the upper septum and the anterior mitral leaflet, which is very thickened and fibrosed from repeated mitral leaflet–septal contact. There was microscopic evidence of extensive myocardial fiber disarray involving both the septum and the free wall of the left ventricle. (From Wigle ED, Rakowski H, Kimball BP, et al. Hypertrophic cardiomyopathy: clinical spectrum and treatment. *Circulation* 1995;92:1680–1692.)

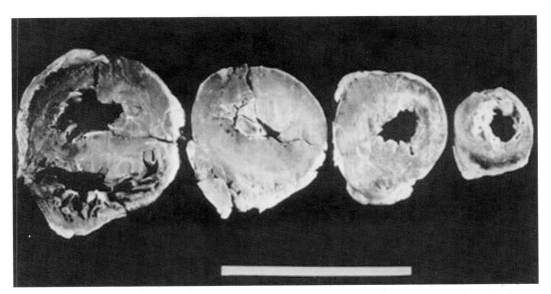

FIG. 15.4. Midventricular hypertrophy. Cross-sectional slices of the heart from a patient who while alive was shown, by hemodynamic, angiographic, and echocardiographic techniques, to have midventricular obstruction. The site of the obstruction was at the level of the papillary muscles, where there was massive hypertrophy (second slice from left). The slice at left is from the base of the heart, and the two slices at the right are from the apex. The apex of the left ventricle was the site of extensive myocardial infarction and aneurysm formation that was evidenced in life by a dyskinetic apical chamber on angiography and by persistent ST segment elevation in leads V_4 to V_6 on the electrocardiogram. The coronary arteries revealed no significant luminal narrowings. The patient died of intractable ventricular arrhythmias. (From Wigle ED, Rakowski H, Kimball BP, et al. Hypertrophic cardiomyopathy: clinical spectrum and treatment. *Circulation* 1995;92:1680–1692.)

have "burnt-out" disease, which is characterized by decreased systolic function and dilated left ventricle. Congestive heart failure is uncommon in sinus rhythm and manifests in these patients when there is severe obstruction, when there is severe systolic or diastolic dysfunction or both, and in the presence of atrial fibrillation. Palpi-

TABLE 15.5. *Types of hypertrophic cardiomyopathy and approximate incidence*

Asymmetric hypertrophy	95%
Ventricular septal hypertrophy	90%
Apical hypertrophy	3%
Midventricular hypertrophy	1%
Rare types	1%
Symmetric (concentric) hypertrophy	5%

From Wigle ED, Rakowski H, Kimball BP, et al. Hypertrophic cardiomyopathy: clinical spectrum and treatment. *Circulation* 1995;92:785–789.

tations are usually due to arrhythmias, of which atrial fibrillation is the commonest. Atrial fibrillation is more commonly associated with mitral regurgitation, increased left atrial size (usually more than 50 mm), and age. Thromboembolism and stroke in these patients have been ascribed to atrial fibrillation. Sudden death cannot be clearly predicted, but risk factors include family history of sudden death, recurrent syncope, and marked hypertrophy of the left ventricular free wall (more than 35 mm).

Clinical examination findings may be normal. The left ventricular apex is hyperdynamic, and the left-sided fourth heart sound may be heard. Auscultation may reveal an S4 gallop, the holosystolic murmur of mitral regurgitation at the apex, and an ejection systolic murmur of dynamic left ventricular ejection along the left

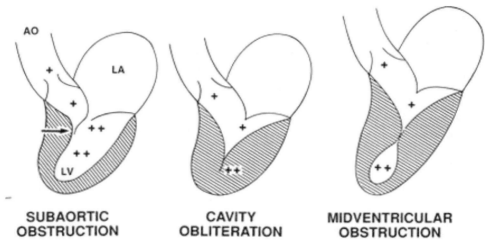

SUBAORTIC OBSTRUCTION   CAVITY OBLITERATION   MIDVENTRICULAR OBSTRUCTION

FIG. 15.5. Diagram showing left ventricular (LV) inflow tract pressure concept. In subaortic obstructive hypertrophic cardiomyopathy (HCM), all LV pressures proximal to the outflow tract obstruction caused by mitral leaflet–septal contact (*arrow*) are elevated, including the inflow tract pressure, just inside the mitral valve. In cavity obliteration and midventricular obstruction, the pressure at the apex of the left ventricle is elevated, but the inflow tract pressure is not. Note that the amount of the LV cavity that is obstructed in subaortic obstructive HCM is greater than in midventricular obstruction (see text). AO, aorta. (Adapted from Wigle ED, Rakowski H, Kimball BP, et al. Hypertrophic cardiomyopathy: clinical spectrum and treatment. *Circulation* 1995;92:1680–1692.)

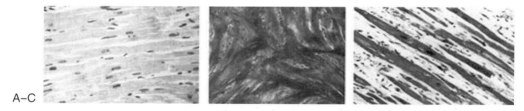

A–C

FIG. 15.6. Histopathology of hypertrophic cardiomyopathy. **A,** The normal architecture of healthy ventricular myocardium shows orderly alignment of myocytes with minimal interstitial fibrosis. **B,** Marked enlargement and disarray of myocytes with increased interstitial fibrosis is evident in hypertrophic cardiomyopathy. [Stains: hematoxylin and eosin (**A**) and Mason trichrome (**B**)]. (From Seidman JG, Seidman C. The genetic basis for cardiomyopathy: from mutation identification to mechanistic paradigms. *Cell* 2001;104:557–567.)

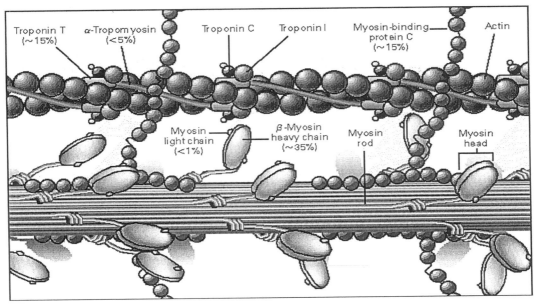

FIG. 15.7. Components of the sarcomere. Cardiac contraction occurs when calcium binds the troponin complex (subunits C, I, and T) and alpha-tropomyosin, making possible the myosin-actin interaction. Actin stimulates adenosine triphosphatase activity in the globular myosin head and results in the production of force along actin filaments. Cardiac myosin-binding protein C, arrayed transversely along the sarcomere, binds myosin and, when phosphorylated, modulates contraction. In hypertrophic cardiomyopathy, mutations may impair these and other protein interactions, which results in effectual contraction of the sarcomere, and produce hypertrophy and disarray of myocytes. Percentages represent the estimated frequency with which a mutation on the corresponding gene causes hypertrophic cardiomyopathy. (From Spirito P, Seidman CE, McKenna WJ, et al. The management of hypertrophic cardiomyopathy. *N Engl J Med* 1997;336:775–785.)

sternal border. The ejection systolic murmur has dynamic characteristics, and the intensity and duration may change with various provocative maneuvers (Table 15.6). Physical signs in obstructive HCM include a bifid arterial pulse, a

TABLE 15.6. *Effects of maneuvers on murmurs of aortic stenosis and hypertrophic cardiomyopathy*

	Valsalva	Squatting	Standing
Preload	↓	↑	↓
Afterload	↓	↑	↓
HCM murmur	↑	↓	↑
AS murmur	↓	↑	↓

AS, aortic stenosis; HCM, hypertrophic cardiomyopathy.

From Grayzel D, Dec GW, Lilly LS. The cardiomyopathies. In: Lilly LS, ed. *Pathophysiology of heart disease,* 2nd ed. Baltimore: Williams & Wilkins, 1997.

double or triple systolic apex beat, and a systolic murmur across the obstruction.

Diagnostic Studies

The diagnosis of HCM is based on patient and family history, physical examination findings, and results of noninvasive tests. The ECG and the echocardiogram are essential for the diagnosis of HCM.

- The *ECG* is usually abnormal in adults. Abnormalities include left ventricular hypertrophy (Fig. 15.8); prominent Q waves in inferior and lateral leads due to thick septum; atrial fibrillation; and ventricular arrhythmias. Ventricular arrhythmias are ominous signs. Atrial enlargement and left axis deviation may

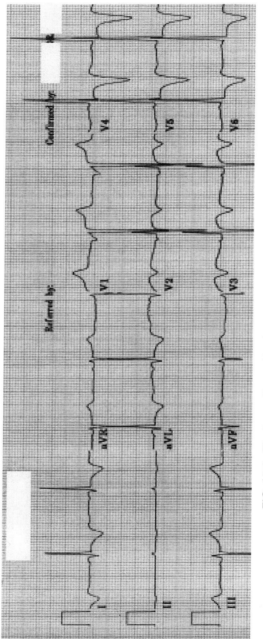

FIG. 15.8. Electrocardiographic changes in hypertrophic cardiomyopathy.

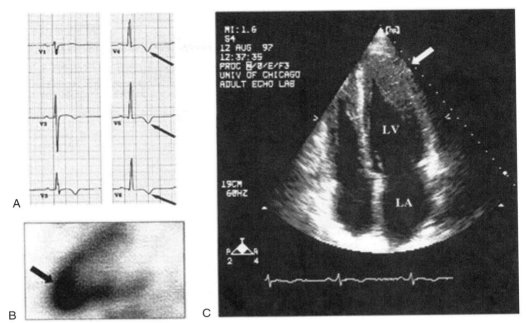

FIG. 15.9. A healthy man was referred for cardiac evaluation because of an abnormal electrocardiogram. The negative T waves (*arrows,* **A**) seen most strikingly along the midlateral precordial leads were present 5 years before this evaluation. Physical examination revealed a displaced apical impulse and a prominent fourth heart sound (S4). Thallium 201 scintigraphic analysis (**B**) demonstrated increased apical count density at rest. Gated tomographic imaging revealed normal overall left ventricular systolic performance, but regional wall motion analysis revealed moderate apical hypokinesis. On two-dimensional echocardiography, an apical four-chamber view of the left ventricle revealed hypertrophy of the apex in an "ace-of-spades" configuration (**C**). The diagnosis was the benign form of hypertrophic cardiomyopathy (HCM) originally described in Japan, apical HCM, and the patient received calcium channel blocker treatment. This apical variant constitutes 25% of cases of HCM in Japan but only 1% to 2% of the cases of HCM in the non-Japanese population. (From Reddy V, Korcarz C, Weinert L, et al. Apical hypertrophic cardiomyopathy. *Circulation* 1998;98:2354.)

precede overt disease in children at risk. Giant negative T waves suggest apical HCM (Fig. 15.9).

- *Echocardiography* (Figs. 15.9 to 15.11) is useful in characterizing the anatomic changes that accompany HCM, particularly left ventricular hypertrophy, asymmetric septal hypertrophy, systolic anterior motion of mitral valve. Ventricular wall thickness of 13 to 15 mm in the absence of hypertension or aortic valvular disease is diagnostic. The Doppler study quantifies outflow gradient and associated mitral regurgitation. This technique is useful in excluding aortic stenosis as an underlying cause for myocardial hypertrophy. Transesophageal studies are useful for determining mitral valve anatomy and, in particular, determining the level of outflow obstruction, which helps the clinician plan, guide, and assess the effects of surgery or percutaneous ablation of the septum.

- *Chest radiographs* may be normal. Abnormalities that may be seen are left ventricular, left atrial, or right atrial enlargement with or without vascular redistribution in the lungs. The aorta is usually small.

- *Stress thallium studies and positron emission tomography* are used to detect underlying myocardial ischemia.

- *Magnetic resonance imaging* is useful for determining left ventricular hypertrophy when two-dimensional echocardiography is unable

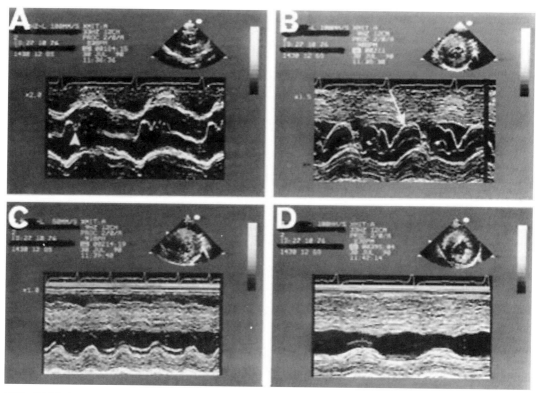

FIG. 15.10. Typical M-mode echocardiogram from a patient with hypertrophic cardiomyopathy, highlighting the four main echocardiographic features of the condition. **A,** Midsystolic closure of the aortic valve (*arrowhead*); **B,** systolic anterior motion of the mitral valve (*arrow*) and asymmetric left ventricular hypertrophy, together with a small, vigorously contracting left ventricle. In frames **C** and **D,** the M-mode beam passes through the septum and posterior wall beyond the mitral valve, at the level of the papillary muscles and apex, demonstrating the large reduction of left ventricular end-systolic dimensions. (From Nihoyannopoulos P, McKenna WJ. Hypertrophic cardiomyopathy. In: Roelandt JRTC, Sutherland GR, Iliceto S, et al., eds. *Cardiac ultrasound.* Edinburgh: Churchill Livingstone, 1993:371–389.)

to obtain satisfactory images. It is particularly useful in apical HCM (Fig. 15.12).

• *Cardiac catheterization and angiography* (Fig. 15.5) is useful for determining coronary anatomy when patients have angina. Measurements of left-sided heart hemodynamics and gradients are required when percutaneous alcohol septal ablation or surgery is being contemplated. Echocardiography has reduced the need for invasive assessment of cardiac hemodynamics.

• The role of invasive *electrophysiologic studies* is controversial, and abnormalities elicited by programmed stimulation have low specificity.

Treatment (41,42)

Nonobstructive Hypertrophic Cardiomyopathy

Pharmacologic Therapy

The pharmacologic management of HCM depends on the anatomic type and the accompanying

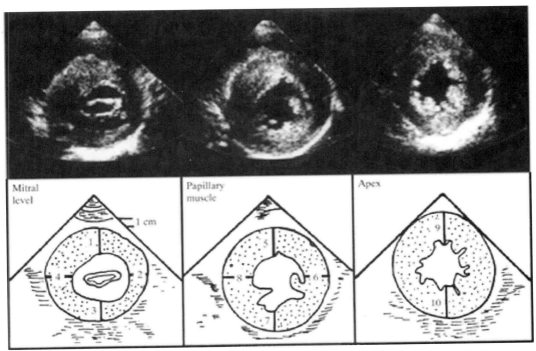

FIG. 15.11. Serial short-axis, cross-sectional views of the left ventricle at three levels: the mitral valve, the papillary muscles, and the apex. (From Prasad K, Atherton J, Smith GC, et al. Echocardiographic pitfalls in the diagnosis of hypertrophic cardiomyopathy. *Heart* 1999;82(Suppl 3):III8–III15.)

hemodynamic changes (Table 15.7). Drugs that are used in the obstructive variety are contraindicated in end-stage HCM accompanied by heart failure; similarly, drugs used for the nonobstructive variety are contraindicated for the obstructive variety.

Normal Systolic Function. In nonobstructive HCM with normal systolic function, calcium channel blockers and beta-adrenergic blockers are preferred when there is impaired diastolic dysfunction, myocardial ischemia, or both. Beta-adrenergic blockers slow the heart rate and thus prolong diastole, which in turn improves diastolic filling. They also reduce myocardial oxygen demand and therefore decrease myocardial ischemia. Verapamil also improves symptoms by improving ventricular filling (43) and myocardial ischemia. It has been preferred when chest pain is

a prominent symptom. Diltiazem has been used occasionally. When patients develop symptoms of heart failure, diuretics may improve symptoms but must be used judiciously because patients with diastolic dysfunction often require relatively high filling pressures to achieve adequate ventricular filling.

Abnormal Systolic Function. In nonobstructive HCM with abnormal systolic function, afterload reduction, diuretics, and digitalis may be used. This is in contrast to obstructive HCM, in which afterload reduction, diuretics, and digitalis are contraindicated because they tend to worsen the obstruction. Also, in nonobstructive HCM, negative inotropic agents and dual-chamber pacing are not indicated. In end-stage nonobstructive HCM, patients should be considered for cardiac transplantation.

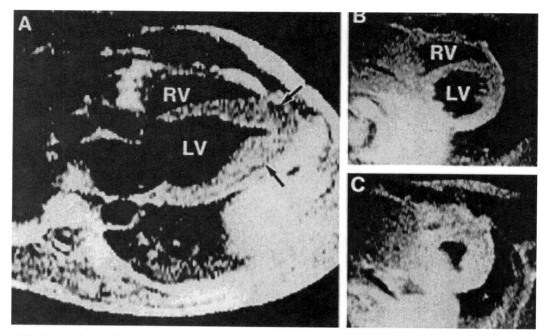

FIG. 15.12. Apical hypertrophy. Magnetic resonance spin-echo images from a patient with apical hypertrophic cardiomyopathy (HCM). **A,** Long-axis four-chamber slice demonstrates localized left ventricular (LV) hypertrophy, involving the apical anterior and inferior walls, and the true apex (*arrows*). Note the characteristic spade-shaped left ventricular cavity at end-diastole, described by Japanese authors and caused by the anterior and inferior wall apical hypertrophy. **B,** Short-axis basal slice showing normal LV wall thickness. **C,** Short-axis apical slice demonstrating circumferential apical hypertrophy. A non–spade-shaped variety of apical HCM has been described, again by Japanese authors, and in these cases, the anterior and inferior apical walls are not involved as they are in **A;** rather, the septal and lateral walls are involved, and this can be picked up only by short-axis magnetic resonance image scanning, as seen in **C.** (From Webb et al. Apical hypertrophic cardiomyopathy: clinical follow-up and diagnostic correlates. *J Am Coll Cardiol* 1990;15:83–90.)

TABLE 15.7. *Treatment obstructive of hypertrophic cardiomyopathy versus nonobstructive hypertrophic cardiomyopathy with impaired systolic function (end-stage hypertrophic cardiomyopathy*

	Obstructive	End-stage
Digoxin	−	+
Diuretics	−	+
Afterload reduction	−	+
Negative inotropes	+	−
Dual chamber pacing	+	−
Surgery	Myomectomy	Transplantation

From Wigle ED, Rakowski H, Kimball BP, et al. Hypertrophic cardiomyopathy: clinical spectrum and treatment. *Circulation* 1995;92:785–789.

Obstructive Hypertrophic Cardiomyopathy

Pharmacologic Therapy

Drugs used to reduce left ventricular outflow obstruction include beta-adrenergic blockers and disopyramide. Drug selection depends on the experience of the clinician. Most clinicians prefer beta blockers as first-line agents, but others have preferred disopyramide, and sometimes both agents have been used. Beta blockers are said to be particularly useful in latent obstruction or mild obstruction but are less effective in severe obstruction. Therefore, other clinicians prefer disopyramide as the drug of choice in treating symptomatic obstructive hypertrophic obstructive cardiomyopathy. Intravenous disopyramide or oral doses up to 600 to 800 mg per day have been shown to reduce or even abolish obstruction. However, the use of the drug is limited by its anticholinergic effects and the fact that its clinical and hemodynamic benefits decrease with time. Disopyramide may shorten the atrioventricular nodal conduction time and may increase ventricular rate during paroxysmal atrial fibrillation; therefore, beta blockers are often initiated simultaneously when the resting heart rate exceeds 70 beats per minute. Calcium channel antagonists, including verapamil, should be avoided when there is a substantial outflow gradient or high pulmonary arterial pressures, because these agents can result in catastrophic hemodynamic consequences.

Dual-Chamber Pacemaker Therapy

Initial nonrandomized, nonblind studies reported that DDD (degenerative disk disease) pacing is effective in reducing subaortic obstruction and improving symptoms, although the mechanism remained unclear. More recent randomized, double-blind studies have not substantiated its benefits, and it has been suggested that it has a placebo effect (44,45). Also, there is no evidence that it reduces mortality or alters the natural history of the disease. Therefore, DDD pacing should be used judiciously in these patients.

Surgical and Nonsurgical Reduction of Septum

Although symptoms are not necessarily due to septal thickening, alcohol ablation of the septum or surgical excision of the septum has been reported to improve symptoms in selected patients.

Surgery. Surgical incision into or excision of a portion of the asymmetrically hypertrophied subaortic portion of the ventricular septum or the Morrow procedure may improve symptoms and provide hemodynamic benefits in many patients (46). These benefits have been proposed to

result from widening of the left ventricular outflow tract and from causing a left intraventricular conduction defect. However, this myotomy/myectomy entails significant morbidity, with the risk of death close to 5%. The mechanism by which the surgery relieves symptoms and improves cardiac function remains unclear. It is recommended that this procedure be reserved for patients with gradients higher than 50 mm HG. It should not be performed in asymptomatic patients or mildly symptomatic patients because its effect on morbidity is not known. Sometimes myotomy/myomectomy may be combined with mitral valve replacement when there is severe mitral regurgitation (47).

Catheter-Based Reduction. Injection of alcohol, via a coronary catheter, into the first major septal coronary artery has been proposed as a means of reducing septal thickness and, consequently, the left ventricular outflow gradient (48). Since its first report, it has been estimated that this technique has been performed in about 800 cases worldwide. Experience with procedure is limited in that long-term follow-up data are not available (49,50). In the short term, it seems to be efficacious. Long-term concerns include (a) increased incidence of bradyarrhythmias, including heart block, caused by disruption of the cardiac conduction system; (b) tachyarrhythmias, including potentially fatal ventricular tachyarrhythmias, because the septal infarction may provide a substrate; and (c) impaired ventricular function caused by thinning of the walls. Finally, because this procedure is easily performed, it has been suggested that it may be performed injudiciously. It has been proposed that this procedure be used with caution and that a registry be established to determine the long-term outcomes of this promising procedure (51,52).

Atrial Fibrillation

The management of atrial fibrillation in these patients is similar to that of other cardiac conditions and includes pharmacologic and electrical cardioversion, atrioventricular nodal ablation with permanent pacemaker in refractory cases, and anticoagulation. Although amiodarone is more effective in restoring sinus rhythm, the relatively young age of these patients makes it desirable to initiate therapy with sotalol. Because the risk of thromboembolism is high in these patients, all patients with atrial fibrillation should be considered for anticoagulation.

Ventricular Tachycardia and Fibrillation

Ventricular tachycardia and fibrillation are restored to sinus rhythm with pharmacologic or electrical cardioversion. Primary prevention with an implantable defibrillator must be considered in patients at high risk for sudden death. The data supporting the use of implantable defibrillators in these patients are based on a large retrospective, multicenter study (53) that found that these devices are highly effective in terminating these arrhythmias and, therefore, have a role in the primary and secondary prevention of sudden death. Cardiac transplantation is an option for patients with refractory ventricular tachyarrhythmias.

Differential Diagnosis

The differential diagnosis includes athlete's heart and aortic stenosis. (Fig. 15.13).

Prognosis

Sudden death occurs in 2% to 4% of adults with HCM per year, and in 4% to 6% of children and adolescents with HCM. Strong indicators of sudden death include a previously aborted cardiac arrest, one or more episodes of sustained ventricular tachycardia, a history of sudden death in two or more young family members, and the magnitude of left ventricular hypertrophy (42). Mutations of troponin T are associated with minor myocardial hypertrophy but also with a high risk of sudden death. Nonsustained ventricular tachycardia on ambulatory monitoring or abnormal blood pressure response to exercise has a low positive predictive value.

Poor prognostic factors include early age at diagnosis, the familial form with known sudden death in first-degree relatives, a history of syn-

cope, the presence of myocardial ischemia, and the presence of ventricular arrhythmias.

Genetic Counseling and Testing

Genetic studies are currently not done, but may be used increasingly in the future to make or confirm the diagnosis. In adults, the diagnosis of HCM is usually established reliably by physical examination and echocardiography. When the clinical diagnosis is certain, determining the precise genetic defect by deoxyribonucleic acid analysis means only a diagnostic confirmation. However, genetic studies do enhance diagnostic reliability in this condition. Molecular studies can play a major role in resolving ambiguous diagnoses, particularly in individuals with a borderline or modest increase in left ventricular wall thickness (e.g., in athletes with left ventricular hypertrophy and in hypertensive patients in whom HCM is suspected) (54).

The availability of genotyping has led to the identification of increasing numbers of children and adults with a preclinical diagnosis of HCM. These subjects have the characteristic genetic mutation but no clinical or phenotypic features of HCM such as left ventricular wall thickening on echocardiogram or cardiac symptoms. On the basis of the current literature, it is likely that most such genotype-positive, phenotype-negative children will develop left ventricular hypertrophy while achieving full body growth and maturation (54).

The absence of left ventricular hypertrophy in genetically affected adults is relatively uncommon and is largely confined to those with nonmyosin mutations, such as those described for cardiac troponin T and, in particular, myosin-binding protein C. The frequency or timing with which these individuals may subsequently develop the HCM phenotype is not known. Currently, the American Heart Association committee on genetic testing concluded that there are no data to justify prohibiting such genotype-positive, phenotype-negative individuals from engaging in most life activities; however, this committee believed that a family history of frequent HCM-related death or

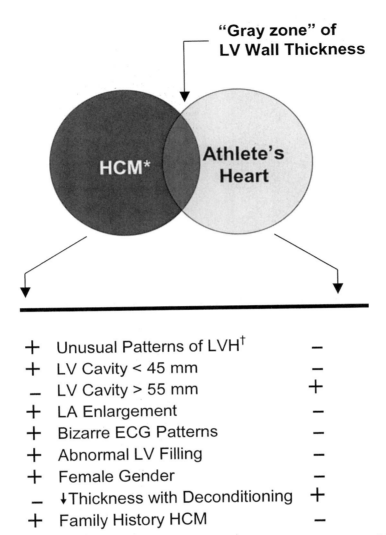

"Gray zone" of LV Wall Thickness

HCM*   Athlete's Heart

+	Unusual Patterns of LVH[†]	—
+	LV Cavity < 45 mm	—
—	LV Cavity > 55 mm	+
+	LA Enlargement	—
+	Bizarre ECG Patterns	—
+	Abnormal LV Filling	—
+	Female Gender	—
—	↓Thickness with Deconditioning	+
+	Family History HCM	—

FIG. 15.13. Chart showing criteria used to distinguish hypertrophic cardiomyopathy (HCM) from athlete's heart when the left ventricular (LV) wall thickness is within the shaded gray zone of overlap, consistent with both diagnoses. *Asterisk* indicates that the condition is assumed to be the nonobstructive form of HCM in this discussion, because the presence of substantial mitral valve systolic anterior motion would confirm, per se, the diagnosis of HCM in an athlete. It may involve a variety of abnormalities, including heterogeneous distribution of left ventricular hypertrophy (LVH), in which asymmetry is prominent, and adjacent regions may be of greatly different thickness, with sharp transitions evident between segments. Also, patterns in which the anterior ventricular septum is spared from the hypertrophic process and the region of predominant thickening may be in the posterior portion of septum or anterolateral or posterior free wall. XX indicates decreased; LA, left atrial. (From Maron BJ, Pelliccia A, Spirito P. Cardiac disease in young trained athletes: insights into methods for distinguishing athlete's heart from structural heart disease, with particular emphasis on hypertrophic cardiomyopathy. *Circulation* 1995;91:1596–1601.)

the documentation of a particularly malignant genotype may justify efforts at risk stratification, including restriction from competitive sports (54).

Hypertrophic Cardiomyopathy of the Elderly

HCM of the elderly (15) may occur with or without a history of hypertension. Clinical and anatomic features resemble that of HCM. Treatment includes control of hypertension and co-morbid factors.

RESTRICTIVE CARDIOMYOPATHY

Definition

Restrictive cardiomyopathy is characterized by abnormally rigid (but not necessarily thickened) ventricles with impaired diastolic filling and without evidence of pericardial disease or systolic dysfunction. The diastolic volume may be normal or decreased. Important causes of restrictive cardiomyopathy are listed in Table 15.2.

Presenting Symptoms and Signs

Typically, affected patients present with symptoms of congestive heart failure, including signs of left- and right-sided failure, low cardiac output (fatigue, decreased exercise tolerance), and systemic congestion that is more prominent than pulmonary congestion (jugular venous distension, peripheral edema, tender liver, ascites). Clinical examination reveals jugular venous distension and prominent x and y descents. A third heart sound is usually heard, and a fourth heart sound may be present. Crackles are heard at both lung bases.

Idiopathic Restrictive Cardiomyopathy

This condition is characterized by marked bi-atrial dilatation without ventricular hypertrophy or enlargement, as determined by echocar-diography. This condition predominantly affects elderly patients, but it occurs in all age groups. It is sometimes familial. Typically, affected patients present with symptoms of systemic and pulmonary venous congestion and atrial fibrillation. The prognosis is poor, and poor prognostic factors include age older than 70 years, male gender, high New York Heart Association class, and a left atrial dimension exceeding 60 mm (55).

Amyloidosis

The histopathologic processes of the different types of amyloid are the same, including Congo red staining of the amyloid fibrils and yellow-green birefringence when the Congo red stain is examined under the polarized microscope. However, there are many types of amyloidosis, and the natural history of cardiac amyloid therefore varies, depending on the type. The classification of amyloidosis is based on the chemical nature of the amyloid fibrils. The three most common types in the United States are immunoglobulin light chain–related (AL), familial transthyretin-associated (ATTR), and AA (secondary) amyloidosis. In AL amyloidosis, the organs commonly involved are kidney and the heart, either together or separately. When the heart is involved, recognized features include rapid onset of heart failure, signs of predominantly right-sided heart failure, low-voltage complexes on heart failure (Fig 15.14), a concentrically thickened left (and often right) ventricle with a normal-to-small cavity shown on echocardiography and mildly reduced or low normal ejection fraction. Doppler echocardiography in these patients shows high-left sided filling pressures as manifested by a small mitral A wave (restrictive pattern). Other features include hepatic infiltration, macroglossia, pulmonary amyloidosis, infiltration of adrenal glands, spontaneous bruising, and autonomic neuropathy. The postural hypotension due to autonomic neuropathy limits the use of angiotensin-converting inhibitors in these patients. In ATTR amyloidosis, the clinical features differ in that autonomic neuropathy and

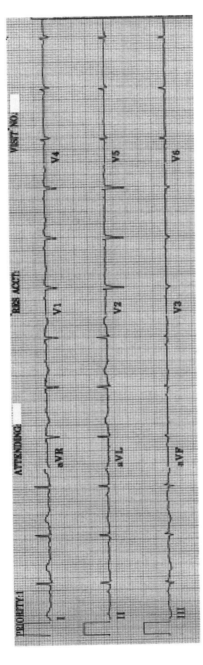

FIG. 15.14. Low-voltage complexes in cardiac amyloidosis.

peripheral neuropathy are more prominent but renal disease is less common and macroglossia does not occur. The extent of myocardial disease depends on the specific transthyretin mutation causing the disease. The ECG is usually normal, but conduction disturbances may occur. The diagnosis is therefore often missed and must be suspected in patients with family history of neurologic disease. In AA (secondary) amyloidosis, cardiac involvement is rare and, when present, rarely causes heart failure. Macroglossia is not a feature, and patients have renal disease, hepatomegaly, splenomegaly, or a combination of the three. The diagnosis is confirmed by tissue biopsy of the organ involved. When the clinical suspicion is high, a positive biopsy of a sample of subcutaneous abdominal fat is sufficient to confirm the diagnosis. The median length of survival in AA amyloidosis is 1 to 2 years, but when there is symptomatic cardiac involvement, the median length of survival is about 6 months. Patients with ATTR amyloidosis may survive up to 15 years, and the prognosis depends on the specific mutation at the time of the disease. In AA amyloidosis, the prognosis depends on the underlying chronic disease. The choice of therapy depends on the underlying cause and the extent of multiorgan involvement. Diuretics are useful for improving symptoms in heart failure initially, but patients may become resistant to this therapy, particularly when there is renal involvement. Beta blockers, calcium channel blockers, and digoxin are contraindicated. A pacemaker may be effective for symptomatic bradycardia, particularly in ATTR amyloidosis. Dose-intensive melphalan with autologous blood–stem cell support is currently undergoing evaluation for AL amyloidosis. There are anecdotal reports of cardiac transplantation in patients with AL amyloidosis, but enthusiasm for this therapy is dampened by the fact that this condition is associated with multiorgan involvement. The definitive treatment for ATTR amyloidosis is liver transplantation. Although this is effective before there is cardiac involvement, this therapy has been shown to worsen cardiac amyloidosis when the heart is involved at the time of liver transplantation. Combined heart and liver transplantation from a single donor has been performed in patients with ATTR amyloidosis when both the heart and liver are involved.

Sarcoidosis

Sarcoidosis causes infiltrative cardiomyopathy and manifests with heart failure. The left ventricular dysfunction may be due to diastolic dysfunction, systolic dysfunction, or infiltration of papillary muscle and may result in mitral regurgitation. The pericardium can also be involved. The ECG shows abnormalities in rhythm, conduction, and repolarization in about half the patients. Echocardiography may show diastolic dysfunction, impaired systolic function, ventricular aneurysms, valvular abnormalities, and pericardial effusion. Myocardial scintigraphy with thallium 201 is often useful in confirming the diagnosis but is not specific. Gallium 67 myocardial scintigraphy is useful for predicting response to steroid therapy. Corticosteroids remain the mainstay of therapy despite the lack of randomized controlled trials. Cyclosporine, however, has proved to be disappointing in the treatment of sarcoidosis. Sarcoidosis has developed in recipients of cardiac transplantation despite long-term cyclosporine therapy. Implantable cardiac defibrillators are useful in the management of potentially lethal ventricular tachyarrhythmias. Cardiac transplantation has been shown to improve prognosis and quality of life in patients who do not have systemic disease and who do not respond to conventional therapy with heart failure medications, corticosteroids, implantable defibrillators, and antiarrhythmic drugs.

Radiation-Induced Cardiac Fibrosis

Radiation delivered to the heart for treatment of malignant lymphoma, breast cancer, or bronchogenic carcinoma can affect the pericardium, the coronary arteries, or the myocardium. When the myocardium is involved, the right ventricle is usually affected, and clinical features are that of restrictive cardiomyopathy. Management is based on symptoms.

Diagnostic Studies

- These studies are used to differentiate radiation-induced cardiac fibrosis from constrictive pericarditis.
- Endomyocardial biopsy is used to different this condition from amyloidosis and hemochromatosis.

- Computed tomography or magnetic resonance imaging reveals thickened pericardium of constrictive pericarditis.

Prognosis

The prognosis is generally poor and depends on the underlying cause.

PRACTICAL POINTS

- Diastolic heart failure is present when an elevated filling pressure is necessary to achieve normal ventricular filling.
- Clinical diagnosis of diastolic heart failure is logistically difficult to establish, and hence the entity is known as congestive heart failure with preserved systolic function.
- It is important to exclude mitral stenosis and constrictive pericarditis before the diagnosis of diastolic dysfunction is established.
- Diastolic heart failure includes a variety of entities.
- Epidemiologic studies suggest that 40% to 50% of patients with clinical heart failure have normal systolic function.
- The majority of the patients with systolic heart failure also have diastolic dysfunction of varying extent.
- It may be impossible to establish whether flash pulmonary edema is caused by transient systolic or diastolic dysfunction.
- There are no randomized clinical trials of patients with diastolic heart failure, and, therefore, the treatment is empirical.

REFERENCES

1. Grossman W. Diastolic dysfunction in congestive heart failure. *N Engl J Med* 1991;325:1557–1564.
2. Grossman W. Defining diastolic dysfunction. *Circulation* 2000;101:2020–2021.
3. Vasan RS, Benjamin EJ, Levy D. Prevalence, clinical features and prognosis of diastolic heart failure: an epidemiologic perspective. *J Am Coll Cardiol* 1995;26:1565–1574.
4. Vasan RS, Larson MG, Benjamin EJ, et al. Congestive heart failure in subjects with normal versus reduced left ventricular ejection fraction: prevalence and mortality in population-based cohort. *J Am Coll Cardiol* 1999;33:1948–1955.
5. Mosterd A, Hoes AW, de Bruyne MC, et al. Prevalence of heart failure and left ventricular dysfunction in the general population: the Rotterdam study. *Eur Heart J* 1999;20:447–455.
6. Kupari M, Lindroos M, Ivivanainen AM, et al. Congestive heart failure in old age: prevalence, mechanisms and 4-year prognosis in the Helsinki Ageing study. *J Intern Med* 1997;241:387–394.
7. Senni M, Tribouilloy CM, Rodeheffer RJ, et al. Congestive heart failure in the community: a study of all incident cases in Olmsted county, Minnesota, in 1991. *Circulation* 1998;98:2282–2289.
8. McDermott MM, Feinglass J, Lee PI, et al. Systolic function, readmission rates, and survival among consecutively hospitalized patients with congestive heart failure. *Am Heart J* 1997;134:728–736.
9. Dauterman KW, Massie BM, Gheorghiade M. Heart failure associated with preserved systolic function: a common and costly clinical entity. *Am Heart J* 1998; 135:S310–S319.
10. Tresch DD, McGough MF. Heart failure with normal systolic function: a common disorder in older people. *J Am Geriatr Soc* 1995;43:1035–1042.
11. Benjamin EJ, Levy D, Anderson KM, et al. Determinants of Doppler indexes of left ventricular diastolic function in normal subjects (the Framingham Heart Study). *Am J Cardiol* 1992;70:508–515.
12. Sagie A, Benjamin EJ, Galderisi M, et al. Reference values for Doppler indexes of left ventricular diastolic filling in the elderly. *J Am Soc Echocardiogr* 1993;6:570–576.
13. Gottdiener JS, Arnold AM, Aurigemma GP, et al. Predictors of congestive heart failure in the elderly: the

Cardiovascular Health Study. *J Am Coll Cardiol* 2000; 35:1628–1637.

14. Davie AP, Francis CM, Caruna L, et al. The prevalence of left ventricular diastolic filling abnormalities in patients with suspected heart failure. *Eur Heart J* 1997;18:981–984.

15. Topol EJ, Traill TA, Fortuin NJ. Hypertensive hypertrophic cardiomyopathy of the elderly. *N Engl J Med* 1985;312:277–283.

16. Weinberg EO, Thienelt CD, Katz SE, et al. Gender differences in molecular remodeling in pressure overload hypertrophy. *J Am Coll Cardiol* 1999;34:264–273.

17. Dodek A, Kassebaum DG, Bristow JD. Pulmonary edema in coronary-artery disease without cardiomegaly: paradox of the stiff heart. *N Engl J Med* 1972;286:1347–1350.

18. Brutsaert DL, Sys SU, Gillebert TC. Diastolic failure: pathophysiology and therapeutic implications. *J Am Coll Cardiol* 1993;22:318–325.

19. Mendes LA, Davidoff R, Cupples LA, et al. Congestive heart failure in patients with coronary artery disease: the genetic paradox. *Am Heart J* 1997;134:207–212.

20. Poirer P, Bogaty P, Garneau C, et al. Diastolic dysfunction in normotensive men with well-controlled type 2 diabetes. *Diabetes Care* 2001;24(1):5–10.

21. Badgett RG, Lucey CR, Mulrow C. Can the clinical examination diagnose left-sided heart failure in adults? *JAMA* 1997;277:1712–1719.

22. Gaasch WH. Diagnosis and treatment of heart failure based on left ventricular systolic or diastolic dysfunction. *JAMA* 1994;271:1276–1280.

23. Nishimura RA, Tajik J. Evaluation of Doppler filling of left ventricle in health and disease: Doppler echocardiography is the clinician's Rosetta stone. *J Am Coll Cardiol* 1997;30:8–18.

24. Mirsky I. Assessment of diastolic function: suggested methods and future considerations. *Circulation* 1984;69:836–841.

25. Shah PM, Pai RG. Diastolic heart failure. *Curr Prob Cardiol* 1992;17:783–788.

26. Cody RJ. The treatment of diastolic heart failure. *Cardiol Clin* 2000;18:589–596.

27. Bonow RO, Udelson JE. Left ventricular diastolic dysfunction as a cause of congestive heart failure: mechanisms and management. *Ann Intern Med* 1992;117:502–510.

28. Swedberg K, Pfeffer M, Granger C, et al. Candesartan in Heart Failure—Assessment of Reduction in Mortality and Morbidity (CHARM): rationale and design. *J Card Fail* 1999;5:276–282.

29. Cleland JG, Tendera M, Adamus J, et al. Perindopril for elderly people with chronic heart failure: the PEP-CHF study. *Eur J Heart Fail* 1999;1:211–217.

30. Gandhi SK, Powers JC, Abdel-Mohsen N, et al. The pathogenesis of acute pulmonary edema associated with hypertension. *N Engl J Med* 2001;344:17–22.

31. Iriarte M, Murga N, Sagastagoitia D, et al. Congestive heart failure from left ventricular diastolic dysfunction in systemic hypertension. *Am J Cardiol* 1993;71:308–312.

32. Kramer K, Kirkman P, Kitzman D, et al. Flash pulmonary edema: association with hypertension and reoccurrence despite coronary revascularization. *Am Heart J* 2000;140:451–455.

33. Spirito P, Maron BJ. Influence of ageing on Doppler echocardiographic indices of left ventricular diastolic function. *Br Heart J* 1988;59:672–679.

34. Cody RJ, Torre S, Clark M, et al. Age-related hemodynamic, renal, and hormonal differences in patients with congestive heart failure. *Arch Intern Med* 1989;149:1023–1028.

35. Schulman SP, Lakatta EG, Fleg JL, et al. Age related decline in left ventricular filling at rest and exercise. *Am J Physiol* 1992;263:H1932–H1938.

36. Cody RJ, Kubo SH, Pickworth KK. Diuretic utilization for the sodium retention of congestive heart failure. *Arch Intern Med* 1994;154:1905–1914.

37. Arrighi JA, Dilsizian V, Perronefilardi P, et al. Improvement of the age-related impairment in left-ventricular diastolic filling with verapamil in the normal human heart. *Circulation* 1994;90:213–219.

38. Weber KT, Sun Y, Campbell SE. Structural remodeling of the heart by fibrous tissue: role of circulating hormones and locally produced peptides. *Eur Heart J* 1995;16(Suppl N):12–18.

39. Leite-Moreiera AF, Correieia-Pinto J. Load as an acute determinant of end-diastolic pressure-volume relation. *Am J Physiol* 2001;280:H51–H59.

40. Maron BJ, Gardin JM, Flack JM, et al. Prevalence of hypertrophic cardiomyopathy in a general population of young adults: echocardiographic analysis of 4111 subjects in the CARDIA study: Coronary Artery Risk Development in (Young) Adults. *Circulation* 1995;92:785–789.

41. Wigle ED, Rakowski H, Kimball BP, et al. Hypertrophic cardiomyopathy: clinical spectrum and treatment. *Circulation* 1995;92:1680–1692.

42. Spirito P, Seidman CE, McKenna WJ, et al. The management of hypertrophic cardiomyopathy. *N Engl J Med* 1997;336:775–785.

43. Bonow RO. Left ventricular diastolic function in hypertrophic cardiomyopathy. *Herz* 1991;16:13–21.

44. Nishimura RA, Trusty JM, Hayes DL, et al. Dual-chamber pacing for hypertrophic cardiomyopathy: a randomized double-blind crossover trial. *J Am Coll Cardiol* 1997;29:435–41.

45. Maron BJ, Nishimura RA, McKenna WJ, et al. Assessment of permanent dual-chamber pacing as a treatment for drug-refractory symptomatic patients with obstructive cardiomyopathy: a double-blind crossover study (M-PATHY). *Circulation* 1999;99:2927–2933.

46. Morrow AG, Lambrew CT, Braunwald E. Idiopathic hypertrophic subaortic stenosis, II: operative and the results of pre- and post-operative hemodynamic evaluations. *Circulation* 1964;30(Suppl IV):120–151.

47. Krajcer Z, Leachman Rd, Cooley DA, et al. Septal myotomy-myomectomy versus mitral valve replacement in hypertrophic cardiomyopathy: ten-year follow-up in 185 patients. *Circulation* 1989;80:157–164.

48. Sigwart U. Non-surgical myocardial reduction for hypertrophic obstructive cardiomyopathy. *Lancet* 1995;346:211–214.

49. Knight C, Kurbaan AS, Seggewiss H, et al. Non-surgical septal reduction for hypertrophic cardiomyopathy: outcome in the first series of the patients. *Circulation* 1997;35:2075–2081.

50. Mazur W, Nagueh SF, Lakkis NM, et al. Regression of left ventricular hypertrophy after non-surgical septal

reduction therapy after hypertrophic obstructive cardiomyopathy. *Circulation* 2001;103:1492–1496.

51. Braunwald E. Induced septal infarction: a new therapeutic strategy for hypertrophic obstructive cardiomyopathy. *Circulation* 1997;95:1981–1982.

52. Spencer III WH, Roberts R. Alcohol septal ablation in hypertrophic obstructive cardiomyopathy: the need for a registry. *Circulation* 2000;102:600–601.

53. Maron BJ, Shen W-K, Link MS, et al. Efficacy of implantable cardioverter-defibrillators for the prevention of sudden death in patients with hypertrophic cardiomyopathy. *N Engl J Med* 2000;342:365–373.

54. Maron BJ, Moller JH, Seidman CE, et al. Impact of laboratory molecular diagnosis on contemporary diagnostic criteria for genetically transmitted cardiovascular diseases: hypertrophic cardiomyopathy, long-QT syndrome, and Marfan syndrome: a statement for healthcare professionals from the Councils on Clinical Cardiology, Cardiovascular Disease in the Young, and Basic Science, American Heart Association. *Circulation* 1998;98:1460–1471.

55. Ammnash NM, Seward JB, Bailey KR, et al. Clinical profile and outcome of idiopathic restrictive cardiomyopathy *Circulation* 2000;101:2490–2496.

16

Paroxysmal Supraventricular Tachycardia

Hakan Oral and Fred Morady

Supraventricular tachycardias arise in or involve at least some part of the atrium or atrioventricular junction. Supraventricular tachycardias develop as a result of abnormal automaticity, triggered activity or, most commonly, reentry. Both atrial flutter and atrial fibrillation are supraventricular tachycardias; however, because of the differences in their mechanisms and clinical manifestations, they are grouped separately from other types of supraventricular tachycardias, commonly referred to as paroxysmal supraventricular tachycardia (PSVT).

USUAL CAUSES AND MECHANISMS OF SUPRAVENTRICULAR TACHYCARDIA

The most common forms of PSVT are atrioventricular nodal reentrant tachycardia (AVNRT), atrioventricular reciprocating tachycardia (AVRT), and atrial tachycardia. Together these constitute more than 95% of all PSVT. Uncommon mechanisms of PSVT include sinus node reentry, junctional ectopic tachycardia, intra-Hisian reentry, and nodoventricular or nodofascicular reentrant tachycardias (Table 16.1). In addition, the symptoms of PSVT sometimes are mimicked by sinus tachycardia.

Atrioventricular Nodal Reentrant Tachycardia

AVNRT is the most common type of PSVT encountered in clinical practice, accounting for approximately two thirds of all cases. AVNRT is more commonly seen in women, with a female-to-male gender ratio of 2:1. It may occur at any age but most commonly manifests during the fourth and fifth decades of life.

AVNRT is caused by reentry. In patients with AVNRT, the atrioventricular junction has two or more functionally discrete pathways. One of these functional pathways, the "fast pathway," conducts impulses rapidly but has a relatively long effective refractory period. The other pathway, "slow pathway," has a slower conduction velocity but a shorter effective refractory period than the fast pathway (1,2). In typical AVNRT, an atrial premature depolarization (APD) conducts to the atrioventricular junction through the atrium. Because it is premature, it may encounter a refractory fast pathway and conduct through only the slow pathway. Because the slow pathway has a longer conduction time, by the time the depolarization travels through the slow pathway and arrives at the compact atrioventricular junction, the fast pathway may have recovered excitability, so that the depolarization travels in a retrograde manner through the fast pathway and back down the slow pathway. If this reentry process continues, a sustained tachycardia occurs (Fig. 16.1) (3–5). Because the fast pathway has a rapid conduction velocity, the ventriculoatrial conduction time during typical AVNRT is very short. Therefore, on the surface electrocardiogram (ECG), retrograde P waves may be buried within the QRS complexes and not be visible or may be partially visible at the end of the QRS complex (Fig. 16.1). P waves are typically inverted in the inferior leads (II, III, and aV_F) and may be manifest as pseudo-S waves, and upright in V_1, leading to a pseudo-r' appearance.

In the atypical form of AVNRT, the fast pathway is utilized as the anterograde limb and the slow pathway as the retrograde limb of the reentrant circuit. Therefore, the ventriculoatrial conduction time is prolonged. The ECG reveals inverted P waves in the inferior leads and a long

TABLE 16.1. *Paroxysmal supraventricular tachycardias*

Mechanism	Prevalence
Atrioventricular nodal reentrant tachycardia	60%
Orthodromic reciprocating tachycardia due to an accessory pathway	30%
Antidromic reciprocating tachycardia due to an accessory pathway	<5%
Atrial tachycardia	10%
Sinus node reentry	<1%
Junctional tachycardia	<1%

RP interval (RP interval exceeds PR interval). Atypical AVNRT accounts for fewer than 10% of cases of AVNRT.

Atrioventricular Reentrant Tachycardia (AVRT)

In normal individuals, the only electrical connections between the atria and the ventricles are the atrioventricular node and the His-Purkinje system. In patients who have an accessory pathway, there is an extra muscular tissue between the atrium and the ventricle. Accessory pathways may conduct electrical impulses in an anterograde or retrograde manner or in both directions. Accessory pathways that conduct only in the retrograde direction are called *concealed* accessory pathways, because no delta waves are present on the ECG. Anterograde conduction over an accessory pathway leads to ventricular preexcitation, with the typical ECG manifestations of a short PR interval and delta waves (Wolf-Parkinson-White pattern). Depending on the relative timing of the activation of the ventricles through the atrioventricular junction, the His bundle, and the accessory pathway, there may be different degrees of ventricular preexcitation, and the delta waves may be subtle or pronounced.

The mechanism of PSVT due to an accessory pathway is reentry. An APD may block in the accessory pathway in an anterograde manner and then activate the ventricle through the atrioventricular node and the His bundle. By the time the impulse reaches the ventricular insertion site of the accessory pathway, the pathway may have regained excitability and may conduct in a retrograde manner, initiating the tachycardia. This type of reentry, in which the atrioventricular node and the His bundle are used as the anterograde limb and the accessory pathway as the

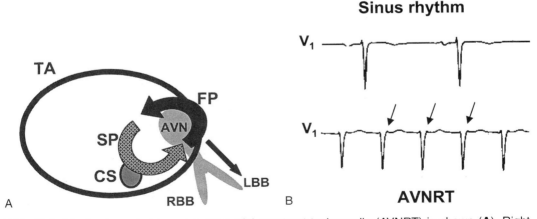

FIG. 16.1. Mechanism of atrioventricular nodal reentrant tachycardia (AVNRT) is shown (**A**). Right atrium and right ventricle are illustrated in the left anterior oblique view. During AVNRT, electrical depolarization conducts in an antegrade manner through the slow pathway (SP, *hatched arrow*) to the compact atrioventricular node (AVN) and in a retrograde manner through the fast pathway (FP, *solid arrow*). **B,** Pseudo-r′ waves caused by retrograde P waves during AVNRT (*arrows*). AVN, atrioventricular node; CS, coronary sinus; FP, fast pathway; LBB: left bundle branch; RBB, right bundle branch; SP, slow pathway; TA: tricuspid annulus.

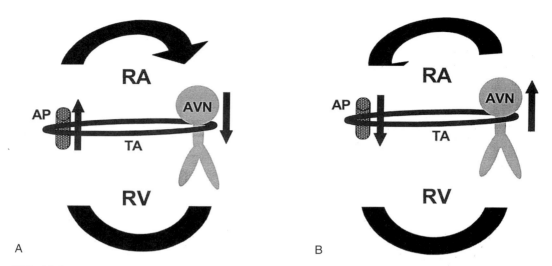

FIG. 16.2. A, Orthodromic reciprocating tachycardia. Electrical impulse propagates in an antegrade manner through the atrioventricular node, His bundle, and bundle branches and conducts in a retrograde manner to the atrium through the accessory pathway. **B,** Antidromic reciprocating tachycardia. Electrical impulse propagates in an antegrade manner through the accessory pathway to the ventricle and conducts in a retrograde manner to the atrium through the His bundle and the atrioventricular node. AP, accessory pathway; AVN, atrioventricular node; LBB, left bundle branch; RA, right atrium; RBB, right bundle branch; RV, right ventricle; TA, tricuspid annulus.

retrograde limb, is called *orthodromic reciprocating tachycardia* (ORT) (Figs. 16.2A, 16.3). Approximately 30% of PSVT arise from orthodromic reciprocating tachycardia (Table 16.1). The type of reentry circuit, in which the accessory pathway is utilized as the anterograde limb and the atrioventricular node–His Purkinje system is utilized as the retrograde limb, is referred to as *antidromic reciprocating tachycardia* (ART) (Figs. 16.2B, 16.4).

The anatomic location of the accessory pathway may be anteroseptal, midseptal, posteroseptal, right free wall, or left free wall. Free-wall sites are subgrouped as anterior, anterolateral, lateral, posterolateral, or posterior in relation to the mitral or tricuspid annulus. Left free-wall pathways account for 60% of all pathways, followed by posteroseptal (30%) and right free-wall pathways (10%). The anteroseptal and midseptal pathways are rare. Multiple accessory pathways exist in 5% of patients with the Wolff-Parkinson-White syndrome. Multiple accessory pathways are more prevalent among patients with congenital heart disease, particularly Ebstein's anomaly.

The most common type of supraventricular tachycardia in patients with an accessory pathway is ORT. ART accounts for fewer than 10% of accessory pathway–mediated PSVTs.

An unusual PSVT is the permanent form of junctional reciprocating tachycardia, an ORT in which a slowly conducting, concealed posteroseptal pathway is used as the retrograde limb of the reentrant circuit. This tachycardia has a long RP interval, with inverted P waves in the inferior leads. It may be incessant and may cause tachycardia-induced cardiomyopathy (Fig. 16.5).

Atrial Tachycardia

Atrial tachycardias account for approximately 10% of all PSVT. In contrast to AVNRT and AVRT, which are caused by reentry, the mechanism of atrial tachycardia may be abnormal automaticity, triggered activity, or reentry, particularly in patients with scarred atrial myocardium. Atrial tachycardia may originate in the right atrium, typically along the crista terminalis, or in the left atrium. In patients with atrial tachycardia,

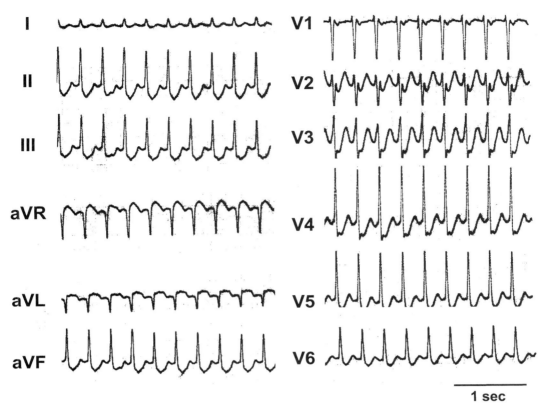

FIG. 16.3. A 12-lead electrocardiogram during paroxysmal supraventricular tachycardia (PSVT) in a patient with a concealed accessory pathway. The mechanism of PSVT was orthodromic reciprocating tachycardia. P waves can easily be visualized in the ST segment, particularly in the inferior leads.

there may be variable atrioventricular conduction, and atrial tachycardia persists even when there is atrioventricular block. In contrast, ORT and ART cannot continue when there is atrioventricular block.

PRESENTING SYMPTOMS AND SIGNS

PSVT has an abrupt onset and termination. The symptoms associated with PSVT depend on the mechanism of the tachycardia, the rate of the tachycardia, and the presence of underlying structural heart disease. Most affected patients experience palpitations. Dyspnea, chest discomfort, lightheadedness, and weakness also are common. Syncope is unusual. In some patients, presyncope and syncope may be caused by a vasodepressor response to the tachycardia.

Incessant forms of PSVT may lead to development of tachycardia-mediated cardiomyopathy. Sudden death due to supraventricular tachycardia is extremely rare. However, sudden death may occur in patients with rapidly conducting accessory pathways. In these patients, very rapid ventricular rates during atrial fibrillation may trigger ventricular fibrillation.

HELPFUL DIAGNOSTIC TESTS AND DIFFERENTIAL DIAGNOSIS

A 12-lead ECG may be helpful in determining the mechanism of PSVT. The P wave and QRS morphologic features and their relation to each other may provide important clues. The hallmark of PSVT is narrow QRS complexes. However, in patients with underlying intraventricular

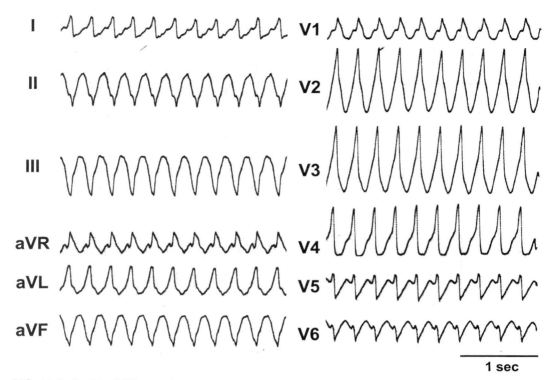

FIG. 16.4. A wide QRS complex tachycardia in a patient with Wolff-Parkinson-White syndrome. Because of ventricular preexcitation over the accessory pathway, QRS complexes are wide. The mechanism of this tachycardia was antidromic reciprocating tachycardia.

conduction delay or bundle branch block, in patients with a rate-related bundle branch block during the tachycardia, or in patients with ventricular preexcitation, PSVT is characterized by wide QRS complexes.

If the P waves are visible, the P wave axis provides information on the site of atrial activation. Negative P waves in leads I and aV_L indicate either a left atrial tachycardia or activation of the left atrium through a left-sided accessory pathway. If the P waves occur in the left half of the RR cycle and are separate from the QRS complex, ORT is more likely than typical AVNRT to be present (Fig. 16.3). During typical AVNRT, P waves usually are buried within the terminal portion of the QRS complexes and often cannot be visualized (Fig. 16.2B).

If there is atrioventricular block during the tachycardia, with more P waves than QRS complexes, atrial tachycardia is very likely to be present. Atrioventricular block during PSVT excludes a tachycardia caused by an accessory pathway. There is one-to-one relationship between the P waves and QRS complexes in most cases of AVNRT; however, two-to-one atrioventricular block can occasionally be observed.

If a record is available, the initiation and termination of a PSVT may provide diagnostic clues. Reproducible initiation of a PSVT with an APD that conducts with a long PR interval may suggest initiation of typical AVNRT, with anterograde conduction over the slow pathway. Termination of a tachycardia with a P wave without a subsequent QRS complex—spontaneously, during carotid sinus massage, or during adenosine administration—makes the presence of atrial tachycardia very unlikely.

In approximately 20% of cases, the mechanism of PSVT cannot be determined from the surface ECG (6). Furthermore, in many patients with PSVT, a 12-lead ECG of the tachycardia is not available. An ambulatory event recorder that is patient activated may be useful in documenting whether PSVT is the cause of symptoms. These

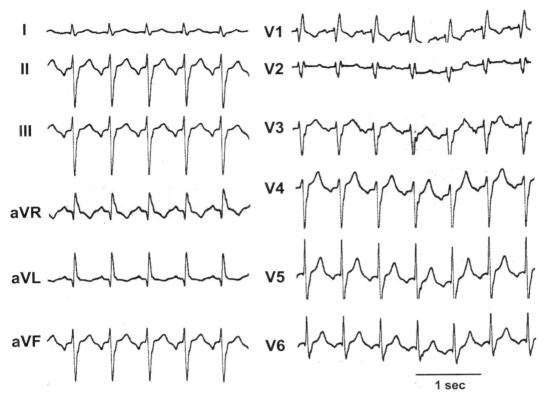

FIG. 16.5. A 12-lead electrocardiogram during paroxysmal supraventricular tachycardia. The mechanism of this tachycardia was permanent form of junctional reciprocating tachycardia, caused by a slowly conducting posteroseptal accessory pathway. The RP interval was longer than the PR interval. P waves were inverted in the inferior leads, II, III, and aV$_F$.

devices can be used for 30 to 60 days. If the symptoms occur on a daily basis, a 24-hour Holter monitor is useful.

An electrophysiologic test is the gold standard for determining the mechanism of PSVT. Once the mechanism has been established, radiofrequency catheter ablation can often be performed during the same procedure.

THERAPY

Acute Management

During PSVT in which the atrioventricular node is part of the reentrant circuit (AVNRT or AVRT), maneuvers or pharmacologic agents that temporarily slow or block atrioventricular conduction may terminate the tachycardia. A Valsalva maneuver or carotid sinus massage should be considered initially in hemodynamically stable patients. Among pharmacologic agents, adenosine has emerged as a useful diagnostic and therapeutic agent (7,8). Adenosine induces transient atrioventricular block and terminates most AVNRTs and AVRTs. Adenosine is contraindicated in patients with reactive airway disease. Adenosine may precipitate atrial fibrillation, and caution is necessary with its use in patients with the Wolff-Parkinson-White syndrome, because atrial fibrillation may be associated with extremely rapid ventricular rates. If adenosine is contraindicated or not available, then intravenous beta blockers such as esmolol, metoprolol, or propranolol or intravenous calcium channel blockers such as verapamil or diltiazem can be used. In patients with atrial fibrillation and the Wolff-Parkinson-White syndrome, intravenous procainamide should be considered as the initial antiarrhythmic agent. Drugs that selectively block atrioventricular conduction should not be used, because they may result in an increase in conduction over the accessory pathway and acceleration of the ventricular rate (9,10). If there is evidence of significant hemodynamic compromise, synchronized direct-current cardioversion should be considered.

Long-Term Therapy

Long-term treatment in patients with PSVT depends on the frequency, duration, and severity of symptoms. In symptomatic patients, radiofrequency catheter ablation is often a first-line therapeutic modality, because of a very favorable risk/benefit ratio. In addition, one study has shown that radiofrequency catheter ablation is the most cost-efficient treatment strategy in patients with PSVT (11). In addition to patient preference, radiofrequency catheter ablation is indicated in patients with frequent episodes of PSVT that are refractory to drugs, in patients with PSVT associated with severe symptoms such as presyncope or syncope, and in patients with the Wolff-Parkinson-White syndrome who have an accessory pathway that is capable of rapid conduction (12).

The efficacy of radiofrequency catheter ablation in curing AVNRT has been reported to be 98% to 100% (13–16). The recurrence rate is less than 2%, and complications such as atrioventricular block are rare (1% or less).

Radiofrequency catheter ablation has been shown to be effective in 85% to 100% of patients with an accessory pathway (12,17–20). The risk of complications such as atrioventricular block or pericardial tamponade is less than 1% (12).

In patients with atrial tachycardia, radiofrequency catheter ablation has a success rate of 80% to 90%. The lower efficacy than for other types of PSVT is attributable in part to an increased propensity for atrial tachycardias to be multifocal (12,21). However, radiofrequency catheter ablation may be appropriate for patients whose condition has been refractory to drug therapy or who prefer catheter ablation over chronic drug therapy.

In patients with symptomatic episodes of PSVT who prefer not to have radiofrequency catheter ablation, medical therapy also is an option. Agents that block atrioventricular nodal conduction—that is, beta blockers or calcium channel blockers—may be useful for AVNRT and ORT (22). However, in patients with the Wolff-Parkinson-White syndrome, these agents may facilitate conduction over the accessory pathway during atrial fibrillation. Class IA (quinidine, procainamide, disopyramide) (23–25), IC (propafenone, flecainide) (26,27), and III (amiodarone, sotalol) (28–31) drugs can be considered for patients whose condition is refractory to beta blockers or calcium channel blockers, for patients with atrial tachycardia, or for patients with the Wolff-Parkinson-White syndrome. The efficacy of these agents in preventing PSVT is unpredictable and variable. Side effects may limit the use of antiarrhythmic drug therapy.

In patients with infrequent and brief episodes of PSVT, no specific drug therapy may be needed. In patients with occasional episodes of PSVT that are long enough or symptomatic enough to warrant therapy, drug therapy can be used on an as-needed basis, instead of on a daily basis. For example, a 20- to 40-mg dose of propranolol taken at the onset of PSVT may lessen the severity of symptoms and shorten the duration of the episode, without causing the side effects that may be associated with daily use of beta blockers.

PRACTICAL POINTS

- AVNRT, AVRT, and atrial tachycardia constitute more than 95% of all PSVT.
- AVNRT is the most common type (60%). The surface ECG may show retrograde P

waves buried at the end of the QRS complex. P waves are typically inverted in the inferior leads (II, III, and aV_F) and may

(continued)

be manifest as pseudo-S waves, and upright in V1, leading to a pseudo-r′ appearance.

- Accessory pathways may conduct electrical impulses in an anterograde manner (manifest), in a retrograde manner (concealed), or in both directions. Anterograde conduction over an accessory pathway leads to ventricular preexcitation, with a short PR interval and delta waves (Wolff-Parkinson-White pattern). Approximately 30% of PSVT is due to accessory pathways. Multiple accessory pathways are more prevalent in patients with congenital heart disease, particularly Ebstein's anomaly.

- Atrial tachycardias account for approximately 10% of all PSVT. In patients with atrial tachycardia, there may be variable atrioventricular conduction, and atrial tachycardia persists even in the presence of atrioventricular block.

- PSVT have an abrupt onset and termination. Most patients experience palpitations. Dyspnea, chest discomfort, lightheadedness, and weakness also are

common. Syncope is unusual. In some patients, presyncope and syncope may be caused by a vasodepressor response to the tachycardia.

- The hallmark of PSVT is narrow QRS complexes. However, in patients with an underlying intraventricular conduction delay or bundle branch block, in patients with a rate-related bundle branch block during the tachycardia, or in patients with ventricular preexcitation, PSVT is characterized by wide QRS complexes.

- In approximately 20% of cases, the mechanism of PSVT cannot be determined from the surface ECG. An electrophysiologic test is the gold standard for determining the mechanism of PSVT. Once the mechanism has been established, radiofrequency catheter ablation can often be performed during the same procedure to eliminate the tachycardia permanently.

- Radiofrequency catheter ablation usually is the most effective and cost-efficient treatment strategy in patients with symptomatic PSVT.

REFERENCES

1. Keim S, Werner P, Jazayeri M, et al. Localization of the fast and slow pathways in atrioventricular nodal reentrant tachycardia by intraoperative ice mapping. *Circulation* 1992;86:919–925.
2. McGuire MA, Bourke JP, Robotin MC, et al. High resolution mapping of Koch's triangle using sixty electrodes in humans with atrioventricular junctional (AV nodal) reentrant tachycardia. *Circulation* 1993;88:2315–2328.
3. Goldberger J, Brooks R, Kadish A. Physiology of "atypical" atrioventricular junctional reentrant tachycardia occurring following radiofrequency catheter modification of the atrioventricular node. *Pacing Clin Electrophysiol* 1992;15:2270–2282.
4. Sung RJ, Styperek JL, Myerburg RJ, et al. Initiation of two distinct forms of atrioventricular nodal reentrant tachycardia during programmed ventricular stimulation in man. *Am J Cardiol* 1978;42:404–415.
5. Lee MA, Morady F, Kadish A, et al. Catheter modification of the atrioventricular junction with radiofrequency energy for control of atrioventricular nodal reentry tachycardia. *Circulation* 1991;83:827–835.
6. Kalbfleisch SJ, el-Atassi R, Calkins H, et al. Differentiation of paroxysmal narrow QRS complex tachycardias using the 12-lead electrocardiogram. *J Am Coll Cardiol* 1993;21:85–89.
7. Camm AJ, Garratt CJ. Adenosine and supraventricular tachycardia. *N Engl J Med* 1991;325:1621–1629.
8. Lerman BB, Belardinelli L. Cardiac electrophysiology of adenosine. Basic and clinical concepts. *Circulation* 1991;83:1499–1509.
9. Gulamhusein S, Ko P, Carruthers SG, et al. Acceleration of the ventricular response during atrial fibrillation in the Wolff-Parkinson-White syndrome after verapamil. *Circulation* 1982;65:348–354.
10. Garratt C, Antoniou A, Ward D, et al. Misuse of verapamil in pre-excited atrial fibrillation. *Lancet* 1989;1: 367–369.
11. Cheng CH, Sanders GD, Hlatky MA, et al. Cost-effectiveness of radiofrequency ablation for supraventricular tachycardia. *Ann Intern Med* 2000;133:864–876.
12. Morady F. Radio-frequency ablation as treatment for cardiac arrhythmias. *N Engl J Med* 1999;340:534–544.
13. Jackman WM, Beckman KJ, McClelland JH, et al. Treatment of supraventricular tachycardia due to atrioventricular nodal reentry, by radiofrequency catheter ablation of slow-pathway conduction. *N Engl J Med* 1992;327:313–318.
14. Kalbfleisch SJ, Strickberger SA, Williamson B, et al. Randomized comparison of anatomic and electrogram

mapping approaches to ablation of the slow pathway of atrioventricular node reentrant tachycardia. *J Am Coll Cardiol* 1994;23:716–723.

15. Haissaguerre M, Gaita F, Fischer B, et al. Elimination of atrioventricular nodal reentrant tachycardia using discrete slow potentials to guide application of radiofrequency energy. *Circulation* 1992;85:2162–2175.

16. Lindsay BD, Chung MK, Gamache MC, et al. Therapeutic end points for the treatment of atrioventricular node reentrant tachycardia by catheter-guided radiofrequency current. *J Am Coll Cardiol* 1993;22:733–740.

17. Calkins H, Langberg J, Sousa J, et al. Radiofrequency catheter ablation of accessory atrioventricular connections in 250 patients. Abbreviated therapeutic approach to Wolff-Parkinson-White syndrome. *Circulation* 1992;85:1337–1346.

18. Jackman WM, Wang XZ, Friday KJ, et al. Catheter ablation of accessory atrioventricular pathways (Wolff-Parkinson-White syndrome) by radiofrequency current. *N Engl J Med* 1991;324:1605–1611.

19. Kay GN, Epstein AE, Dailey SM, et al. Role of radiofrequency ablation in the management of supraventricular arrhythmias: experience in 760 consecutive patients. *J Cardiovasc Electrophysiol* 1993;4:371–389.

20. Swartz JF, Tracy CM, Fletcher RD. Radiofrequency endocardial catheter ablation of accessory atrioventricular pathway atrial insertion sites. *Circulation* 1993;87:487–499.

21. Lesh MD, Van Hare GF, Epstein LM, et al. Radiofrequency catheter ablation of atrial arrhythmias. Results and mechanisms. *Circulation* 1994;89:1074–1089.

22. Winniford MD, Fulton KL, Hillis LD. Long-term therapy of paroxysmal supraventricular tachycardia: a randomized, double-blind comparison of digoxin, propranolol and verapamil. *Am J Cardiol* 1984;54:1138–1139.

23. Bauernfeind RA, Wyndham CR, Dhingra RC, et al. Serial electrophysiologic testing of multiple drugs in patients with atrioventricular nodal reentrant paroxysmal tachycardia. *Circulation* 1980;62:1341–1349.

24. Wu D, Hung JS, Kuo CT, et al. Effects of quinidine on atrioventricular nodal reentrant paroxysmal tachycardia. *Circulation* 1981;64:823–831.

25. Brugada P, Wellens HJ. Effects of intravenous and oral disopyramide on paroxysmal atrioventricular nodal tachycardia. *Am J Cardiol* 1984;53:88–92.

26. Pritchett EL, McCarthy EA, Wilkinson WE. Propafenone treatment of symptomatic paroxysmal supraventricular arrhythmias. A randomized, placebo-controlled, crossover trial in patients tolerating oral therapy. *Ann Intern Med* 1991;114:539–544.

27. Henthorn RW, Waldo AL, Anderson JL, et al. Flecainide acetate prevents recurrence of symptomatic paroxysmal supraventricular tachycardia. The Flecainide Supraventricular Tachycardia Study Group. *Circulation* 1991;83:119–125.

28. Wellens HJ, Brugada P, Abdollah H. Effect of amiodarone in paroxysmal supraventricular tachycardia with or without Wolff-Parkinson-White syndrome. *Am Heart J* 1983;106:876–880.

29. Kopelman HA, Horowitz LN. Efficacy and toxicity of amiodarone for the treatment of supraventricular tachyarrhythmias. *Prog Cardiovasc Dis* 1989;31:355–366.

30. Kunze KP, Schluter M, Kuck KH. Sotalol in patients with Wolff-Parkinson-White syndrome. *Circulation* 1987;75:1050–1057.

31. Singh BN, Deedwania P, Nademanee K, et al. Sotalol. A review of its pharmacodynamic and pharmacokinetic properties, and therapeutic use. *Drugs* 1987;34:311–349.

17

Atrial Fibrillation and Atrial Flutter

Frank Pelosi, Jr., and Fred Morady

Atrial fibrillation is the most common cardiac arrhythmia necessitating hospitalization in the United States (1). Although not immediately life-threatening, atrial fibrillation is associated with significant rates of morbidity and mortality. Furthermore, recurrences of arrhythmia and complications from therapy present a challenge for both the patient and the clinician.

USUAL CAUSES

The most widely accepted explanation of the mechanism of atrial fibrillation centers on the presence of multiple self-sustaining waves of atrial depolarization, or *wavelets,* triggered by premature atrial depolarization or rapidly firing foci of arrhythmogenic activity (2,3) (Table 17.1). Despite the termination of the initiating trigger, the wavelets interact in such a way as to allow atrial fibrillation to sustain itself and, over time, alter the electrophysiologic and structural properties of the atrium. Although atrial fibrillation can be *paroxysmal,* or self-terminating, these changes allow atrial fibrillation to become *persistent* until therapeutic intervention terminates the arrhythmia or to become *permanent,* whereby efforts to restore sinus rhythm become futile.

Approximately 1% to 2% of the general population has atrial fibrillation; however, the prevalence of atrial fibrillation increases with age from less than 1% among persons younger than 50 years up to 9% for those older than 80 years (4,5). There is no distinct preponderance with regard to gender.

Atrial fibrillation has a significant association with structural heart disease. Twenty-five percent of patients with atrial fibrillation also have concomitant coronary artery disease (5). Although only about 10% of all myocardial infarctions are associated with atrial fibrillation, its presence is associated with a mortality rate of up to 40% (6). One third of patients undergoing coronary artery bypass grafting experience atrial fibrillation, usually around the third postoperative day. Although it usually terminates spontaneously, postoperative atrial fibrillation adds to hospital length of stay and cost.

The association of atrial fibrillation and valvular heart disease is well established. Rheumatic valvular disease greatly increases the chance of developing atrial fibrillation and quadruples the risk of thromboembolic complications. Of the patients with left ventricular dysfunction, approximately one in five have atrial fibrillation (7). This arrhythmia can also be part of the initial presentation of acute pericarditis and rare cardiac tumors, such as atrial myxoma.

Other cardiac arrhythmias, such as those related to the Wolff-Parkinson-White syndrome, can be associated with atrial fibrillation. Fortunately, ablation of the extranodal accessory pathway that causes this syndrome also eliminates atrial fibrillation in 90% of cases (8). Other arrhythmias associated with atrial fibrillation include atrial tachycardia, atrioventricular nodal reentrant tachycardias, and bradyarrhythmias such as sick sinus syndrome and other sinus node dysfunction.

Atrial fibrillation is associated with otherwise noncardiac systemic diseases. Systemic hypertension is found in 45%, and diabetes mellitus in 10%, of patients with atrial fibrillation (5). Although associated thyroid disease accounts for about 2% of cases of atrial fibrillation, it is one of a few reversible causes of this arrhythmia and should not be overlooked (9). The presence of atrial fibrillation and chronic obstructive

TABLE 17.1. *Cardiac and noncardiac conditions associated with atrial fibrillation*

Cardiac diseases associated with atrial fibrillation
Coronary artery disease
Dilated cardiomyopathy
Hypertrophic cardiomyopathy
Valvular heart disease
  Rheumatic
  Nonrheumatic
Cardiac arrhythmias
  Atrial tachycardia
  Atrial flutter
  Atrioventricular nodal reentrant tachycardia
  Wolf-Parkinson-White syndrome
  Sick sinus syndrome
Pericarditis
Noncardiac disease associated with atrial fibrillation
Systemic hypertension
Diabetes mellitus
Hyperthyroidism
Pulmonary diseases
  Chronic obstructive pulmonary disease
  Primary pulmonary hypertension
  Acute pulmonary embolism

Adapted from Pelosi F, Morady F. Evaluation and management of atrial fibrillation. *Med Clin North Am* 2001;85:225–244.

pulmonary disease is associated with an increased rate of mortality. Patients with acute pulmonary embolism can initially present with atrial fibrillation.

No apparent cause can be identified in approximately 3% of patients with atrial fibrillation (10). This *lone atrial fibrillation* is not associated with a high thromboembolic risk in younger age groups, but as a person ages or develops other associated conditions, that risk may increase.

SIGNS AND SYMPTOMS

The presenting symptoms of atrial fibrillation can be quite variable. Palpitations, fatigue, or dyspnea with exertion are common. Atrial fibrillation can exacerbate symptoms of cardiac ischemia in the presence of underlying coronary artery disease. Loss of atrial contractile function during atrial fibrillation lowers cardiac output and can lead to congestive heart failure in patients with left ventricular dysfunction. Atrial fibrillation rarely causes syncope; therefore, syncope attributed to such a diagnosis should be called

into question. Asymptomatic events can occur in otherwise symptomatic patients with atrial fibrillation; therefore, depending on symptoms alone to determine the duration of atrial fibrillation is insufficient (11).

History and physical examination of a patient with atrial fibrillation should first be directed at determining the degree of clinical compromise (Table 17.2). The pulse is classically described as "irregularly irregular," but a very rapid ventricular rate may make this difficult to detect. Blood pressure is typically normal, and hypotension is rare in the absence of left ventricular outflow tract obstruction. The examiner should look for signs of congestive heart failure such as pulmonary rales, a third heart sound (S3), or peripheral edema. Cardiac auscultation may reveal cardiac murmurs, right ventricular lift, or displaced point of maximum impulse suggestive of structural heart disease.

HELPFUL TESTS

Electrocardiography is the most helpful means of establishing a diagnosis of atrial fibrillation. The electrocardiogram is characterized by an irregular ventricular rate with no clear pattern ("irregularly irregular"), although this can be obscured by rapid rates (Fig. 17.1). Replacement of the normal P waves with disorganized, fibrillatory atrial activity is the hallmark of atrial fibrillation but can be concealed by artifact or rapid ventricular rates. In the presence of complete atrioventricular block, the ventricular rate can be regular. The diagnosis of atrial flutter is made by the presence of *flutter waves,* a more organized atrial activity appearing as a regular sawtooth pattern of atrial activity best seen in the inferior limb leads II, III, and aV$_F$ (Fig. 17.2). Ventricular rates are typically regular at a fixed ratio to the flutter rate (e.g., 2:1, 3:1); however, variable block in the atrioventricular node can result in variable ventricular rates. Atrial tachycardia is distinguished by the presence of distinct P waves of regular rates but of an abnormal morphologic pattern or axis. The presence of ST segment or T wave abnormalities suggests ongoing ischemia. Prolongation of the QRS duration can

TABLE 17.2. *Components of clinical evaluation of atrial fibrillation*

Component	Findings
History	Determine duration of atrial fibrillation
	Determine severity of symptoms
	Palpitation
	Fatigue
	Dyspnea, particularly upon exertion
	Lightheadedness
	Identify symptoms of ischemia or congestive heart failure (CHF)
Physical examination	
Vital signs	Pulse: rate and irregularity
	Blood pressure
Neck	Jugular venous distention
Pulmonary	Rales suggestive of CHF
Cardiac	S3 gallop suggestive of CHF
	Presence of murmurs suggestive of valvular disease
Abdominal	Hepatomegaly suggesting right-sided heart failure
Extremities	Peripheral edema suggestive of CHF
Laboratory tests	Hematocrit (anemia), thyroid-stimulating hormone (thyroid disease)
	Cardiac enzymes if ischemia is suspected
Electrocardiography	Confirm atrial fibrillation
	Identify ischemia, left ventricular preexcitation, preexcitation syndromes
	(Wolff-Parkinson-White syndrome)
Echocardiography	Left ventricular function, valvular function, outflow obstruction, cardiac chamber size
Exercise testing	Identify cardiac ischemia
	Determine adequacy of rate control
Ambulatory monitoring	Determine adquacy of rate control
	Correlate symptoms with arrhythmia

be suggestive of distal conduction system disease, left ventricular hypertrophy, or preexcitation syndromes such as Wolff-Parkinson-White syndrome.

Chest radiography can identify abnormalities in cardiac silhouette or confirm the presence of pulmonary congestion.

Echocardiography has emerged as a helpful tool for identifying associated structural heart disease and guiding management in patients with atrial fibrillation. Associated conditions such as valvular heart disease or cardiomyopathy can be revealed, which has significant impact on treatment decisions. The presence of large atria can be interpreted as a sign of a low likelihood of maintenance of normal rhythm over the long term (12).

Because of the association of coronary artery disease with atrial fibrillation, exercise testing should be strongly considered for patients with new-onset atrial fibrillation, particularly in those with coronary risk factors or anginal symptoms. Exercise testing can also be used to determine the adequacy of ventricular rate control during initial presentation and therapy.

COMPLICATIONS

Although not immediately life-threatening, atrial fibrillation has several complications associated with increased rates of morbidity and mortality. In some patients with the Wolff-Parkinson-White syndrome and rapidly conducting extranodal pathways that bypass the atrioventricular node, unabated atrioventricular conduction during atrial fibrillation with ventricular preexcitation can lead to ventricular fibrillation and sudden death (Fig. 17.3). For this reason, radiofrequency ablation of the extranodal pathway is recommended when ventricular preexcitation during atrial fibrillation is present. Atrial fibrillation with rapid ventricular rates associated with left ventricular outflow tract obstruction or mitral stenosis can lead to hypotension and rapid clinical deterioration. Similar complications can occur with atrial flutter with rapid ventricular rates.

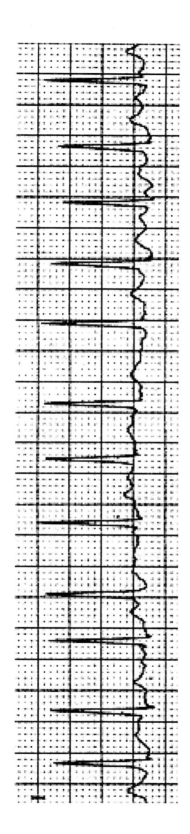

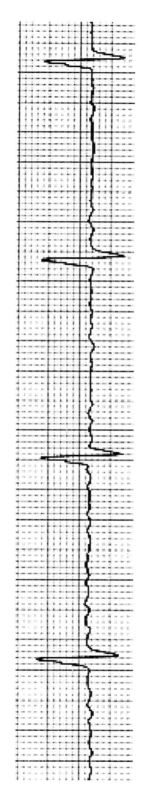

FIG. 17.1. Top: A patient with atrial fibrillation; note the fibrillatory atrial activity. **Bottom:** Atrial fibrillation with complete heart block. Although atrial fibrillation is clearly present, complete heart block with a junctional escape rhythm results in a regular ventricular rhythm.

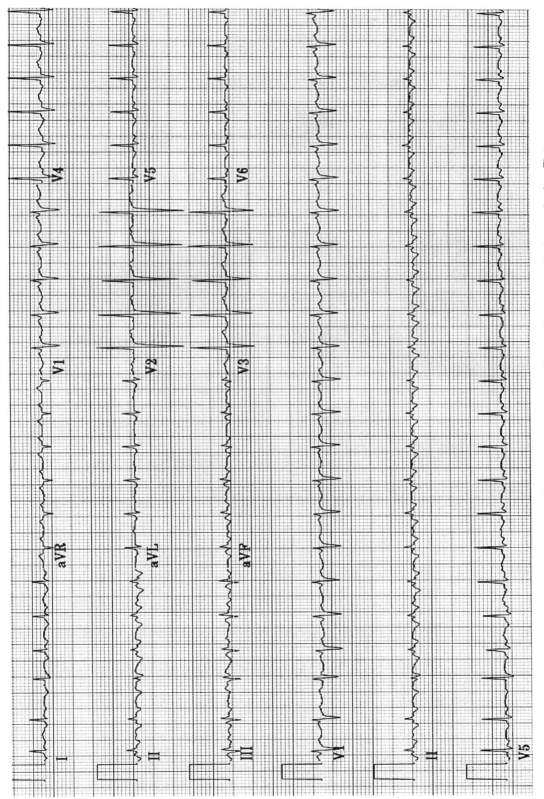

FIG. 17.2. A 12-lead electrocardiogram showing atrial flutter and 2:1 atrioventricular conduction. Flutter waves appear as a sawtooth pattern best seen in leads II, III, and aV$_F$.

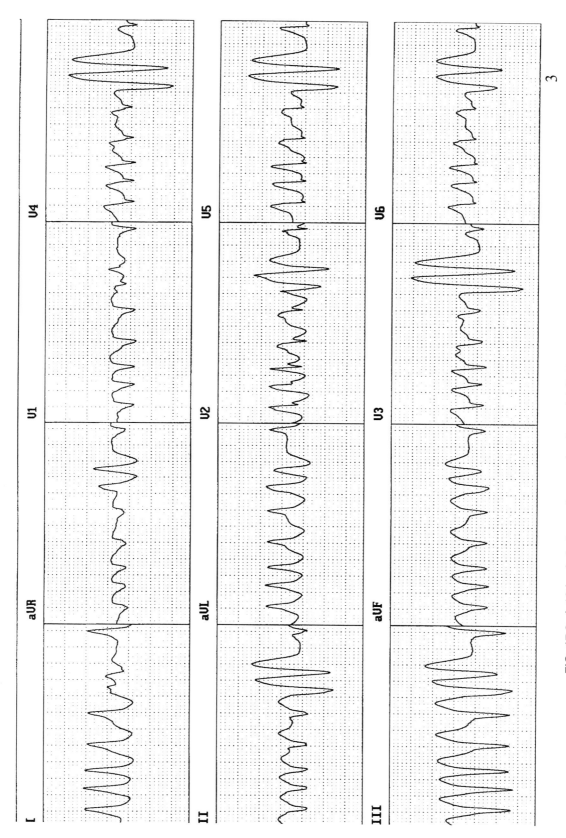

FIG. 17.3. A 12-lead electrocardiogram showing atrial fibrillation with ventricular preexcitation in a patient with Wolff-Parkinson-White syndrome. Note the long QRS duration

Uncontrolled rapid ventricular rates can lead to a cardiomyopathy induced by the persistent tachycardias (13,14).

Of the more common complications of atrial fibrillation, the most devastating is that of thromboembolism, especially stroke. Stroke attributed to atrial fibrillation is associated with death or severe debilitation at a rate twice that of stroke from other causes (15,16). The incidence of stroke increases with age, thereby making recovery more difficult for those afflicted. Large multicenter trials have established clinical variables with nonrheumatic atrial fibrillation that are independently associated with stroke (17). These variables are age older than 65 years, history of previous stroke, transient ischemic attack or peripheral thromboembolism, left ventricular dysfunction, or systemic hypertension. Echocardiographic predictors, such as left atrial size and left ventricular hypertrophy, have also been reported (12).

THERAPY

The management goals of atrial fibrillation or flutter are directed at three objectives: (a) prevention of thromboembolic events, (b) control of accelerated ventricular rates, and (c) restoration and maintenance of sinus rhythm.

The presence of atrial fibrillation confers a risk of thromboembolic events four times that of the general population in selected groups (18). This risk is multiplied even further in the presence of mitral stenosis. Multiple clinical trials have demonstrated that warfarin significantly reduces the risk of stroke (18–23). The American College of Chest Physicians has published guidelines for anticoagulation for those with nonrheumatic atrial fibrillation (Table 17.3) (24). In general, those without any high or moderate risk factors can be treated with aspirin. For those with any high risk factors, anticoagulation with warfarin dose-adjusted to an International Normalization Ratio of 2 to 3 is recommended. For those with a single moderate risk factor (age 65 to 75 years, presence of coronary artery disease, presence of diabetes mellitus), either aspirin or warfarin can be used. Those with more than one moderate risk factor are considered to be at high risk, and warfarin is recommended. Atrial fibrillation as short as 48 hours in duration can lead to the development of intracardiac thrombi and thromboembolic complications. Therefore, thorough documentation of the onset of atrial fibrillation must be pursued to establish duration of the arrhythmia.

Although atrial flutter has been presumed to carry a lower risk of thromboembolic complications, accumulating evidence indicates that patients with atrial flutter have a greater thromboembolic risk than those with normal rhythm, and an antithrombotic strategy similar to that for atrial fibrillation is favored (25,26).

Most of the symptoms of atrial fibrillation, including those attributed to ischemia or congestive heart failure, can be relieved with control of rapid ventricular rates. Rapid ventricular rates may be suspected if the average heart rate exceed 80 beats per minute or if there is a greater than expected rise in heart rate with low-level activities.

Control of ventricular rates is directed primarily at slowing conduction of the atrioventricular node. Many agents are available both in oral

TABLE 17.3. *Recommendations for anticoagulation for patients with atrial fibrillation and flutter*

Low risk (no RF)	Moderate risk (one moderate RF)	High risk (more than one moderate RF or one or more high RF)
Aspirin, 325 mg/day	Warfarin* or aspirin	Warfarin*

RF, risk factor.
*Dose adjusted to an International Normalization Ratio of 2–3.
Moderate risk factors: age 65–75 years, diabetes mellitus, coronary artery disease.
High risk factors: age >75 years, prior thromboembolic events, systemic hypertension, poor left ventricular systolic function.

and intravenous formulations. In order to rapidly control ventricular rates, an agent is commonly administered intravenously and converted to an oral form once rates have been stabilized. Secondary causes of rapid rates, such as anemia, congestive heart failure, ischemia, or thyrotoxicosis, should be managed. Beta blockers are preferred for patients with coronary artery disease and cardiomyopathy but must be used carefully because of their negative inotropic effects. Calcium channel blockers, such as verapamil and diltiazem, can also be used for short-term therapy, but the safety of long-term use in the presence of coronary artery disease or cardiomyopathy has not been established. Calcium channel blockers in the dihydropyridine group, such as nifedipine, have no role in controlling accelerated ventricular rates. Although digoxin is commonly used to control ventricular rates, its effect on atrioventricular nodal conduction is indirect and can be overcome by clinical states associated with increased adrenergic tone, such as exertion or congestive heart failure. It is beneficial in patients with left ventricular dysfunction, but it is otherwise a relatively poor choice for ventricular rate control of atrial fibrillation.

If medical therapy fails to control ventricular rates adequately, nonpharmacologic therapy in the form of ablation of the atrioventricular node is available. This is performed by means of a catheter-based approach from the right femoral vein. Radiofrequency energy is applied to the atrioventricular node until complete heart block is achieved. A permanent pacemaker is then necessary to maintain appropriate heart rates at rest and during exertion. This therapy has been shown to improve symptoms and quality of life for individuals with atrial fibrillation and symptomatic rapid ventricular rates (27–29). Modification of atrioventricular node was once a promising ablation technique for reducing ventricular rates, but the high numbers of patients requiring pacemakers make this procedure impractical, and it is rarely used (30).

The same agents used to control ventricular rates in the presence of atrial fibrillation are also used for atrial flutter. However, with the emergence of radiofrequency ablation as curative therapy for atrial flutter, ablation of atrioventricular

node is reserved for patients in whom both medical and ablative therapy have failed.

The restoration of sinus rhythm has immediate impact on control of ventricular rates and prevention of thromboembolic events. Although restoration of sinus rhythm can usually be achieved with electrical or pharmacologic cardioversion, maintenance of sinus rhythm is far more challenging.

The conversion of atrial fibrillation to sinus rhythm, known as cardioversion, is most commonly achieved with the use of direct current electrical energy delivered as a synchronized shock through an external defibrillator. This method restores sinus rhythm in approximately 85% of cases (31). Newer defibrillators in which biphasic defibrillation waveforms are used have demonstrated improved success rates. The procedure is performed while the patient is adequately sedated to control discomfort. An external defibrillator is used with defibrillator patches placed in the sternal-apical or anterior-posterior configurations. Direct current energy is usually delivered at 200 joules and increased to up to 360 joules if conversion of sinus rhythm is not achieved. Although conversion to sinus rhythm is usually achieved quickly, recovery of atrial function may take several weeks. For this reason, the high risk of thromboembolic complications persists; therefore, several weeks of adequate anticoagulation is required. An International Normalization Ratio of 2 to 3 must be maintained for 21 days before cardioversion and continued for at least 4 weeks after cardioversion.

There are some situations in which adequate anticoagulation before cardioversion is not possible or feasible. If the physician suspects that atrial fibrillation is life-threatening, cardioversion to sinus rhythm can be performed if the possible benefits outweigh the risks. The use of transesophageal echocardiography to identify thrombus in the left atrial appendage has emerged as a useful tool for safely performing cardioversion; however, continuous anticoagulation for the ensuing 28 days is necessary to prevent complications as atrial function improves (32). Because atrial function appears to be preserved during atrial fibrillation of short duration, anticoagulation before and after cardioversion for atrial

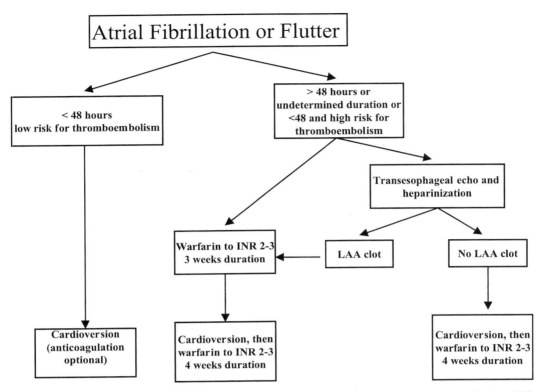

FIG. 17.4. A suggested algorithm for anticoagulation before cardioversion for atrial fibrillation. INR, International Normalization Ratio; LAA, left atrial appendage. (Modified from Pelosi F, Morady F. Evaluation and management of atrial fibrillation. *Med Clin North Am* 2000;85:225–244.)

fibrillation lasting less than 48 hours is optional for patients at low risk (26). A suggested algorithm for anticoagulation before and after cardioversion is found in Fig. 17.4. For patients with atrial flutter, the same precautions as those for atrial fibrillations should be pursued (24,26).

Pharmacologic agents to perform cardioversion are also used and obviate the need for sedation. The agent most commonly used is the Class III antiarrhythmic agent ibutilide, which can convert atrial fibrillation in as high as 64% of cases and higher for those with atrial fibrillation (33). The previously mentioned regimen of anticoagulation should be used, because the risk of thromboembolic complications after cardioversion is not related to the method. Ibutilide is very useful as a facilitator to improve efficacy of direct-current cardioversion, improving efficacy of cardioversion to as high as 100% (34). Ibutilide is also associated with a 3% to 10% risk of

polymorphic ventricular tachycardia (torsades de pointes) and should not be used in patients with prolonged QT intervals on electrocardiogram or severe left ventricular dysfunction (34). All patients receiving ibutilide should be monitored for several hours. Other antiarrhythmic agents used to convert atrial fibrillation acutely have included procainamide, quinidine, flecainide, propafenone, and amiodarone.

Preventing recurrences of atrial fibrillation after cardioversion has been the most daunting challenge in the management of this arrhythmia. Pharmacologic therapy has been the standard for decades, but recurrence of atrial fibrillation with these agents has been as high as 50%. Some antiarrhythmic agents, such as flecainide, moricizine, and propafenone, are contraindicated in patients with structural heart disease, because of associated increased rates of mortality from drug-induced proarrhythmia (35,36).

Certain Vaughn Williams Class III antiarrhythmics, such as amiodarone and sotalol, can be used in patients with structural heart disease and are effective in maintaining sinus rhythm (37–39). Dofetilide is relatively new Class III antiarrhythmic and has been studied in patients with structural heart disease. Although no significant increase in mortality was shown, 3% of patients experienced ventricular proarrhythmia in the first 72 hours of treatment (40). Therefore, dofetilide therapy should be initiated under inpatient telemetric monitoring

Nonpharmacologic therapies have emerged to restore and maintain sinus rhythm. Implantable atrial defibrillators allow cardioversion to sinus rhythm by either a patient-activated or an automatic mechanism. Cardioversion to sinus rhythm quickly after atrial fibrillation onset has been associated with reduced atrial fibrillation burden over several months (41). Implanted permanent pacemakers with the capability to pace both atria or with antitachycardia pacing algorithms have been introduced, with mixed initial results (42,43).

The role of arrhythmogenic foci arising from pulmonary veins has been the subject of intense investigation (44,45). Catheter-based radiofrequency ablation of these suspected triggers of atrial fibrillation have resulted in complete cures in certain subsets of patients. Also, ablative therapy has been applied to fascicles of conductive tissue located between the pulmonary veins and the left atrium to electrically "isolate" the triggers from the rest of the left atrium. Although they are quite promising, it is as yet unclear how prominent a role these foci have for patients suffering from atrial fibrillation.

The maze procedure is a surgical technique to prevent the propagation of atrial wavelets attributed to the maintenance of atrial fibrillation (46). Incisions are made in various sections of both atria via an open thoracotomy, with reported cure rates of as high as 90% (47). Complications of such an approach, including sinus node dysfunction that necessitates a permanent pacemaker in 4% of cases, compel the clinician to consider the risks and benefits of this treatment for an arrhythmia that is not immediately life-threatening. Catheter-based techniques to reproduce this procedure have produced disappointing results.

In contrast to atrial fibrillation, radiofrequency ablation has emerged as a promising curative therapy for atrial flutter. The mechanism of typical atrial flutter is a single, large reentrant circuit involving a narrow band of atrial tissue between the septal leaflet of tricuspid valve and the inferior vena cava (48). This tricuspid valve *isthmus* is the target site of ablative therapy. With a catheter-based technique, a line of radiofrequency applications is formed across the isthmus until conduction across this area is completely blocked. The creation of conduction block results in a cure rate of up to 90% with few complications, eliminating the need for antiarrhythmics or anticoagulants (49). Radiofrequency ablation may someday become first-line therapy for atrial flutter, as it is for other supraventricular tachycardias.

PROGNOSIS

The overall prognosis of atrial fibrillation is favorable in the absence of other cardiac disease. In patients with structural heart disease, the presence of atrial fibrillation complicates management and is associated with increased rates of mortality. Without treatment, the risk of stroke is 4% to 6% per year in patients with associated risk factors. Exacerbation of congestive heart failure or the development of cardiomyopathy from chronically elevated ventricular rates can have an adverse effect on survival.

Various therapeutic agents such as anticoagulants and antiarrhythmics carry their own risks and can adversely affect survival. Complications of anticoagulation including major bleeding, which affects 2% of patients per year; therefore, careful monitoring of warfarin therapy is necessary. As previously mentioned, some antiarrhythmics carry the risk of dangerous ventricular proarrhythmias.

FOLLOW-UP

Patients being treated for atrial fibrillation require follow-up depending on the treatment provided. In those requiring warfarin, the

International Normalized Ratio should be monitored weekly in preparation for cardioversion for 21 days before and 4 weeks after cardioversion. Once a stable dose of warfarin is established, the International Normalized Ratio should be checked monthly.

Patients taking antiarrhythmic drugs should be monitored every 4 to 6 months. Because of possible adverse effects, patients on amiodarone should have baseline thyroid-stimulating hormone measurements, liver function tests, and chest radiography every 4 to 6 months. Pulmonary function tests with assessment of diffusion capacity should be obtained at baseline and when symptoms of amiodarone pulmonary toxicity, such as dyspnea, are suspected. In those taking sotalol or dofetilide, renal function should be assessed regularly, because elevated drug levels as a result of reduced renal clearance could lead to life-threatening proarrhythmia. With these agents, regular electrocardiograms should be obtained to assess for abnormal QT prolongation; if the corrected QT interval is greater than 500 milliseconds, the drugs should be stopped. For those taking Class IC drugs, such as flecainide or propafenone, patients should be monitored clinically, and these drugs should be stopped if structural heart disease develops or the duration of the QRS complex prolongs by more than 50% during therapy.

PRACTICAL POINTS

- Atrial fibrillation is the most common cardiac arrhythmia necessitating hospitalization in the United States
- It is associated with significant morbidity, the most serious complication being stroke.
- It is most commonly associated with structural heart disease and with old age.
- The primary goals of treatment of atrial fibrillation are prevention of thromboembolic complications, control of accelerated ventricular rates, and restoration and maintenance of normal sinus rhythm.
- With new understanding of the physiologic basis of atrial fibrillation comes the emergence of nonpharmacologic approaches to treatment.

REFERENCES

1. Bialy D, Lehmann MH, Schumacjer DN, et al. Hospitalization for arrhythmias in the United States: importance of atrial fibrillation. *J Am Coll Cardiol* 1992; 19:41A(abstr 716-4).
2. Moe GK, Abildskov JA. Atrial fibrillation as a self-sustaining arrhythmia independent of a focal discharge. *Am Heart J* 1959;58:59–70.
3. Allessie MA, Lammers WJEP, Bonke FIM, et al. Experimental evaluation of Moe's multiple wavelet hypothesis of atrial fibrillation. Orlando, FL: Grune & Stratton, 1985:265–275.
4. Hiss RG, Lamb LE. Electrocardiographic features in 122,043 individuals. *Circulation* 1962;25:947.
5. Kannel WB, Abbott RD, Savage DD, et al. Epidemiologic features of chronic atrial fibrillation: the Framingham study. *N Engl J Med* 1982;306:1018–1022.
6. Sakata K, Kurihara H, Iwamori K, et al. Clinical and prognostic significance of atrial fibrillation in acute myocardial infarction. *Am J Cardiol* 1997;80:1522–1527.
7. Middlekauff HR, Stevenson WG, Stevenson LW. Prognostic significance of atrial fibrillation in advanced heart failure: a study of 390 patients. *Circulation* 1991;84:40–48.
8. Haissaguerre M, Fischer B, Labbe T, et al. Frequency of recurrent atrial fibrillation after catheter ablation of overt accessory pathways. *Am J Cardiol* 1992;69:493–497.
9. Krahn AD, Klein GJ, Kerr CR, et al. How useful is thyroid function testing in patients with recent-onset atrial fibrillation? The Canadian Registry of Atrial Fibrillation Investigators. *Arch Intern Med* 1996;156:2221–2224.
10. Kopecky SL, Gersh BJ, McGoon MD, et al. The natural history of lone atrial fibrillation. A population-based study over three decades. *N Engl J Med* 1987;317:669–674.
11. Page RL, Wilkinson WE, Clair WK, et al. Asymptomatic arrhythmias in patients with symptomatic paroxysmal atrial fibrillation and paroxysmal supraventricular tachycardia. *Circulation* 1994;89:224–227.
12. Vaziri SM, Larson MG, Benjamin EJ, et al. Echocardiographic predictors of nonrheumatic atrial fibrillation. *Circulation* 1994;89:724–730.
13. Grogan M, Smith HC, Gersh BJ, et al. Left ventricular dysfunction due to atrial fibrillation in patients initially

believed to have idiopathic dilated cardiomyopathy. *Am J Cardiol* 1992;69:1570–1573.

14. Packer DL, Bardy GH, Worley SJ, et al. Tachycardia-induced cardiomyopathy: a reversible form of left ventricular dysfunction. *Am J Cardiol* 1986;57:563–570.

15. Wolf PA, Mitchell JB, Baker CS, et al. Impact of atrial fibrillation on mortality, stroke, and medical costs. *Arch Intern Med* 1998;158:229–234.

16. Lin HJ, Wolf PA, Kelly-Hayes M, et al. Stroke severity in atrial fibrillation. The Framingham study. *Stroke* 1996;27:1760–1764.

17. Predictors of thromboembolism in atrial fibrillation: I. Clinical features of patients at risk. The Stroke Prevention in Atrial Fibrillation Investigators. *Ann Intern Med* 1992;116:1–5.

18. Stroke Prevention in Atrial Fibrillation Study. Final results. *Circulation* 1991;84:527–539.

19. Secondary prevention in non-rheumatic atrial fibrillation after transient ischaemic attack or minor stroke. EAFT (European Atrial Fibrillation Trial) Study Group. *Lancet* 1993;342:1255–1262.

20. Connolly SJ, Laupacis A, Gent M, et al. Canadian Atrial Fibrillation Anticoagulation (CAFA) Study. *J Am Coll Cardiol* 1991;18:349–355.

21. Ezekowitz MD, Bridgers SL, James KE, et al. Warfarin in the prevention of stroke associated with nonrheumatic atrial fibrillation. Veterans Affairs Stroke Prevention in Nonrheumatic Atrial Fibrillation Investigators. *N Engl J Med* 1992;327:1406–1412. [Erratum, *N Engl J Med* 1993;328:148.]

22. Petersen P, Boysen G, Godtfredsen J, et al. Placebo-controlled, randomised trial of warfarin and aspirin for prevention of thromboembolic complications in chronic atrial fibrillation. The Copenhagen AFASAK study. *Lancet* 1989;1:175–179.

23. Singer DE, Hughes RA, Gress DR, et al. The effect of aspirin on the risk of stroke in patients with non-rheumatic atrial fibrillation: the BAATAF Study. *Am Heart J* 1992;124:1567–1573.

24. Albers GW, Dalen JE, Laupacis A, et al. Antithrombotic therapy in atrial fibrillation. *Chest* 2001;119:194S–206S.

25. Lanzarotti CJ. Thromboembolism in chronic atrial flutter: is the risk underestimated? *J Am Coll Cardiol* 1997;30:1506–1511.

26. Fuster V, Ryden LE, Asinger RW, et al. ACC/AHA/ESC guidelines for the management of patients with atrial fibrillation: executive summary. A report of the American College of Cardiology/American Heart Association Task Force on Practice Guidelines and the European Society of Cardiology Committee for Practice Guidelines and Policy Conferences (Committee to Develop Guidelines for the Management of Patients with Atrial Fibrillation). *Circulation* 2001;104:2118–2150.

27. Kay GN, Ellenbogen KA, Giudici M, et al. The Ablate and Pace Trial: a prospective study of catheter ablation of the AV conduction system and permanent pacemaker implantation for treatment of atrial fibrillation. APT Investigators. *J Interv Card Electrophysiol* 1998;2:121–135.

28. Lee SH, Chen SA, Tai CT, et al. Comparisons of quality of life and cardiac performance after complete atrioventricular junction ablation and atrioventricular junction modification in patients with medically refractory atrial fibrillation. *J Am Coll Cardiol* 1998;31:637–644.

29. Natale A, Zimerman L, Tomassoni G, et al. AV node ablation and pacemaker implantation after withdrawal of effective rate-control medications for chronic atrial fibrillation: effect on quality of life and exercise performance. *Pacing Clin Electrophysiol* 1999;22:1634–1639.

30. Morady F, Hasse C, Strickberger SA, et al. Long-term follow-up after radiofrequency modification of the atrioventricular node in patients with atrial fibrillation. *J Am Coll Cardiol* 1997;29:113–121.

31. Mittal S, Ayati S, Stein KM, et al. Transthoracic cardioversion of atrial fibrillation: comparison of rectilinear biphasic versus damped sine wave monophasic shocks. *Circulation* 2000;101:1282–1287.

32. Manning WJ, Silverman DI, Gordon SP, et al. Cardioversion from atrial fibrillation without prolonged anticoagulation with use of transesophageal echocardiography to exclude the presence of atrial thrombi. *N Engl J Med* 1993;328:750–755.

33. Ellenbogen KA, Stambler BS, Wood MA, et al. Efficacy of intravenous ibutilide for rapid termination of atrial fibrillation and atrial flutter: a dose-response study. *J Am Coll Cardiol* 1996;28:130–136. [Erratum, *J Am Coll Cardiol* 1996;28:1082.]

34. Oral H, Souza JJ, Michaud GF, et al. Facilitating transthoracic cardioversion of atrial fibrillation with ibutilide pretreatment. *N Engl J Med* 1999;340:1849–1854.

35. Effect of the antiarrhythmic agent moricizine on survival after myocardial infarction. The Cardiac Arrhythmia Suppression Trial II Investigators. *N Engl J Med* 1992;327:227–233.

36. Echt DS, Liebson PR, Mitchell LB, et al. Mortality and morbidity in patients receiving encainide, flecainide, or placebo. The Cardiac Arrhythmia Suppression Trial. *N Engl J Med* 1991;324:781–788.

37. Duytschaever M, Haerynck F, Tavernier R, et al. Factors influencing long term persistence of sinus rhythm after a first electrical cardioversion for atrial fibrillation. *Pacing Clin Electrophysiol* 1998;21:284–287.

38. Julian DG, Prescott RJ, Jackson FS, et al. Controlled trial of sotalol for one year after myocardial infarction. *Lancet* 1982;1:1142–1147.

39. Roy D, Talajic M, Dorian P, et al. Amiodarone to prevent recurrence of atrial fibrillation. Canadian Trial of Atrial Fibrillation Investigators. *N Engl J Med* 2000;342:913–920.

40. Torp-Pedersen C, Moller M, Bloch-Thomsen PE, et al. Dofetilide in patients with congestive heart failure and left ventricular dysfunction. Danish Investigations of Arrhythmia and Mortality on Dofetilide Study Group. *N Engl J Med* 1999;341:857–865.

41. Tse HF, Lau CP, Yu CM, et al. Effect of the implantable atrial defibrillator on the natural history of atrial fibrillation. *J Cardiovasc Electrophysiol* 1999;10:1200–1209.

42. Levy T, Walker S, Rochelle J, et al. Evaluation of bi-atrial pacing, right atrial pacing, and no pacing in patients with drug refractory atrial fibrillation. *Am J Cardiol* 1999;84:426–429.

43. Saksena S, Delfaut P, Prakash A, et al. Multisite electrode pacing for prevention of atrial fibrillation. *J Cardiovasc Electrophysiol* 1998;9:S155–S162.

44. Haissaguerre M, Jais P, Shah DC, et al. Spontaneous initiation of atrial fibrillation by ectopic beats originating in the pulmonary veins. *N Engl J Med* 1998;339:659–666.

45. Jais P, Haissaguerre M, Shah DC, et al. A focal source of atrial fibrillation treated by discrete radiofrequency ablation. *Circulation* 1997;95:572–576.

46. Cox JL, Boineau JP, Schuessler RB, et al. Electrophysiologic basis, surgical development, and clinical results of the maze procedure for atrial flutter and atrial fibrillation. *Adv Card Surg* 1995;6:1–67.

47. Cox JL, Boineau JP, Schuessler RB, et al. Five-year experience with the maze procedure for atrial fibrillation. *Ann Thorac Surg* 1993;56:814–823. [Discussion, *Ann Thorac Surg* 1993;56:823–824.]

48. Lee SH, Tai CT, Yu WC, et al. Effects of radiofrequency catheter ablation on quality of life in patients with atrial flutter. *Am J Cardiol* 1999;84:278–283.

49. Movsowitz C, Callans DJ, Schwartzman D, et al. The results of atrial flutter ablation in patients with and without a history of atrial fibrillation. *Am J Cardiol* 1996;78:93–96.

18

Ventricular Tachycardia

Bradley P. Knight and Fred Morady

USUAL CAUSES

There are many causes of ventricular tachycardia (Table 18.1). However, ventricular tachycardia usually occurs in patients with underlying structural heart disease. Myocardial disease and scarring cause abnormal cardiac impulse formation and propagation, which can lead to ventricular tachycardia. In developed countries, the most common cause of structural heart disease is coronary artery disease. In patients with coronary artery disease, ventricular fibrillation and polymorphic ventricular tachycardia usually are caused by acute ischemia, whereas sustained monomorphic ventricular tachycardia usually is caused by reentry around a scar from a previous myocardial infarction.

Other intrinsic causes of ventricular tachycardia include nonischemic, dilated cardiomyopathy; hypertensive heart disease; valvular heart disease; hypertrophic cardiomyopathy; and infiltrative disorders such as sarcoidosis. The likelihood of developing ventricular tachycardia is proportional to the degree of ventricular dysfunction. Arrhythmogenic right ventricular dysplasia is an infiltrative disorder, predominantly of the right ventricle, that is characterized by fatty infiltration and fibrosis and may be a cause of cardiac arrest in apparently healthy individuals.

Ventricular tachycardia and fibrillation can also occur in individuals without any apparent structural heart disease. Idiopathic ventricular tachycardia most often arises in the outflow tract of the right ventricle or the left posterior fascicle in the left ventricle.

A molecular abnormality of one of the cardiac membrane ion channels can also result in ventricular tachycardia. More than 170 mutations of genes have been identified as causes of congenital long QT syndrome (LQTS). Mutations of the potassium channel genes, KvLQT1 and HERG, and the sodium channel gene, SCN5A, account for most cases. Each LQTS subtype has been associated with a specific T wave abnormality (1). Polymorphic ventricular tachycardia occurs in these patients as a result of early afterdepolarizations. Brugada's syndrome is caused by a sodium channel defect, is manifested as incomplete right bundle branch block with ST segment elevation in leads V_1 to V_3 (Fig. 18.1), and can lead to ventricular fibrillation (2).

Extrinsic causes of ventricular tachycardia include drugs and electrolyte abnormalities. Many cardiac and noncardiac drugs block the potassium channel Ikr. Blockade of the potassium current leads to prolongation of repolarization (Fig. 18.2) and can lead to a polymorphic ventricular tachycardia known as torsades de pointes. Commonly prescribed drugs that prolong the QT interval are listed in Table 18.2. A complete list can be found on the World Wide Web at *www.torsades.org*. Factors that predispose to torsades de pointes include female gender, bradycardia, hypokalemia, the administration of more than one QT interval–prolonging drug, and decreased drug clearance. Digitalis toxicity can cause ventricular tachycardia by causing delayed afterdepolarizations.

PRESENTING SYMPTOMS AND SIGNS

Patients who develop sustained ventricular tachycardia can present with cardiac arrest, syncope, presyncope, congestive heart failure, chest pain, or palpitations. Sudden death occurs in approximately 400,000 persons in the Unites States annually and is usually caused by ventricular fibrillation. Patients with nonsustained ventricular

TABLE 18.1. *Causes of ventricular tachyarrhythmias*

Structural causes
  Coronary artery disease
  Dilated nonischemic cardiomyopathy
  Hypertensive heart disease
  Valvular heart disease
  Hypertrophic cardiomyopathy
  Infiltrative diseases
  Arrhythmogenic right ventricular dysplasia
  Congenital heart disease
  Chagas' disease
  Myocarditis
Primary electrical causes
  Idiopathic ventricular tachycardia
  Idiopathic ventricular fibrillation
  Congenital long QT syndrome
  Brugada's syndrome
  Wolf-Parkinson-White syndrome
Extrinsic causes
  Drugs
  Hypokalemia
  Hypomagnesemia
  Hypoxemia
  Chest trauma
  Asynchronous shock during cardioversion
  Central nervous system abnormality

tachycardia are usually asymptomatic but can have palpitations or syncope.

Examination of a patient who is having sustained ventricular tachycardia may reveal pulselessness, unconsciousness, pulmonary edema, or signs of shock. When ventricular tachycardia is hemodynamically tolerated, there may be signs of tachycardia and atrioventricular dissociation.

HELPFUL TESTS

The most useful test in a patient with a sustained ventricular tachycardia is an electrocardiogram. A recording of atrial activity during a sustained wide–QRS complex tachycardia with an esophageal electrode can help establish the presence of atrioventricular dissociation. A recording from a temporary atrial epicardial pacing electrode is valuable in patients who have recently undergone cardiac surgery. Patients with sustained ventricular tachycardia or ventricular fibrillation must also undergo a careful physical examination, review of medications, and measurement of electrolytes and cardiac enzymes. Most patients should undergo coronary angiography and left ventriculography.

The prognosis of a patient with asymptomatic, nonsustained ventricular tachycardia depends on the presence or absence of ventricular dysfunction. Therefore, patients with nonsustained ventricular tachycardia should undergo testing to evaluate ventricular function and to exclude ischemia. Patients with preserved ventricular function have a good prognosis and usually do not need further testing. On the other hand, patients with significant ventricular dysfunction are at an increased risk of dying suddenly and should undergo further evaluation. Electrophysiologic testing can be done to risk-stratify patients with coronary artery disease, prior myocardial infarction, and left ventricular dysfunction who experience nonsustained ventricular tachycardia. Patients with sustained ventricular tachycardia inducible during programmed electrical stimulation are at high risk for cardiac arrest and appear to benefit from implantation of a prophylactic cardiac defibrillator (3–5). Electrophysiologic testing has no value in the risk stratification of patients with a nonischemic cardiomyopathy.

Noninvasive tests that have been used to risk-stratify patients with nonsustained ventricular tachycardia include signal-averaged electrocardiography, measurement of heart rate variability, and assessment of T wave alternans. Their clinical utility appears to be limited.

DIFFERENTIAL DIAGNOSIS

Ventricular tachycardia is defined as three or more consecutive ventricular complexes at a rate greater than 100 beats per minute and can be categorized on the basis of the morphologic features of the QRS complexes: as monomorphic ventricular tachycardia, polymorphic ventricular tachycardia, or ventricular fibrillation. A ventricular arrhythmia is considered sustained when it requires termination, when it results in symptoms, or when it lasts longer than 30 seconds.

When faced with an apparent wide–QRS complex tachycardia, it is important to first exclude electrocardiographic artifact (6). Artifact can be recognized when portions of the baseline QRS complexes are visible within the suspected wide–QRS complex tachycardia at intervals that are

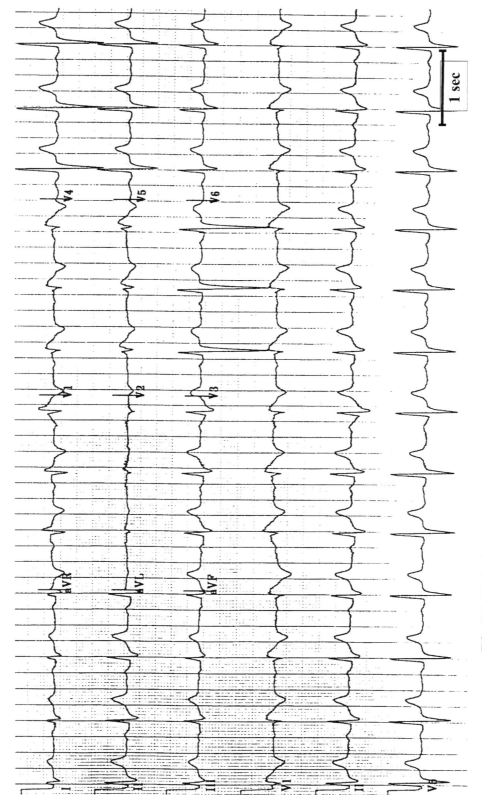

FIG. 18.1. Twelve-lead electrocardiogram of a patient with Brugada's syndrome. Note the incomplete right bundle branch block with ST segment elevation and T wave inversion in leads V_1 to V_2. Two of the patient's brothers had died suddenly.

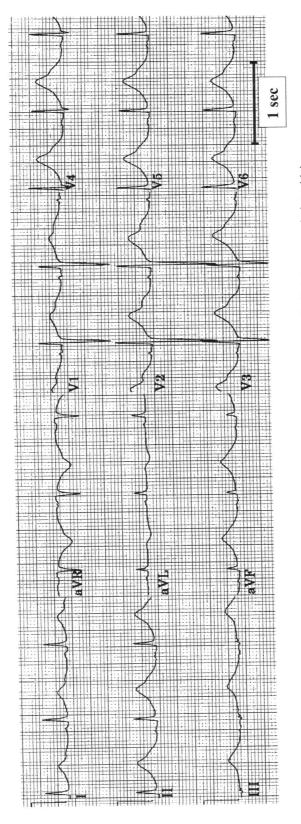

FIG. 18.2. Electrocardiogram recorded from a patient who was treated with intravenous haloperidol, showing sinus rhythm with marked prolongation of the QT interval.

TABLE 18.2. *List of commonly used medications that prolong the QT interval*

Cardiac drugs
  Procainamide
  Quinidine
  Disopyramide
  Sotalol
  Ibutilide
  Dofetilide
  Amiodarone
  Probucol
Noncardiac drugs
  Tricyclic antidepressants
  Phenothiazines
  Haloperidol
  Risperidone
  Halothane
  Terfenadine
  Astemizole
  Cisapride
  Pentamidine
  Macrolide antibiotics

similar to the cycle length of the baseline rhythm (Fig. 18.3). Other clues that suggest artifact include a disturbance of the baseline before the onset, a QRS complex that follows termination of the apparent tachycardia earlier than would be expected, and witnessed body movements during the recording. Sinus tachycardia with ST segment elevation can also manifest as a pseudo–wide–QRS complex tachycardia. A 12-lead electrocardiogram identifies ST segment elevation as the cause of the apparent wide QRS complexes (Fig. 18.4).

Monomorphic Ventricular Tachycardia

Monomorphic ventricular tachycardia must be distinguished from supraventricular tachycardia with bundle branch block aberration. Other, less common causes of a regular, wide–QRS complex tachycardia include antidromic atrioventricular reentrant tachycardia that occurs through an accessory pathway and ventricular pacing. Antidromic atrioventricular reentrant tachycardia often is indistinguishable from ventricular tachycardia.

Differentiation of ventricular tachycardia from supraventricular tachycardia with aberrancy is important because of the implications for immediate and long-term treatment. Clinical and electrocardiographic factors must be considered when a wide–QRS complex tachycardia is present. An important principle is that when there is any uncertainty regarding the diagnosis, it is safest to assume that a wide–QRS complex tachycardia is ventricular tachycardia. A history of myocardial infarction or congestive heart failure has a positive predictive value of greater than 95% for ventricular tachycardia (7). The presence of hemodynamic stability and minimal symptoms should not influence the differentiation of ventricular tachycardia from supraventricular tachycardia with aberration (8).

Electrocardiographic findings that support a diagnosis of ventricular tachycardia are summarized in Table 18.3 and can be remembered by the alphabetical mnemonic: "ABCDEF." The principle of each criterion is that when the QRS morphologic pattern does not have features of a typical left or right bundle branch block pattern, the rhythm is most likely ventricular tachycardia. However, there are many exceptions to these rules. Atrioventricular dissociation ("A") is the most helpful criterion. Unfortunately, atrioventricular dissociation is not present in about one quarter of ventricular tachycardias because there is 1:1 ventriculoatrial conduction, and it is often difficult to identify unless the tachycardia rate is relatively slow. Signs of atrioventricular dissociation include P waves that are independent of the QRS complexes, capture beats, and fusion beats (Fig. 18.5). The broader ("B") the QRS complex is, the more likely it is that the rhythm is ventricular tachycardia (Fig. 18.6). A QRS duration exceeding 160 milliseconds for left bundle branch morphologic patterns and exceeding 140 milliseconds for right bundle branch morphologic patterns supports a diagnosis of ventricular tachycardia. An RS interval (the time from the onset of the R wave to the nadir of the

TABLE 18.3. *Electrocardiographic findings that support a diagnosis of ventricular tachycardia*

Atrioventricular dissociation
Broad
Concordance
Deviation of axis
Effect of maneuvers
Features of the QRS complex

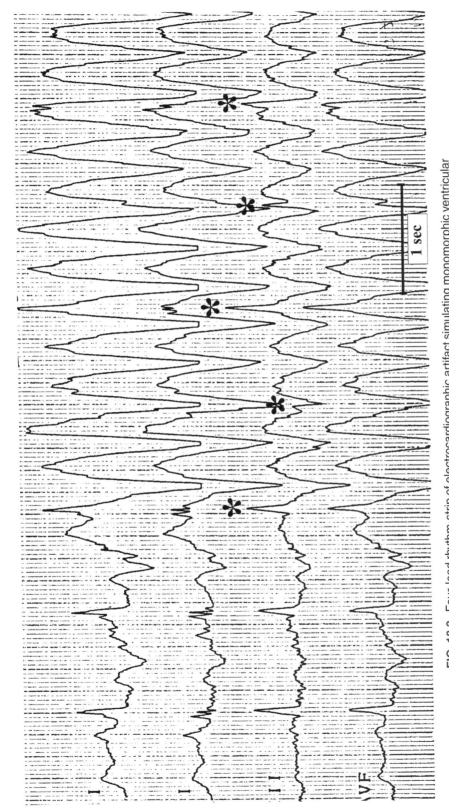

FIG. 18.3. Four-lead rhythm-strip of electrocardiographic artifact simulating monomorphic ventricular tachycardia. A diagnosis of artifact can be made on the basis of identification of portions of QRS complexes (denoted with *asterisks*) at intervals that correspond to the baseline sinus cycle length. Note the unstable baseline before the onset of the apparent tachycardia.

291

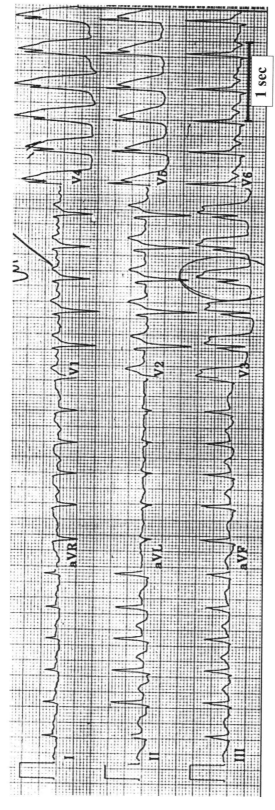

FIG. 18.4. Twelve-lead electrocardiogram recorded in a patient with an acute anterior myocardial infarction. A single, modified chest lead recording from the same patient appeared to demonstrate a wide–QRS complex tachycardia that was actually sinus tachycardia with prominent ST segment elevation.

292

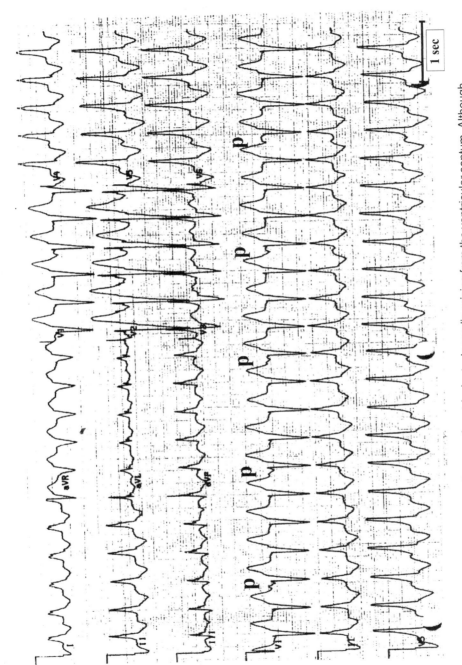

FIG. 18.5. Electrocardiogram of ventricular tachycardia arising from the ventricular septum. Although the QRS duration is relatively short, there is evidence of atrioventricular dissociation consistent with ventricular tachycardia. P waves are marked with the letter "p."

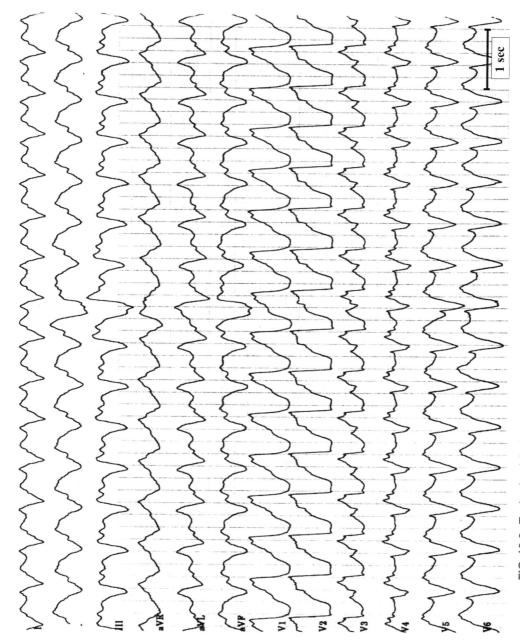

FIG. 18.6. Twelve-lead rhythm strip of ventricular tachycardia at a rate just below 100 beats per minute. The very wide QRS complex is more consistent with ventricular tachycardia than with supraventricular tachycardia with aberrancy.

S wave) in the precordial leads that exceeds 100 milliseconds is consistent with ventricular tachycardia (9). Concordance ("C") is defined as the presence of QRS complexes that are all upright or all inverted in the precordial leads and is a sign of ventricular tachycardia. Bundle branch block patterns do not demonstrate concordance because they usually have at least one biphasic complex in the precordial leads. Deviation ("D") of the axis in a direction that is not typical for a bundle branch block pattern, such as right axis deviation with a left bundle branch block pattern, suggests ventricular tachycardia.

The effect ("E") of certain maneuvers can also be helpful. Vagal maneuvers or adenosine can unmask an underlying atrial tachycardia by causing transient atrioventricular block (Fig. 18.7) or can terminate an atrioventricular node–dependent supraventricular tachycardia (Fig. 18.8). Ventricular tachycardia is probably present when the administration of adenosine has no effect or causes ventriculoatrial dissociation during tachycardia (10).

Certain morphologic features ("F") of the QRS complex are seen more commonly with ventricular tachycardia than with aberrancy. For example, when the QRS complex has a right bundle branch block pattern in lead V_1, an R wave that is taller than the R' (Fig. 18.9) or a monophasic or biphasic QRS complex suggests ventricular tachycardia. When the QRS complex has a left bundle branch block pattern in lead V_1, an R wave that is wider than 40 milliseconds or a qS pattern favors ventricular tachycardia.

Electrocardiographic features that support a diagnosis of a supraventricular arrhythmia with aberrancy include initiation of the tachycardia by a premature atrial depolarization or an initiation that is associated with a long-short sequence (Ashman's phenomenon). When a patient has a documented narrow–QRS complex tachycardia that is the same rate as the wide–QRS complex tachycardia, the likelihood that the wide–QRS complex rhythm is due to aberrancy is high.

Subtypes of monomorphic ventricular tachycardia include bundle branch reentry, accelerated idioventricular rhythm, paroxysmal ventricular tachycardia, and repetitive monomorphic ventricular tachycardia. The most common type of repetitive monomorphic ventricular tachycardia arises from the right ventricular outflow tract and has a left bundle, inferior axis morphologic pattern (Fig. 18.10). Ventricular flutter is a subtype of monomorphic ventricular tachycardia, occurs at a rate of 200 to 300 beats per minute, resembles a sine wave, and results in hemodynamic collapse.

Bidirectional ventricular tachycardia is an uncommon ventricular tachycardia characterized by QRS complexes that have a right bundle branch block pattern with an alternating polarity in the frontal plane (Fig. 18.11). Bidirectional ventricular tachycardia is usually a result of digitalis toxicity but also may be idiopathic.

Polymorphic Ventricular Tachycardia

Polymorphic ventricular tachycardia is characterized by QRS complexes that vary in morphologic pattern. The term *torsades de pointes* refers to polymorphic ventricular tachycardia that occurs in the setting of an abnormally long QT interval and that has a pattern of QRS complexes that appear to twist around the isoelectric line.

Ventricular Fibrillation

Ventricular fibrillation is present when there are irregular undulations of varying contour and amplitude (Fig. 18.12). It is important to exclude asystole when the fibrillatory waves are small in amplitude.

COMPLICATIONS

The complications of ventricular tachycardia are caused by insufficient cardiac output and include death, shock, loss of consciousness, and injury. There are additional complications associated with the treatment of ventricular tachycardia. Complications from antiarrhythmic drug therapy include acquired LQTS, ventricular proarrhythmia, heart block, and organ toxicity. Complications from implantation of a defibrillator include

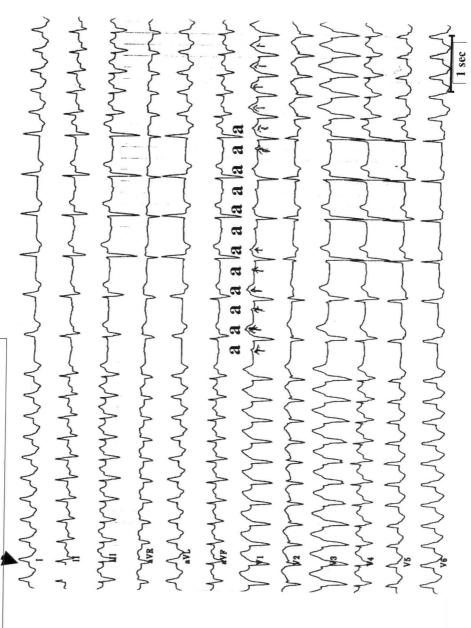

Intravenous Adenosine

infection, pneumothorax, lead failure, inappropriate shocks for supraventricular tachycardias, premature battery depletion, and device failure (11).

THERAPY

Acute Management

The acute management of a patient with a ventricular tachyarrhythmia should follow the Advanced Cardiovascular Life Support (ACLS) guidelines (12) (Fig. 18.13). The most effective method for restoring sinus rhythm is an unsynchronized, direct-current electrical shock to the chest. Patients with ventricular fibrillation or pulseless ventricular tachycardia should undergo basic cardiopulmonary resuscitation. A precordial thump may also be delivered while the resuscitation team is awaiting arrival of a defibrillator. As soon as a defibrillator is available, three attempts at defibrillation should be delivered in succession until sinus rhythm is restored. The recommended energy levels in using a standard defibrillator are 200 joules, followed by 200 or 300 joules, and then 360 joules. If a 360-joule shock is ineffective, drugs should be administered in a stepwise manner, followed by repeat attempts at defibrillation. Traditionally, epinephrine, 1 mg, is given every 3 to 5 minutes; however, a one-time dose of vasopressin, 40 U, is an alternative in the ACLS guidelines.

Intravenous antiarrhythmic drugs that can be used for refractory ventricular tachyarrhythmias include lidocaine, procainamide, and amiodarone. Bretylium is no longer recommended because amiodarone has been found to be as effective as bretylium and associated with less hypotension (13). In a randomized clinical trial of intravenous amiodarone for resuscitation after out-of-hospital cardiac arrest due to ventricular fibrillation, amiodarone increased survival to hospital admission from 33% to 43%, in comparison with placebo (14). However, the trial did not have sufficient statistical power to detect a difference in survival to hospital discharge.

After defibrillation, contributing factors such as ischemia, hypoxemia, hypokalemia, hypomagnesemia, or extreme bradycardia should be corrected. Patients who undergo conversion from polymorphic ventricular tachycardia and are found to have a long QT interval should be treated to prevent recurrent ventricular tachycardia. The ACLS guidelines recommend magnesium, overdrive pacing, isoproterenol, phenytoin, or lidocaine.

Treatment of sustained monomorphic ventricular tachycardia depends on the clinical status of the patient. If the ventricular tachycardia is not hemodynamically tolerated, immediate cardioversion is appropriate. If the patient is hemodynamically stable, pharmacologic conversion may be attempted. Intravenous amiodarone and lidocaine are reasonable first choices. Intravenous procainamide has been shown to be more effective than intravenous lidocaine for sustained monomorphic ventricular tachycardia, but in the ACLS guidelines, it is not recommended when cardiac function is impaired. Synchronized electrical cardioversion should be performed if pharmacologic attempts fail. Adequate sedation or anesthesia should precede a shock for patients who are conscious. Overdrive pacing with a temporary transvenous pacemaker can also be used to terminate sustained monomorphic ventricular tachycardia, but it is rarely indicated.

External defibrillator technology has evolved. Conventional defibrillators deliver a direct-current shock as a damped sine wave. Biphasic defibrillation waveforms that have been used in implantable defibrillators for years have been

---

FIG. 18.7. Twelve-lead rhythm strip of a wide–QRS complex tachycardia that is caused by an atrial tachycardia with left bundle branch block aberration. Intravenous adenosine is administered during tachycardia and results in transient 2:1 atrioventricular block. During atrioventricular block, the underlying atrial tachycardia is visible (denoted with the letter "a") at the same rate as the wide–QRS complex tachycardia. The QRS complex becomes narrow when the ventricular rate slows.

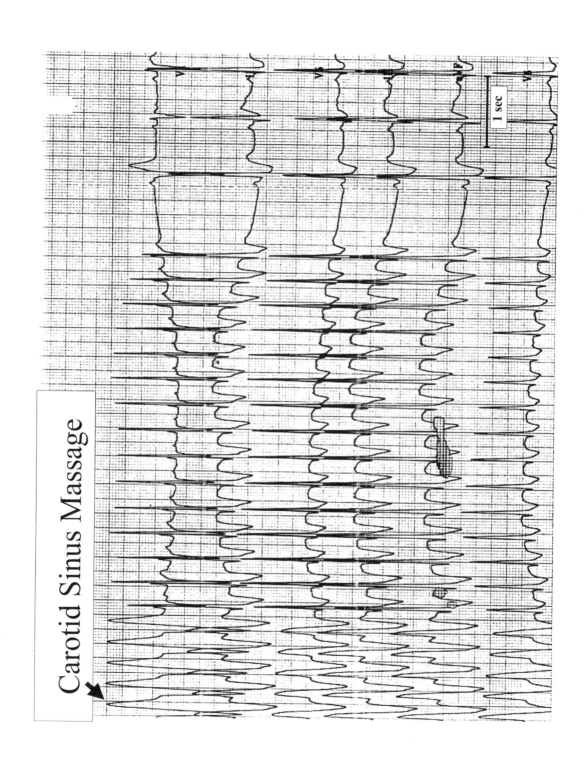

Carotid Sinus Massage

1 sec

incorporated into external defibrillators. Biphasic waveforms are more effective than a standard waveform and are able to successfully defibrillate with lower energy requirements (15). Because there are currently various manufacturers of biphasic defibrillators, each with subtle waveform differences, it is difficult to provide energy recommendations that are comparable with those of a standard defibrillator. If a clinician has access to a biphasic defibrillator, it is important to know which energy levels have efficacy equal to the doses that are recommended by the ACLS guidelines. Automatic external defibrillators are safe and effective and, because they are increasingly available for use by nonmedical personnel, have the potential to dramatically increase survival from cardiac arrest (16).

Long-Term Management

Patients who have experienced an episode of sustained ventricular tachycardia or ventricular fibrillation are at risk of having a recurrence unless there is a clear-cut and correctable cause. Patients who have had a cardiac arrest in the setting of an acute transmural myocardial infarction, severe hypokalemia, or hypoxemia are usually considered to be at relatively low risk for recurrence. However, studies have suggested that patients considered to have "reversible" causes of cardiac arrest may still carry an unacceptable risk for cardiac arrest (17).

Long-term management of patients with ventricular tachyarrhythmias can be divided into drug therapy, device therapy, and ablation. Occasionally, all three therapies are necessary to manage a patient with ventricular tachycardia. In general, the most effective pharmacologic therapy for secondary prevention of sustained ventricular arrhythmias is oral amiodarone. Its efficacy may be related to its ability to block sodium, potassium, and calcium channels, as well as beta-adrenergic receptors. Amiodarone appears to be less likely to cause ventricular proarrhythmia in patients with structural heart disease than is pure sodium or potassium channel blockers.

Implantable defibrillators have been available since the late 1980s and are highly effective at preventing death from ventricular tachycardia or ventricular fibrillation. Three large, randomized, controlled trials have compared antiarrhythmic drugs (primarily amiodarone) to implantable defibrillators for secondary prevention of symptomatic ventricular arrhythmias. In the largest trial, the Antiarrhythmic Versus Implantable Defibrillator (AVID) trial, defibrillator therapy resulted in a 31% reduction in overall mortality at 3 years of follow-up in comparison with amiodarone (18). The Canadian Implantable Defibrillator Study (CIDS) found a 20% relative risk reduction in all-cause mortality and a 33% reduction in arrhythmic mortality with implantable cardioverter-defibrillator therapy in comparison with amiodarone (19). In the Cardiac Arrest Study Hamburg (CASH), therapy with a defibrillator was associated with a 23% reduction of all-cause mortality when compared with treatment with amiodarone or metoprolol (20). It is generally accepted that defibrillator implantation is first-line therapy for patients with sustained ventricular tachycardia or cardiac arrest unless a contraindication is present.

The American College of Cardiology and the American Heart Association have published guidelines for implantation of cardiac defibrillators (21). The complete guidelines are available on the World Wide Web at *www.americanheart.org* and are summarized in Table 18.4.

FIG. 18.8. Six-lead rhythm strip of a wide–QRS complex tachycardia that is caused by orthodromic atrioventricular reentrant tachycardia with left bundle branch block aberration. Carotid sinus massage results in slowing of the supraventricular tachycardia and resolution of the aberration. The tachycardia then terminates. The first sinus beat is associated with ventricular preexcitation.

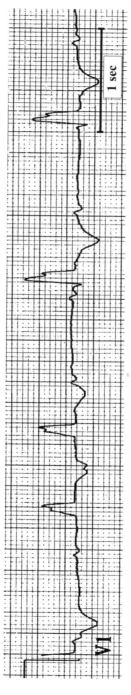

FIG. 18.9. A rhythm strip recorded from lead V$_1$ of sinus rhythm with right bundle branch block and first-degree atrioventricular block (first two QRS complexes), followed by complete atrioventricular block and a ventricular escape rhythm (last two QRS complexes). This recording demonstrates the morphologic differences between QRS complexes that are a result of right bundle branch block aberration (R wave smaller than R′ wave) and QRS complexes that are left ventricular in origin (R wave taller than R′ wave).

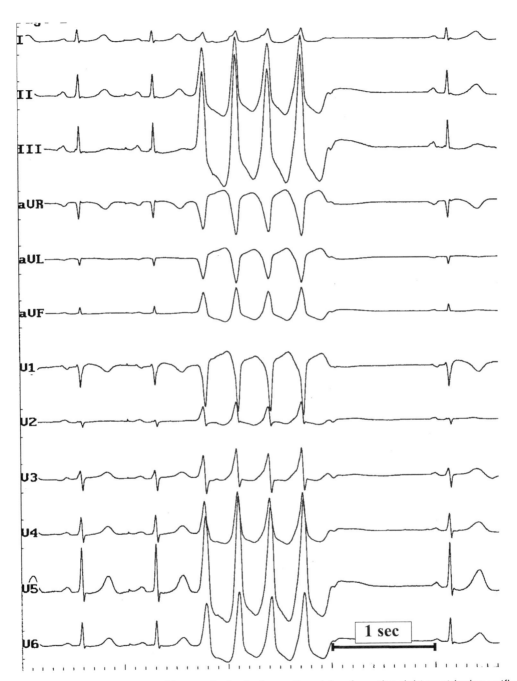

FIG. 18.10. Example of idiopathic ventricular tachycardia arising from the right ventricular outflow tract. Note the four beats of ventricular tachycardia with left bundle branch block and inferior axis morphologic pattern.

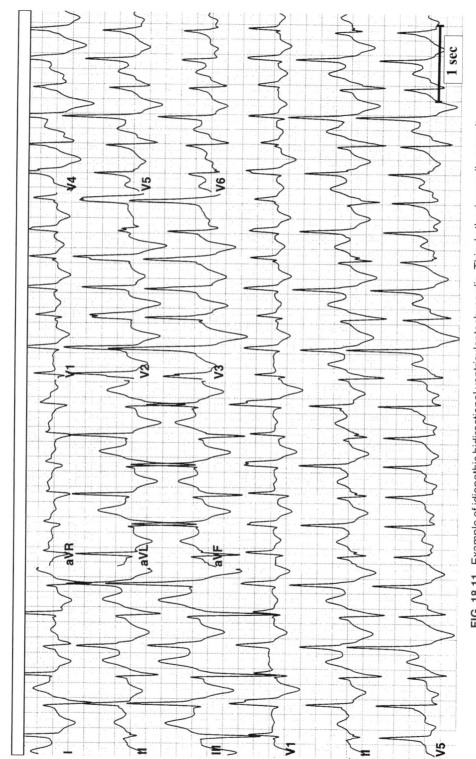

FIG. 18.11. Example of idiopathic bidirectional ventricular tachycardia. This rhythm is usually a result of digitalis toxicity. Note the right bundle branch block morphologic pattern and an alternating QRS axis in the inferior leads.

TABLE 18.4. *Indications and contraindications for implantable defibrillator therapy*

Class I indications*
1. Cardiac arrest due to VF or VT not due to a transient or reversible cause
2. Spontaneous sustained VT in association with structural heart disease
3. Syncope of undetermined origin with clinically relevant, hemodynamically significant sustained VT or VF induced on electrophysiologic study when drug therapy is ineffective, not tolerated, or not preferred
4. Nonsustained VT with coronary disease, prior MI, LV dysfunction, and inducible VF or sustained VT on electrophysiologic study that is not suppressible by a Class I antiarrhythmic drug
5. Spontaneous sustained VT in patients who do not have structural heart disease that is not amenable to other treatment

Class II indications*
1. Patients with LV ejection fraction of less than or equal to 30%, at least one month post myocardial infarction and three months post coronary artery revascularization surgery
2. Cardiac arrest presumed to be due to VF when EP testing is contraindicated
3. Severe symptoms attributable to sustained VT while awaiting transplantation
4. Familial or inherited conditions with a high risk for life-threatening ventricular tachyarrhythmias, such as long QT syndrome or hypertrophic cardiomyopathy
5. Nonsustained VT with coronary artery disease, prior MI, and LV dysfunction, and inducible sustained VT or VF on electrophysiologic study
6. Recurrent syncope of undetermined etiology in the presence of ventricular dysfunction and inducible ventricular arrhythmias on electrophysiologic study when other causes of syncope have been excluded
7. Syncope of unexplained etiology or family history of unexplained sudden cardiac death in association with typical or atypical right bundle-branch block and ST-segment elevations (Brugada syndrome)
8. Syncope in patients with advanced structural heart disease in which thorough invasive and noninvasive investigation has failed to define a cause

Contraindications
1. Syncope of undetermined cause in a patient without inducible VT and without structural heart disease
2. Incessant VT or VF
3. VF or VT resulting from arrhythmias amenable to surgical or catheter ablation
4. Ventricular tachyarrhythmias due to a transient or reversible disorder
5. Significant psychiatric illnesses
6. Terminal illnesses with projected life expectancy 6 months
7. Patients with CAD, LV dysfunction, and prolonged QRS duration in the absence of spontaneous or inducible VT who are undergoing coronary bypass surgery
8. NYHA Class IV drug–refractory CHF in patients not candidates for transplantation

CAD, coronary artery disease; CHF, congestive heart failure; EP, electrophysiologic; LV, left ventricular; MI, myocardial infarction; NYHA, New York Heart Association; VF, ventricular fibrillation; VT, ventricular tachycardia.

*A Class I indication refers to a condition for which there is evidence that defibrillator therapy is beneficial. A Class II indication refers to a condition for which there is conflicting evidence and/or a divergence of opinion.

Adapted from Hayes RA, et. al. ACC/AHA/NASPE 2002 guideline update for implantation of cardiac devices: summary article: a report of the American College of Cardiology/American Heart Association Task Force on Practical Guidelines (ACC/AHA/NASPE committee to update the 1998 pacemaker guidelines)

The use of defibrillators for primary prevention of sudden death remains controversial. Certain cardiac conditions are associated with a high risk of cardiac arrest. However, it is not clear at this time how high that risk needs to be to justify implantation of a costly device.

Patients with nonsustained ventricular tachycardia and prior myocardial infarction represent a group at high risk for sudden death. Previously, these patients were treated with antiarrhythmic drugs to suppress ventricular ectopy in an attempt to reduce the likelihood of sustained ventricular tachycardia. However, trials such as Cardiac Arrhythmia Suppression Trial (CAST) found that pharmacologic therapy with sodium channel blockers resulted in a higher mortality rate than did placebo (22). Empirical amiodarone for patients with an ischemic cardiomyopathy and for patients who have suffered a recent myocardial infarction may reduce the likelihood of a cardiac-related death but has not been shown to reduce overall mortality rates (23–25). Defibrillator therapy is currently recommended for patients with coronary artery disease, impaired ventricular function, asymptomatic nonsustained ventricular tachycardia, and sustained ventricular tachycardia that is inducible with programmed stimulation (4).

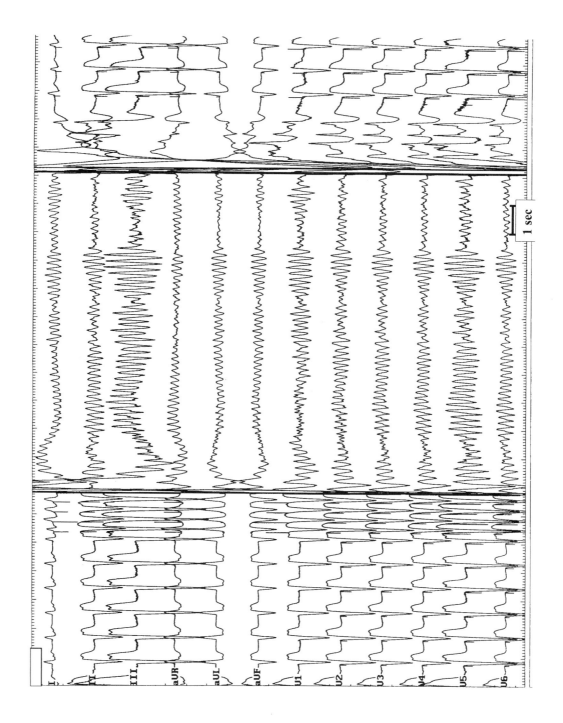

1 sec

For patients with nonischemic dilated cardiomyopathy and nonsustained ventricular tachycardia, results of some trials have suggested a reduction in mortality with amiodarone. The AMIOdarone Versus Implantable defibrillator Trial (AMIOVIRT) found that patients with dilated cardiomyopathy and nonsustained ventricular tachycardia have comparable mortality rates when treated with either amiodarone or a defibrillator (26).

Defibrillator therapy should also be considered for primary prevention of sudden death in patients with congenital LQTS associated with syncope and those with hypertrophic cardiomyopathy associated with syncope, family history of sudden death, or severe hypertrophy.

Studies are currently being conducted to determine whether defibrillator therapy reduces overall mortality rate among patients who have moderate to severe ventricular dysfunction in the absence of any other high-risk features (27). The MADIT II study recently found that defibrillator therapy was associated with a 30% reduction in mortality for patients with prior myocardial infarction and a left ventricular ejection fraction < 0.30 (27.5). Primary prevention of sudden death requires efforts to reduce coronary artery disease and control hypertension, identification of high-risk patients, improved therapy for congestive heart failure, and improvements in public access to defibrillation.

Currently available implantable transvenous defibrillators can be implanted by an electrophysiologist into the pectoral position, are as small as 32 cc, are fully programmable, provide retrievable intracardiac electrograms, are capable of dual-chamber pacing and antitachycardia pacing, and can deliver a 30-joule biphasic shock within 10 seconds of the beginning of fibrillation (28).

Catheter ablation is a treatment option for some patients who have sustained monomorphic ventricular tachycardia. Ideal candidates for ablation are patients with idiopathic ventricular tachycardia (29) or bundle branch reentry. Catheter ablation is also effective in patients with prior myocardial infarction (30,31) but is rarely used as sole therapy. In general, ventricular tachycardias must be hemodynamically tolerated in order to be treated with catheter ablation, because mapping is usually performed during tachycardia. However, newer techniques are available for the ablation of poorly tolerated ventricular tachycardia (32). Ablation is useful as adjunctive therapy for patients who have experienced multiple defibrillator therapies (33).

PROGNOSIS AND FOLLOW-UP

Most patients with ventricular tachycardia have underlying structural heart disease, and their prognosis is closely related to the severity of ventricular dysfunction (34). One study of defibrillator recipients found that the number of fixed nuclear perfusion defects was the only independent predictor of mortality (35). Patients with idiopathic ventricular tachycardia generally have a good prognosis.

Patients with implantable defibrillators require careful follow-up to assess the battery status, integrity of leads, and stability of defibrillation energy requirements. Support groups are beneficial for this group of patients (36). Patients receiving long-term amiodarone need surveillance testing to monitor for organ toxicity, including thyroid and liver function tests every 6 months and a chest radiograph every 6 to 12 months (37). A baseline ophthalmologic examination is also recommended. More frequent assessment is indicated if symptoms develop.

FIG. 18.12. Twelve-lead rhythm strip recorded during testing of an implantable defibrillator. The initial rhythm is atrial fibrillation with ventricular pacing. The device induces ventricular fibrillation by delivering four ventricular pacing stimuli, followed by a low-energy shock that is synchronous with the T wave. The defibrillator detects the tachycardia, charges the capacitors, and delivers a 21-joule biphasic shock. The shock successfully defibrillates the patient but is initially followed by four beats of polymorphic ventricular tachycardia.

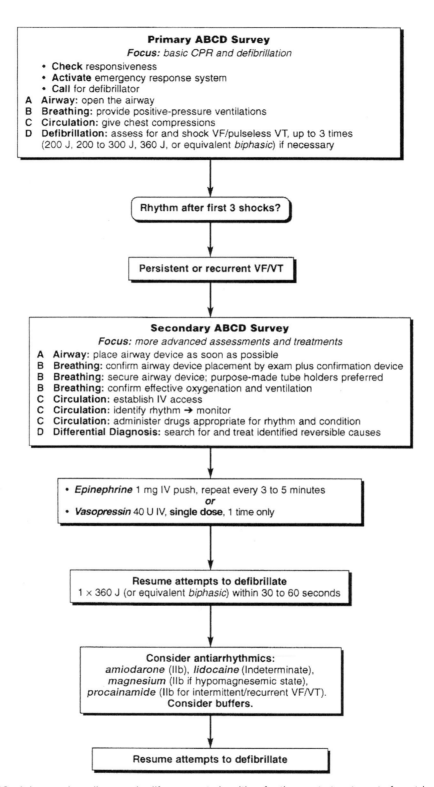

FIG. 18.13. Advanced cardiovascular life support algorithm for the acute treatment of ventricular fibrillation or pulseless ventricular tachycardia. (From Guidelines 2000 for Cardiopulmonary Resuscitation and Emergency Cardiovascular Care. *Circulation* 2000;102(Suppl):I1–I384.)

PRACTICAL POINTS

- Ventricular tachycardia is defined as three or more consecutive ventricular complexes at a rate greater than 100 beats per minute.
- A ventricular arrhythmia is considered sustained when intervention is required for termination, when it results in symptoms, or when it lasts longer than 30 seconds.
- Ventricular tachycardia usually occurs in patients with underlying structural heart disease
- Patients with significant ventricular dysfunction are at increased risk of dying

suddenly and should undergo further evaluation.
- The most useful test in a patient with a sustained ventricular tachycardia is an electrocardiogram.
- Electrophysiologic testing has no value in the risk stratification of patients with a nonischemic cardiomyopathy.
- The acute management of a patient with a ventricular tachyarrhythmia should follow the ACLS guidelines.
- Long-term management of patients with ventricular tachyarrhythmias includes drug therapy, device therapy, and ablation.

REFERENCES

1. Zang L, Timothy KW, Vincent GM, et al. Spectrum of ST–T-wave patterns and repolarization parameters in congenital long-QT syndrome. ECG findings identify genotype. *Circulation* 2000;102:2849–2855.
2. Brugada J, Brugada R, Brugada P. Right bundle-branch block and ST-segment elevation in leads V1 through V3: a marker for sudden death in patients without demonstrable structural heart disease. *Circulation* 1998;97:457–460.
3. Buxton AE, Lee KL, Fisher JD, et al. A randomized study of the prevention of sudden death in patients with coronary artery disease. Multicenter Unsustained Tachycardia Trial. *N Engl J Med* 1999;341:1882–1890.
4. Moss AJ, Hall WJ, Cannom DS, et al. Improved survival with an implanted defibrillator in patients with coronary disease at high risk for ventricular arrhythmia. *N Engl J Med* 1996;335:1933–1940.
5. Buxton AE, Lee KL, DiCarlo L, et al. Electrophysiologic testing to identify patients with coronary artery disease who are at risk for sudden death. Multicenter Unsustained Tachycardia Trial Investigators. *N Engl J Med* 2000;342:1937–1945.
6. Knight BP, Pelosi F, Michaud GF, et al. Clinical consequences of electrocardiographic artifact mimicking ventricular tachycardia. *N Engl J Med* 1999;341:1270–1274.
7. Baerman JM, Morady F, DiCarlo LA Jr, et al. Differentiation of ventricular tachycardia from supraventricular tachycardia with aberration: value of the clinical history. *Ann Emerg Med* 1987;16:40–43.
8. Morady F, Baerman JM, DiCarlo LA Jr, et al. A prevalent misconception regarding wide-complex tachycardias. *JAMA* 1985;254:2790–2792.
9. Brugada P, Brugada J, Mont L, et al. A new approach to the differential diagnosis of a regular tachycardia with a wide QRS complex. *Circulation* 1991;83:1649–1659.
10. Knight BP, Zivin A, Souza J, et al. Use of adenosine in patients hospitalized in a university medical center. *Am J Med* 1998;105:275–280.
11. Kron J, Herre J, Renfroe GE, et al., for the AVID Investigators. Lead- and device-related complications in the Antiarrhythmics Versus Implantable Defibrillators trial. *Am Heart J* 2001;141:92–98.
12. Guidelines 2000 for Cardiopulmonary Resuscitation and Emergency Cardiovascular Care. *Circulation* 2000;102(Suppl):I1–I384.
13. Kowey PR, Levine JH, Herre JM, et al. Randomized, double-blind comparison of intravenous amiodarone and bretylium in the treatment of patients with recurrent, hemodynamically destabilizing ventricular tachycardia or fibrillation. The Intravenous Amiodarone Multicenter Investigators Group. *Circulation* 1995;92:3255–3263.
14. Kudenchuk PJ, Cobb LA, Copass MK, et al. Amiodarone for resuscitation after out-of-hospital cardiac arrest due to ventricular fibrillation. *N Engl J Med* 1999;341:871–878.
15. Mittal S, Ayati S, Stein KM, et al. Comparison of a novel rectilinear biphasic waveform with a damped sine wave monophasic waveform for transthoracic ventricular defibrillation. ZOLL Investigators. *J Am Coll Cardiol* 1999;34:1595–1601.
16. Kerber RE, Becker LB, Bourland JD, et al. Automatic external defibrillators for public access defibrillation: recommendations for specifying and reporting arrhythmia analysis algorithm performance, incorporating new waveforms, and enhancing safety. A statement for health professionals from the American Heart Association Task Force on Automatic External Defibrillation, Subcommittee on AED Safety and Efficacy. *Circulation* 1997;95:1677–1682.
17. Anderson JL, Hallstrom AP, Epstein AE, et al. Design

and results of the antiarrhythmics vs. implantable defibrillators (AVID) registry. The AVID Investigators. *Circulation* 1999;99:1692–1699.

18. A comparison of antiarrhythmic-drug therapy with implantable defibrillators in patients resuscitated from near-fatal ventricular arrhythmias. The Antiarrhythmics versus Implantable Defibrillators (AVID) Investigators. *N Engl J Med* 1997;337:1576–1583.

19. Connolly SJ, Gent M, Roberts RS, et al. Canadian implantable defibrillator study (CIDS): a randomized trial of the implantable cardioverter defibrillator against amiodarone. *Circulation* 2000;101:1297–1302.

20. Kuck KH, Cappato R, Siebels J, et al. Randomized comparison of antiarrhythmic drug therapy with implantable defibrillators in patients resuscitated from cardiac arrest: the Cardiac Arrest Study Hamburg (CASH). *Circulation* 2000;102:748–754.

21. Gregoratos G, Abrams J, Epstein AE, et. al. ACC/AHA/NASPE 2002. Guidelines update for implantation of cardiac pacemakers and antiarrhythmia devices: summary article: a report of the American College of Cardiology/American Heart Association Task Force on Practical Guidelines (ACC/AHA/NASPE commitee to update the 1998 pacemaker guidelines). *Circulation.* 2002;106:2145–2161.

22. Echt DS, Liebson PR, Mitchell LB, et al. Mortality and morbidity in patients receiving encainide, flecainide, or placebo. The Cardiac Arrhythmia Suppression Trial. *N Engl J Med* 1991;324:781–788.

23. Singh SN, Fletcher RD, Fisher SG, et al. Amiodarone in patients with congestive heart failure and asymptomatic ventricular arrhythmia. Survival Trial of Antiarrhythmic Therapy in Congestive Heart Failure. *N Engl J Med* 1995;333:77–82.

24. Julian DG, Camm AJ, Frangin G, et al. Randomized trial of effect of amiodarone on mortality in patients with left-ventricular dysfunction after recent myocardial infarction: EMIAT. European Myocardial Infarct Amiodarone Trial Investigators. *Lancet* 1997;349:667–674.

25. Cairns JA, Connolly SJ, Roberts R, et al. Randomised trial of outcome after myocardial infarction in patients with frequent or repetitive ventricular premature depolarisations: CAMIAT. Canadian Amiodarone Myocardial Infarction Arrhythmia Trial Investigators. *Lancet* 1997;349:675–682.

26. Strickberger SA. *AMIOVIRT (Amiodarone vs. Implantable defibrillator in patients with nonischemic cardiomyopathy and asymptomatic nonsustained ventricular tachycardia).* Presented at the Clinical Trials Results Session of the Scientific Sessions of the American Heart Association, November 15, 2000.

27. Klein H, Auricchio A, Reek S, et al. New primary prevention trials of sudden cardiac death in patients with left ventricular dysfunction: SCD-HEFT and MADIT-II. *Am J Cardiol* 1999;83:91D–97D.

27.5. Moss AJ, Zareba W, Hall WJ, et. al. For the multicenter automatic defibrillator in patients with myocardial infarction and reduced ejection fraction. *N Engl J Med* 2002;346:877–883.

28. Strickberger SA, Hummel JD, Daoud E, et al. Implantation by electrophysiologists of 100 consecutive cardioverter defibrillators with nonthoracotomy lead systems. *Circulation* 1994;90:868–872.

29. Flemming MA, Oral H, Kim MH, et al. Electrocardiographic predictors of successful ablation of tachycardia or bigeminy arising in the right ventricular outflow tract. *Am J Cardiol* 1999;84:1266–1268.

30. Morady F, Harvey M, Kalbfleisch SJ, et al. Radiofrequency catheter ablation of ventricular tachycardia in patients with coronary artery disease. *Circulation* 1993;87:363–372.

31. Bogun F, Bahu M, Knight BP, et al. Comparison of effective and ineffective target sites that demonstrate concealed entrainment in patients with coronary artery disease undergoing radiofrequency ablation of ventricular tachycardia. *Circulation* 1997;95:183–190.

32. Strickberger SA, Michaud GF, et al. Mapping and ablation of ventricular tachycardia guided by virtual electrograms using a noncontact, computerized mapping system. *J Am Coll Cardiol* 2000;35:414–421.

33. Strickberger SA, Man KC, Daoud EG, et al. A prospective evaluation of catheter ablation of ventricular tachycardia as adjuvant therapy in patients with coronary artery disease and an implantable cardioverter-defibrillator. *Circulation* 1997;96:1525–1531.

34. Kim SG, Fisher JD, Choue CW, et al. Influence of left ventricular function on outcome of patients treated with implantable defibrillators. *Circulation* 1992;85:1304–1310.

35. Gioia G, Bagheri B, Gottlieb CD, et al. Prediction of outcome of patients with life-threatening ventricular arrhythmias treated with automatic implantable cardioverter-defibrillators using SPECT perfusion imaging. *Circulation* 1997;95:390–394.

36. Dickerson SS, Posluszny M, Kennedy MC. Help seeking in a support group for recipients of implantable cardioverter defibrillators and their support persons. *Heart Lung* 2000;29:87–96.

37. Goldschlager N, Epstein AE, Naccarelli G, et al. Practical guidelines for clinicians who treat patients with amiodarone. Practice guidelines. *Arch Intern Med* 2000;160:1741–1748.

19

Bradycardia

Bradley P. Knight and William H. Kou

USUAL CAUSES OF BRADYCARDIA

Causes of bradycardia can be divided into intrinsic and extrinsic causes and are listed in Table 19.1. Because the cardiac conduction system is composed of specialized cardiac myocytes, common myocardial diseases such as ischemia, infarction, hypertension, surgical trauma, degeneration due to age, and dilated cardiomyopathies can result in bradycardia. Less common pathologic causes of bradycardia include infiltrative disorders, collagen vascular diseases, familial conduction system diseases, and infections such as endocarditis or Lyme disease. Part of the atrioventricular conduction system is a narrow electrical corridor without redundancy. Therefore, a small pathologic lesion can result in profound bradycardia. Occasionally, bradycardia is caused by idiopathic degeneration of the conduction tissue. Bradycardia can also be a result of intentional or unintentional catheter ablation of the sinus node or atrioventricular junction.

Congenital heart block tends to occur in children of women with autoimmune diseases and results from transplacental transfer of maternal anti-Ro and/or anti-La antibodies. Sinus bradycardia may be associated with congenital complete heart block (1).

Extrinsic causes of bradycardia include hypervagotonia, drugs, hypoxemia, central nervous system disease, thyroid disease, and electrolyte abnormalities. Sleep is normally accompanied by marked bradycardia, especially in young patients. One report added partial complex seizures to the long list of functional causes of bradycardia (2).

An abnormal increase in vagal tone is responsible for the bradycardia seen during vasodepressor syncope, carotid sinus hypersensitivity, and cough and micturition syncope, although adrenergic withdrawal can also be a factor. Careful identification of reversible causes can lead to prevention of unnecessary therapy. For example, tracheostomy can correct the bradycardia associated with sleep apnea (3).

PRESENTING SYMPTOMS AND SIGNS

Patients with bradycardia have a broad spectrum of symptoms and signs. Because symptoms are usually nonspecific, it is important to be as certain as possible that the symptoms are secondary to bradycardia. Patients with persistent bradycardia can present with symptoms that progress gradually, such as fatigue, dizziness or exercise intolerance, or can present with symptoms that occur suddenly, such as syncope, congestive heart failure, or cardiac arrest. Patients with paroxysmal bradycardia usually present with palpitations, dizzy spells, presyncope, syncope, or seizures, depending on the escape rhythm and the degree of cerebral perfusion during the bradycardia. Many patients with bradycardia are asymptomatic.

Bradycardia is often accompanied by a bounding pulse and a large pulse pressure. When complete heart block is present, the physical examination can reveal signs of atrioventricular dissociation such as cannon A waves in the neck veins and variable atrioventricular valve closure sounds. In affected elderly patients, confusion is occasionally the sole manifestation of bradycardia.

HELPFUL TESTS

Proper characterization of a bradycardia often helps identify the cause. For example, transient atrioventricular block that occurs at the same time as transient sinus slowing is diagnostic

TABLE 19.1. *Causes of bradycardia*

Intrinsic causes
  Coronary artery disease
  Hypertensive heart disease
  Dilated cardiomyopathy
  Infiltrative diseases
  Collagen vascular diseases
  Surgical trauma
  Catheter ablation
  Infections
  Genetic conduction diseases
  Idiopathic degeneration
Extrinsic causes
  Drugs
  Neurocardiogenic syncope
  Increased vagal tone
  Carotid sinus hypersensitivity
  Hypothyroidism
  Neurologic disorders
  Hyperkalemia

of a vagal cause and does not require further evaluation. However, when an intrinsic cause is suspected, further testing is usually warranted, to exclude underlying structural heart disease.

An electrocardiographic recording is necessary to establish a diagnosis of bradycardia. Simple palpation of the pulse can lead to an erroneous diagnosis of bradycardia in the setting of atrial or ventricular bigeminy. A 12-lead electrocardiogram should be obtained for all patients with symptoms suggestive of bradycardia.

For patients with daily symptoms suggestive of bradycardia, an ambulatory Holter monitor can be helpful for characterizing the rhythm. For patients with less frequent symptoms, a continuous-loop recorder collects data better than does a Holter monitor. Continuous-loop recorders can be worn for several weeks and can be used to transmit a rhythm strip over the phone after a patient has symptoms (4). An implantable loop recorder is also available for patients who have infrequent symptoms but is usually reserved for patients with recurrent, unexplained syncope (5).

A formal exercise treadmill test can be helpful in establishing a diagnosis of chronotropic incompetence. However, a simple recording of the cardiac rhythm before and immediately after a short walk or stair climbing is often sufficient and saves the expense of formal exercise testing.

Maneuvers or medications that increase the sinus rate, such as ambulation or atropine, are useful tests in the setting of second-degree atrioventricular block. If the atrioventricular block worsens when the sinus rate increases, the conduction block is usually pathologic, related to an intrinsic abnormality of the His-Purkinje system.

Electrophysiologic testing can be useful in the evaluation of patients with symptoms suggestive of bradycardia (6). Measurement of the sinus node recovery time—the time between cessation of rapid atrial pacing and the first spontaneous atrial depolarization from sinus node—is a useful test of sinus node function. Intracardiac recordings are valuable in patients with atrioventricular block when the surface electrocardiogram is not sufficient to determine the level of block. Intracardiac His bundle recordings can reveal whether atrioventricular block is at or below the level of the atrioventricular node. If the level of atrioventricular block is below the atrioventricular node, placement of a pacemaker is often indicated. Early studies suggested that electrophysiologic testing should be performed in patients with bundle branch block to determine whether the patient is at risk for developing higher degree atrioventricular block (7). However, the predictive value in this setting is low. Therefore, electrophysiologic testing is currently not indicated for the evaluation of asymptomatic patients with isolated bundle branch block.

Patients with unexplained syncope and bundle branch block should undergo electrophysiologic testing to exclude inducible ventricular tachycardia before paroxysmal bradycardia is assumed to be the cause of syncope, especially in the setting of left ventricular dysfunction (8).

DIFFERENTIAL DIAGNOSIS

Bradyarrhythmias can be categorized as those caused by dysfunction of the sinus node and those caused by dysfunction of the atrioventricular conduction system. The characteristics of each bradyarrhythmia are described in the following sections. Proper characterization of the bradyarrhythmia is important because it helps determine the cause, prognosis, and treatment.

Tissues that constitute the cardiac conduction system have the ability to depolarize spontaneously. The intrinsic spontaneous rate of depolarization usually decreases in the anatomic direction of normal impulse propagation. The dominant pacemaker normally arises from within the sinus node complex and suppresses spontaneous depolarization of the distal conduction tissue. During bradycardia, these latent pacemaker cells are unmasked and give rise to the dominant rhythm. Escape beats and rhythms are also described as follows.

Sinus Node Dysfunction

Abnormal sinus node function can result from abnormal automaticity or from sinus node exit block, and it manifests as sinus bradycardia, sinus pauses, or chronotropic incompetence. Sinus node dysfunction is often referred to as sick sinus syndrome and is the most common indication for a pacemaker. Patients with sinus node dysfunction often have associated atrial disease, which results in atrial tachyarrhythmias. This common association is referred to as the *tachycardia-bradycardia syndrome.*

Sinus Bradycardia

Sinus bradycardia is defined as a sinus rhythm with a rate less than 60 beats per minute (bpm) (Figs. 19.1, 19.2). The traditional cutoff rate of 60 bpm is arbitrary, and many asymptomatic persons with heart rates below 60 bpm should not be considered abnormal. Some authors have argued that sinus rhythm rates as low as 46 bpm in men and 51 in women should be considered normal (9). Young patients and trained athletes often have marked sinus bradycardia because of elevated vagal tone. Sinus bradycardia is also observed normally during sleep.

Sinus Pause

A sinus pause is present when the length of a pause is not a multiple of the baseline sinus cycle length (Fig. 19.3). In contrast, sinoatrial (SA) exit block is diagnosed when there is a pause and the length of the pause is equal to a multiple of the

baseline sinus cycle length. As with atrioventricular blocks, SA block can be categorized as first-, second-, or third-degree block. First-degree SA block is caused by a delay in transmission of SA depolarization to the atrial tissue and can be diagnosed only with specialized intracardiac recordings. Second-degree SA block is manifested as a sinus pause and results from intermittent failure of conduction from the sinus node to the surrounding atrial muscle. Second-degree SA block can be categorized in the Wenckebach classification system as type I or type II. Type I SA block is manifested as gradual shortening of the sinus cycle length followed by a pause that is not equal to the preceding PP interval (Fig. 19.4). Type II SA block is characterized by a constant sinus cycle length followed by a sinus pause that is equal to the preceding PP interval. High-grade SA block is present when the pause is equal to a multiple of the preceding PP interval.

An excessively long pause is often called *sinus arrest* and can be caused by third-degree SA exit block or decreased automaticity (Fig. 19.5).

Chronotropic Incompetence

Chronotropic incompetence is present when the heart rate does not increase sufficiently with exertion. It can be considered relative bradycardia. There are several proposed definitions for chronotropic incompetence, including failure to reach a heart rate that is either 85% of, or two standard deviations below, the age-predicted maximum heart rate (220 bpm minus years of age). However, patients who have clinically relevant chronotropic incompetence usually demonstrate an obvious inability to increase the heart rate appropriately with activity.

Atrioventricular Conduction Disturbances

Atrioventricular block can occur at the level of the atrioventricular node, within the His bundle, or distal to the His bundle. Atrioventricular block can also be a result of intraatrial conduction block, in which case the sinus node impulse does not reach the atrioventricular node, but this is rare. Atrioventricular block is categorized as first-, second-, or third-degree. Identification of

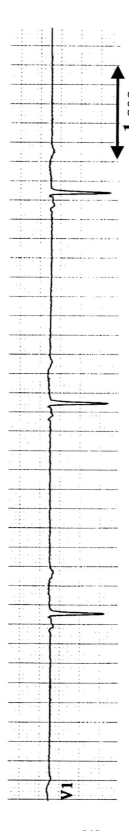

FIG. 19.1. Rhythm strip from lead V₁, showing marked sinus bradycardia. The sinus rate is 27 beats per minute.

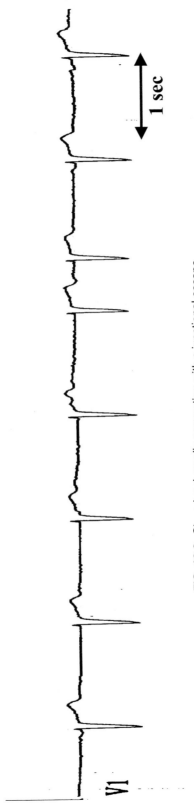

FIG. 19.2. Sinus bradycardia competing with a junctional escape.

313

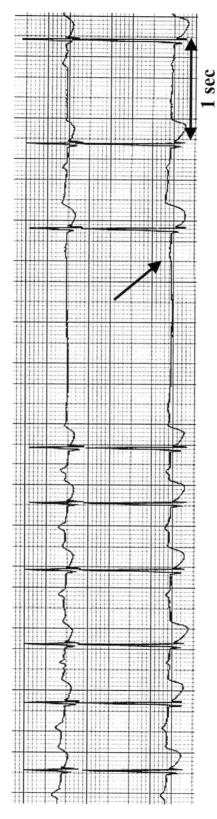

FIG. 19.3. Two-lead rhythm strip of a sinus pause with an atrial escape beat. Note that the morphologic pattern of the first P wave after the sinus pause differs from the sinus P waves (*arrow*).

1 sec

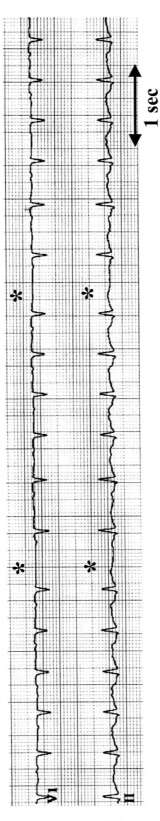

FIG. 19.4. Rhythm strip from leads V$_1$ and II of second-degree, type I sinoatrial exit block. Note the progressive shortening in the PP interval, followed by a sinus pause (*asterisk*). The duration of the sinus pause is less than twice the sinus cycle length. The pattern repeats itself.

315

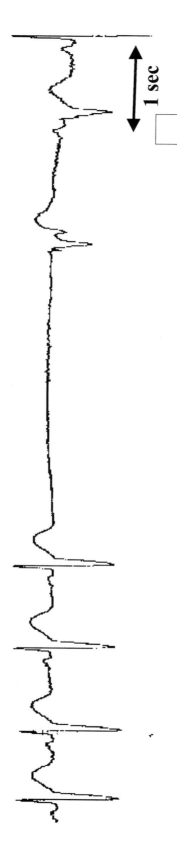

FIG. 19.5. Sinus arrest. There is a ventricular escape beat before the sinus rhythm recovers.

the level and type of block is important, because they are related to the prognosis and therapy.

The atrioventricular conduction system serves to prevent rapid atrial rhythms from conducting to the ventricle on a 1:1 basis. Therefore, pathologic atrioventricular block must be distinguished from atrioventricular block that results from normal refractoriness (Fig. 19.6).

First-Degree Atrioventricular Block

First-degree atrioventricular block itself does not result in bradycardia but is often associated with other bradycardic rhythms and may be a precursor of higher degree atrioventricular block. First-degree atrioventricular block is caused by conduction delay from the atrium to the ventricle and is manifested as a prolonged PR interval (more than 200 milliseconds in the adult). The level of conduction delay is usually within the atrioventricular node but can be lower in the conduction system. An associated bundle branch block suggests that the first-degree atrioventricular block is caused by conduction delay below the atrioventricular node (Fig. 19.7). In rare instances, patients with dual atrioventricular nodal pathways can have a prolonged PR interval when atrioventricular conduction occurs via the "slow" atrioventricular nodal pathway (Fig. 19.8).

Second-Degree Atrioventricular Block

Second-degree atrioventricular block is present when there is intermittent failure of atrioventricular conduction, and it can be categorized as Mobitz type I (Wenckebach) or Mobitz type II atrioventricular block. The names Mobitz and Wenckebach continue to be used to describe the types of second-degree atrioventricular block. Karel Frederik Wenckebach, using arterial and jugular venous pressure recordings, first described type I atrioventricular block in 1899 (10). John Hay, also using pressure recordings, reported a patient with type II atrioventricular block in 1906 (11). Woldemar Mobitz used electrocardiographic recordings to classify the two types of atrioventricular block (12).

During sinus rhythm with type I atrioventricular block, there is progressive prolongation of the PR interval before atrioventricular block (Fig. 19.9). Although the PR interval gradually lengthens with each sinus beat, the amount by which the PR interval lengthens with each sinus beat actually decreases. Therefore, in classic Wenckebach atrioventricular block, the RR interval progressively decreases before atrioventricular block. This pattern often repeats itself and results in so-called grouped beating. However, this classic atrioventricular Wenckebach pattern is present in fewer than half of Wenckebach atrioventricular blocks. In the absence of progressive prolongation of the PR interval, a diagnosis of Wenckebach atrioventricular block can be made when the PR interval of the first conducted beat is shorter than the PR interval of the last conducted beat before the block. During type II atrioventricular block, the PR interval remains constant before and after atrioventricular block (Fig. 19.10).

Type I atrioventricular block is a more benign conduction disturbance than is type II and usually does not necessitate pacemaker therapy. Wenckebach atrioventricular block is usually caused by block in the atrioventricular node secondary to increased vagal tone, but in rare instances, it can occur in the His-Purkinje system. Because type II atrioventricular block is usually associated with conduction system disease, it tends to be progressive and to necessitate pacemaker therapy. The presence of a bundle branch block is suggestive of type II atrioventricular block. Type I atrioventricular block occurs more commonly during inferior myocardial infarction, is transient, and does not require temporary pacing, whereas type II atrioventricular block occurs more commonly during anterior myocardial infarction, necessitates pacing, and is associated with a high rate of mortality.

When 2:1 atrioventricular block is present, two consecutive PR intervals are not available for comparison (Figs. 19.11, 19.12). Distinguishing atrioventricular nodal block from His-Purkinje block may not be straightforward in this situation. Clues that suggest that the level of block is in the atrioventricular node include a narrow QRS complex and prolonged PR interval during the conducted beats, slowing of the sinus rate during atrioventricular block, and documented Wenckebach block when lower degree atrioventricular

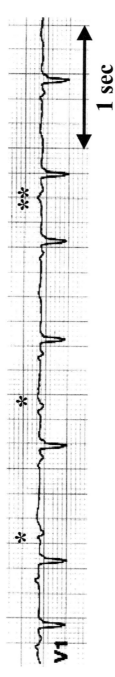

FIG. 19.6. Sinus rhythm with premature atrial depolarizations that result in atrioventricular block when the coupling interval is short (*asterisk*) but are conducted to the ventricle when the coupling interval is longer (*double asterisk*). This is an example of functional, nonpathologic atrioventricular block.

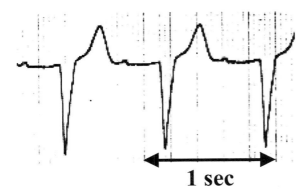

1 sec

FIG. 19.7. First-degree atrioventricular block. The PR interval is 280 milliseconds long, and there is an associated left bundle branch block.

block is present (Figs. 19.13, 19.14). When two or more consecutive P waves fail to be conducted to the ventricle, high-grade atrioventricular block is present. The same clues during 2:1 atrioventricular block can help determine the level of block during high-grade atrioventricular block.

Complete Atrioventricular Block

Third-degree, or complete, atrioventricular block occurs when no atrial activity is conducted to the ventricles. During complete heart block, atrioventricular dissociation is present, and the ventricular escape rhythm is slower than the atrial rhythm (Figs. 19.15, 19.16). Isorhythmic atrioventricular dissociation is a rare arrhythmia that occurs when two independent atrial and ventricular foci discharge at a similar rate, and it is characterized by a P wave that migrates in and out of the QRS complexes with successive beats (Fig. 19.17). Either slowing of the dominant atrial pacemaker or acceleration of a subsidiary junctional or ventricular pacemaker results in this rhythm. Common causes include increased vagal tone and medications. It may be difficult to determine whether atrioventricular conduction is intact.

Escape Rhythms

Escape beats and rhythms that are associated with bradycardias arise from the atrium (Fig. 19.3), the atrioventricular junction (Figs. 19.2, 19.15), and the ventricle (Figs. 19.5, 19.14, 19.16). The escape rhythm usually arises from conduction

tissue just below the level of block. Therefore, block in the atrioventricular node is usually associated with a narrow ventricular escape rhythm between 40 and 60 bpm that is responsive to autonomic tone, whereas block in the His-Purkinje system is usually associated with a wide ventricular escape rhythm less than 40 bpm. Occasionally, there is no escape rhythm, and asystole is present.

COMPLICATIONS

Complications associated with bradycardia include syncope, physical injury, cardiac arrest, bradycardia-dependent ventricular tachycardia, and complications from pacemaker therapy. Early pacemaker complications include bleeding, pneumothorax, cardiac perforation, and brachial plexus injury. Long-term complications related to pacing therapy include infection, venous thrombosis, skin erosion, device migration, and lead failure. The weakest link in the pacing system is the leads, because they are susceptible to insulation failure and conductor fracture. Pacemaker generator failure is rare, but premature battery depletion does occur.

THERAPY

The management of bradycardia can be divided into acute and long-term management.

Acute Management

When patients present with bradycardia that is associated with serious signs and symptoms, the

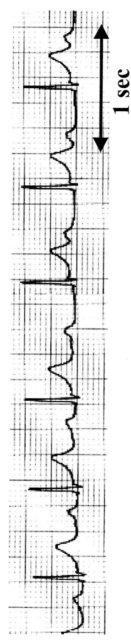

FIG. 19.8. Rhythm strip obtained from a patient who had just been laid supine from a sitting position. The first three PR intervals are normal. Then the PR interval increases to approximately 400 milliseconds. This tracing can be explained by the presence of dual atrioventricular nodal pathways.

1 sec

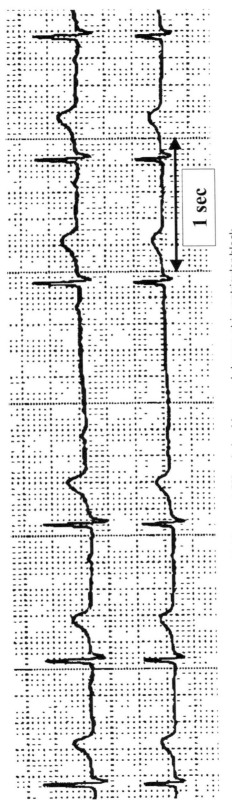

FIG. 19.9. Mobitz type I (Wenckebach) second-degree atrioventricular block.

321

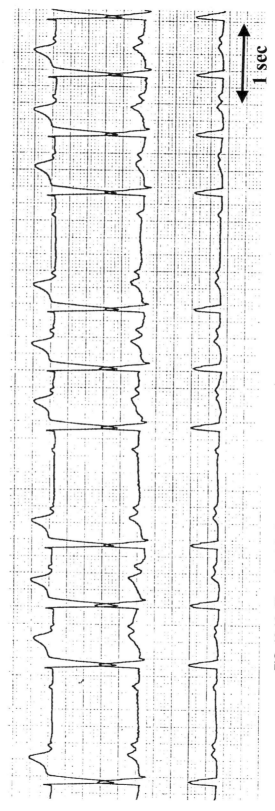

FIG. 19.10. Three-lead rhythm strip of Mobitz type II, second-degree atrioventricular block. There is a constant PR interval before the block sinus beats. The PR interval is prolonged with the conducted beats, and there is an intraventricular conduction delay.

322

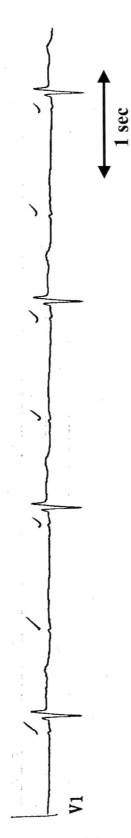

FIG. 19.11. Rhythm strip from lead V$_1$ showing 2:1 atrioventricular block. The slow sinus rate and narrow QRS complex suggest that the level of atrioventricular block is within the atrioventricular node.

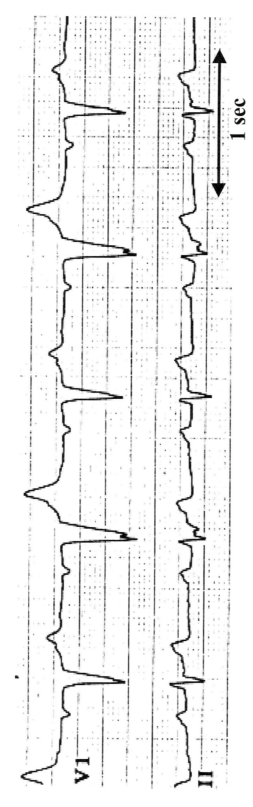

FIG. 19.12. Rhythm strip from lead V_1 showing 2:1 atrioventricular block. The alternating QRS morphologic pattern is consistent with alternating degrees of left bundle branch block and suggests that the level of atrioventricular block is within the His-Purkinje conduction system.

324

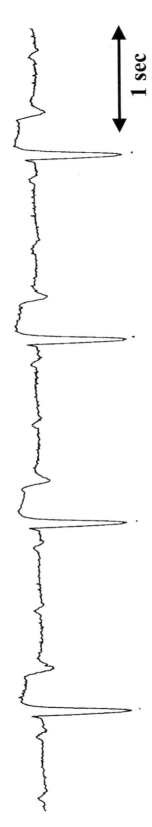

FIG. 19.13. High-grade atrioventricular block with a 3:1 conduction ratio.

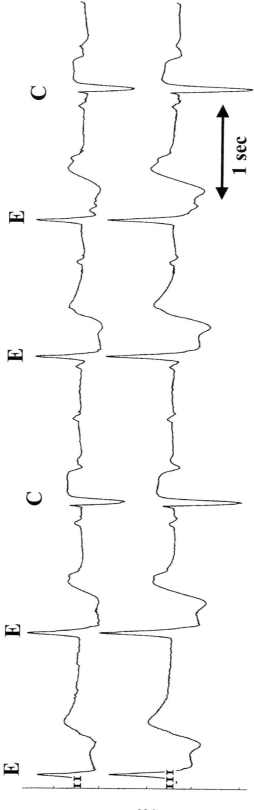

FIG. 19.14. Sinus tachycardia and high-grade atrioventricular block. The morphologic pattern of the conducted beats (C) differs from that of the ventricular escape beats (E).

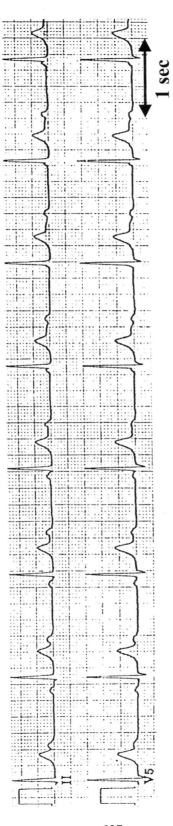

FIG. 19.15. Rhythm strip from leads II and V₅ showing third-degree atrioventricular block with a junctional escape. There is atrioventricular dissociation.

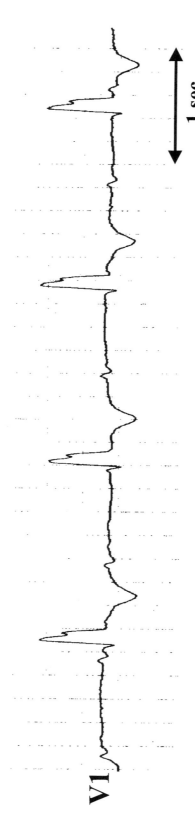

FIG. 19.16. Third-degree atrioventricular block with a ventricular escape. There is atrioventricular dissociation.

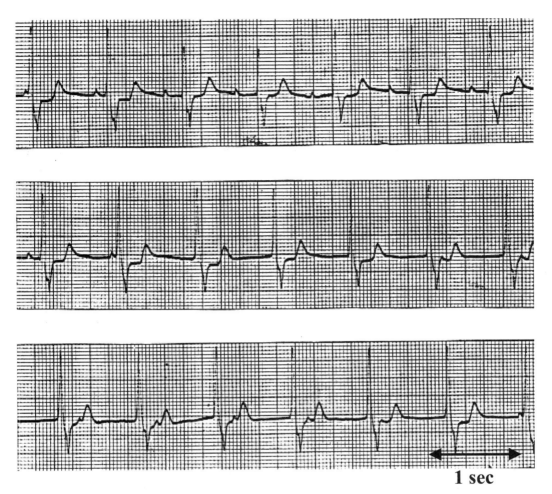

FIG. 19.17. Continuous rhythm strip showing isorhythmic atrioventricular dissociation. The atrial rate is slightly variable and competing with a fixed junctional rhythm. The result is a P wave that migrates in and out of the QRS complexes with successive beats. Atrioventricular conduction is probably intact because the third RR interval is approximately 40 milliseconds shorter than the other RR intervals.

acute management should follow the Advanced Cardiovascular Life Support (ACLS) guidelines (Fig. 19.18). Atropine at a dose of 0.5 to 1.0 mg should be administered in most cases. However, in some situations, atropine may worsen the bradycardia. When there is intermittent atrioventricular block below the atrioventricular node, atropine can increase the sinus rate and result in higher-grade atrioventricular block and, therefore, a slower ventricular rate. Dopamine and epinephrine can be used in refractory cases of symptomatic bradycardia associated with hy-

potension. Isoproterenol is a strong positive chronotropic agent but is no longer included in the ACLS algorithm because of its potential for causing cardiac ischemia. Reversible causes of bradycardia should be identified and corrected.

A temporary transvenous pacemaker should be inserted as soon as possible in patients with bradycardia who continue to be symptomatic despite pharmacologic therapy. Transcutaneous pacing has the advantage of being applied quickly at the bedside, in comparison with transvenous pacing, and is available in most

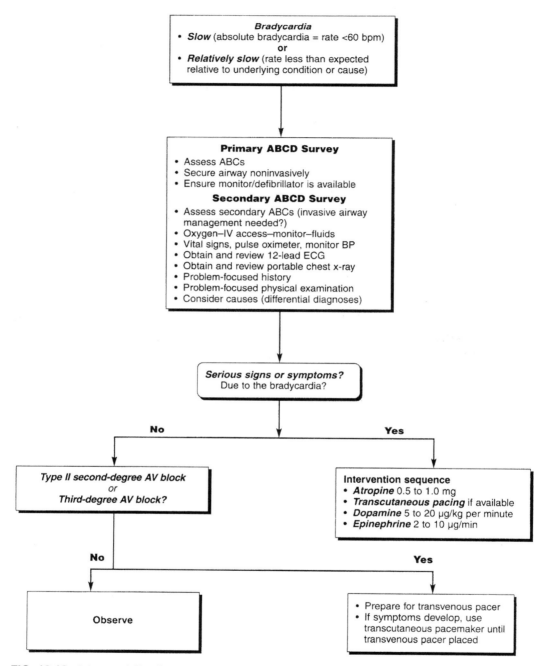

FIG. 19.18. Advanced Cardiovascular Life Support (ACLS) algorithm for the acute management of bradycardia.

external defibrillators. However, external pacing does not always result in ventricular capture, is often poorly tolerated by the patient, and should be used only to stabilize the patient while a transvenous pacer is being inserted.

Long-Term Management

Because there is no well-tolerated, effective, long-term pharmacologic therapy for bradycardia, most patients with persistent symptomatic bradycardia require implantation of a permanent pacemaker.

The American College of Cardiology and the American Heart Association have published guidelines for implantation of cardiac pacemakers (14). A Class I indication refers to a condition for which there is evidence that pacing is beneficial, and a Class II indication refers to a condition for which there is conflicting evidence, a divergence of opinion, or both. A summary of the indications is listed in Table 19.2. These indications focus on the presence or absence of symptoms. In general, patients with symptoms caused by an inadequate heart rate should undergo pacemaker implantation.

There are also a few circumstances when patients who do not have symptoms should undergo prophylactic pacemaker implantation. These situations include an HV interval exceeding 100 milliseconds and documented Mobitz II atrioventricular block. In addition, there are miscellaneous conditions in which pacing therapy can benefit patients, either by changing the cardiac contraction sequence (e.g., in patients with hypertrophic obstructive cardiomyopathy) or by preventing pauses (e.g., in patients with the long QT syndrome). Multisite atrial pacing reduces intraatrial conduction delay and is being evaluated in patients to prevent atrial fibrillation. Multisite ventricular pacing improves hemodynamics and symptoms in patients who have congestive heart failure and a left bundle branch block and is being evaluated as long-term therapy.

It is important to understand pacemaker nomenclature. Pacing modes are described using the NBG code (North American Society of Pacing and Electrophysiology; British Pacing and Electrophysiology Group). The first letter in the code refers to the chamber that is paced (A, atrium; V, ventricle; D, dual), the second letter refers to the chamber sensed (A, atrium; V, ventricle; D, dual; or O, none), and the third letter refers to the response to sensing (T, triggered; I, inhibit; D, dual; or O, none). The letter R is added as a fourth letter in the code if the mode is rate responsive. Common pacing modes include VVI for ventricular demand pacing; AAI for atrial demand pacing; DDD for dual-chamber, demand, atrial-tracking, pacing; and VOO for asynchronous ventricular pacing.

TABLE 19.2. *Indications for permanent pacemaker implantation*

Patients with symptoms due to inadequate heart rate or conduction delay
Documented symptomatic bradycardia
  Sinus bradycardia
  Second-degree AV block
  Third-degree AV block
Syncope presumed due to bradycardia
  Carotid sinus hypersensitivity
  Abnormal sinus node or AV conduction at EP testing
  Medically refractory vasodepressor syncope
  Chronic bifascicular or trifascicular block*
Chronotropic incompetence
Pacemaker syndrome due to first-degree AV block*
Patients without symptoms but at risk for severe bradycardia
Asymptomatic third-degree AV block and average awake rate < 40 bpm
Transient third-degree AV block during acute MI and associated BBB
Asymptomatic third-degree AV block and average awake rate ≥ 40 bpm*
HV > 100 msec or infranodal block at the time of EP testing*
Documented Mobitz II AV block or Mobitz I below the AV node*
Miscellaneous indications
Dilated cardiomyopathy and severe first-degree AV block (PR interval, > 300 msec)*
Hypertrophic cardiomyopathy with LV outflow tract gradient*
Sustained pause-dependent ventricular tachycardia
High-risk patients with congenital long-QT syndrome*

AV, atrioventricular; BBB, bundle branch block; EP, electrophysiologic; HV, His-ventricular interval; LV, left ventricular; MI, myocardial infarction.
  Indications not marked by an asterisk are Class I indications.
  A Class I indication refers to a condition for which there is evidence that pacing is beneficial. A Class II indication refers to a condition for which there is conflicting evidence and/or a divergence of opinion.
  *Class II indication.

There continues to be debate regarding the appropriate pacing mode for patients who need a pacemaker. In general, most patients who need a pacemaker should undergo implantation of a dual-chamber device, unless persistent atrial fibrillation or atrial flutter is present. Because the additional atrial lead required for physiologic pacing is associated with additional costs and perioperative complications, studies have been conducted to quantify the benefit of physiologic pacing. A prospective, randomized clinical trial found that physiologic pacing reduced the incidence of atrial fibrillation but did not significantly reduce rates of stroke, mortality, or hospitalization for heart failure in comparison with ventricular pacing (15). This study may have underestimated the benefit of physiologic pacing, because the follow-up period was only 3 years. Other studies have found the incidence of pacemaker syndrome, characterized by palpitations, fatigue, presyncope, and syncope in patients with a ventricular pacemaker, to be as high as 26% (16).

A single-chamber, rate-responsive atrial pacemaker is a reasonable option for patients with sinus node dysfunction and normal atrioventricular conduction. The rate of development of atrioventricular block in these patients is low.

Patients with sinus node dysfunction or with persistent atrial fibrillation and atrioventricular block are usually treated with a rate-responsive pacemaker. Most rate-responsive pacemakers use sensors that detect body movement and increase the pacing rate accordingly. Sensors that are based on minute ventilation are more physiologic and have been combined with motion sensors to maximize the benefits of rate-responsive pacing.

Pacemaker technology has dramatically improved over the past few decades. Advances include improved sensor technology, automatic gain control, improved diagnostics, automatic assurance of capture, dynamic adjustment of pacing intervals and refractory periods, and the ability to automatically switch to a nonatrial tracking mode in response to intermittent atrial tachyarrhythmias to prevent unnecessary rapid ventricular pacing. Improved pacemaker lead technology has led to high-impedance and steroid-eluting leads that result in lower capture thresholds and therefore increased battery longevity. Future leads will also be isodiametric, to allow for easier extraction.

PROGNOSIS AND FOLLOW-UP

The prognosis of a patient with bradycardia depends largely on the nature of the bradycardia and the presence of structural heart disease. Patients with second-degree atrioventricular block are less likely to progress to complete heart block if the level of block is nodal rather than infranodal. Patients with reversible causes and no structural heart disease have a good prognosis.

Pacemaker therapy can significantly improve quality of life. However, pacemakers do not prolong survival, except for pacemaker-dependent patients. In one study, the 5- and 10-year survival rates among pacemaker recipients older than 65 years with heart block and coexisting heart disease were 31% and 11%, respectively (17). In evaluating patients who are candidates for pacing therapy, it is important to remember that many have severe underlying structural heart disease. Implantation of a prophylactic defibrillator with pacing capabilities rather than a pacemaker alone may reduce mortality among pacemaker recipients who are at high risk for sudden death (18).

Patients treated with a permanent pacemaker need careful follow-up. Patients should be seen in clinic every 4 to 6 months to determine the battery status, to check pacing thresholds and sensing, to test the lead impedance, and to identify any clinical problems. Transtelephonic monitoring can be used to supplement clinic visits to confirm adequate battery status and ventricular capture. Patients apply a magnet to the pacemaker, which results in asynchronous pacing at a model-specific rate that relates to the battery status. Battery longevity ranges from 7 to 10 years and can be improved by minimizing the pacing output and avoiding unnecessary stimulation. Stored diagnostic tests, including histograms, are often useful when patients have symptoms suggestive of pacemaker malfunction or arrhythmias.

PRACTICAL POINTS

- Bradycardia is associated with a wide spectrum of symptoms ranging from syncope to exercise intolerance.
- Documentation and characterization of the rhythm during bradycardia are helpful in determining the origin, prognosis, and therapy.
- A continuous-loop recorder is a better test than a Holter monitor for evaluating a patient with infrequent symptoms suggestive of bradycardia.
- An implantable loop recorder is currently available as an alternative to prolonged monitoring with an external loop recorder.
- Causes of bradycardia can be divided into sinus node dysfunction or atrioventricular conduction disturbances.
- Atrioventricular block that is associated

with slowing of the sinus rate is caused by an increase in vagal tone and usually does not indicate a need for pacing.
- The ACLS guidelines are useful during the acute management of symptomatic bradycardia.
- Long-term management of symptomatic bradycardia requires implantation of a permanent pacemaker.
- The American College of Cardiology/American Heart Association guidelines provide accepted indications for pacemaker implantation.
- Implantation of a prophylactic defibrillator with pacing capabilities rather than a pacemaker alone should be considered for patients who require pacing and who are at high risk for sudden cardiac death.

REFERENCES

1. Mazel JA, El-Sherif N, Buyon J, et al. Electrocardiographic abnormalities in a murine model injected with IgG from mothers of children with congenital heart block. *Circulation* 1999;99:1914–1918.
2. Locatelli ER, Varghese JP, Shuaib A, et al. Cardiac asystole and bradycardia as a manifestation of left temporal lobe complex partial seizure. *Ann Intern Med* 1999;130:581–583.
3. Tilkian AG, Guilleminault C, Schroeder JS, et al. Sleep-induced apnea syndrome. Prevalence of cardiac arrhythmias and their reversal after tracheostomy. *Am J Med* 1977;63:348–358.
4. Fogel RI, Evans JJ, Prystowsky EN. Utility and cost of event recorders in the diagnosis of palpitations, presyncope and syncope. *Am J Cardiol* 1977;70;207–208.
5. Krahn AD, Klein GJ, Yee R, et al. Use of an extended monitoring strategy in patients with problematic syncope. Reveal Investigators. *Circulation* 1999;99:406–410.
6. Fisher JD. Role of electrophysiologic testing in the diagnosis and treatment of patients with known and suspected bradycardias and tachycardias. *Prog Cardiovasc Dis* 1981;24:25–90.
7. Scheinman MM, Peters RW, Suave MJ, et al. Value of the H-Q measurement in patients with bundle branch block and the role of prophylactic permanent pacing. *Am J Cardiol* 1982;50:1316–1322.

8. Morady F, Higgins J, Peters RW, et al. Electrophysiology testing in bundle branch block and unexplained syncope. *Am J Cardiol* 1984;54:587–591.
9. Spodick DH. Normal sinus heart rate: appropriate rate thresholds for sinus tachycardia and bradycardia. *South Med J* 1996;89:666–667.
10. Upshaw CB Jr, Silverman ME: The Wenckebach phenomenon: A salute and comment on the centennial of its original description. *Ann Intern Med* 1999;130:58–63.
11. Hay J. Bradycardia and cardiac arrhythmia produced by depression of certain of the functions of the heart. *Lancet* 1906;1:139–140.
12. Mobitz W. Uber die unvollstandige Storung der Erregungsuberleitung zwischen vorhof und kammer des menschllichen herzens [Concerning partial block of conduction between the atria and ventricles of the human heart]. *Z Ges Exp Med* 1924;41:180–237.
13. Guidelines 2000 for Cardiopulmonary Resuscitation and Emergency Cardiovascular Care. *Circulation* 2000;102(Suppl):I1–I384.
14. Gregoratos G, Abrams J, Epstein AE, et al. ACC/AHA/NASPE 2002 Guideline update guidelines for implantation of cardiac pacemakers and antiarrhythmia devices. A report of the American College of Cardiology/American Heart Association Task Force on Practice Guidelines (Committee to update the 1998 Pacemaker Guidelines). *Circulation* 2002;106:2145–2161.

15. Connolly SJ, Kerr CR, Gent M, et al. Effects of physiologic pacing versus ventricular pacing on the risk of stroke and death due to cardiovascular causes. *N Engl J Med* 2000;342:1385–1391.

16. Lamas GA, Orav EJ, Stambler BS, et al. Quality of life and clinical outcomes in elderly patients treated with ventricular pacing as compared with dual-chamber pacing. *N Engl J Med* 1998;338:1097–1104.

17. Shen WK, Hammill SC, Hayes DL, et al. Long-term survival after pacemaker implantation for heart block in patients > 65 years. *Am J Cardiol* 1994;74:560–564.

18. Moss AJ, Hall WJ, Cannom DS, et al. Improved survival with an implantable defibrillator in patients with coronary artery disease at high risk for ventricular arrhythmia. *N Engl J Med* 1996;335:1933–1940.

20

Infective Endocarditis

Ragavendra R. Baliga and Sunil Das

DEFINITION

Infective endocarditis is an infection (usually bacterial) of the lining of heart (usually the valves) or the vascular endothelium. The disease may have either an acute and fulminating course or a subacute and insidious course, which is known as subacute bacterial endocarditis. The annual incidence of endocarditis in the United States is approximately 15,000 to 20,000 new cases, and this number continues to rise.

Valves that are damaged or congenitally abnormal as a result of such causes as rheumatic valvular disease, mitral regurgitation due to mitral valve prolapse, and calcific aortic stenosis are more prone to endocarditis [native valve endocarditis (NVE)]. Mitral valve NVE is more common than aortic valve NVE. It can involve normal valves in immunocompromised patients and intravenous drug abusers. It is also associated with many congenital heart diseases, including ventricular septal defect and persistent ductus arteriosus. Prosthetic Dacron grafts in the vasculature, prosthetic valves, and other synthetic material are all susceptible to infection. Prosthetic valve endocarditis is more common in aortic valves than in mitral valves and often necessitates surgery for a cure. NVE, however, is more sensitive to antibiotic therapy and carries a better chance for medical cure (1,2).

USUAL CAUSES

Infective endocarditis is usually caused by bacteria, and the three most common bacteria include *Streptococcus viridans, Staphylococcus aureus,* and *Enterococcus faecalis.* Another cause is *Staphylococcus epidermidis.* Gram-negative bacteria, although a common cause of septicemia, do not cause endocarditis. Important fungal causes include *Histoplasma, Brucella, Candida,* and *Aspergillus* species. *Coxiella burnetii* is a rickettsia that causes endocarditis.

S. viridans, an alpha-hemolytic streptococcus, is responsible for about half the cases. These bacteria are normal commensals of the pharynx and upper respiratory tract. Dental procedures such as cleaning or extraction, bronchoscopy, or tonsillectomy result in infection in susceptible individuals. In one study, it was the commonest organism in intravenous drug abusers (3).

S. aureus can cause both acute and subacute endocarditis. It is common in intravenous drug abusers and in patients with central venous catheters such as Swan-Ganz catheters, temporary pacemaker wires, parenteral feeding lines, or central lines for administering chemotherapy (4).

Coagulase negative staphylococci (*S. epidermidis*), fungi (*Histoplasma, Candida, Aspergillus*), and *Brucella* species are organisms that commonly cause infection in patients with prosthetic valves, intravenous drug abusers, and alcoholic persons.

E. faecalis is found in the perineal region and feces. Genitourinary procedures, pelvic surgery, pelvic infections, and prostatic disease in older men are predisposing factors for this infection.

Streptococcus bovis is present in the bowel and is associated with carcinoma of the colon.

C. burnetii is a rickettsia that is is widespread in both domestic and farm animals. It spreads to humans through aerosols, dust, and unpasteurized milk.

HACEK organisms (*Haemophilus parainfluenzae, Haemophilus aphrophilus, Actinobacillus [Haemophilus] actinomycetemcomitans,*

*Cardiobacterium hominis, Eikenella*species, and *Kingella* species).

Other causative bacteria include *Streptococcus pyogenes* and *Neisseria, Pseudomonas,* and *Brucella* species.

PRESENTING SYMPTOMS AND SIGNS

Mode of Presentation

Acute Endocarditis

The onset usually dates to a preceding suppurative infection or to intravenous drug abuse. Persistent fever, new heart murmurs, vasculitis, hemorrhagic petechiae, embolic phenomena and metastatic abscesses, and development of heart failure are suggestive of acute endocarditis. *S. aureus* is usually implicated in acute endocarditis.

Subacute Endocarditis

The onset of illness is insidious, and the date of onset is usually unclear. Patients present with systemic symptoms such as fever, malaise, anorexia, weight loss, rigors, arthralgia, symptoms of heart failure, or embolism. Heart failure results from destruction of valve or rupture of chordae, and in these cases, the onset may be more fulminant. Embolic phenomena include stroke, pulseless limbs, pulmonary infarctions, or renal infarctions. Thus, a combination of heart murmur, anemia, hematuria, and renal failure should raise the suspicion of subacute endocarditis.

Prosthetic Valve Endocarditis

There are two modes of onset: The first has an *early* onset, develops soon after surgery, and is caused by infection of the prosthesis at surgery. The second has a *late* onset and is caused by infection of the valve as a result of persistent bacteremia. Infection of the valve ring occurs in both types. Vegetations can interfere with valve function, and myocardial abscesses can interfere with cardiac conduction system.

Symptoms

Nonspecific symptoms of inflammation, including intermittent fever, malaise, anorexia, weight loss, and rigors, may occur. Fever may be absent in moribund or immunocompromised individuals. Some patients also complain of myalgia and arthralgia. Endocarditis must always be suspected in a patient with a heart murmur and fever. Progressive cardiac failure is another presenting feature, and the onset of heart failure can be dramatic when there is destruction of a valve. Emboli form vegetations that can result in a pulseless limb, stroke, renal infarction, or pulmonary infarction. Loin pain and arthralgia occur due to immune complex deposition.

Signs

Cardiac Findings

The change in the character of an existing murmur or the development of a new murmur must raise the suspicion of infective endocarditis. In some instances, the only finding may be a "trivial" aortic regurgitation. In right-sided endocarditis, murmurs are not present.

Vascular lesions: Such lesions include petechiae, Roth's spots, Janeway's lesions, subungual splinter hemorrhages, and Osler's nodes (Fig. 20.1). Petechial or mucosal hemorrhages are caused by vasculitis and are typically small and red with a pale center. They are seen on the conjunctiva or pharyngeal mucosa. Those seen on the retina are called Roth's spots. Janeway's lesions are flat, small, erythematous macules that are not tender and seen mainly on the hypothenar and thenar eminences. These lesions blanch with pressure. Osler's nodes are painful, tender, hard, subcutaneous swellings that occur in the palms, soles, toes, and fingers.
Clubbing of fingers: Clubbing of fingers typically occurs in persons with subacute bacterial endocarditis. This is, however, a late manifestation and is rarely seen nowadays.
Splenomegaly: Splenomegaly is a feature of subacute endocarditis, and usually the spleen is mildly enlarged.

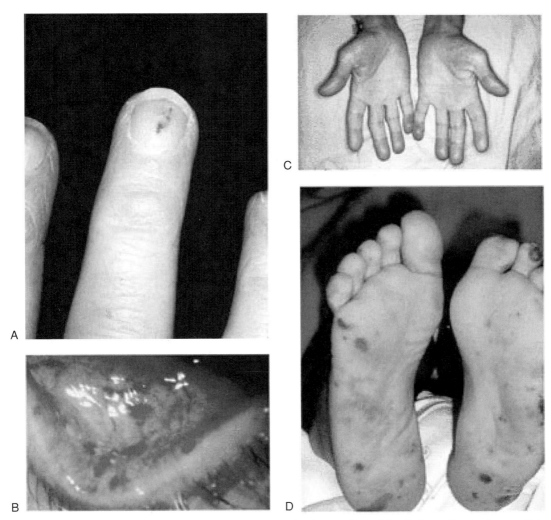

FIG. 20.1. Common peripheral manifestations of infective endocarditis. Splinter hemorrhages (**A**) are normally seen under the fingernails or toenails. They are usually linear and red for the first 2 to 3 days and brownish thereafter. **B,** Conjunctival petechiae. Osler's nodes (**C**) are tender subcutaneous nodules, often in the pulp of the digits or the thenar eminence. Janeway's lesions (**D**) are nontender erythematous, hemorrhagic, or pustular lesions, often on the palms or soles. (From Mylonakis E, Calderwood SB. Infective endocarditis in adults. *N Engl J Med* 2001;345:1318–1330.)

Renal manifestations: Microscopic hematuria is almost always present. Frank hematuria is suggestive of renal infarction caused by emboli. Acute glomerulonephritis and renal abscesses are other manifestations.

Arthritis: Arthritis of major joints has been reported frequently.

Embolic phenomena: Stroke can be caused by emboli to the middle cerebral artery and its branches. Vegetations can embolize and result in infarction of a limb, pulmonary infarction, and coronary infarctions. Mycotic aneurysms can occur anywhere on the vascular tree; when cerebral vessels are affected, there may be cerebral hemorrhage. Extracranial mycotic aneurysms are usually asymptomatic until they rupture or leak. These can occur in intrathoracic or intraabdominal vessels.

HELPFUL TESTS

Laboratory Tests

Blood: Typically, affected patients have normocytic normochromic anemia. There usually is an increase in neutrophils, and thrombocytopenia occurs in some patients. Markers of inflammation, including the erythrocyte sedimentation rate and C-reactive protein, are increased. There may hemolysis with paraprosthetic leaks.

Liver function tests: There be mild derangement of liver function test results, particularly a raised alkaline phosphatase level.

Immunoglobulin: There is an increase in serum immunoglobulin levels.

Complement: Both total complement and C3 complement levels are decreased as a result of immune complex formation.

Urine: Microscopic hematuria is an almost constant phenomenon, and proteinuria may occur.

Blood cultures: Blood cultures are positive in about 75% of cases and are helpful in identifying the suspected pathogen and its susceptibility to antimicrobial agents. At least three separate sets of cultures, 1 hour apart from separate venipuncture samplings, should be taken. Each set equals one aerobic bottle and one anaerobic bottle. Special cultures may be required for HACEK organisms and *Bartonella, Legionella, Brucella,* and *Histoplasma* species. The administration of antibiotics before obtaining blood cultures may reduce the yield of isolated pathogens by 35% to 40%. Polymerase chain reaction testing on blood is useful when the suspected pathogens are *Tropheryma whippleii* or *Bartonella* species.

Serologic tests: Serologic tests may be required when uncommon organisms, including *Coxiella, Chlamydia, Candida, Bartonella,* and *Brucella* species, are suspected.

Chest radiograph: Chest radiography is useful for documenting emboli in right-sided endocarditis or for confirming evidence of cardiac failure.

Electrocardiogram: Electrocardiography may show defects in cardiac conduction or, in rare cases, myocardial infarction caused by emboli.

Echocardiography: Figure 20.2 and Table 20.1 show the recommendations for the use of echocardiography.

Transthoracic echocardiography: Four major echocardiographic features of infective endocarditis are typical vegetations, abscesses, new prosthetic valve dehiscence, or new regurgitation, which must be interpreted in combination with other clinical features(5) (Fig. 20.3). Transthoracic echocardiography cannot exclude the diagnosis of infective endocarditis, and in a fifth of the cases, vegetations may not be detected because of obesity, chest wall abnormalities, or chronic obstructive pulmonary disease. For vegetations, this procedure has good specificity (98%), but sensitivity is only 60% (6–8). The procedure is useful in detecting vegetations larger than 2 mm in diameter, particularly on right-sided valves that are close to the anterior portion of the chest (9). It is not useful in excluding prosthetic valve endocarditis, perforation of leaflets, fistulae, or periannular abscess (8,10); therefore, a negative study result in a suspected case does not rule out negative endocarditis. The other limitation is that a positive study result does not rule out major complications.

Transesophageal echocardiography: This procedure is the investigation of choice and more accurately identifies infective endocarditis, particularly of prosthetic valves (Figs. 20.4, 20.5). For prosthetic valve endocarditis, the sensitivity is 86% to 94% and specificity is 88% to 100%. Abscesses of the aortic root, a serious complication, are only reliably excluded by this procedure. It has a specificity of 94%, and sensitivity varies from 76% to 100% for perivalvular infection because the esophageal transducer allows examination of the root of the aorta and basal part of the ventricular septum, where most such complications occur. However, the technique is not 100% sensitive for other infection, and in such situations, the diagnosis may have to be made on

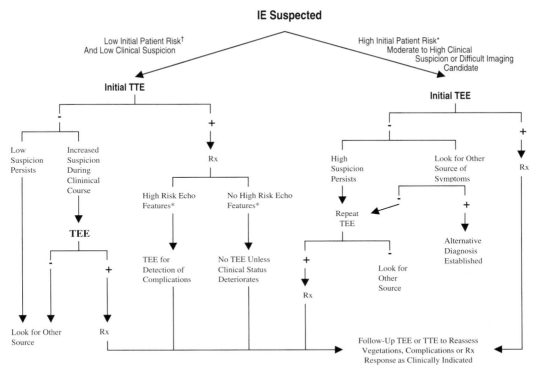

FIG. 20.2. American College of Cardiology/American Heart Association approach to the diagnostic use of echocardiography. *High-risk echocardiographic features include large or mobile vegetations, valvular insufficiency, suggestion of perivalvular extension, or secondary ventricular dysfunction (see text). For example, a patient with fever and a previously known heart murmur and no other stigmata of infective endocarditis. †High initial risks include prosthetic heart valves, many congenital heart diseases, previous endocarditis, new murmur, heart failure, or other stigmata of endocarditis. Rx, antibiotic treatment for endocarditis. From Bayer, et. al. Diagnosis and management of infective endocarditis and its complications. *Circulation* 1998;98:2936–2948.

clinical grounds (6). False-negative findings result from prior embolization of vegetations, small size of vegetations, or inadequate views to detect small abscesses. Another limitation is that prosthetic valve shadows may not allow complete visualization; therefore, multiple views and planes must be studied in order to decrease the number of false-negative findings. Also, a combination of transthoracic and transesophageal techniques may have to be used to obtain accurate images; when both studies yield negative results, the negative predictive value approaches 95%. The American College of Cardiology/American Heart Association (ACC/AHA) committee recommends (11) that when clinical suspicion of infective endocardi-

tis is high and the transesophageal study result is negative, a repeat study should be considered within 7 to 10 days to demonstrate previously undetected vegetations or abscesses. After a course of therapy, vegetations may persist in 59% of the patients, and this is not correlate with subsequent complications; however, any increase in the size of the vegetations with therapy heralds late complications, independent of persistent bacteremia or clinical features of infective endocarditis (12,13).

DIAGNOSIS

The Duke Criteria are used to make either a definite diagnosis or a possible diagnosis, or to

TABLE 20.1. *ACC/AHA recommendations for echocardiography in infective endocarditis in native valves*

Class I: There is evidence and/or general agreement that echocardiography is useful and effective

Native valves
 Detection and characterization of valvular lesions, their hemodynamic severity, and/or ventricular compensation*
 Detection of vegetations and characterization of lesions in patients with congenital heart disease in whom infective endocarditis is suspected
 Detection of associated abnormalities (e.g., abscesses, shunts)*
 Reevaluation studies in complex endocarditis (e.g., virulent organism, severe hemodynamic lesion, aortic valve involvement, persistent fever or bacteremia, clinical change, or symptomatic deterioration)*
 Evaluation of patients with high clinical suspicion of culture-negative endocarditis

Prosthetic valves
 Detection and characterization of valvular lesions, their hemodynamic severity, and/or ventricular compensation*
 Detection of associated abnormalities (e.g., abscesses, shunts)*
 Reevaluation studies in complex endocarditis (e.g., virulent organism, severe hemodynamic lesion, aortic valve involvement, persistent fever or bacteremia, clinical change, or symptomatic deterioration)
 Evaluation of bacteremia with a known source*

Class IIa: The weight of evidence/opinion is in favor of usefulness/efficacy
 Evaluation of bacteremia with a known source*
 Risk stratification in established endocarditis*

Class IIb: Usefulness/efficacy is less well established by evidence/opinion
 Routine reevaluation in uncomplicated endocarditis during antibiotic therapy

Class III: There is evidence and/or general agreement that echocardiography is not useful and in some cases may be harmful
 Evaluation of fever and nonpathologic murmur without evidence of bacteremia

---

*TEE may provide incremental value to TTE
ACC/AHA, American College of Cardiology/American Heart Association; TEE, transesophageal echocardiography; TTE, transthoracic echocardiography.

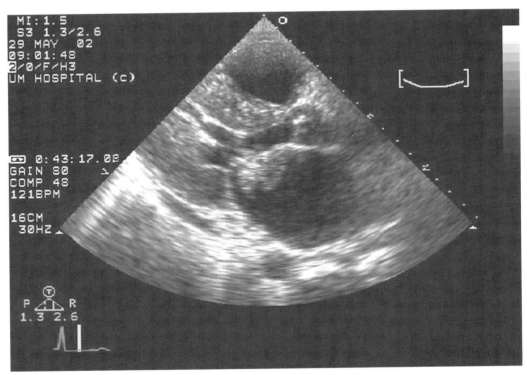

FIG. 20.3. Two-dimensional echocardiogram showing vegetations on mitral valve endocarditis.

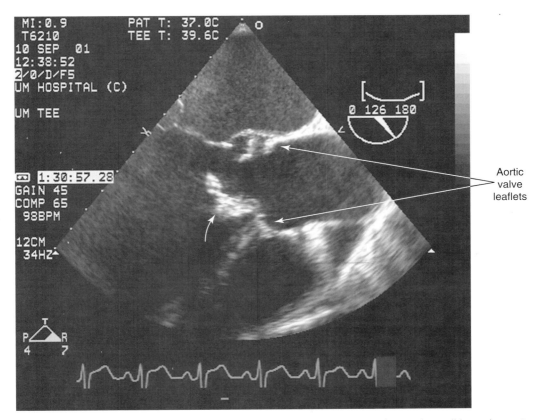

FIG. 20.4. Transesophageal echocardiogram in a patient with aortic valve endocarditis and vegetations. Vegetations attached to the aortic valve leaflets (*arrows*) can be identified; their presence was subsequently confirmed by surgery. LA, left atrium; LV, left ventricle.

reject the diagnosis, of infective endocarditis (Table 20.2). A definite diagnosis requires isolation of the causative microorganism, a histologic diagnosis, or the presence of clinical criteria. Clinical criteria are defined specifically in Table 20.2; a definite diagnosis of infective endocarditis requires the presence of two major criteria, one major and three minor criteria, or five minor criteria. A possible diagnosis includes findings that fall short of definite but not "rejected." The diagnosis is rejected when there is a firm alternative diagnosis for the clinical manifestations, when clinical manifestations resolve with a 4-day course

of antibiotic therapy, or when pathologic evidence of infective endocarditis is absent at surgery or autopsy, after a 4-day course of antibiotic therapy. Major criteria include positive blood cultures and documentation of endocardial vegetations by echocardiography. Minor criteria include predisposing heart conditions or intravenous drug use, temperature of 38.0°C, major arterial emboli, septic pulmonary infarctions, mycotic aneurysm, intracranial hemorrhage, conjunctival hemorrhages, Janeway's lesions, glomerulonephritis, Osler's nodes, Roth's spots, and rheumatoid factor (see Table 20.3 for details).

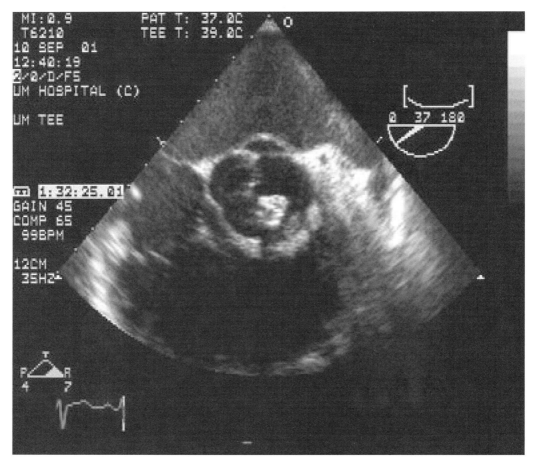

FIG. 20.5. Aortic valve endocarditis.

TABLE 20.2. *Duke criteria*

Definite IE
Pathologic criteria
  Microorganisms: demonstrated by culture or histologic study in a vegetation, in a vegetation that has
    embolized, or in an intracardiac abscess, or
  Pathologic lesions: vegetation or intracardiac abscess present, confirmed by histologic study showing active
    endocarditis
Clinical criteria, with specific definitions listed in Table 20.3
  Two major criteria, or
  One major and three minor criteria, or
  Five minor criteria
Possible IE
Findings consistent with IE that fall short of "Definite" but not "Rejected"
Rejected
Firm alternative diagnosis for manifestations of endocarditis, or
Resolution of manifestations of endocarditis with antibiotic therapy for 4 days, or
No pathologic evidence of IE at surgery or autopsy, after antibiotic therapy for 4 days

  IE, infective endocarditis.

TABLE 20.3. *Duke criteria*

Major criteria
Positive blood culture for IE
   Typical microorganism consistent with IE from two separate blood cultures:
      Viridans streptococci, *Streptococcus bovis,* or HACEK group, or
      Community-acquired *Staphylococcus aureus* or enterococci, in the absence of a primary focus
   Microorganisms consistent with IE from persistently positive blood cultures defined as
      Two positive cultures of blood samples drawn >12 hours apart, or
      All of three or a majority of four separate cultures of blood (with first and last sample drawn 1 hour apart)
Evidence of endocardial involvement
   Positive echocardiogram for IE defined as
      Oscillating intracardiac mass on valve or supporting structures, in the path of regurgitant jets, or on
         implanted material in the absence of an alternative anatomic explanation, or
      Abscess, or
      New partial dehiscence of prosthetic valve
   New valvular regurgitation (worsening or changing of preexisting murmur not sufficient)
Minor criteria
Predisposition: predisposing heart condition or intravenous drug use
Fever: temperature 38.0°C
Vascular phenomena: major arterial emboli, septic pulmonary infarctions, mycotic aneurysm, intracranial
   hemorrhage, conjunctival hemorrhages, and Janeway's lesions
Immunologic phenomena: glomerulonephritis, Osler's nodes, Roth's spots, and rheumatoid factor
Microbiologic evidence: positive blood culture but does not meet a major criterion as noted previously, or
   serologic evidence of active infection with organism consistent with IE
Echocardiographic findings: consistent with IE but do not meet a major criterion as noted previously

HACEK, combination of *Haemophilus parainfluenzae, Haemophilus aphrophilus, Actinobacillus actinomycetem-comitans, Cardiobacterium hominis, Eikenella corrodens,* and *Kingella kingae;* IE, infective endocarditis.

THERAPY

The management of a patient with infective endocarditis is a multidisciplinary approach with the involvement of the cardiologist, an infectious disease specialist, and a cardiothoracic surgeon.

Pharmacologic Therapy

Bactericidal antibiotics, selected on the basis of blood culture results and sensitivity, should be administered for at least 6 weeks (Tables 20.4 to 20.10). In febrile patients with suspected endocarditis, immediate antibiotic treatment is not necessary (unless there are signs of toxicity); a delay of 48 to 72 hours will allow efforts to identify the organism. When the infecting organism is not isolated, patients may be treated empirically. In acute endocarditis, the antibiotics included should cover for *Staphylococcus* species; in subacute endocarditis, they should cover for *S. viridans.* In most instances, a broad-spectrum combination of gentamicin and penicillin is used, and the choice of antibiotics is adjusted when patients do not respond.

Surgical Therapy

Surgery is indicated in the following situations (Table 20.11):

- Progressive heart failure.
- Worsening renal function.
- Embolization.
- Failure of medical treatment to control infective process (possible abscess formation), indicated by continuing fever for more than 10 days, rising C-reactive protein concentration, and worsening nephritis.
- Indications of abscess formation, such as conduction abnormalities, cavity on echocardiography, or prosthetic valve dehiscence.
- Hemodynamic deterioration; for example, pulmonary edema or increasing cardiomegaly.
- Infection by organisms that are difficult to eradicate, such as *S. aureus, Candida* species, and *Aspergillus* species.
- Infection of a prosthetic valve or of a prosthetic material.
- Recurrent embolization or enlarging, large vegetations while patient is on effective antimicrobial therapy.

TABLE 20.4. *Native valve endocarditis involving penicillin-susceptible* Streptococci viridans *and* Streptococcus bovis (*minimum inhibitory concentration,* $\leq$0.1 μg/mL)[a]

Antibiotic	Dosage and route	Duration (weeks)	Comments
Aqueous crystalline penicillin G sodium or	12–18 million U/24 hr IV either continuously or in six equally divided doses	4	Preferred in most patients older than 65 yr and in those with impairment of the eighth nerve or renal function
Ceftriaxone sodium	2 g once daily IV or IM[b]	4	
Aqueous crystalline penicillin G sodium	12–18 million U/24 hr IV either continuously or in six equally divided doses	2	When obtained 1 hr after a 20- to 30-min IV infusion or IM injection, serum concentration of gentamicin of approximately 3 μg/mL
With gentamicin sulfate[c]	1 mg/kg IM or IV every 8 hr	2	
Vancomycin hydrochloride[d]	30 mg/kg per 24 hr IV in two equally divided doses, not to exceed 2 g/24 hr unless serum levels are monitored	4	Vancomycin therapy is recommended for patients allergic to beta-lactams; peak serum concentrations of vancomycin should be obtained 1 hr after completion of the infusion and should be in the range of 30–45 μg/mL for twice-daily dosing

IM, intramuscular; IV, intravenous.
[a]Dosages recommended are for patients with normal renal function. For nutritionally variant streptococci, see Table 24.
[b]Patients should be informed that IM injection of ceftriaxone is painful.
[c]Dosing of gentamicin on a mg/kg basis produces higher serum concentrations in obese patients than in lean patients. Therefore, in obese patients, dosing should be based on ideal body weight (ideal body weight for men is 50 kg + 2.3 kg/in. >5 ft; ideal body weight for women is 45.5 kg + 2.3 kg/in. >5 ft). Relative contraindications to use gentamicin are age >65 yr, renal impairment, or impairment of the eighth nerve. Other potentially nephrotoxic agents (e.g., nosteroidal antiinflammatory drugs) should be reduced in patients with impaired renal function.
[d]Vancomycin given on a mg/kg basis produces higher serum concentration in obese patients than in lean patients. Therefore, in obese patients, dosing should be based on ideal body weight. Each dose of vancomycin should be infused over $\geq$1 hr to reduce the risk of histamine-release "red man" syndrome (15).

TABLE 20.5. *Native valve endocarditis involving* Streptococci viridans *and* Streptococcus bovis *relatively resistant to penicillin G (minimum inhibitory concentration,* >0.1 μg/mL *and* <0.5 μg/mL)[a]

Antibiotic	Dosage and route	Duration (weeks)	Comments
Aqueous crystalline penicillin G sodium	18 million U/24 hr IV either continuously or in six equally divided doses	4	Cefazolin or other first-generation cephalosporins may be substituted for penicillin in patients whose penicillin hypersensitivity is not of the immediate type
With gentamicin sulfate[b]	1 mg/kg IM or IV every 8 hr	2	
Vancomycin hydrochloride[c]	30 mg/kg per 24 hr IV in two equally divided doses, not to exceed 2 g/24 hr unless serum levels are monitored	4	Vancomycin therapy is recommended for patients allergic to beta-lactams

IM, intramuscular; IV, intravenous.
[a]Dosages recommended are for patients with normal renal function.
[b]For specific dosing adjustment and issues concerning gentamicin (obese patients, relative contraindications), see Table 22 footnotes.
[c]For specific dosing adjustment and issues concerning vancomycin (obese patients, length of infusion), see Table 20.4 footnotes.
From Wilson et al. Antibiotic treatment of adults with infective endocarditis due to streptococci, enterococci, staphylocci, and hacek organisms: American Heart Association. *Jama* 1995;274:1706–1713.

TABLE 20.6. *Standard therapy for endocarditis due to enterococci[a]*

Antibiotic	Dosage and route	Duration (weeks)	Comments
Aqueous crystalline penicillin G sodium	18–30 million U/24 hr IV either continuously or in six equally divided doses	4–6	
With gentamicin sulfate[b]	1 mg/kg IM or IV every 8 hr	4–6	4-wk therapy recommended for patients with symptoms <3 mo in duration; 6-wk therapy recommended for patients with symptoms >3 mo in duration
Ampicillin sodium	12 g/24 hr IV either continuously or in six equally divided doses	4–6	
With gentamicin sulfate[b]	1 mg/kg IM or IV every 8 hr	4–6	
Vancomycin hydrochloride[c]	30 mg/kg per 24 hr IV in two equally divided doses, not to exceed 2 g/24 hr unless serum levels are monitored	4–6	Vancomycin therapy is recommended for patients allergic to beta-lactams; cephalosporins are not acceptable alternatives for patients allergic to penicillin
With gentamicin sulfate[b]	1 mg/kg IM or IV every 8 hr	4–6	

IM, intramuscular; IV, intravenous.

[a]All enterococci causing endocarditis must be tested for antimicrobial susceptibility in order to select optimal therapy. This table is for endocarditis due to gentamicin- or vancomycin-susceptible enterococci, *Streptococci viridans* with minimum inhibitory concentration of >0.5 μg/mL, nutritionally variant *S. viridans*, or prosthetic valve endocarditis cause by *S. viridans* or *Streptococci bovis*. Antibiotic dosages are for patients with normal renal function.

[b]For specific dosing adjustment and issues concerning gentamicin (obese patients, relative contraindications), see Table 20.4 footnotes.

[c]For specific dosing adjustment and issues concerning vancomycin (obese patients, length of infusion), see Table 20.4 footnotes.

From Wilson et al.

TABLE 20.7. *Endocarditis due to* Staphylococcus *in the absence of prosthetic material[a]*

Antibiotic	Dosage and route	Duration	Comments
Methicillin-susceptible staphylococci			
Regimens for non–beta-lactam–allergic patients	2 g IV every 4 hr	4–6 wk	Benefit of additional aminoglycosides has not been established
Nafcillin sodium or oxacillin sodium			
With optional addition of gentamicin sulfate[b]	1 mg/kg IM or IV every 8 hr	3–5 d	
Regimens for beta-lactam–allergic patients	2 g IV every 8 hr	4–6 wk	Cephalosporins should be avoided in patients with immediate-type hypersensitivity to penicillin
Cefazolin (or other first-generation cephalosporins in equivalent dosages)			
With optional addition of gentamicin[b]	1 mg/kg IM or IV every 8 hr	3–5 d	
Vancomycin hydrochloride[c]	30 mg/kg per 24 hr IV or two equally divided doses, not to exceed 2 g/24 hr unless serum levels are monitored	4–6 wk	Recommended for patients allergic to penicillin
Methicillin-resistant staphylococci			
Vancomycin hydrochloride[c]	30 mg/kg per 24 hr IV in two equally divided doses, not to exceed 2 g/24 hr unless serum levels are monitored	4–6 wk	

IM, intramuscular; IV, intravenous.

[a]For treatment of endocarditis due to penicillin-susceptible staphylococci (minimum inhibitory concentration $\leq$ 0.1 μg/mL), aqueous crystalline penicillin G sodium (Table 22, first regimen) can be used for 4–6 wk instead of nafcillin or oxacillin. Shorter antibiotic courses have been effective in some drug addicts with right-sided endocarditis due to *Staphylococcus aureus*.

[b]For specific dosing adjustment and issues concerning gentamicin (obese patients, relative contraindications), see Table 20.4 footnotes.

[c]For specific dosing adjustment and issues concerning vancomycin (obese patients, length of infusion), see Table 20.4 footnotes.

From Wilson et al.

TABLE 20.8. *Endocarditis due to* Staphylococcus *in the presence of a prosthetic value or other prosthetic material*[a]

Antibiotic	Dosage and route	Duration (weeks)	Comments
Regimen for methicillin-resistant staphylococci			
Vancomycin hydrochloride[b]	30 mg/kg per 24 hr IV in two or four equally divided doses, not to exceed 2 g/24 hr unless serum levels are monitored	≥ 6	
With rifampin[c]	300 mg orally every 8 hr	≥ 6	Rifampin increases the amount of warfarin sodium required for antithrombotic therapy
And with gentamicin sulfate[d,e]	1.0 mg/kg IM or IV every 8 hr	2	
Regimens for methicillin-resistant staphylococci			
Nafcillin sodium or oxacillin sodium	2 g IV every 4 hr 1 mg/kg IM or IV every 8 hr	≥ 6	First-generation cephalosporins or vancomycin should be used in patients allergic to beta-lactam
With rifampin[c]	300 mg orally every 8 hr	≥ 6	Cephalosporins should be avoided in patients with immediate-type hypersensitivity to penicillin or with methicillin-resistant staphylococci
And with gentamicin sulfate[d,e]	1.0 mg/kg IM or IV every 8 hr	2	

IM, intramuscular; IV, intravenous.

[a]Dosages recommended are for patients with normal renal function.

[b]For specific dosing adjustment and issues concerning vancomycin (obese patients, length of infusion), see Table 22 footnotes.

[c]Rifampin plays a unique role in the eradication of staphylococcal infection involving prosthetic material; combination therapy is essential to prevent rifampin resistance.

[d]For specific dosing adjustment and issues concerning gentamicin (obese patients, relative contraindications), see Table 20.4 footnotes.

[e]Use during initial 2 wk.

From Wilson et al.

TABLE 20.9. *Therapy for endocarditis due to HACEK microorganisms* (Haemophilus parainfluenzae, Haemophilus aphrophilus, Actinobacillus actinomycetemcomitans, Cardiobacterium hominis, Eikenella corrodens, *and* Kingella kingae)[a]

Antibiotic	Dosage and route	Duration (weeks)	Comments
Ceftriaxone sodium[b]	2 g once daily IV or IM[b]	4	Cefotaxime sodium or other third-generation cephalosporins may be substituted
Ampicillin sodium[c]	12 g/24 hr IV either continuously or in six equally divided doses	4	
With gentamicin sulfate[d]	1 mg/kg IM or IV every 8 hr	4	

IM, intramuscular; IV, intravenous.

[a]Antibiotic dosages are for patient with normal renal functions.

[b]Patients should be informed that IM injection of ceftriaxone is painful. For patients unable to tolerate beta-lactam therapy, consult text.

[c]Ampicillin should not be used if laboratory test show beta-lactamase production.

[d]For specific dosing adjustment and issues concerning gentamicin (obese patients, relative contraindications), see Table 20.4 footnotes.

From Wilson et al.

TABLE 20.10. *Fungal endocarditis and culture-negative endocarditis[a]*

Agent	Dosage and route	Duration (weeks)
Fungal endocarditis[a]	1 mg/kg per day IV (total dose, 2.0–2.5 g)	6–8
	150 mg/kg per day PO in four divided doses	6–8
Amphotericin B with or without flucytosine		
Culture-negative endocarditis[b]		
Vancomycin plus gentamicin	15 mg/kg IV every 12 hr	6
	1 mg/kg IM or IV every 8 hr	6

IM, intramuscular; IV, intravenous; PO, per os (oral).
[a]Recommendations for fungal endocarditis were not part of the American Heart Association recommendations on infective endocarditis.
[b]Proposed regimen for culture-negative, presumed bacterial endocarditis.

TABLE 20.11. *ACC/AHA recommendations for surgery in infective endocarditis[a]*

Class I: There is evidence and/or general agreement that surgery is useful and effective
Native valves
  Acute aortic regurgitation or mitral regurgitation with heart failure
  Acute aortic regurgitation with tachycardia and early close of the mitral valve
  Fungal endocarditis
  Evidence of annular or aortic abscess, sinus or aortic true or false aneurysms
  Evidence of valve dysfunction and persistent infection after a prolonged period (7 to 10 days) of appropriate antibiotic therapy, as indicated by presence of fever, leukocytosis, and bacteremia, provided there are no noncardiac causes for infection
Prosthetic valves
  Early prosthetic valve endocarditis (first 2 months or less after surgery)
  Heart failure with prosthetic valve dysfunction
  Fungal endocarditis
  Staphylococcal endocarditis not responding to antibiotic therapy
  Evidence of paravalvular leak, annular or aortic abscess, sinus or aortic true or false aneurysm, fistula formation, or new-onset conduction disturbances
  Infection with gram-negative organisms or organisms with a poor response to antibiotics
Class IIa: The weight of evidence/opinion is in favor of usefulness/efficacy
Native valves
  Recurrent emboli after appropriate antibiotic therapy
  Infection with gram-negative organisms with a poor response to antibiotics in patients with evidence of valve dysfunction
Prosthetic valves
  Persistent bacteremia after a prolonged course (7 to 10 days) of appropriate antibiotic therapy without noncardiac causes for bacteremia
  Recurrent peripheral emboli despite therapy
Class IIb: Usefulness/efficacy is less well established by evidence/opinion
Native valves
  Mobile vegetations >10 mm
Prosthetic valves
  Vegetation of any size on or near the prosthesis
Class III: There is evidence and/or general agreement that surgery is not useful and in some cases may be harmful
  Early infections of the mitral valve that can probably to be repaired
  Persistent pyrexia- and leukocytosis-negative blood cultures

[a]Criteria also apply to repaired mitral and aortic allograft or autograft valves. For endocarditis defined by clinical criteria with or without laboratory verification, there must be evidence that function of a cardiac valve is impaired.

TABLE 20.12. *ACC/AHA recommendations for endocarditis prophylaxis*

Class I: There is evidence and/or general agreement that a given procedure or treatment is useful and effective

High-risk category
  Prosthetic heart valves, including bioprosthetic homograft and allograft valves
  Previous bacterial endocarditis
  Complex cyanotic congenital heart disease (e.g., single-ventricle states, transposition of the great arteries, tetralogy of Fallot)
  Surgically constructed systemic-pulmonary shunts or conduits
Moderate-risk category
  Most other congenital cardiac malformations (other than those listed previously or later)
  Acquired valvular dysfunction (e.g., rheumatic heart disease)
  Hypertrophic cardiomyopathy[a]
  MVP with auscultatory evidence of valvular regurgitation and/or thickened leaflets[b]

Class III: Conditions for which there is evidence and/or general agreement that the procedure/treatment is not useful and in some cases may be harmful

Low- or negligible-risk category
  Isolated secundum atrial septal defect
  Surgical repair of atrial septal defect, ventricular septal defect, or patent ductus arteriosus (without residua >6 mo)
  Previous coronary artery bypass graft surgery
  MVP without valvular regurgitation[b]
  Physiologic, functional, or innocent heart murmurs[c]
  Previous Kawasaki's disease without valvular dysfunction
  Cardiac pacemakers and implanted defibrillators

ACC/AHA, American College of Cardiology/American Heart Association; MVP, mitral valve prolapse.

[a]This committee recommends prophylaxis in hypertrophic cardiomyopathy only when there is latent or resting obstruction.

[b]Patients with MVP without regurgitation require additional clinical judgment. Indications for antibiotic prophylaxis in MVP are discussed in section III.D.2. of these guidelines. Patients who do not have mitral regurgitation (MR) but do have echocardiographic evidence of thickening and/or redundancy of the valve leaflets and especially men >2 45 years may be at increased risk for bacterial endocarditis. In addition, approximately one third of patients with MVP without MR at rest may have exercise-induced MR. Some patients may exhibit MR at rest on one occasion and not on others. There are no data available to address this latter issue and, at present, the decision must be left to clinical judgment, taking into account the nature of the invasive procedure, the previous history of endocarditis, and the presence or absence of valve thickening and/or redundancy.

[c]In patients with echocardiographic evidence of physiologic MR in the absence of a murmur and with structurally normal valves, prophylaxis is not recommended. The committee also does *not* recommend prophylaxis for physiologic tricuspid and pulmonary regurgitation detected by Doppler imaging in the absence of a murmur, as such findings occur in a large number of normal individuals and the risk of endocarditis is extremely low. Recommendations regarding Doppler echocardiography for purposes of antibiotic prophylaxis in patients who have received anorectic drugs are given in section III.H. of these guidelines.

Adapted from Dajani AS, Taubert KA, Wilson W, et al. Prevention of bacterial endocarditis: recommendations of the American Heart Association. *Circulation* 1997;96:358–366.

Once the need for surgery is established, early surgery is preferable.

PROGNOSIS

Poor prognostic factors include the following:

- Age: In older patients, endocarditis is typically more difficult to treat; elderly patients are poor candidates for surgery, frequently have comorbid conditions, and are more likely develop renal insufficiency.
- Comorbid conditions, including chronic renal or liver disease and immunocompromised states such as acquired immunodeficiency syndrome.
- Prosthetic valve infection, in contrast to native valve infection.
- Right-sided endocarditis.
- Complications such as cardiac failure, embolic phenomena, or persistent pyrexia.

Echocardiographic predictors of poor prognosis include the following:

- Larger vegetations: The increased size is associated with increased risk of emboli and,

TABLE 20.13. *Endocarditis prophylaxis regimens for dental, oral, respiratory tract, and esophageal procedures*

Situation	Agent	Regimen[a]
Standard general prophylaxis	Amoxicillin	Adults: 2.0 g; children: 50 mg/kg orally 1 hr before procedure
Unable to take oral medications	Ampicillin	Adults: 2.0 g IM or IV; children: 50 mg/kg IM or IV within 30 min before procedure
Allergic to penicillin	Clindamycin	Adults: 600 mg; children: 20 mg/kg orally 1 hr before procedure
	or	
	Cephalexin[b] or cephadroxil[b]	Adults: 2.0 g; children: 50 mg/kg orally 1 hr before procedure
	or	
	Azithromycin or clarithromycin	Adults: 500 mg; children: 15 mg/kg orally 1 hr before procedure
Allergic to penicillin and unable to take oral medications	Clindamycin	Adults: 600 mg; children: 20 mg/kg IV within 30 min before procedure
	or	
	cefazolin[b]	Adults: 1.0 g; children: 25 mg/kg IM or IV within 30 min before procedure

[a]Total children's dose should not exceed adult dose.

[b]Cephalexin should not be used in individuals with intermediate-type hypersensitivity reaction (urticaria, angioedema, or anaphylaxis) to penicillins.

From Dajani AS, Taubert KA, Wilson W, et al. Prevention of bacterial endocarditis: recommendations of the American Heart Association. *Circulation* 1997;96:358–366.

consequently, need for surgery. It is not associated with increased mortality.

- Destruction or dehiscence of the valve.
- Abscesses of valve ring.
- Fistulae.

Microbiologic predictors of prognosis include the following:

- Low morbidity: infection with *S. viridans.*
- High morbidity: *Staphylococcus,* fungi, and nosocomial infection.

Clinical situations constituting high risk for complications for infective endocarditis (11) include the following:

- Prosthetic cardiac valves.
- Left-sided infective endocarditis.
- *S. aureus*–caused infective endocarditis.
- Fungal infective endocarditis.
- Previous infective endocarditis.
- Prolonged clinical symptoms (3 months or longer).
- Cyanotic or complex congenital heart disease.
- Presence of systemic-to-pulmonary shunts.
- Poor clinical response to antimicrobial therapy.

PROPHYLAXIS

The ACC/AHA guidelines recommend antibiotic prophylaxis in patients with cardiac conditions whose risk of infective endocarditis is significantly higher than that of the general population (14) and particularly in individuals with a substantially higher rate of morbidity and mortality as a consequence of the infection. In Table 20.12, these cardiac conditions are stratified as high, moderate and negligible risk. High-risk conditions include the presence of prosthetic heart valves; complex cyanotic congenital heart diseases; previous history of endocarditis, even in the absence of other cardiac disease; and surgically constructed systemic pulmonary shunts and conduits. Moderate-risk conditions include (a) uncorrected congenital conditions, such as ventricular septal defect, ostium primum atrial septal defect, patent ductus arteriosus, bicuspid aortic valve, and coarctation of the aorta, and (b) acquired conditions, such as valvular heart disease due to rheumatic heart disease, mitral valve prolapse, and hypertrophic cardiomyopathy. Endocarditis is not recommended for patients with secundum atrial septal defect, those who have undergone previous coronary artery bypass grafting, those with

TABLE 20.14. *Endocarditis prophylaxis for nondental procedures*

Endocarditis prophylaxis recommended
Respiratory tract
    Tonsillectomy/adenoidectomy
    Surgical operations involving respiratory mucosa
    Bronchoscopy with rigid bronchoscope
Gastrointestinal tract (prophylaxis for high-risk patients; optimal for moderate risk)
    Sclerotherapy for esophageal varices
    Esophageal stricture dilation
    Endoscopic retrograde cholangiography with biliary obstruction
    Biliary tract surgery
    Surgical operations involving intestinal mucosa
Genitourinary tract
    Prostatic surgery
    Cystoscopy
    Urethral dilation
Endocarditis prophylaxis not recommended
Respiratory tract
    Endotracheal intubation
    Bronchoscopy with a flexible bronchoscope, with or without biopsy[a]
    Tympanostomy tube insertion
Gastrointestinal tract
    Transesophageal echocardiography[a]
    Endoscopy with or without gastrointestinal biopsy[a]
Genitourinary tract
    Vaginal hysterectomy[a]
    Vaginal delivery[a]
    Caesarian section[a]
    In uninfected tissue:
        Urethral catheterization
        Uterine dilation and curettage
        Therapeutic abortion
        Sterilization procedures
        Insertion or removal of intrauterine devices
Other
    Cardiac catheterization, including balloon angioplasty
    Implementation of cardiac pacemakers, implantable defibrillators, and coronary stents
    Incision or biopsy of surgically scrubbed skin
    Circumcision

---

[a]Prophylaxis is optional for high-risk patients.
From Dajani AS, Taubert KA, Wilson W, et al. Prevention of bacterial endocarditis: recommendations of the American Heart Association. *Circulation* 1997;96:358–366.

mitral valve prolapse without regurgitation, those with physiologic or functional heart murmur, or those who have had previous rheumatic heart disease without valvular dysfunction. Antibiotic prophylaxis is recommended in procedures (including dental and oral procedures and respiratory, gastrointestinal, and genitourinary procedures) known to induce bacteremias and endocarditis. The ACC/AHA guidelines specifically identify procedures in which antibiotic prophylaxis is required and those in which it is not (Tables 20.12). The choice of antibiotic (Tables 20.13 to 20.15) also depends on the type of procedure, and antibiotic prophylaxis is limited to high- and moderate-risk cardiac conditions. When patients are taking an antibiotic recommended for prophylaxis for a procedure, a drug from a different antibiotic class should be used for prophylaxis. Antibiotic prophylaxis is also recommended in surgical procedures involving infected tissues that may result in bacteremia. Patients undergoing elective cardiac surgery should undergo dental evaluation to reduce the risk of late postoperative endocarditis. Finally, physicians should exercise their own clinical judgment in the choice of antibiotic and the number of doses that are to be administered in any given patient.

TABLE 20.15. *Endocarditis prophylactic regimens for genitourinary/gastrointestinal (excluding esophageal) procedures*

Situation	Agents[a]	Regimen[b]
High-risk patients	Ampicillin plus gentamicin	Adults: ampicillin, 2.0 g IM or IV, plus gentamicin, 1.5 mg/kg (not to exceed 120 mg) within 30 min of starting procedure; 6 hr later, ampicillin, 1 g IM/IV or amoxicillin, 1 g orally Children: ampicillin, 50 mg/kg IM or IV (not to exceed 2.0 g), plus gentamicin, 1.5 mg/kg within 30 min of starting the procedure; 6 hr later, ampicillin, 25 mg/kg IM/IV, or amoxicillin, 25 mg/kg orally
High-risk patients allergic to ampicillin/amoxicillin	Vancomycin plus gentamicin	Adults: vancomycin, 1.0 g IV over 1–2 hr, plus gentamicin, 1.5 mg/kg IV/IM (not to exceed 120 mg); complete injection/infusion within 30 min of starting procedure Children: vancomycin, 20 mg/kg IV over 1–2 hr, plus gentamicin, 1.5 mg/kg IV/IM complete injection/infusion within 30 min of starting procedure
Moderate-risk patients	Amoxicillin or ampicillin	Adults: amoxicillin, 2.0 g orally 1 hr before procedure, or ampicillin, 2.0 g IM/IV within 30 min of starting procedure Children: amoxicillin, 50 mg/kg orally 1 hr before procedure, or ampicillin, 50 mg/kg IM/IV within 30 min of starting procedure
Moderate-risk patients allergic to ampicillin/amoxicillin	Vancomycin	Adults: vancomycin, 1.0 g IV over 1–2 hr, complete infusion within 30 min of starting procedure Children: vancomycin, 20 mg/kg IV over 1–2 hr; complete infusion within 30 min of starting procedure

[a]No second dose of vancomycin or gentamicin is recommended.
[b]Total children's dose should not exceed adult dose.
From Dajani AS, Taubert KA, Wilson W, et al. Prevention of bacterial endocarditis: recommendations of the American Heart Association. *Circulation* 1997;96:358–366.

PRACTICAL POINTS

- Infective endocarditis is usually caused by bacteria, and the three most common bacteria are *S. viridans, S. aureus,* and *E. faecalis.*

- Persistent fever, new heart murmurs, vasculitis, hemorrhagic petechiae, embolic phenomena and metastatic abscesses, and development of heart failure are suggestive of acute endocarditis. *S. aureus* is usually implicated in acute endocarditis.

- A combination of heart murmur, anemia, hematuria, and renal failure should raise the suspicion of subacute endocarditis.

- Fever may be absent in moribund or immunocompromised individuals.

- The change in the character of an existing murmur or the development of a new murmur must raise the suspicion of infective endocarditis. In some instances, the only finding may be a "trivial" aortic regurgitation. In right-sided endocarditis, murmurs are not present.

- The management of a patient with infective endocarditis is a multidisciplinary approach with the involvement of a cardiologist, an infectious disease specialist, and a cardiothoracic surgeon.

- The ACC/AHA guidelines recommend antibiotic prophylaxis in patients with cardiac conditions whose risk of infective endocarditis is significantly higher than that of the general population.

REFERENCES

1. Dismukes WE-, Karchmer AW, Buckley MJ, et al. Prosthetic valve endocarditis: an analysis of 38 cases. *Circulation* 1973;48:365–377.
2. Baumgartner WA, Miller DC, Reitz BA, et al. Surgical treatment of prosthetic valve endocarditis. *Ann Thorac Surg* 1983;35:87–104.
3. Netzer RO, Zollinger E, Seiler C, et al. Infective endocarditis: clinical spectrum presentation and outcome. An analysis of 212 cases 1980–1995. *Heart* 2000;84:25–30.
4. Fowler VG Jr, Sanders LL, Kong LK, et al. Infective endocarditis due to *Staphylococcus aureus*: 59 prospectively identified cases with follow-up. *Clin Infect Dis* 1999;28:106–114.
5. Durack DT, Lukes AS, Bright DK. New criteria for diagnosis of infective endocarditis: utilization of specific echocardiographic findings: Duke Endocarditis Service. *Am J Med* 1994;96:200–209.
6. Shively BK, Gurule FT, Roldan CA, et al. Diagnostic value of transesophageal compared with transthoracic echocardiography in infective endocarditis. *J Am Coll Cardiol* 1991;18:391–397.
7. Mugge A, Daniel WG, Frank G, et al. Echocardiography in infective endocarditis: reassessment of prognostic implications of vegetation size determined by the transthoracic and the transesophageal approach. *J Am Coll Cardiol* 1989;14:631–638.
8. Shapiro SM, Young E, De Guzman S, et al. Transesophageal echocardiography in diagnosis of infective endocarditis. *Chest* 1994;105:377–382.
9. Roy P, Tajik AJ, Guiliani ER, et al. Spectrum of echocardiographic findings in bacterial endocarditis. *Circulation* 1976;53:474–482.
10. Daniel WG, Mugge A, Grote J, et al. Comparison of transthoracic and transesophageal echocardiography for detection of abnormalities of prosthetic and bioprosthetic valves in the mitral and aortic positions. *Am J Cardiol* 1993;71:210–215.
11. Bayer AS, Bolger AF, Taubert KA, et al. Diagnosis and management of infective endocarditis. *Circulation* 1998;98:2936–2948.
12. Vuille C, Nidorf M, Weyman AE, et al. Natural history of vegetations during successful medical treatment of endocarditis. *Am Heart J* 1994;128:1200–1209.
13. Rohmann S, Erbel R, Darius H, et al. Prediction of rapid versus prolonged healing of infective endocarditis by monitoring vegetation size. *J Am Soc Echocardiogr* 1991;4:465–474.
14. Dajani AS, Taubert KA, Wilson W, et al. Prevention of bacterial endocarditis: recommendations of the American Heart Association. *Circulation* 1997;96:358–366.
15. Wilson WR, et al. Antibiotic treatment of adults with infective endocarditis due to streptococci, eterococci, staphylocci, and hacek organisms: American Heart Association. *Jama* 1995;275:1706–1713.

21

Mitral Regurgitation

David S. Bach, Mark R. Starling, and Steven F. Bolling

USUAL CAUSES

The mitral apparatus is a complex structure comprising the anterior and posterior mitral leaflets, the left atrium and mitral valve annulus, the subvalvular chordae tendineae and papillary muscles, and, because of its affect on mitral valve function, the left ventricle (1). Disease or geometric change involving any of these structures can result in mitral regurgitation. In general, the causes of mitral regurgitation can be divided into two categories: anatomic and functional. Anatomic mitral regurgitation is caused by abnormal anatomy of the mitral leaflets, papillary muscles, or chordae, whereby mitral regurgitation can be attributed to a mechanical abnormality that precludes valve competency. In contrast, functional mitral regurgitation is caused by changes in the size or geometry of either the left ventricle or the left atrium and mitral annulus, whereby mitral regurgitation is caused by incomplete coaptation of anatomically normal or nearly normal leaflets.

Chronic Mitral Regurgitation

Chronic mitral regurgitation caused by anatomic abnormalities of the mitral leaflets can be caused by congenital disease, rheumatic disease, myxomatous degeneration, connective tissue diseases, infective endocarditis, or annular calcification (Table 21.1). Congenitally cleft anterior leaflet usually occurs as part of an endocardial cushion defect, with accompanying primum atrial septal defect, paramembranous ventricular septal defect, and abnormalities of the tricuspid valve. The mitral valve is the valve most commonly affected valve in rheumatic heart disease, with thickening and sclerosis of leaflet and subvalvular tissue, resulting in stenosis, regurgitation, or both. Myxomatous degeneration of the mitral valve occurs in the setting of the mitral valve prolapse syndrome (also known as Barlow's syndrome), in which redundant leaflet tissue and elongation of chordae tendineae are associated with premature valve degeneration and chordal rupture. In the mitral valve prolapse syndrome, mitral regurgitation can be caused by complete or partial leaflet flail or by pathologic prolapse without flail. Connective tissue diseases associated with mitral regurgitation include systemic lupus erythematosus, rheumatoid arthritis, ankylosing spondylitis, and scleroderma. Valvular involvement in connective tissue diseases is variable, but about half of patients with systemic lupus erythematosus have some mitral regurgitation, and approximately one fourth have significant regurgitation. Mitral regurgitation caused by infective endocarditis can occur because of direct interference of a vegetation with leaflet coaptation or, more commonly, because of tissue destruction with leaflet erosion or perforation, or with chordal rupture and complete or partial leaflet flail. Finally, mitral annular calcification is common among elderly patients as well as among patients with diseases associated with dystrophic calcification, such as end-stage renal insufficiency. Although mitral regurgitation is commonly seen in association with mitral annular calcification, it is not usually severe. Mitral regurgitation caused by leaflet thickening has been described in conjunction with anorectic drug use, although the importance of this is unclear.

Functional mitral regurgitation is caused by alteration of left ventricular size or geometry or, less commonly, alteration of mitral annular geometry that results in restriction of mitral leaflet motion and incomplete mitral leaflet coaptation. As such, significant functional mitral

TABLE 21.1. *Causes of mitral regurgitation*

Chronic mitral regurgitation, anatomic
  Congenital
  Rheumatic
  Myxomatous degeneration
  Connective tissue diseases
  Infective endocarditis
  Annular calcification
  Prosthetic valve dysfunction
Chronic mitral regurgitation, functional
  Dilated cardiomyopathy
  Coronary artery disease
Acute mitral regurgitation
  Infective endocarditis
  Myxomatous degeneration with chordal rupture
  Acute myocardial infarction with papillary muscle
    rupture
  Acute myocardial infarction with infarct expansion
  Prosthetic valve dysfunction

regurgitation occurs in the setting of normal or nearly normal leaflet anatomy. Functional mitral regurgitation can occur in the setting of nonischemic or ischemic cardiomyopathy. In addition, alteration of left ventricular geometry caused by relatively small inferior or posterolateral myocardial infarction can result in restrictive mitral leaflet motion with incomplete leaflet coaptation and significant regurgitation.

Ischemic mitral regurgitation is mitral regurgitation that results from underlying coronary artery disease. Ischemic mitral regurgitation can be caused by mechanical disruption of the mitral apparatus, such as papillary muscle rupture complicating acute myocardial infarction. More commonly, ischemic mitral regurgitation is functional mitral regurgitation that occurs in the setting of coronary artery disease. Specifically, most ischemic mitral regurgitation is caused by prior myocardial infarction with unfavorable left ventricular remodeling or left ventricular dilation that causes incomplete mitral leaflet coaptation. Ischemic mitral regurgitation can be dynamic, most often as a function of varying left ventricular loading conditions with dynamic changes in left ventricular size and geometry. In addition, transient ischemia involving a papillary muscle or an adjacent region of the left ventricle also may be able to cause dynamic mitral regurgitation.

Finally, mitral regurgitation can occur as a result of mechanical or bioprosthetic valve dysfunction. Mild transvalvular regurgitation is normal and an anticipated finding with many mechanical prostheses, as well as with some constructed pericardial bioprostheses. In addition, small amounts of paraprosthetic regurgitation are common with any mitral valve prosthesis. Larger paravalvular leaks can cause significant regurgitation, which is of potential clinical importance either because of hemodynamic significance or because of the severity of associated hemolysis. Pathologic transvalvular prosthetic regurgitation can occur in association with either mechanical or tissue prostheses. Significant valvular regurgitation with a mechanical valve is suggestive of entrapment or dysfunction of the occluder; significant regurgitation in association with a bioprosthesis is suggestive of leaflet fracture.

Acute Mitral Regurgitation

Acute severe mitral regurgitation is caused by infective endocarditis, myxomatous disease with chordal rupture, acute myocardial infarction with either papillary muscle rupture or infarct expansion and leaflet restriction, or prosthetic valve dysfunction.

PRESENTING SYMPTOMS AND SIGNS

Symptoms

Mitral regurgitation results in left ventricular volume overload with ejection of left ventricular volume into both the high-impedance aorta and the compliant, low-impedance left atrium. In chronic mitral regurgitation, left atrial dilation maintains low left atrial and pulmonary venous pressures. Compensatory left ventricular dilation results in increases in left ventricular end-diastolic volume, ejection fraction, and stroke volume, thereby maintaining forward cardiac output (2). Patients typically remain asymptomatic during this phase of compensated mitral regurgitation, which may last for years. Prolonged left ventricular volume overload eventually leads to left ventricular systolic dysfunction and pulmonary congestion, with an increase in left ventricular end-systolic volume and decreases in ejection fraction and forward cardiac output. Because left ventricular emptying does not rely on overcoming high aortic pressure, left ventricular stroke volume remains elevated, and ejection fraction remains within the normal range despite progressive left ventricular systolic dysfunction (3–6). Late in the course of disease, the left ventricular ejection fraction falls below normal. At some time during the course of chronic severe mitral regurgitation, patients develop symptoms of fatigue and exertional dyspnea, followed by more overt symptoms of congestive heart failure. However, symptoms are typically insidious in onset, and patients often fail to recognize the gradual fatigue and subtle exercise limitations associated with chronic severe mitral regurgitation.

In acute severe mitral regurgitation, limited left atrial distensibility results in an acute increase in left atrial and pulmonary venous pressures with resulting pulmonary edema. Although increased preload associated with acute severe mitral regurgitation results in a modest increase in total left ventricular stroke volume (5), the absence of compensatory left ventricular dilation results in reduced forward stroke volume. Compensatory tachycardia is typically insufficient to maintain forward cardiac output. In this setting, patients with acute severe mitral regurgitation are almost always symptomatic, with fulminant symptoms of pulmonary edema.

Signs

Physical examination of patients with chronic severe mitral regurgitation may reveal a hyperactive precordium and lateral displacement of the left ventricular apical impulse because of ventricular enlargement. A late systolic left parasternal lift caused by left atrial expansion may be present; this, in conjunction with an apical heave, results in a rocking motion of the precordium. An apical systolic thrill may be evident. The first heart sound is usually normal, although it may be encompassed by the systolic murmur and difficult to appreciate. An S3 is often present because of the large regurgitant volume reentering the left ventricle across a fixed mitral orifice, and is not necessarily indicative of ventricular failure. The classic murmur of mitral regurgitation is a loud, blowing holosystolic murmur that may obliterate S1 and S2. The murmur is usually loudest at the apex with radiation to the axilla or the back, although it is often audible throughout the precordium. Mitral regurgitation caused by leaflet flail is usually eccentric, and the murmur associated with posterior leaflet flail radiates anteriorly to the left sternal border. Because of the proximity of the ascending aorta immediately anterior to the roof of the left atrium, the murmur of an anteriorly directed mitral regurgitation jet can be transmitted to the carotid arteries. The large volume of blood crossing the mitral valve in diastole causes turbulent flow in patients with severe regurgitation, sometimes causing a diastolic rumble, despite the absence of mitral stenosis. In contrast, the systolic murmur in patients with acute severe mitral regurgitation may be decrescendo rather than holosystolic, because of early equilibration of left atrial and left ventricular pressures. In acute severe mitral regurgitation, the apical left ventricular impulse is not displaced, and an S3 and S4 are common.

The Mitral Valve Prolapse Syndrome

The mitral valve prolapse syndrome can occur without associated mitral regurgitation, although progression of mitral regurgitation is common over the course of the disease. Patients with the mitral valve prolapse syndrome may have symptoms of palpitations or atypical chest pain (7,8). Physical examination reveals a characteristic midsystolic nonejection click that moves later in systole with maneuvers such as squatting that increase left ventricular preload. In patients with mitral valve prolapse without leaflet flail, mitral regurgitation, if present, occurs late in systole, and the accompanying murmur occurs only in the portion of systole after the midsystolic click.

HELPFUL TESTS

In general, echocardiography with Doppler imaging is an ideal modality for the assessment of the presence, etiology, severity, and impact of mitral regurgitation (Table 21.2). Transthoracic imaging usually allows for sufficient assessment of mitral valve anatomy and the severity of mitral regurgitation, as well as assessment of left atrial

TABLE 21.2. *Echocardiographic imaging in mitral regurgitation*

Transthoracic echocardiography
  Baseline evaluation to quantify mitral regurgitation
  Baseline evaluation to quantify left ventricular
    systolic function
  Delineation of mechanism of mitral regurgitation
  Annual or semiannual surveillance of left ventricular
    systolic function
  Establish cardiac status after change in symptoms
  Evaluation after mitral valve replacement or repair
Transesophageal echocardiography
  Evaluation of mitral regurgitation in patients with
    nondiagnostic transthoracic echocardiogram
  Assessment of suspected prosthetic valve
    dysfunction
  Preoperative assessment of suitability for mitral
    valve repair
  Intraoperative assessment of mitral valve repair

Adapted from Bonow RO, Carabello B, de Leon AC Jr, et al. Guidelines for the management of patients with valvular heart disease: executive summary. A report of the American College of Cardiology/American Heart Association Task Force on Practice Guidelines (Committee on Management of Patients with Valvular Heart Disease). *J Am Coll Cardiol* 1998;32:1486–1588.

and left ventricular size and systolic function. Anterior and posterior mitral leaflet anatomy and the submitral apparatus are usually well visualized on transthoracic imaging. Left ventricular size and overall left ventricular systolic function can be assessed and quantified, and left ventricular wall motion abnormalities associated with coronary artery disease may be evident. Color flow Doppler imaging allows semiquantitative assessment of mitral regurgitation severity (9,10), as well as assessment of jet characteristics that may help with determination of the cause of regurgitation (11). Highly eccentric jets are usually indicative of leaflet flail, although an eccentric jet also can be seen with leaflet restriction in the setting of ischemic mitral regurgitation (12). Evidence of concomitant valve disease or pulmonary hypertension also may be visible.

Transesophageal echocardiography provides superb visualization of mitral valve anatomy, including the mitral leaflets and subvalvular apparatus (13). Transesophageal echocardiographic imaging essentially always allows visualization of mitral anatomy sufficient to define the cause of regurgitation and is instrumental in the as-

sessment of mitral anatomy in anticipation of possible mitral valve repair. In addition, transesophageal echocardiography is indicated in order to evaluate suspected prosthetic mitral regurgitation (14), which can be underestimated on transthoracic imaging. Finally, intraoperative transesophageal echocardiography is used to evaluate the suitability for and results after surgical mitral valve repair.

Other tests that may be useful in patients with mitral regurgitation include electrocardiogram (ECG), chest radiograph, cardiac catheterization, and stress testing. The ECG and chest radiograph may reveal evidence of left atrial or left ventricular enlargement in patients with chronic mitral regurgitation. Later, the ECG may disclose atrial arrhythmias, including atrial fibrillation. Although cardiac catheterization with left ventriculography allows assessment of left ventricular ejection fraction and semiquantitative assessment of mitral regurgitation severity, both are usually available with noninvasive imaging. Coronary angiography is useful for assessment of coronary anatomy in patients at risk for coronary disease who are undergoing mitral valve surgery and in patients in whom an ischemic cause of mitral regurgitation is suspected. Exercise stress testing is useful for objectively defining exercise tolerance. Inasmuch as symptoms in chronic mitral regurgitation are slowly progressive, many patients do not recognize the insidious decrease in exercise tolerance that occurs over years. In addition, Doppler studies during exercise can sometimes disclose worsening of mitral regurgitation that is less significant at rest (15).

DIFFERENTIAL DIAGNOSIS

Symptoms of fatigue and exertional dyspnea are nonspecific and potentially referable to a long list of cardiac and noncardiac causes. The murmur of mitral regurgitation can be differentiated from that of aortic stenosis by its holosystolic nature and by its blowing, rather than harsh, quality. The murmur of tricuspid insufficiency is usually loudest at the lower left sternal border and should be augmented with inspiration. Echocardiographic imaging should be diagnostic, although mitral regurgitation can be dynamic and therefore can vary in severity during different conditions of loading (16). In some instances, functional mitral regurgitation can appear less significant on left ventriculography if the patient has taken nothing by mouth for several hours, as is customary before invasive testing, or if loading conditions are altered during invasive testing with the use of nitroglycerin. Finally, catheter-induced mitral regurgitation can occur if the left ventricular catheter interferes with otherwise normal mitral valve function, typically caused by catheter entanglement in the chordae tendineae.

Myxomatous degeneration of the mitral valve can be expressed in one of three ways: billowing, prolapse, or flail. Mitral valve *billowing* implies that the body of the valve extends above the plane of the annulus in systole, but the zone of leaflet coaptation is preserved, and there is usually with no associated regurgitation. Mitral valve *prolapse* occurs when the free edge of a leaflet extends above the plane of the annulus in systole, usually with associated regurgitation. Partial or complete leaflet *flail* is loss of continuity between the leaflet and one or more chordae, usually with significant associated regurgitation. Finally, the diagnosis of mitral valve prolapse on echocardiography should be distinguished from normal variants that can occur in the setting of dehydration and a hypercontractile left ventricle (17). In addition, significant enlargement of the right ventricle can affect the shape of the mitral valve annulus and cause an appearance of mitral valve prolapse in the absence of any myxomatous tissue degeneration.

COMPLICATIONS

Chronic severe mitral regurgitation results in left ventricular dilation and eventually in progressive systolic dysfunction with resulting congestive heart failure. Atrial arrhythmias, including atrial fibrillation, occur more often over time among patients with untreated mitral regurgitation. By one estimate, the linearized rates of acquired chronic atrial fibrillation or congestive heart failure among patients with medically treated severe mitral regurgitation are approximately 2.2% and

8.2%, respectively (18). As with any valve disease, patients with mitral regurgitation are at risk of infective endocarditis.

It is important to recognize that left ventricular systolic dysfunction precedes a detectable decrease below normal in left ventricular ejection fraction (3–6), because early systolic dysfunction is masked by the ability of the left ventricle to empty into the low-impedance left atrium. Therefore, delaying surgical intervention until the presence of symptoms or overt left ventricular systolic dysfunction clearly carries a risk of permanent left ventricular systolic dysfunction and congestive heart failure, as well as dramatically increasing surgical risks and worsening the rate of postoperative survival (19–22).

THERAPY

Medical Therapy

Medical therapy for chronic mitral regurgitation is limited. As with other valvular heart disease, appropriate antibiotic prophylaxis should be used (23). Antibiotic prophylaxis should be given to patients with mitral valve prolapse in the presence of a click-murmur complex on physical examination or if there is a click on physical examination and echocardiographic evidence of mitral valve prolapse and mitral regurgitation. In addition, antibiotic prophylaxis should be considered in the absence of mitral regurgitation if there is evidence of myxomatous degeneration on echocardiography. Afterload-reducing agents can decrease the severity of functional mitral regurgitation (24–26). As with all patients with left ventricular dysfunction, afterload reducing agents should be used in patients with cardiomyopathy and secondary mitral regurgitation. In addition, afterload-reducing agents may be useful in the treatment of asymptomatic patients with chronic severe mitral regurgitation, although the long-term benefit of therapy has not been fully tested (27).

For patients with acute severe mitral regurgitation, medical therapy is intended to decrease the severity of mitral regurgitation and thereby increase forward cardiac output and minimize pulmonary venous congestion. Nitroprusside is useful alone in normotensive patients with acute severe mitral regurgitation (28,29) or in combination with an inotropic agent in patients with hypotension. Intraaortic balloon counterpulsation is a useful adjunct for patients with acute severe mitral regurgitation and hypotension or pulmonary edema.

Surgical Intervention

Surgical intervention is the definitive therapy for mitral regurgitation and includes the alternatives of mitral valve repair and mitral valve replacement with or without chordal preservation. Mitral valve replacement without chordal preservation results in loss of ventricular systolic shortening and decreased postoperative left ventricular systolic function, with lower functional class and impaired survival (30–34). Mitral valve repair minimizes the use of prosthetic material, obviating the need for long-term anticoagulation and reducing the risk of endocarditis. Repair is often associated with more favorable hemodynamics in comparison with valve replacement, and there is no risk of prosthetic valve failure. Furthermore, mitral valve repair is associated with better preservation of left ventricular systolic function and improved survival in comparison with mitral valve replacement (35–39). However, mitral repair is a more technically demanding procedure, requiring substantial surgical expertise, and may not be feasible for all valves. Despite being a more technically demanding procedure with longer extracorporeal circulation times, mitral valve repair is associated with lower rates of operative and subsequent mortality than is valve replacement, and it avoids or minimizes many of the pitfalls associated with prosthetic valves, including thromboembolic risk, long-term anticoagulation, endocarditis risk, hemolysis, and structural and nonstructural prosthesis dysfunction. Avoiding many of the pitfalls associated with prosthetic valves allows consideration for surgical intervention with mitral valve repair earlier in the course of disease, reducing the risk of developing atrial arrhythmias, occult left ventricular systolic dysfunction, and congestive heart failure (18). Finally, preservation of left ventricular

shape and systolic function with mitral valve repair makes surgical intervention feasible among patients with severely impaired left ventricular systolic function (40), for whom the risk of mitral valve replacement may be prohibitive (27). Mitral valve repair should therefore be considered the surgical procedure of choice if valve structure is amenable to reconstruction and if appropriate surgical expertise is available.

Mitral valve surgery is indicated for patients with severe mitral regurgitation and either symptoms of heart failure or evidence of left ventricular systolic dysfunction, defined as left ventricular ejection fraction less than 60% or left ventricular end-systolic diameter of 45 mm or more (27) (Table 21.3). Although severe left ventricular systolic dysfunction before surgery is associated with increased rates of operative and later mortality, symptomatic patients should nonetheless be considered for surgical intervention. Asymptomatic patients with normal left ventricular size and systolic function and a good likelihood of successful valve repair may benefit from early surgical intervention with the goal of preventing the sequelae of chronic mitral regurgitation, including the risks of atrial fibrillation,

---

TABLE 21.3. *Surgery for severe mitral regurgitation*

Acute severe mitral regurgitation
  Congestive heart failure or hemodynamic compromise
  Absence of symptoms, if repair likely
Chronic mitral regurgitation
  NYHA Class II, III, or IV symptoms with normal left ventricular size and systolic function
  Any left ventricular systolic dysfunction
  Evidence of atrial fibrillation or pulmonary hypertension
  Any left ventricular enlargement, if repair likely
  Severe left ventricular systolic dysfunction, if chordal preservation likely
  Consideration, if repair likely, despite absence of symptoms, left ventricular dilation, or systolic dysfunction

NYHA, New York Heart Association.
Adapted from Bonow RO, Carabello B, de Leon AC Jr, et al. Guidelines for the management of patients with valvular heart disease: executive summary. A report of the American College of Cardiology/American Heart Association Task Force on Practice Guidelines (Committee on Management of Patients with Valvular Heart Disease). *J Am Coll Cardiol* 1998;32:1486–1588.

congestive heart failure, and death associated with delayed surgical intervention (18). Asymptomatic patients with severe mitral regurgitation and evidence of progressive left ventricular dilation or with atrial fibrillation of recent onset and patients with new severe mitral regurgitation similarly should be considered for early mitral valve repair.

The presence of ischemic mitral regurgitation is a marker of poor prognosis (41–43). Similarly, residual mitral regurgitation after surgical coronary revascularization is associated with a significantly decreased rate of survival over the first few postoperative years (41,44–46). Although some investigators and clinicians prefer the use of mitral valve replacement, our experience is that ischemic mitral regurgitation caused by restrictive mitral leaflet motion is usually amenable to repair by a simple annuloplasty technique (47). In light of the feasibility of mitral valve repair or replacement and the dire impact on survival of residual mitral regurgitation after coronary revascularization, aggressive intervention is warranted to address ischemic mitral regurgitation at the time of coronary bypass grafting.

PROGNOSIS

Acute severe mitral regurgitation is a fulminant disease, typically accompanied by hypotension and congestive heart failure with pulmonary edema. In contrast, chronic mitral regurgitation is indolent in its course. Patients typically remain asymptomatic until late in the course of disease. However, the onset of symptoms often occurs after the onset of permanent left ventricular systolic dysfunction. Because surgical risk and long-term morbidity and mortality rates increase after the onset of left ventricular systolic dysfunction (19–22), intervention should occur before the onset of either symptoms or left ventricular systolic dysfunction. As noted previously, early mitral valve repair may avoid significant risks of atrial fibrillation, congestive heart failure, and death associated with delayed surgical intervention (18). Finally, the presence of ischemic mitral regurgitation is a marker of poor prognosis and should be aggressively treated at the time of coronary artery bypass surgery (41–46).

FOLLOW-UP

Asymptomatic patients with mild mitral regurgitation and normal left ventricular systolic function should undergo periodic assessment, including assesment for symptoms and physical examination on approximately a yearly basis (27). After the initial documentation of mild mitral regurgitation, echocardiographic imaging should be repeated if there are new symptoms or evidence on physical examination of worsened regurgitation. Periodic assessment with echocardiography and Doppler imaging to evaluate for change in mitral regurgitation severity is advisable, because the severity of mitral regurgitation is difficult to assess reliably on physical examination. Patients with moderate mitral regurgitation should undergo yearly assessment, including history documentation, physical examination, and echocardiographic imaging to assess for new symptoms or signs of heart failure and to monitor left ventricular size and function. Asymptomatic patients with severe mitral regurgitation should undergo assessment with history documentation, physical examination, and echocardiography every 6 to 12 months, with more frequent testing if symptoms develop, if there is echocardiographic evidence of progressive left ventricular dilation, or if there is any evidence of a decrease in left ventricular systolic function. Among patients with chronic mitral regurgitation, accurate quantitative assessment of left ventricular size and systolic function are important as a baseline to which future study results can be compared.

Because preoperative left ventricular systolic function is an important predictor of postoperative survival, patients should be referred for surgical intervention before the onset of left ventricular systolic dysfunction (27). As noted previously, the left ventricular ejection fraction remains within the normal range in patients with chronic severe mitral regurgitation after the onset of left ventricular systolic dysfunction. Therefore, ejection fraction alone is a poor measure of left ventricular systolic function in patients with mitral regurgitation, and any evidence of change in left ventricular size or systolic function should be considered in evaluating the timing of surgical intervention.

PRACTICAL POINTS

- Mitral regurgitation is a common condition with multiple potential causes.

- Causes include diseases of the mitral valve leaflets, the subvalvular apparatus, and the left ventricle.

- The disease has an indolent course; symptoms occur late.

- Echocardiography with Doppler imaging is the test of choice for confirming diagnosis and further characterizing disease.

- Transesophageal echocardiography is useful if transthoracic imaging is nondiagnostic or with prosthetic valves.

- Patients should be referred for surgical intervention before the onset of symptoms or left ventricular systolic dysfunction (left ventricular ejection fraction less than 60%).

- Surgical intervention should aim to preserve subvalvular apparatus.

- Mitral repair is the procedure of choice if feasible.

REFERENCES

1. Perloff JK, Roberts WC. The mitral apparatus: functional anatomy of mitral regurgitation. *Circulation* 1972;46:227–239.

2. Zile MR, Gaasch WH, Carroll JD, et al. Chronic mitral regurgitation: predictive value of preoperative echocardiographic indexes of left ventricular function and wall stress. *J Am Coll Cardiol* 1984;3:235–242.

3. Schuler G, Peterson KL, Johnson A, et al. Temporal response of left ventricular performance to mitral valve surgery. *Circulation* 1979;59:1218–1231.

4. Carabello BA, Nolan SP, McGuire LB. Assessment of preoperative left ventricular function in patients with mitral regurgitation: value of the end-systolic wall stress–end-systolic volume ratio. *Circulation* 1981;64:1212–1217.

5. Carabello BA. Mitral regurgitation: basic pathophysiologic principles. Part 1. *Mod Concepts Cardiovasc Dis* 1988;57:53–58.

6. Starling MR, Kirsh MM, Montgomery DG, et al. Impaired left ventricular contractile function in patients with long-term mitral regurgitation and normal ejection fraction. *J Am Coll Cardiol* 1993;22:239–250.

7. Crawford MH, O'Rourke RA. Mitral valve prolapse syndrome. In: Isselbacher KJ, Adams RD, Braunwaid E, eds. *Harrison's principles of internal medicine: update I.* New York: McGraw-Hill, 1981:91–152.

8. Fontana ME, Sparks EA, Boudoulas H, et al. Mitral valve prolapse and the mitral valve prolapse syndrome. *Curr Probl Cardiol* 1991;16:309–375.

9. Spain MG, Smith MD, Grayburn PA, et al. Quantitative assessment of mitral regurgitation by Doppler color flow imaging: angiographic and hemodynamic correlations. *J Am Coll Cardiol* 1989;13:585–590.

10. Cape EG, Yoganathan AP, Weyman AE, et al. Adjacent solid boundaries alter the size of regurgitant jets on Doppler color flow maps. *J Am Coll Cardiol* 1991;17:1094–1102.

11. Stewart WJ, Currie PJ, Salcedo EE, et al. Evaluation of mitral leaflet motion by echocardiography and jet direction by Doppler color flow mapping to determine the mechanisms of mitral regurgitation. *J Am Coll Cardiol* 1992;20:1353–1361.

12. Levi GS, Bolling SF, Bach DS. Eccentric mitral regurgitation jets among patients having sustained inferior wall myocardial infarction. *Echocardiography* 2001;18:97–103.

13. Castello R, Fagan LJ, Lenzen P, et al. Comparison of transthoracic and transesophageal echocardiography for assessment of left-sided valvular regurgitation. *Am J Cardiol* 1991;68:1677–1680.

14. Bach DS. TEE evaluation of prosthetic valves. *Cardiol Clin* 2000;18:751–771.

15. Tischler MD, Battle RW, Saha M, et al. Observations suggesting a high incidence of exercise-induced severe mitral regurgitation in patients with mild rheumatic mitral valve disease at rest. *J Am Coll Cardiol* 1995;25:128–133.

16. Bach DS, Deeb GM, Bolling SF. Accuracy of intraoperative transesophageal echocardiography for estimating the severity of functional mitral regurgitation. *Am J Cardiol* 1995;76:508–512.

17. Lax D, Eicher M, Goldberg SJ. Mild dehydration induces echocardiographic signs of mitral valve prolapse in healthy females with prior normal cardiac findings. *Am Heart J* 1992;124:1533–1540.

18. Ling LH, Enriquez-Sarano M, Seward JB, et al. Clinical outcome of mitral regurgitation due to leaflet flail. *N Engl J Med* 1996;335:1417–1423.

19. Phillips HR, Levine FH, Carter JE, et al. Mitral valve replacement for isolated mitral regurgitation: analysis of clinical course and late postoperative left ventricular ejection fraction. *Am J Cardiol* 1981;48:647–654.

20. Crawford MH, Souchek J, Oprian CA, et al. Determinants of survival and left ventricular performance after mitral valve replacement: Department of Veterans Affairs Cooperative Study on Valvular Heart Disease. *Circulation* 1990;81:1173–1181.

21. Enriquez-Sarano M, Tajik AJ, Schaff HV, et al. Echocardiographic prediction of survival after surgical correction of organic mitral regurgitation. *Circulation* 1994;90:830–837.

22. Wisenbaugh T, Skudicky D, Sareli P. Prediction of outcome after valve replacement for rheumatic mitral regurgitation in the era of chordal preservation. *Circulation* 1994;89:191–197.
23. Dajani AS, Taubert KA, Wilson W, et al. Prevention of bacterial endocarditis: recommendations by the American Heart Association. *Circulation* 1997;96:358–366.
24. Schon HR, Schroter G, Barthel P, et al. Quinapril therapy in patients with chronic mitral regurgitation. *J Heart Valve Dis* 1994;3:303–312.
25. Devlin WH, Starling MR. Outcome of valvular heart disease with vasodilator therapy. *Compr Ther* 1994;20:569–574.
26. Dujardin KS, Enriquez-Sarano M, Bailey KR, et al. Effect of losartan on degree of mitral regurgitation quantified by echocardiography. *Am J Cardiol* 2001;87:570–576.
27. Bonow RO, Carabello B, de Leon AC Jr, et al. Guidelines for the management of patients with valvular heart disease: executive summary. A report of the American College of Cardiology/American Heart Association Task Force on Practice Guidelines (Committee on Management of Patients with Valvular Heart Disease). *J Am Coll Cardiol* 1998;32:1486–1588.
28. Chatterjee K, Parmley WW, Swan HJ, et al. Beneficial effects of vasodilator agents in severe mitral regurgitation due to dysfunction of the subvalvular apparatus. *Circulation* 1973;48:684–690.
29. Yoran C, Yellin EL, Becker RM, et al. Mechanism of reduction of mitral regurgitation with vasodilator therapy. *Am J Cardiol* 1979;43:773–777.
30. David TE, Uden DE, Strauss HD. The importance of the mitral apparatus in left ventricular function after correction of mitral regurgitation. *Circulation* 1983;68:II76–II82.
31. David TE, Burns RJ, Bacchus CM, et al. Mitral valve replacement for mitral regurgitation with and without preservation of chordae tendineae. *J Thorac Cardiovasc Surg* 1984;88:718–725.
32. Hennein HA, Swain JA, McIntosh CL, et al. Comparative assessment of chordal preservation versus chordal resection during mitral valve replacement. *J Thorac Cardiovasc Surg* 1990;99:828–836.
33. Rozich JD, Carabello BA, Usher BW, et al. Mitral valve replacement with and without chordal preservation in patients with chronic mitral regurgitation: mechanisms for differences in postoperative ejection performance. *Circulation* 1992;86:1718–1726.
34. Horskotte D, Schulte HD, Bircks W, et al. The effect of chordal preservation on late outcome after mitral valve replacement: a randomized study. *J Heart Valve Dis* 1993;2:150–158.
35. Duran CG, Pomar JL, Revuelta JM, et al. Conservative operation for mitral insufficiency: critical analysis supported by postoperative hemodynamic studies of 72 patients. *J Thorac Cardiovasc Surg* 1980;79:326–337.
36. Yacoub M, Halim M, Radley-Smith R, et al. Surgical treatment of mitral regurgitation caused by floppy valves: repair versus replacement. *Circulation* 1981;64:II210–II216.
37. Goldman ME, Mora F, Guarino T, et al. Mitral valvuloplasty is superior to valve replacement for preservation of left ventricular function: an intraoperative two-dimensional echocardiographic study. *J Am Coll Cardiol* 1987;10:568–575.
38. Tischler MD, Cooper KA, Rowen M, et al. Mitral valve replacement versus mitral valve repair: a Doppler and quantitative stress echocardiographic study. *Circulation* 1994;89:132–137.
39. Enriquez-Sarano M, Schaff HV, Orszulak TA, et al. Valve repair improves the outcome of surgery for mitral regurgitation: a multivariate analysis. *Circulation* 1995;91:1022–1028.
40. Bolling SF, Pagani FD, Deeb GM, et al. Intermediate term outcome of mitral reconstruction in cardiomyopathy. *J Thorac Cardiovasc Surg* 1998;115:381–386.
41. Hickey MStJ, Smith R, Muhlbaier LH, et al. Current prognosis of ischemic mitral regurgitation: implications for future management. *Circulation* 1988;78(Suppl I):I51–I59.
42. Lamas GA, Mitchell GF, Flaker GC, et al. Clinical significance of mitral regurgitation after acute myocardial infarction. *Circulation* 1997;96:827–833.
43. Grigioni F, Enriquez-Sarano M, Zehr KJ, et al. Ischemic mitral regurgitation: long-term outcome and prognostic implications with quantitative Doppler assessment. *Circulation* 2001;103:1759–1764.
44. Pinson CW, Cobanoglu A, Metzdorff MT, et al. Late surgical results for ischemic mitral regurgitation. *J Thorac Cardiovasc Surg* 1984;88:663–672.
45. Sheikh KH, Bengtson JR, Rankin JS, et al. Intraoperative transesophageal Doppler color flow imaging used to guide patient selection and operative treatment of ischemic mitral regurgitation. *Circulation* 1991;84:594–604.
46. Hausmann H, Siniawski H, Hetzer R. Mitral valve reconstruction and replacement for ischemic mitral insufficiency: seven years' follow up. *J Heart Valve Dis* 1999;8:536–542.
47. Bolling SF, Deeb GM, Bach DS. Mitral valve reconstruction in elderly ischemic patients. *Chest* 1996;109:35–40.

22

Aortic Regurgitation

David S. Bach, Michael J. Shea, and G. Michael Deeb

USUAL CAUSES

The aortic valve comprises three semilunar aortic cusps, the sinuses of Valsalva, and the sinotubular junction. Aortic regurgitation is caused by acquired or congenital abnormalities of the aortic valve cusps or by acquired abnormalities of the aortic root that affect the competence of what may be anatomically normal cusps. In general, aortic regurgitation caused by aortic root disease necessitates dilation at the level of the sinotubular junction; isolated aortic annular dilation is unlikely to occur, owing to the dense surrounding fibrous tissue.

Chronic Aortic Regurgitation

Chronic aortic regurgitation can be caused by congenital or acquired abnormalities (Table 22.1). The most common congenital abnormality of the aortic valve associated with aortic regurgitation is bicuspid aortic valve; fenestrations of the aortic valve cusps are a less frequent cause. Acquired causes of chronic aortic regurgitation resulting from predominant disease of the valve cusps include calcific degeneration, rheumatic disease, infective endocarditis, myxomatous degeneration, and chronic anorectic drug use. Less common etiologies of aortic regurgitation caused by abnormalities of the cusps include discrete subaortic stenosis and aortic cuspal prolapse caused by perimembranous ventricular septal defect.

Aortic root disease resulting in chronic aortic regurgitation can be idiopathic, associated with bicuspid aortic valve, or caused by systemic hypertension, cystic medial necrosis with or without other features of Marfan's syndrome, or aortic dissection. Other, less commonly encountered causes of aortic root disease include connec-

tive tissue diseases such as Reiter's syndrome, ankylosing spondylitis, and rheumatoid arthritis. Luetic (syphilitic) aortitis is still described as a potential cause of aortic root disease but, in effect, is no longer encountered clinically in the United States.

Finally, dysfunction of a mechanical or bioprosthetic aortic valve prosthesis can result in aortic regurgitation. Mild transvalvular regurgitation is an anticipated finding with most mechanical prostheses, and small amounts of paraprosthetic regurgitation are common with any prosthesis. Larger paravalvular leaks can be of clinical importance either because of their hemodynamic significance or because of associated hemolysis. Significant valvular regurgitation with a mechanical prosthesis suggests entrapment or dysfunction of the occluder; significant regurgitation in association with a bioprosthesis suggests leaflet fracture.

Acute Aortic Regurgitation

Acute severe aortic regurgitation is caused by infective endocarditis, aortic dissection, nonpenetrating (or, in rare cases, penetrating) chest trauma, or prosthetic valve dysfunction.

PRESENTING SYMPTOMS AND SIGNS

Symptoms

Patients with chronic aortic regurgitation usually remain asymptomatic for years or decades. During this compensated phase, the left ventricular volume overload of aortic regurgitation is accommodated through increases in left ventricular volume and chamber compliance and through both eccentric and concentric hypertrophy. Increased stroke volume maintains normal forward cardiac output, and increased left ventricular compliance

TABLE 22.1. *Causes of aortic regurgitation*

Chronic aortic regurgitation, related to valve cusps
    Congenital (bicuspid aortic valve, fenestrations)
    Calcific degeneration
    Rheumatic
    Infective endocarditis
    Myxomatous degeneration
    Anorectic drugs
    Prosthetic valve dysfunction
Chronic aortic regurgitation, related to ascending aorta
    Idiopathic aortic root dilation
    Root dilation related to bicuspid aortic valve
    Root dilation secondary to hypertension
    Cystic medial necrosis (including Marfan's syndrome)
    Aortic dissection
Acute aortic regurgitation
    Infective endocarditis
    Aortic dissection
    Nonpenetrating chest trauma
    Prosthetic valve dysfunction

be nocturnal) and symptoms of right-sided congestive heart failure with ascites and peripheral edema.

Acute severe aortic regurgitation usually occurs in the setting of infective endocarditis, acute aortic dissection or, more rarely, after blunt chest trauma. Patients typically exhibit symptoms referable to the underlying disease, including fever with infective endocarditis or chest or back pain with aortic dissection. In the absence of the compensatory mechanisms present in chronic aortic regurgitation, acute severe aortic regurgitation is poorly tolerated hemodynamically, and patients frequently present with pulmonary edema or cardiogenic shock.

maintains normal filling pressures with maintained preload reserve. The increase in chamber size results in increased wall stress, with compensatory hypertrophy in response to increased afterload. During this period, myocardial contractility and left ventricular ejection fraction remain normal. Symptoms during this phase of compensated chronic aortic regurgitation may include a sensation of pounding in the chest, palpitations, or head pounding, caused by increased stroke volume and a wide pulse pressure.

Eventually, persistent volume and pressure overload exhaust left ventricular preload reserve; in addition, hypertrophy may become inadequate for increased afterload. At this point, further increases in afterload result in decreased left ventricular ejection fraction. Exertional dyspnea is typically the first manifestation of left ventricular decompensation, with later development of orthopnea and paroxysmal nocturnal dyspnea.

Initially, left ventricular systolic dysfunction is caused by pure afterload excess and is reversible after aortic valve replacement. Later, depressed myocardial contractility causes progressive and irreversible systolic dysfunction. In addition, inadequate coronary flow reserve in the setting of left ventricular hypertrophy, along with decreased perfusion pressure associated with low diastolic pressures, can result in coronary insufficiency. Symptoms of more advanced disease eventually include angina pectoris (which may

Signs

Physical findings in patients with chronic severe aortic regurgitation reflect the combination of increased stroke volume and widened pulse pressure. Findings can be extensive, and there may be no other single lesion so rich with associated eponyms (Table 22.2). In general appearance,

TABLE 22.2. *Selected physical findings and eponyms associated with severe chronic aortic regurgitation*

Physical finding	Eponym
Bobbing motion of the torso or the head	de Musset's sign
Systolic pulsation of the uvula	Müller's sign
Exaggerated systolic distension and diastolic collapse of arterial pulses	Water-hammer pulse, Corrigan's pulse
Capillary pulsation visible in nail bed with distal compression	Quincke's pulse
Brief, loud systolic sound on auscultation of large arteries	Pistol shot pulse
Booming systolic and diastolic sounds on auscultation of femoral artery	Traube's sign
Systolic murmur with light proximal pressure of stethoscope; diastolic murmur with distal pressure	Duroziez's sign
Diastolic murmur radiating to left ventricular apex	Austin-Flint murmur

patients can exhibit a bobbing motion of the torso or the head (de Musset's sign) synchronous with the heartbeat. Systolic pulsation of the uvula may be visible (Müller's sign). Arterial pulses are unusually prominent, with exaggerated systolic distension and exaggerated diastolic collapse on palpation (water-hammer or Corrigan's pulse). Palpation of the carotid arteries reveals a bisferiens, or double-peaking, pulse. Capillary pulsation may be visible in the nail beds when the distal nail is softly compressed (Quincke's pulse). Auscultation of large arteries may reveal a brief, loud systolic (pistol shot) sound. Auscultation of the femoral artery reveals booming systolic and diastolic sounds (Traube's sign); light pressure of the stethoscope proximally reveals a systolic murmur, with a diastolic murmur when pressure is applied distally (Duroziez's sign). The systolic blood pressure is typically elevated, and the diastolic blood pressure is often very low, revealing a wide pulse pressure.

The left ventricular apical impulse is enlarged and displaced as a result of left ventricular enlargement, and it may be visible. A systolic thrill may be evident along the base of the heart or in the carotid arteries, caused by the large left ventricular stroke volume. On auscultation, the aortic component of S2 may be diminished or absent. An S3 is common and is not indicative of congestive heart failure. The murmur of aortic regurgitation is a high-pitched, blowing decrescendo diastolic murmur, loudest at the left or right upper sternal border. Held end-expiration with the patient upright and leaning forward and the stethoscope diaphragm held firmly against the chest aids in the auscultation of soft murmurs of aortic regurgitation. The aortic regurgitant jet may result in vibration of the anterior mitral valve leaflet, resulting in a low-pitched diastolic rumble at the cardiac apex (Austin Flint murmur) that can mimic mitral stenosis, albeit without presystolic accentuation. A systolic ejection murmur, often louder and more easily heard than the diastolic murmur, is caused by the large stroke volume and is not indicative of aortic stenosis.

Many of the typical physical findings associated with chronic aortic regurgitation are absent in patients with acute severe aortic regurgitation. Because the left ventricle is not dilated in acute aortic regurgitation, stroke volume is not increased, pulse pressure is not widened, and the associated peripheral arterial manifestations are absent. Tachycardia is typical, in a compensatory attempt to maintain forward cardiac output without the benefit of increased stroke volume. Premature closure of the mitral valve may be associated with decreased intensity of S1. The diastolic murmur in acute, severe aortic regurgitation is often shorter and softer than that associated with chronic aortic regurgitation, because diastolic pressure equilibration between the ascending aorta and left ventricle occurs earlier in diastole. Although chronic severe aortic regurgitation usually can be diagnosed on physical examination, the detection of acute severe regurgitation is less certain.

HELPFUL TESTS

Echocardiography with Doppler imaging is an ideal modality for the assessment of the presence, etiology, severity, and impact of aortic regurgitation (Table 22.3). Echocardiography is indicated for patients with suspected aortic regurgitation to

TABLE 22.3. *Echocardiographic imaging in aortic regurgitation (AR)*

Transthoracic echocardiography
Baseline evaluation to assess presence, severity of AR
Baseline evaluation to quantify left ventricular size and systolic function
Delineation of etiology of aortic regurgitation, evaluate proximal aortic root
Annual surveillance of left ventricular size and systolic function in patients with severe aortic regurgitation
Establish cardiac status after change in symptoms
Evaluation after aortic valve replacement
Transesophageal echocardiography
Evaluation of AR in patients with nondiagnostic transthoracic echocardiogram
Assessment of suspected prosthetic valve dysfunction
Evaluation of thoracic aorta, aortic dissection

Adapted from Bonow RO, Carabello B, de Leon AC Jr, et al. Guidelines for the management of patients with valvular heart disease: executive summary. A report of the American College of Cardiology/American Heart Association Task Force on Practice Guidelines (Committee on Management of Patients with Valvular Heart Disease). *J Am Coll Cardiol* 1998;32:1486–1588.

confirm the presence of and to establish the severity and cause of regurgitation. The dimensions, mass, and systolic function of the left ventricle should be determined, as well as the size and anatomy of the aortic root. Because absolute and subsequent change in left ventricular dimensions directly affect management, accurate quantification is important both on baseline measurement and on subsequent examinations.

Transthoracic echocardiography allows assessment of aortic valve structure and may establish the cause of aortic regurgitation with evidence of congenital abnormalities, calcific or rheumatic disease, or findings suggestive of infective endocarditis. In addition, the proximal 2 to 3 cm of ascending aorta can usually be visualized on transthoracic imaging, allowing assessment for gross dilation of the aortic root. In the absence of Doppler imaging, aortic regurgitation is suggested by diastolic fluttering of the anterior mitral valve leaflet, and acute severe regurgitation is associated with premature closure of the mitral valve. Doppler imaging allows reliable detection and semiquantification of aortic regurgitation (1,2). Aortic regurgitation severity is estimated by the size of the regurgitant jet in relation to the left ventricular outflow tract (3), as well as deceleration characteristics of regurgitant flow (4,5). Diastolic flow reversal in the descending thoracic aorta is a marker of severe aortic regurgitation. Transesophageal echocardiographic imaging allows optimal assessment of aortic valve structure, as well as definitive assessment of anatomy of the thoracic aorta. Transesophageal imaging is indicated if aortic dissection (6,7) or prosthetic valve dysfunction (8) is suspected.

Neither electrocardiography nor chest radiography is accurate in the detection or estimation of severity of aortic regurgitation. However, the electrocardiogram may reveal evidence of left ventricular hypertrophy or interventricular conduction delay, and the chest radiograph may reveal cardiomegaly, dilation of the aortic root, or evidence of pulmonary venous congestion.

Other tests that may be useful in patients with aortic regurgitation include radionuclide ventriculography, stress testing, and cardiac catheterization. Radionuclide ventriculography is a useful noninvasive means for the assessment of left ventricular size and function if these data are not available on echocardiographic imaging or if there is discordance between clinical data and data from echocardiographic imaging. Cardiac catheterization with coronary angiography allows assessment of coronary anatomy among patients at risk for coronary artery disease for whom surgical intervention is planned. Aortic regurgitation severity and aortic root size can be assessed with root angiography, although these data are usually available with noninvasive testing.

Exercise testing is useful for assessing functional capacity and symptoms in patients with significant aortic regurgitation and equivocal symptoms. Furthermore, exercise testing is valuable as a means of objectively assessing baseline and change in functional capacity among patients with moderate or severe aortic regurgitation. Change in left ventricular ejection fraction with exercise has been used as an indication for surgical intervention, although there are no definitive data to support the incremental diagnostic or prognostic value.

DIFFERENTIAL DIAGNOSIS

Early symptoms of exertional dyspnea associated with chronic aortic regurgitation are non-specific and potentially referable to many cardiac and noncardiac causes. Symptoms of more advanced congestive heart failure can similarly have many cardiac causes. Symptoms of angina pectoris can obviously be suggestive of coronary artery disease.

The decrescendo diastolic murmur of aortic regurgitation can be differentiated from that of mitral stenosis if it is predominantly localized at the left or right upper sternal border. The Austin Flint murmur, with radiation to the left ventricular apex, can be differentiated from a murmur of mitral stenosis in patients in sinus rhythm by its lack of presystolic accentuation. Mitral stenosis and aortic regurgitation can be reliably differentiated by echocardiographic imaging.

COMPLICATIONS

Chronic severe aortic regurgitation results in left ventricular dilation and, eventually, in progressive systolic dysfunction with consequent congestive heart failure. Initially, left ventricular systolic dysfunction is caused by pure afterload excess and is reversible after surgical intervention. Later in the course of disease, myocardial contractility is impaired, and this impairment is responsible for progressive and irreversible left ventricular systolic dysfunction. As is the case with any valve disease, patients with aortic regurgitation are at risk of infective endocarditis.

THERAPY

Medical Therapy

Patients with aortic regurgitation should receive appropriate antibiotic prophylaxis (9). Asymptomatic patients with chronic severe aortic regurgitation benefit from long-term vasodilator therapy with angiotensin-converting enzyme inhibitors or long-acting nifedipine; afterload-reducing therapy is associated with a delay in the need for aortic valve replacement and with improved left ventricular size and function after surgery (10–15). In general, asymptomatic patients with severe aortic regurgitation and normal left ventricular systolic function should receive long-term vasodilator therapy, with a goal to titrate the dose upward until there is a decrease in systolic blood pressure or until the development of side effects (16). In addition, vasodilator therapy may be useful among patients with systolic hypertension and any degree of aortic regurgitation, among patients with persistent left ventricular systolic dysfunction after aortic valve replacement, and as short-term therapy before aortic valve replacement to improve hemodynamics among patients with left ventricular dysfunction and severe heart failure (16). However, medical therapy is not an alternative to surgery for patients with severe aortic regurgitation and evidence of left ventricular systolic dysfunction or for patients with aortic regurgitation and symptoms of heart failure.

Patients with acute severe aortic regurgitation typically suffer hemodynamic compromise with fulminant pulmonary edema and cardiogenic shock. Medical therapy should be directed at aggressive afterload reduction with intravenous nitroprusside or nitroglycerin. Inotropic agents such as dopamine or dobutamine may also help improve forward flow. Diuretics are useful in the management of pulmonary edema. Regurgitant volume decreases with an increasing heart rate, owing to a shorter diastolic interval. Therefore, maintaining a rapid heart rate by temporary cardiac pacing or beta-adrenergic agonists is useful among patients with acute severe aortic regurgitation and hemodynamic compromise. Intraaortic balloon counterpulsation is contraindicated.

Aortic Valve Replacement

Surgical intervention with aortic valve replacement is the definitive therapy for aortic regurgitation. Aortic valve repair is possible in some patients, although its use is limited to younger patients with noncalcific abnormalities of the aortic cusps or annulus, typically of congenital or myxomatous origin (17). Inasmuch as most adult patients requiring surgical intervention for aortic regurgitation are older and have significant associated calcification of the aortic valve annulus and cusps and of the wall of the ascending aorta, valve repair plays a much smaller role for the aortic valve than for the mitral valve.

Aortic valve replacement is indicated for patients with severe aortic regurgitation and symptoms of angina or heart failure or with evidence of left ventricular systolic dysfunction (defined as left ventricular ejection fraction of less than 50% at rest) (Table 22.4). The risk entailed by surgery increases with progressive left ventricular systolic dysfunction or advanced symptoms, although functional status and prognosis are improved with aortic valve replacement despite preexisting severe left ventricular systolic dysfunction (18,19). Surgical indications for asymptomatic patients with severe aortic regurgitation and normal left ventricular systolic function are more problematic and a topic of controversy. On the basis of a review of available literature, the American College of Cardiology/American Heart Association (ACC/AHA) (16) recommends surgical intervention for asymptomatic patients with

TABLE 22.4. *Surgery for severe aortic regurgitation*

Acute severe aortic regurgitation
  Symptoms or hemodynamic compromise
Chronic severe aortic regurgitation
  Functional class II, III or IV and preserved LV
    systolic function
  Symptoms of angina pectoris, with or without
    coronary artery disease
  Any LV systolic dysfunction, with or without symptoms
  Evidence of significant LV dilation, taken in context
    of patient body size and previous assessment of
    chamber size
  Patients undergoing bypass surgery, surgery on
    other heart valves, or surgery of the ascending
    aorta

Adapted from Bonow RO, Carabello B, de Leon AC Jr, et al. Guidelines for the management of patients with valvular heart disease: executive summary. A report of the American College of Cardiology/American Heart Association Task Force on Practice Guidelines (Committee on Management of Patients with Valvular Heart Disease). *J Am Coll Cardiol* 1998;32:1486–1588.

preserved left ventricular systolic function only if there is evidence of marked left ventricular chamber dilation (diastolic diameter exceeding 75 mm or systolic diameter exceeding 55 mm). However, if aortic valve replacement is performed by a surgeon with extensive experience in valve surgery and using state-of-the-art valve substitutes, then the published guidelines may be excessively conservative and may lead to poor postoperative outcomes among at least a subset of patients.

The decision to defer aortic valve replacement for patients with severe aortic regurgitation is based on the balance between the risks and benefits of intervention; the benefits of intervention are, in essence, synonymous with avoidance of the natural history of disease and of the risks of delayed intervention. This balance favors delayed intervention among asymptomatic patients either if the operative mortality rate is high or if there is substantial postoperative morbidity or mortality associated with earlier intervention. Current operative techniques allow performance of aortic valve replacement with low rates of operative morbidity and mortality among compensated patients. In addition, state-of-the-art valve substitutes appear to provide for more durable prostheses with better hemodynamics and higher

rates of postoperative survival than those that were used in the published reports on which the ACC/AHA guidelines are based (20,21). In addition, there is evidence that the existing criteria for aortic valve replacement are associated with excessively high rates of postoperative mortality among women in comparison with men (22), probably because of smaller body habitus and failure to normalize threshold values for surgical intervention to patient body size. Although strict criteria have not been developed and tested, it may be prudent to consider aortic valve replacement earlier if severe aortic regurgitation and evidence of moderate or progressive left ventricular dilation are present, and if surgery can be performed by experienced physicians with state-of-the-art valve substitutes.

Finally, patients with severe aortic regurgitation who require coronary artery bypass grafting, surgery on other heart valves, or surgery on the thoracic aorta should also undergo aortic valve replacement. Surgical considerations for primary aortic root disease are discussed in Chapters 29 and 30.

PROGNOSIS

Prognosis is poor among symptomatic patients with severe aortic regurgitation treated with medical therapy alone. According to natural history data that predate the era of surgical aortic valve replacement, the presence of angina pectoris or symptoms of congestive heart failure were associated with mortality rates of more than 10% and more than 20% per year, respectively (23–25). Thus, without surgical intervention, symptomatic aortic regurgitation appears to be associated with a prognosis as dire as that for symptomatic aortic stenosis. Asymptomatic patients with impaired left ventricular systolic function typically develop symptoms within 2 to 3 years of diagnosis (26–28); the estimated rate of developing symptoms is approximately 25% per year (16).

The prognosis of asymptomatic patients with normal left ventricular systolic function has been evaluated in seven independent series (12,29–35) that were summarized in the ACC/AHA Guidelines on the Management of Patients with Valvular Heart Disease (16). These data revealed a 4.3% annual rate of progression to the development of either symptoms or left ventricular systolic dysfunction. Asymptomatic left ventricular systolic dysfunction occurred at a rate of 1.3% per year. Sudden death among patients with compensated severe aortic regurgitation is rare but has been reported, with a mortality rate of less than 0.2% per year. In general, asymptomatic patients with moderate or severe aortic regurgitation should be able to participate in normal physical activity (including mild-intensity exercise), although weightlifting and other isometric exercises should be avoided.

Age and left ventricular diameter in systole are predictors of adverse outcome. In one multivariate analysis, death or development of symptoms or left ventricular dysfunction occurred within 8 years of diagnosis among 19% of patients with left ventricular systolic diameter of more than 50 mm, among 6% of patients with left ventricular systolic diameter of 40 to 50 mm, and in no patient with left ventricular systolic diameter of less than 40 mm (32). It is important to note that, of asymptomatic patients who developed adverse outcomes of death or left ventricular systolic dysfunction in the previously cited studies (30–33,35), more than 25% had no prior development of symptoms. Furthermore, surgical risk increases after the development of either left ventricular systolic dysfunction or marked chamber dilation. Inasmuch as the disease can progress and the prognosis worsens without the development of symptoms, there is some inherent risk in delaying surgical intervention among patients who do not yet meet conventional criteria.

The prognosis after aortic valve replacement appears to improve substantially. However, as noted previously, women do not fare as well as men after aortic valve replacement for aortic regurgitation (22), possibly because the disease in women is more advanced at the time of surgical intervention.

FOLLOW-UP

Asymptomatic patients with mild aortic regurgitation and normal left ventricular size and systolic function should undergo periodic assessment, including history and physical examination, on approximately a yearly basis (16). After the initial documentation of mild aortic regurgitation, echocardiographic imaging should be repeated if there are new symptoms or evidence of worsened regurgitation on physical examination. Because the severity of regurgitation and even moderate change in left ventricular size are difficult to assess reliably on physical examination, echocardiography with Doppler imaging should be repeated periodically (approximately every 2 to 3 years) to evaluate for change in an otherwise stable patient.

At the time of an initial diagnosis of moderate or severe aortic regurgitation, asymptomatic patients should undergo (a) quantitation of left ventricular size and systolic function with echocardiographic imaging and (b) evaluation of functional status by history or exercise testing. If surgery is not indicated, then patients should undergo serial assessment for the development of new symptoms and for changes in functional status, the severity of regurgitation, and left ventricular size and systolic function. If the chronicity and stability of aortic regurgitation is not known, then patients should undergo reevaluation, including echocardiographic imaging, after 2 to 3 months. After the stability of the regurgitant lesion has been established, the frequency of subsequent reevaluations and repeated noninvasive testing should be based on the severity of aortic regurgitation, the presence and severity of left ventricular dilation on echocardiography, evidence of progression or change on previous studies, and the reliability of the assessment of functional stability. It is important to recognize that a sedentary lifestyle in many patients precludes the reliable assessment of functional status without the use of periodic exercise testing. In general, stable, asymptomatic patients with severe aortic regurgitation should be reevaluated approximately yearly or more frequently as indicated according to the criteria just described. Finally, in addition to routine testing, patients should undergo reassessment if there are new symptoms or a change in functional status.

PRACTICAL POINTS

- Aortic regurgitation has multiple potential causes, including diseases of aortic valve cusps and the ascending aorta.

- Chronic volume overload eventually leads to left ventricular dilation and systolic dysfunction.

- The disease has an indolent course; symptoms occur late.

- Symptoms include exertional dyspnea, followed by symptoms of overt congestive heart failure or angina pectoris or both.

- Echocardiography with Doppler imaging is the test of choice for confirming diagnosis and for quantifying and further characterizing regurgitation and its impact on left ventricular size and systolic function.

- Transesophageal echocardiography is useful if transthoracic imaging is nondiagnostic, with aortic root disease, and with prosthetic valves.

- The prognosis is favorable in the absence of symptoms, in patients with good functional capacity, and in patients with normal left ventricular size and systolic function.

- Patients should be referred for surgical intervention if any symptoms, left ventricular systolic dysfunction, or significant left ventricular dilation is present.

REFERENCES

1. Feigenbaum H. Acquired valvular heart disease. In: Feigenbaum H, ed. *Echocardiography,* 5th ed. Philadelphia: Lea & Febiger, 1994:239–349.

2. Otto CM. Valvular regurgitation: diagnosis, quantitation, and clinical approach. In: Otto CM, ed. *Textbook of clinical echocardiography,* 2nd ed. Philadelphia: WB Saunders, 2000:265–300.

3. Perry GJ, Helmcke F, Nanda NC, et al. Evaluation of aortic insufficiency by Doppler color flow mapping. *J Am Coll Cardiol* 1987;9:952–959.

4. Teague SM, Heinsimer JA, Anderson JL, et al. Quantification of aortic regurgitation utilizing continuous wave Doppler ultrasound. *J Am Coll Cardiol* 1986;8:592–599.

5. Labovitz AJ, Ferrara RP, Kern MJ, et al. Quantitative evaluation of aortic insufficiency by continuous wave Doppler echocardiography. *J Am Coll Cardiol* 1986;8:1341–1347.

6. Nienaber CA, von Kodolitsch Y, Nicolas V, et al. The diagnosis of thoracic aortic dissection by noninvasive imaging procedures. *N Engl J Med* 1993;328:1–9.

7. Cigarroa JE, Isselbacher EM, DeSanctis RW, et al. Diagnostic imaging in the evaluation of suspected aortic dissection: old standards and new directions. *N Engl J Med* 1993;328:35–43.

8. Bach DS. TEE evaluation of prosthetic valves. *Cardiol Clin* 2000;18:751–771.

9. Dajani AS, Taubert KA, Wilson W, et al. Prevention of bacterial endocarditis: recommendations by the American Heart Association. *Circulation* 1997;96:358–366.

10. Greenberg B, Massie B, Bristow JD, et al. Long-term vasodilator therapy of chronic aortic insufficiency: a randomized double-blinded, placebo-controlled clinical trial. *Circulation* 1988;78:92–103.

11. Scognamiglio R, Fasoli G, Ponchia A, et al. Long-term nifedipine unloading therapy in asymptomatic patients with chronic severe aortic regurgitation. *J Am Coll Cardiol* 1990;16:424–429.

12. Scognamiglio R, Rahimtoola SH, Fasoli G, et al. Nifedipine in asymptomatic patients with severe aortic regurgitation and normal left ventricular function. *N Engl J Med* 1994;331:689–694.

13. Wisenbaugh T, Sinovich V, Dullabh A, et al. Six month pilot study of captopril for mildly symptomatic, severe isolated mitral and isolated aortic regurgitation. *J Heart Valve Dis* 1994;3:197–204.

14. Lin M, Chiang HT, Lin SL, et al. Vasodilator therapy in chronic asymptomatic aortic regurgitation: enalapril versus hydralazine therapy. *J Am Coll Cardiol* 1994;24:1046–1053.

15. Schon HR, Dorn R, Barthel P, et al. Effects of 12 months quinapril therapy in asymptomatic patients with chronic aortic regurgitation. *J Heart Valve Dis* 1994;3:500–509.

16. Bonow RO, Carabello B, de Leon AC Jr, et al. Guidelines for the management of patients with valvular heart disease: executive summary. A report of the American College of Cardiology/American Heart Association Task Force on Practice Guidelines (Committee on Management of Patients with Valvular Heart Disease). *J Am Coll Cardiol* 1998;32:1486–1588.

17. Duran CMG. Present status of reconstructive surgery for aortic valve disease. *J Card Surg* 1993;8:443–452.

18. Bonow RO, Picone AL, McIntosh CL, et al. Survival and functional results after valve replacement for aortic regurgitation from 1976 to 1983: impact of preoperative left ventricular function. *Circulation* 1985;72:1244–1256.

19. Bonow RO, Dodd JT, Maron BJ, et al. Long-term se-rial changes in left ventricular function and reversal of ventricular dilatation after valve replacement for chronic aortic regurgitation. *Circulation* 1988;78:1108–1120.

20. David TE, Puschmann R, Ivanov J, et al. Aortic valve replacement with stentless and stented porcine valves: a case-match study. *J Thorac Cardiovasc Surg* 1998;116:236–241.

21. Del Rizzo DF, Abdoh A, Cartier P, et al. The ef-fect of prosthetic valve type on survival after aortic valve surgery. *Semin Thorac Cardiovasc Surg* 1999; 11(Suppl 1):1–8.

22. Klodas E, Enriquez-Sarano M, Tajik AJ, et al. Surgery for aortic regurgitation in women: contrasting indica-tions and outcome compared with men. *Circulation* 1996;94:2472–2478.

23. Hegglin R, Scheu H, Rothlin M. Aortic insufficiency. *Circulation* 1968;38:77–92.

24. Spagnuolo M, Kloth H, Taranta A, et al. Natural his-tory of rheumatic aortic regurgitation: criteria predictive of death, congestive heart failure, and angina in young patients. *Circulation* 1971;44:368–380.

25. Rapaport E. Natural history of aortic and mitral valve disease. *Am J Cardiol* 1975;35:221–227.

26. Henry WL, Bonow RO, Rosing DR, et al. Observa-tions on the optimum time for operative intervention for aortic regurgitation. II. Serial echocardiographic evalua-tion of asymptomatic patients. *Circulation* 1980;61:484–492.

27. McDonald IG, Jelinek VM. Serial M-mode echocardiog-raphy in severe chronic aortic regurgitation. *Circulation* 1980;62:1291–1296.

28. Bonow RO. Radionuclide angiography in the manage-ment of asymptomatic aortic regurgitation. *Circulation* 1991;84:I296–I302.

29. Bonow RO, Rosing DR, McIntosh CL, et al. The natu-ral history of asymptomatic patients with aortic regurgi-tation and normal left ventricular function. *Circulation* 1983;68:509–517.

30. Scognamiglio R, Fasoli G, Dalla Volta S. Progression of myocardial dysfunction in asymptomatic patients with severe aortic insufficiency. *Clin Cardiol* 1986;9:151–156.

31. Siemienczuk D, Greenberg B, Morris C, et al. Chronic aortic insufficiency: factors associated with progres-sion to aortic valve replacement. *Ann Intern Med* 1989;110:587–592.

32. Bonow RO, Lakatos E, Maron BJ, et al. Serial long-term assessment of the natural history of asymptomatic patients with chronic aortic regurgitation and normal left ventricular systolic function. *Circulation* 1991;84:1625–1635.

33. Tornos MP, Olona M, Permanyer-Miralda G, et al. Clin-ical outcome of severe asymptomatic chronic aortic re-gurgitation: a long-term prospective follow-up study. *Am Heart J* 1995;130:333–339.

34. Ishii K, Hirota Y, Suwa M, et al. Natural history and left ventricular response in chronic aortic regurgitation. *Am J Cardiol* 1996;78:357–361.

35. Borer JS, Hochreiter C, Herrold EM, et al. Prediction of indications for valve replacement among asymptomatic or minimally symptomatic patients with chronic aortic regurgitation and normal left ventricular performance. *Circulation* 1998;97:525–534.

23

Mitral Stenosis

Mani A. Vannan

DEFINITION

The normal mitral valve has an area of 4 to 6 cm^2, and turbulent flow across the stenosed valve occurs when the area is less than 2 cm^2. In general, in "tight" mitral stenosis, the valve area is less than 1 cm^2 and the gradient across the valve is more than 10 mm HG. The normal functioning of the mitral valve is dependent on the coordinated action of the mitral valve annulus, the valve leaflets (anterior or aortic, and posterior or mural), the chordae tendineae, and the left ventricular (LV) papillary muscles. In most patients with mitral stenosis (MS), there is an increase in pulmonary artery pressure proportional to the elevation in left atrial (LA) pressure. This is called passive pulmonary hypertension (PHT). Some patients with severe MS manifest elevated pulmonary artery pressures disproportional to the increase in LA pressure. This so-called reactive pulmonary hypertension has been postulated to occur to protect the pulmonary capillary bed from excessive engorgement and pulmonary edema at times of increased venous return to the obstructed LA (e.g., during exercise). This explanation remains controversial, and it is unclear why it occurs only in some patients with severe MS and does not seem to be related to the duration of LA hypertension (1–3). The cost of increased pulmonary vascular resistance (PVR) in reactive PHT by opposing RV emptying leads to RV hypertrophy and eventually to dilatation and failure, with consequent worsening of tricuspid regurgitation and other signs of right-sided heart failure.

USUAL CAUSES

Rheumatic fever is by far the most common cause of MS; in acute rheumatic fever, foci of fibrinoid necrosis occur within the cusps or along the chordae on which friable vegetations (verrucae) are seated along the lines of closure. The tiny and translucent verrucae result from the precipitation of fibrin at the sites of erosion and inflammation of endocardial surfaces where the leaflets impinge on each other. As mitral valve involvement progresses to its chronic and symptomatic phase, the acute inflammatory process organizes into a deforming fibrosis, causing thickening of the valve cusps, accompanied by calcific deposits that further aggravate the fibrosis and make the valve ring rigid. The valve may assume a funnel-like shape, further promoting commissural fusion and thickening, retraction, and fusion of the chordae. Chordal fusion with or without retraction contributes to the "buttonhole" or "fishmouth" configuration of the valve. Thus, depending on the predominant site, commissural, cuspal, and chordal fusion all play a role in the development of inflow obstruction. Other, more uncommon causes of MS are listed in Table 23.1.

SYMPTOMS

The age at onset of symptoms is typically between 25 and 45 years (4–6) (Table 23.2). In the western hemisphere, however, it is not unusual for MS to manifest for the first time in the fifth or sixth decade of life. The predominant symptoms are exertional dyspnea, orthopnea, and paroxysmal nocturnal dyspnea, which may be

TABLE 23.1. *Causes of Mitral Stenosis*

Rheumatic fever
Congenital
Severe mitral annular calcification
Carcinoid, malignant sarcoid, gout
Systemic lupus erythematosus
Methysergide therapy
Rheumatoid arthritis
Whipple's disease
Amyloid
Hurler's, Fabry's, and Morteaux-Lamy diseases
Lutembacher's syndrome (atrial septal defect + mitral stenosis)
Left atrial myxoma
Cor triatriatum
Left atrial ball-valve thrombus

accompanied by cough and wheezing. Hemoptysis is an infrequent presenting feature. Features of forward failure such as fatigue and cachexia occur late in the course of events. Systemic emboli usually are seen with severe stenosis; however, they may occur in patients with mild valvular restriction. In some cases, signs of embolism may occur before dyspnea and may be the first clues to the underlying disease. Atrial fibrillation may be the initial clinical problem, especially in older patients (6).

SIGNS

The general appearance of the patient includes ruddy cheeks, also known as "mitral facies" (Table 23.3). This is due to livedo reticularis of the malar area as a result of systemic

TABLE 23.2. *Clinical features of mitral stenosis (MS)*

These can be broadly classified into those that reflect the severity of mitral valve obstruction and those that are manifestations of the disease process irrespective of the severity
Related to degree of stenosis
  Dypnea and orthopnea
    Stiff lung due to PV hypertension that causes fluid transudation
  Pulmonary edema
    Usually occurs when PV pressure exceeds 25 mm HG
    Can occur in noncritical MS during rapid AF or tachycardia (fever, pregnancy)
  Hemoptysis
    Pink frothy sputum of pulmonary edema (alveolar capillary rupture)
    Blood-stained sputum complicating chronic bronchitis (mucosal edema)
    Pulmonary infarction, a complication of with RV failure
    Sudden hemorrhage of pulmonary apoplexy (rupture of bronchial veins)
Unrelated to degree of stenosis
  Atrial fibrillation
    ~ 40% of symptomatic MS have AF (intermittent or pesistent)
    Commoner in older age groups (80% incidence in patients older than 50 yr)
    Frequent in those with LA size > 40 mm (>50% incidence)
    Marker of poor prognosis; 10-year survival rate, 25%, in comparison with 46% in SR
    Potential consequences are pulmonary edema and systemic embolization
    May be paroxysmal or persistent and multifactorial in origin
  Systemic embolization
    Rate of embolization between 10% and 20% (many go undetected)
    Cerebral embolization accounts for up to 70% of episodes
    Older age and presence of AF are predisposing factors
    Almost all embolizations occur in the first year of AF
    Unrelated to LA size but the probability is greater in marked LA enlargement
  RV failure
    Elevated neck veins, peripheral edema, and hepatomegaly
    Progressing to ascites, cirrhosis, and cachexia
    Hoarse voice (recurrent laryngeal nerve palsy; Ortner's syndrome)
  Infective endocarditis
    Uncommon in pure MS (only 5% of deaths over 10 years)
    Usually occurs when there is concurrent MR or AF
    Antibiotic prophylaxis is recommended in pure MS

AF, atrial fibrillation; LA, left ventricular; PV, pulmonary venous; RV, right ventricular; SR, sinus rhythm; MR, mitral regurgitation.

TABLE 23.3. *Auscultatory findings in mitral stenosis*

Typical findings
  Accentuated and delayed first heart sound
    Excessive rigidity and immobility can diminish or obliterate S1
  Opening snap
    Due to sudden tensing of the chordae and leaflets
    Intensity reflects leaflet mobility (louder means pliable valve)
    Usually heard at the apex
    OS-A2 interval directly related to severity of mitral stenosis
  Middiastolic murmur
    Low-pitched rumble best heard in end-expiration and left lateral position
    End-expiration and left lateral recumbent posture also accentuates intensity
    Duration not intensity correlates with severity of obstruction
Other findings
  Systolic murmurs
    Soft systolic murmurs at the LSE and apex are frequent do not signify MR apical pansystolic murmur signifies MR
    LV S3 and soft S1 or OS indicate severe MR in the presence of MR murmur pansystolic murmur at LSE indicates TR (accentuates with inspiration)
  Diastolic murmurs high-pitched, decrescendo diastolic murmur at LSE of PR (Graham-Steell murmur) due to dilatation of PV ring in severe pulmonary hypertension

LSE, left sternal edge; LV, left ventricular; MR, mitral regurgitation; PR, pulmonic regurgitation; PV, pulmonary venous; TR, tricuspid regurgitation.

TABLE 23.4. *Transthoracic echocardiography in mitral stenosis*

Anatomic findings
  Leaflet thickening retraction, and calcification
  Commissural fusion and calcification
  Doming of the anterior mitral leaflet, indicating pliability
  Thickening and fusion of chordae
  Dilated LA and LAA
Hemodynamics
  Method of choice (over TEE)
  Gradients and Doppler valve area
  Planimetry of geometric valve area
  Estimation of pulmonary pressure
  Exercise hemodynamics

LA, left atrium; LAA, left atrial appendage; TEE, transesophageal echocardiography.

vasoconstriction and decreased cardiac output. The JVD may reveal a prominent *a wave,* signifying a vigorous right atrial contraction if significant pulmonary hypertension or tricuspid stenosis is present. If the rhythm is atrial fibrillation (AF), the X descent disappears, and the JVD reveals only a common *c-v wave* in systole. Precordial palpation may reveal an inconspicuous left ventricle. An enlarged right ventricle can displace the left ventricle posteriorly and produce a prominent apex. Prominent left parasternal pulsations are palpated in patients who have right ventricular hypertrophy, and a loud second pulmonic heart sound (P2) may be palpable in the second left intercostal area in patients with pulmonary hypertension. A palpable first heart sound at the apex is suggestive of a pliable anterior leaflet. The findings on precordial auscultation (Table 23.4) correlate with the underlying state of the valve leaflets and structures "upstream" to the diseased valve—that is, the left atrium, the right ventricle, the tricuspid valve, and the right atrium.

USEFUL DIAGNOSTIC TESTS

Chest Radiograph

In a patient with hemodynamically significant MS, the frontal chest radiograph may be normal, except for the appearance of an enlarged left atrial appendage. However, LA enlargement is almost always evident on lateral and oblique views. An extreme enlargement of the LA indicates coexistent mitral regurgitation. Roentgenographic signs of LA dilatation are straightening of the left heart border (mitralization), elevation of the left main bronchus with a widening of the carinal angle, double atrial shadow, and backward displacement of the esophagus by the enlarged atrium.

Other radiographic findings include prominence of the left pulmonary artery and dilatation of the pulmonary veins in the upper lobe of the lungs. In severe MS, all structures "upstream" to the mitral valve—both atria, pulmonary arteries and veins, right ventricle, and superior vena cava—are prominent. Pulmonary congestion, edema, and increased vascularity of the upper lobes caused by redistribution of blood flow to those regions are all markers of pulmonary venous hypertension. Later in the course of this process, generalized haziness and Kerley's B lines (transverse, dense, opaque bands 1 to 2 cm in length at the bases, caused by interlobular septal edema) are seen when the LA pressure exceeds 20 mm HG. In rare cases, hemosiderotic nodules may be visible, and signs of pulmonary infarction may be also seen.

Electrocardiogram

In patients in normal sinus rhythm, the P wave is tall in lead II, which suggests LA enlargement. It may become upright in V_1 when MS is complicated by severe pulmonary hypertension or tricuspid stenosis, both of which cause RA enlargement. In patients presenting with AF, coarse fibrillation waves greater than 0.1 mV in amplitude in V1 are typically seen, which is consistent with LA dilatation. With severe pulmonary hypertension, right axis deviation and right ventricular hypertrophy are seen. The angle of the QRS axis in the frontal plane often correlates with the severity of the valvular obstruction and pulmonary vascular resistance in cases of pure MS. A mean QRS axis of more than 60 degrees indicates a valve area less than 1.3 cm^2.

Echocardiography

Two-dimensional transthoracic echocardiography (TTE) is the diagnostic test of choice for MS (7–10). It provides anatomic and hemodynamic information that is used to assess the severity of obstruction and plan the appropriate management strategy. Any combination of the features listed in Table 23.4 can be found in MS by TTE. The indications for transesophageal echocardiography (TEE) are usually limited to situations in which a poor transthoracic acoustic window precludes a proper anatomic assessment; it is also used for exclusion of LA or left atrial appendage clot before percutaneous mitral commissurotomy (PMC), better definition of severity of coexistent mitral regurgitation, and in cases of suspected endocarditis (11,12). Occasionally, TEE may be done to visualize the submitral apparatus from the transgastric window or to planimetry the anatomic mitral valve area from the gastroesophageal location. Hemodynamic evaluation is best done by TTE with

a combination of valve area and gradients derived from Doppler imaging and anatomic valve area measured from two-dimensional echocardiography (Figs. 23.1 and 23.2). Three-dimensional echocardiography offers a promising new approach for measuring the anatomic orifice area (13) (Fig 23.2). Stress hemodynamics are indicated when the resting gradient and the severity of the symptoms are discordant. The preferred method of stress testing is upright or supine bicycle exercise. Both mitral valve gradient and tricuspid regurgitation (TR) are assessed at rest and at peak exercise (14–16). PMC or surgery is indicated in patients with peak pulmonary artery systolic pressure exceeding 60 mm HG, a peak mean gradient exceeding 15 mm HG, or in those pulmonary capillary wedge pressure higher than 25 mm HG. Intervention may be also indicated in patients with doubling of the resting mitral valve gradient at peak exercise or in selected patients with clear exacerbation of symptoms regardless of peak hemodynamics. Although lung disease, LV dysfunction, and deconditioning may be the causes of dyspnea in the latter group of patients, it is not known whether this population, who also have mild to moderate MS, do indeed benefit symptomatically from PMC. Both TTE and TEE have been used to guide and assess the results of balloon valvotomy. TEE for this purpose of guiding interventions necessitates anesthesia, in which case intracardiac echocardiography may be used to guide the intervention (Fig. 23.4); this involves only local anesthesia and light conscious sedation at the most.

Cardiac Catheterization

Invasive hemodynamic measurements are not necessary to make the diagnosis of MS in most cases. The combination of symptoms, signs, and noninvasive tests and imaging results is usually diagnostic. However, there may be specific circumstances (Table 23.5) in which invasive hemodynamic measurements can complement noninvasive assessment of severity of MS. Transvalvular gradients and flow are used to derive MV area with the Gorlin formula (Fig. 23.3) (17–19). Table 23.5 also lists other indications for

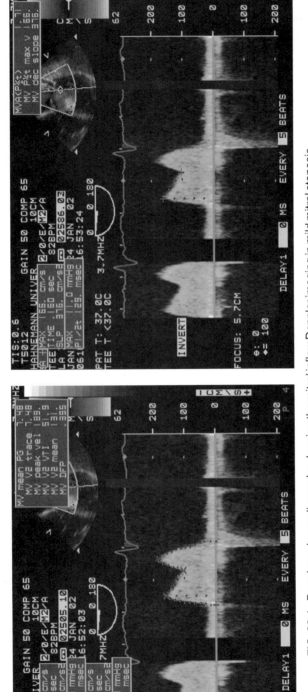

FIG. 23.1. Doppler echocardiography showing the mitral inflow Doppler imaging in mild mitral stenosis. Tracing the spectral profile of the inflow provides automated calculation of pressure half-time ($P\frac{1}{2}$, in milliseconds) and peak and mean gradients with the use of the simplified Bernoulli equation of $4V^2$. Valve area is calculated as $P\frac{1}{2}/220$ (in milliseconds).

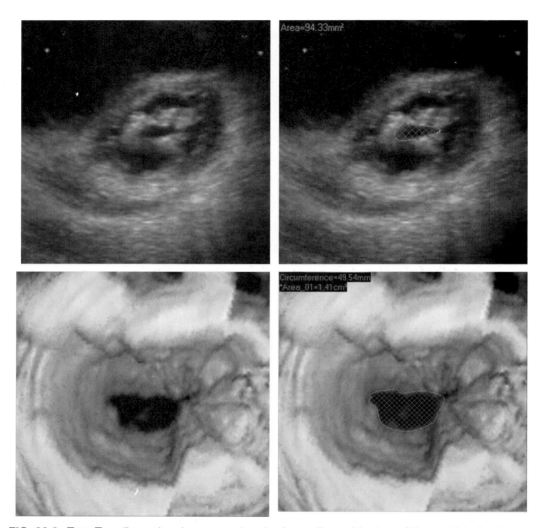

FIG. 23.2. Top, Two-dimensional cross-sectional echocardiographic view of the restricted mitral orifice in severe mitral stenosis. It also shows valve leaflet thickening and commissural fusion. Planimetry of the orifice yields a valve area (0.9 cm²). **Bottom,** The unroofed three-dimensional echocardiographic view (surgical orientation) of mitral stenosis from another patient. It also shows nodular thickening of the anterior and posterior leaflets and commissural fusion. Planimetry yields a three-dimensional valve area of 1.4 cm².

cardiac catheterization in patients with MS. Clearly, PMC mandates cardiac catheterization.

prevention of thromboembolism, treatment of AF, and prevention or treatment of endocarditis.

TREATMENT

Medical Therapy

Medical therapy is aimed primarily at amelioration of symptoms of mitral inflow obstruction,

Physical Exertion

Avoidance of undue physical exertion and administration of diuretics are usually effective in relief of symptoms of dyspnea. However, in

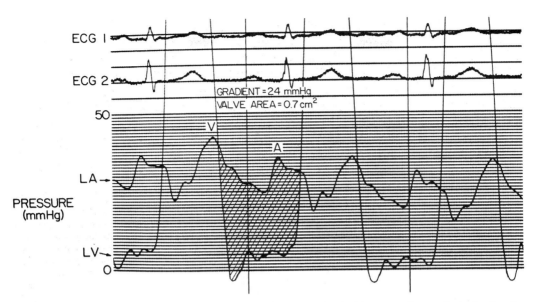

FIG. 23.3. Left atrial and left ventricular pressure tracing obtained from cardiac catheterization in a patient with severe mitral stenosis. (From Pepine CJ, ed. *Diagnostic and therapeutic catheterization.* Baltimore: Williams and Wilkins, 1989: 404.)

patients in whom symptoms are associated with resting or exertional tachycardia, beta blockers or calcium channel blockers may be of additional benefit. Limiting physical exertion helps prevent pulmonary edema caused by sudden steep increase in pulmonary venous pressure, although this is relevant only in significant inflow obstruction. In addition, there is some concern regarding the adverse effects of recurrent exertion augmenting pulmonary vascular pressures and its effect on the right ventricle. However, these concerns are largely unproven, and in most patients, symptom-limited physical activity should be permitted (22). Digoxin is only recommended if there is evidence of right or left ventricular dysfunction.

Anticoagulation

Long-term oral warfarin (Coumadin) is indicated for patients with paroxysmal or persistent atrial fibrillation and when there has been a prior embolic event. Although there are no prospective randomized studies of benefits of anticoagulation in mitral stenosis, retrospective data suggest

a four- to 15-fold decrease in systemic and pulmonary embolism. It is uncertain whether there is any benefit to be had from long-term warfarin in the absence of atrial fibrillation or simply when there is marked enlargement of the left atrium. Also, there is no correlation between the absence of detectable thrombus in the left atrium and the risk of embolism. LA thrombus is seen in only 15% to 20% of patients with a prior history of embolism, which suggests that there may be other sources of embolism (6,23).

Antiarrhythmic Therapy

Control of the ventricular response in atrial fibrillation is achieved by digoxin, beta blockers, or calcium channel blockers; the latter two agents are especially useful in controlling exertional tachycardia. Amiodarone and other group IA or IC agents may be used preventively in recurrent paroxysmal AF. When there is hemodynamic instability associated with rapid ventricular response, direct-current cardioversion can be used to restore sinus rhythm. Warfarin is indicated, as mentioned previously, and intravenous heparin is indicated in an acute

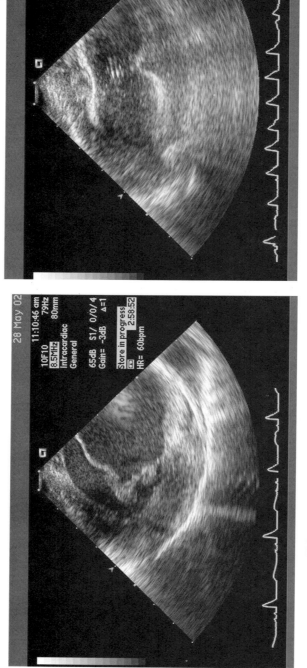

FIG. 23.4. Intracardiac echocardiography guidance of percutaneous mitral commissurotomy. **Left,** Thickened and restricted mitral valve; **Right,** Inflated balloon across the mitral valve.

TABLE 23.5. *Cardiac catheterization in mitral stenosis*

Diagnostic and hemodynamic
    Coronary arteriography is patients over 55 years of age (before surgery)
    Direct-measurement of LA pressure in difficult clinical situations
    Evaluation of combined valvular lesions
    Assessment of MR
    Measurement of PVR in reactive pulmonary hypertension
    Therapeutic (PMC)

LA, left atrial; MR, mitral regurgitation; PMC, percutaneous mitral commissurotomy; PVR, pulmonary vascular resistance.

episode of AF if electrical cardioversion is considered. PMC in recurrent or new-onset AF in absence of symptoms is sometimes performed, but this is a Class IIb indication in the American College of Cardiology/American Heart Association task force recommendations (24).

Operative and Interventional Therapy

Definitive therapy of MS comprises measures that relieve inflow obstruction. These methods include both nonsurgical and surgical methods.

Percutaneous Mitral Commissurotomy

This is the procedure of choice in young patients with favorable mitral valve anatomy and no significant mitral regurgitation. The usual technique uses a single (Inoue) balloon, a double-balloon, or a metallic dilator similar to the Tubb dilator used during surgical commissurotomy. Metallic dilators in commissurotomy have the advantage of being reusable, which is an important consideration in developing countries, but there are no randomized trials comparing it to the balloon technique. In several trials, PMC has been shown to produce favorable immediate and long-term outcomes in comparison with surgical commissurotomy (25–27). These randomized trials of about 400 relatively young patients (about 30 years of age) and optimal valvular anatomy demonstrated comparable acute hemodynamic benefit from either strategy. However, during long-term follow-up of 3 to 7 years, PMC and

open surgical commissurotomy showed symptomatic benefit superior to that from closed surgical commissurotomy (rates of freedom from reintervention, about 90% vs. 50%). When unfavorable mitral valve anatomy is included, PMC results in about 50% to 60% rates of survival free of such events as repeat PMC, valve surgery, and death (28–32). The cumulative experience since 1982 has allowed the understanding of the predictors of good outcome. Both immediate and long-term results are determined by favorable mitral valve anatomy, which is classified by various echocardiographic scores (33–36). Regardless of which scoring system is used, the most important anatomic determinants of poor results are the presence of significant commissural calcification, marked commissural fusion and distortion, and more than mild mitral regurgitation (36–38). In addition, there are a number of clinical predictors of suboptimal outcome and contraindications, as shown in Table 23.6.

Symptomatic mitral stenosis is the usual indication for PMC, but, as shown in later sections, it may also be indicated in asymptomatic inflow obstruction when the valve anatomy is favorable. Valvular anatomy is frequently unfavorable in western populations (39), and although PMC remains controversial in these

TABLE 23.6. *Clinical predictors of suboptimal outcome after percutaneous mitral commissurotomy and contraindications*

Predictors of poor outcome
    Older age
    Advanced functional class
    Small mitral valve area
    Previous history of commissurotomy
    Tricuspid regurgitation
    Nonuse of Inoue balloon
Contraindications
    Left atrial thrombus
    Severe mitral regurgitation
    Commissural and subvalvular fusion or calcification (MGH score, 9–16; USC score, 3–4)
    Significant coronary artery disease necessitating CABG
    Severe concomitant aortic or tricuspid valvular stenosis or regurgitation
    Left atrial appendage thrombus

CABG, coronary artery bypass graft; MGH, Massachussets General Hospital; USC, University of Southern California

TABLE 23.7. *Indications for percutaneous mitral commissurotomy*

Favorable valvular anatomy
Symptomatic mitral stenosis (NYHA Classes III and IV)
Asymptomatic mitral stenosis or NYHA functional
  Class I and II
  History of previous thromboembolism
  Dense left atrial spontaneous echocardiographic
    contrast
  Before major noncardiac surgery
  Recurrent atrial fibrillation
  Previous aortic valve replacement
  Pulmonary hypertension (>50 mm HG at rest or
    >60 mm at exercise)
  Pregnancy
  Anticoagulants contraindicated
Unfavorable valvular anatomy
Advanced age
Previous surgical commissurotomy
Previous aortic valve replacement
Persistent symptoms in pregnancy
Pregnancy
Anticoagulants contraindicated

NYHA, New York Heart Association.

patients, it may be considered as an option under certain circumstances (Table 23.7).

In 80% to 95% of patients with favorable anatomy who undergo PMC, the valve area doubles to about 2.0 cm^2, and the mean gradient decreases by 50% to 60%. Thus, a successful PMC is defined as that which results in a valve area greater than 1.5 cm^2 (greater than $1 \text{ cm}^2/\text{m}^2$) or a final LA pressure of less than 18 mm HG. The most frequent complications (40) are severe mitral regurgitation (up to 10%) and residual atrial septal defect. Mitral regurgitation is the result of leaflet tears and occurs mostly in the setting of unfavorable anatomy. It seldom necessitates surgical intervention. Small interatrial shunts with a Qp:Qs ratio of less than 1.5 are seen on transesophageal echocardiography in 40% to 80% of cases. Larger shunts can be seen in fewer than 5% of patients undergoing a single-balloon procedure and about 10% of those undergoing a double-balloon procedure. More serious complications, such as perforation of the left ventricle that causes hemopericardium and thromboembolism, are reported in 0.5% to 3% of procedures. The rate of mortality from PMC in centers with skilled operators is less than 1%. Thus, PMC can be done successfully 90% of the time with a complication rate of less than 3% and with a long-term benefit rate in excess of 80% in carefully selected patients.

Surgery

Mitral valve commissurotomy involves mechanical splitting of fused commissures to increase the valve area. Closed valvotomy (no direct vision of the mitral valve apparatus) has largely been abandoned because of significant rate of reoperations. Open mitral commissurotomy (OMC) has also been replaced by valve replacement techniques. However, OMC may be indicated in place of PMC in symptomatic (NYHA Classes III and IV) patients with favorable anatomy and when PMC is not available or not possible because of perisistent LA thrombus despite adequate anticoagulation. When valve anatomy is favorable, OMC is sometimes indicated for patients with recurrent embolization who are receiving adequate anticoagulation, despite lack of significant symptoms. Randomized studies of PMC and OMC have shown comparable results (25–27). Mitral valve replacement (MVR) is the procedure of choice in symptomatic MS when there is significant valve calcification, fibrosis, subvalvular disease, or significant mitral regurgitation. PMC or OMC under these circumstances produces suboptimal results. MVR results in excellent symptomatic relief, although it is accompanied by potential risks of prosthetic heart valves such as thromboembolism, endocarditis, and mechanical dysfunction (2% to 6% per year). Bioprosthesis may be an option in older patients, although structural failure of these valves (approximately 50% at 10 years) continues to pose a considerable problem. Although MVR is recommended in symptomatic MS, it is not advisable to postpone surgery until symptoms progress to NYHA Class IV. In fact, MVR is sometimes recommended for patients with severe pulmonary hypertension (pulmonary artery systolic pressure exceeding 60 mm HG) even when patients are only mildly symptomatic (24).

SPECIAL CONSIDERATIONS

Pregnancy

Asymptomatic mild to moderate MS is usually well tolerated throughout pregnancy. Patients with mild symptoms (NYHA Classes I and II), usually require no more than diuretics and beta blockers in doses titrated against improvement of symptoms. In the last trimester, particular care should be paid to effects of diuretics on placentouteral perfusion and the potential dampening effects of beta blockers on myometrial contractions. The usual dilemma is the choice of appropriate anticoagulation strategy. Most authorities do not recommend warfarin; instead, they choose subcutaneous heparin. The risk of fetal malformations with warfarin has been estimated to be between 4% and 10%, and it seems to be related to dose and timing of exposure (exposure during 6 to 12 weeks of gestation poses the greatest risk). Even if warfarin is used at any time during pregnancy, it is usually discontinued by the 36th week to prevent adverse fetal and maternal hemorrhage in case of complicated labor. Low-molecular-weight heparin, which does not cross the placental barrier, offers an alternative to unfractionated heparin for subcutaneous administration. In comparison with unfractionated heparin, it has the advantages of predictable bioavailability, less need for frequent monitoring of clotting parameters, and lower risk of thrombocytopenia and osteoporosis. However, data on its efficacy in preventing arterial thromboembolism are scant at best; therefore, caution must be used when it is selected as the agent of choice. When unfractionated heparin is used, the goal is to maintain the activated partial thromboplastin time at two to three times control levels. In the absence of specific contraindications, heparin or warfarin, or both, can be commenced within 6 hours of delivery even in mothers who elect to breast-feed. Symptomatic patients (NYHA Classes III and IV) with severe MS should undergo percutaneous balloon mitral valvuloplasty (PBMV) before pregnancy. In rare instances in which symptoms worsen despite maximal medical therapy during pregnancy, PMC may be performed under fluoroscopic guidance with appropriate pelvic or abdominal shielding or under echocardiographic guidance. Although small individual experience of emergency PMC during pregnancy has yielded excellent maternal outcome and almost no fetal complications, it is still a procedure best resorted to in experienced centers and when medical options have truly failed.

Surgical commissurotomy for similar indications has been done, but PBMV has largely supplanted this (41–43).

Combined Valvular Lesions

When aortic regurgitation (AR) coexists with MS, it is usually mild and of rheumatic origin. The pathophysiologic impact of severe AR (nonrheumatic and rheumatic causes are equally common) in the setting of severe MS is modified by the LV inflow obstruction. Signs of hyperdynamic circulation are lacking, and the LV dilation is blunted. The PHT of mitral valve inflow seen by Doppler imaging is affected by significant AR and cannot be used to estimate valve area. Although symptoms dictate the need to intervene, a more accurate assessment of the lesions may be necessary when the clinical picture is uncertain. This often requires combined echocardiographic and invasive hemodynamic assessments. If double-valve replacement is not advised, PMC is usually done with follow-up of AR. Double-valve replacement is then done later when clinically appropriate. Aortic stenosis (AS) in the setting of severe MS is almost always rheumatic in origin and poses the problem of obtaining a proper evaluation of the severity of outflow tract obstruction. The inflow restriction reduces flow and thus reduces gradient across the aortic valve. PMC of severe MS may allow a more reliable assessment of AS severity. If PMC is not appropriate, hemodynamic assessments of the severity of the combined lesion usually require data from echocardiography and cardiac catheterization. Planimetery of anatomic aortic valve area during TEE is an alternative method of assessing the aortic valve in low-flow situations. Tricuspid valve disease in the setting of MS is usually TR associated with PHT, and when the valve anatomy is preserved, TR usually improves after PMC. However, improvement in TR is unpredictable, and in the setting of right-heart failure and annular dilatation, tricuspid valve annuloplasty at the time of mitral valve surgery is recommended. Echocardiography is usually sufficient for evaluating the severity and the cause of TR. Other valve lesions such as tricuspid stenosis and pulmonary stenosis can coexist with MS, and they are almost always rheumatic in origin.

A single technique for assessing the severity of MS is insufficient when these two lesions are present. Thus, combined invasive and noninvasive assessments are necessary, and the decision to intervene is based on these data and the clinical picture.

PROGNOSIS

Untreated symptomatic mitral stenosis carries a 10-year mortality rate between 60% and 85%, and at 20 years, about 80% of affected patients are dead regardless of whether they were symptomatic initially (4,20,21). Of those whose disease was categorized as New York Heart Association (NYHA) functional Class IV, none survived 10 years. Most common causes of death were congestive heart failure and thromboembolism. It is also noteworthy that even among survivors, functional class had deteriorated in nearly all of them; only about 4% reported no change in symptoms.

PRACTICAL POINTS

- Rheumatic fever is the most cause of MS even in the absence of a clear prior clinical history.
- Characteristic symptoms and signs enable accurate bedside diagnosis in most patients with MS.
- Warfarin is mandatory even in the absence of a clinical embolic episode when AF complicates MS.
- Echocardiography provides diagnostic anatomic and hemodynamic information in most patients with MS.

- Cardiac catheterization is usually indicated for therapeutic intervention (PMC).
- Symptomatic MS without definitive treatment (PMC or surgery) carries a dismal prognosis.
- PMC is feasible in most patients with symptomatic MS and yields clinical results comparable with those of OMC.
- Valve replacement is usually reserved for patients who are symptomatic and unable to undergo PMC or in whom PMC has failed.

REFERENCES

1. Jordon SC. Development of pulmonary hypertension in mitral stenosis. *Lancet* 1965;2:322.
2. Wood P. An appreciation of mitral stenosis. Part II. Investigations and results. *BMJ* 1954;1:1113.
3. Doyle AE, et al. Pulmonary vascular patterns in pulmonary hypertension. *Br Heart J* 1957;19:353.
4. Olesen KH. The natural history of 271 patients with mitral stenosis under medical treatment. *Br Heart J* 1962;24:349–357.
5. Selzer A, Cohn KE. Natural history of mitral stenosis: a review. *Circulation* 1972;45:878–890.
6. Wood P. An appreciation of mitral stenosis: part I. *BMJ* 1954;1:1051–1063.
7. Wann LS, Weyman AE, Feigenbaum H, et al. Determination of mitral valve area by cross-sectional echocardiography. *Ann Intern Med* 1978;88:337–341.
8. Hatle L, Angelsen B, Tromsdal A. Noninvasive assessment of atrioventricular pressure half-time by Doppler ultrasound. *Circulation* 1979;60:1096–1104.
9. Nishimura RA, Rihal CS, Tajik AJ, et al. Accurate measurement of transmitral gradient in patients with mitral stenosis: a simultaneous catheterization and Doppler echocardiographic study. *J Am Coll Cardiol* 1994;24:152–158.
10. Thomas JD, Wilking GT, Choong CY, et al. Inaccuracy of mitral pressure half-time immediately after percutaneous mitral valvotomy: dependence on transmitral gradient and left atrial and ventricular compliance. *Circulation* 1988;78:980–993.
11. Mugge A, Daniel WG, Haverich A, et al. Diagnosis of noninfective cardiac mass by two-dimensional echocardiography: comparison of the transthoracic and transesophageal approaches. *Circulation* 1991;83:70.
12. Schweizer P, Bardos P, Erbel R, et al. Detection of left atrial thrombi by echocardiography. *Br Heart J* 1981;45:148.
13. Sutaria N, Northridge D, Masani N, et al. Three dimensional echocardiography for the assessment of mitral valve disease. *Heart* 2000;84(Suppl II):II19.
14. Kasalicky J, Hurych J, Widimsky R, et al. Left heart hemodynamics at rest and during exercise in patients with mitral stenosis. *Br Heart J* 1968;30:188–195.
15. Leavitt JI, Coats MH, Falk RH. Effects of exercise on transmitral gradient and pulmonary artery pressure in patients with mitral stenosis or a prosthetic mitral valve:

a Doppler echocardiographic study. *J Am Coll Cardiol* 1991;17:1520–1526.

16. Cheriex EC, Pieters FA, Janssen JH, et al. Value of exercise Doppler-echocardiography in patients with mitral stenosis. *Int J Cardiol* 1994;45:219–226.

17. Gorlin R, Gorlin SG. Hydraulic formula for calculation of stenotic mitral valve, other cardiac valves, and central circulatory shunts. *Am Heart J* 1951;41:1–29.

18. Hammermeister KE, Murray JA, Blackmon JR. Revision of Gorlin constant for calculation of mitral valve area from left heart pressures. *Br Heart J* 1972;35:392–396.

19. Cohen MV, Gorlin R. Modified orifice equation for the calculation of mitral valve area. *Am Heart J* 1972;84:839–840.

20. Rowe JC, Bland EF, Sprague HB. The course of mitral stenosis without surgery: ten and twenty year perspectives. *Ann Intern Med* 1960;52:741–749.

21. Rapaport E. Natural history of aortic and mitral valve disease. *Am J Cardiol* 1975;29:469.

22. Chetlin MD, Douglas PS, Parmley WW. 26th Bethesda conference: recommendations for determining eligibility for competition in athletes with cardiovascular abnormalities. Task force 2: acquired valvular heart disease. *J Am Coll Cardiol* 1994;24:874–880.

23. Coulshed N, Epstein EJ, McKendrick CS, et al. Systemic embolization in mitral valve disease. *Br Heart J* 1970;32:26–34.

24. Bonow R, Carabello B, de Leon AC Jr, et al. ACC/AHA Task Force Report ACC/AHA Guidelines for the management of patients with valvular heart disease: executive summary. A report of the American College of Cardiology/American Heart Association Task Force on Practice Guidelines (Committee on Management of Patients with Valvular Heart Disease). *J Am Coll Cardiol* 1998;32:1486–1588. Patel JJ, Shama D, Mitha AS, et al. Balloon valvuloplasty versus closed commissurotomy for pliable mitral stenosis: a prospective hemodynamic study. *J Am Coll Cardiol* 1991;18:1318.

25. Arora R, Nair M, Kaltra GS, et al. Immediate and long-term results of balloon and surgical closed mitral valvotomy: a randomized comparative study. *Am Heart J* 1993;125:1091.

26. Reyes VP, Raju BS, Wynne J, et al. Percutaneous balloon valvuloplasty compared with open surgical commissurotomy for mitral stenosis. *N Engl J Med* 1994;331:961.

27. Turi ZG, Reyes VP, Raju BS, et al. Percutaneous balloon versus surgical closed commissurotomy for mitral stenosis: a prospective, randomized trial. *Circulation* 1991;83:1179.

28. Palacios IF, Tuzcu ME, Weyman AE, et al. Clinical follow-up of patients undergoing percutaneous mitral balloon valvotomy. *Circulation* 1995;91:671.

29. Multicenter experience with balloon mitral commissurotomy. NHLBI Balloon Valvuloplasty Registry Report on immediate and 30-day follow-up results. *Circulation* 1992;85:448.

30. Feldman T. Hemodynamic results, clinical outcomes, and complications of Inoue balloon mitral valvotomy. *Cathet Cardiovasc Diagn* 1994;Suppl 2:2.

31. Cohen DJ, Kuntz RE, Gordon SP, et al. Predictors of long-term outcome after percutaneous balloon mitral valvoplasty. *N Engl J Med* 1992;327:1329.

32. Orrange SE, Kawanishi DT, Lopez BM, et al. Actuarial outcome after catheter balloon commissurotomy in patients with mitral stenosis. *Circulation* 1997;95:382.

33. Abascal VM, Wilkins GT, Choong CY, et al. Echocardiographic evaluation of mitral structure and function in patients followed for at least 6 months after percutaneous balloon mitral valvuloplasty. *J Am Coll Cardiol* 1998;12:606–615.

34. Reid CL, McKay CR, Chandraratna PA, et al. Mechanism of increase in mitral valve area and influence of anatomic features in double-balloon catheter balloon valvuloplasty in adults with rheumatic mitral stenosis: a Doppler and two-dimensional echocardiographic study. *Circulation* 1987;76:628–636.

35. Reid CL, McKay CR, Chandraratna PA, et al. Influence of mitral valve morphology on double balloon catheter valvuloplasty in patients with mitral stenosis: analysis of factors predicting immediate and 3 month results. *Circulation* 1989;80:515–524.

36. Vahanian A. Balloon valvuloplasty. *Heart* 2001;85:223–238.

37. Fatkin D, Roy P, Morgan JJ, et al. Percutaneous balloon mitral valvotomy with the Inoue single-balloon catheter: commissural morphology as a determinant of outcome. *J Am Coll Cardiol* 1993;21:390–397.

38. Cannan CR, Nishimura RA, Redder GS, et al. Echocardiographic assessment of commissural calcium: a simple predictor of outcome after percutaneous mitral balloon valvotomy. *J Am Coll Cardiol* 1997;29:175–180.

39. Carroll JD, Feldman T. Percutaneous mitral balloon valvotomy and the new demographics of mitral stenosis. *JAMA* 1993;270:1731–1736.

40. Complications and mortality of percutaneous balloon mitral commissurotomy: a report from the National Heart, Lung and Blood Institute Balloon Valvuloplasty Registry. *Circulation* 1992;85:2014.

41. Iung B, Cromier B, Elias J, et al. Usefulness of percutaneous balloon commissurotomy for mitral stenosis during pregnancy. *Am J Cardiol* 1994;73:398.

42. Oto MA, Kabukcu M, Ovunc K, et al. Percutaneous balloon valvuloplasty for severe mitral valve stenosis in pregnancy: four case reports. *J Vasc Dis* 1997;48:463.

43. Patel JJ Mitha AS, Hassen F, et al. Percutaneous balloon mitral valvotomy in pregnant patients with tight mitral stenosis. *Am Heart J* 1993;125:1106–1109.

24

Aortic Stenosis

Ragavendra R. Baliga, Mauro Moscucci, Michael J. Shea, and G. Michael Deeb

DEFINITION

Valvular aortic stenosis is the most common valve lesion in adults in industrialized nations, and calcified aortic stenosis is the valve lesion most commonly considered for valve replacement in the United States, particularly in the elderly. The normal aortic valve has three leaflets and has an area of 2 to 3 cm^2. Aortic stenosis is often not apparent until the valve orifice area is reduced by 50%. In general, patients are asymptomatic until the valve area is less than 1 cm^2. The onset of symptoms is associated with a 2-year survival rate of less than 50% (Fig. 24.1). In contrast, adults with asymptomatic aortic stenosis have an excellent clinical prognosis.

USUAL CAUSES

Aortic stenosis is usually acquired and occurs in previously normal valves (Table 24.1). Seventy percent of affected patients suffer from calcific stenosis (60% bicuspid, 10% tricuspid), 15% from rheumatic stenosis, and 15% from other forms of stenosis. Acquired aortic stenosis occurs a result of arteriosclerotic degeneration and calcification of the aortic leaflets and usually manifests in the sixth, seventh, and eighth decades. According to the Helsinki Ageing study, almost 3% of the individuals aged between 75 and 86 years have critical aortic stenosis (1).

Approximately 1% of the population have bicuspid aortic valves (Figs. 24.2, 24.3). Individuals with bicuspid aortic valves are more likely to develop aortic stenosis than are individuals with normal valves, and in such instances, the condition manifests in the third and fourth decades. The bicuspid aortic valve is the most common pathologic finding in symptomatic patients who are younger than 65 years (2). Bicuspid aortic

valve is four times more common among men than among women. About one fifth of the patients with bicuspid aortic valves have associated cardiac abnormalities such as patient ductus arteriosus or coarctation of the aorta (3). The bicuspid aortic valve is not stenosed at birth, but it has a single fused commissure, which results in an eccentrically oriented orifice. These anatomic characteristics, when subjected to hemodynamic stress, may result in thickening and calcification of the valve leaflets, rendering them immobile. Many of these patients have associated abnormalities of the medial layer of the aorta above the bicuspid valve, predisposing to dilatation of the aortic root.

In developing countries, rheumatic fever is a common cause of aortic stenosis, and usually the valve is also regurgitant. The stenosis occurs in a previously normal valve and is characterized by the fusion of the commissures, followed by secondary calcification and contraction of leaflets and annulus. In these patients, the mitral valve is also almost always affected.

Aortic stenosis can coexist with other congenital cardiovascular defects such as coarctation of aorta, in which the valve is often bicuspid (e.g., as in Turner's syndrome); hypoplastic left heart syndrome; corrected transposition of great arteries; ventricular septal defect with or without pulmonary stenosis; and coarctation of aorta with a patent ductus arteriosus.

SYMPTOMS

Many patients with aortic stenosis are asymptomatic. Symptoms usually manifest when the valve area is less than 50% (normal valve area is 2 to 3 cm^2). Typical symptoms of aortic stenosis include angina, syncope, and shortness of breath.

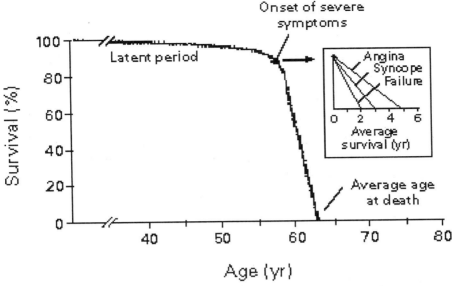

FIG. 24.1. Natural history of aortic stenosis. Asymptomatic patients with aortic stenosis have a normal life span. However, once symptoms develop, the risk of mortality is substantially increased. Of patients in whom the aortic valve is not replaced, about half die within 5 years after angina develops, and half die within 3 years after the onset of syncope; patients with dyspnea/heart failure die within only 2 years after these develop. Up to 20% of patients with severe congestive aortic stenosis die during childhood, mainly because of progressive heart failure. [Adapted from Ross J Jr, Braunwald E. Aortic stenosis. *Circulation* 1968;38(Suppl V):V-61.]

Angina occurs in about 70% of patients and, when coronary arteries are normal, results from a combination of increased myocardial oxygen demand and reduced coronary flow reserve caused by increased left ventricular mass. In one study, about one fourth of the patients with severe aortic

---

TABLE 24.1. *Usual causes of left ventricular outflow tract obstruction*

Aortic valvular stenosis
Arteriosclerotic degeneration and calcification of valve
Congenital (usually bicuspid valve)
Rheumatic fever
Atherosclerosis: marked hypercholesterolemia as in homozygous type II hyperlipoproteinemia can result in massive deposition of atheroma on the valve, aortic valve, and coronary arteries
Supravalvular narrowing (Williams' syndrome)
Subvalvular diaphragm or ridge
Hypertrophic cardiomyopathy (see page 245)
Discrete fibromuscular ring
Tunnel subaortic stenosis
Anomalous attachment of the anterior mitral valve leaflet

---

stenosis had angiographically significant coronary artery disease (4).

Syncope occurs in about 25% of patients and often occurs during or immediately after exercise (see Chapter 5). Exertional syncope has been attributed to the fact that cardiac output is restricted by the stenosed valve, when peripheral resistance falls on exercise. Impaired vasodepressor response is a second explanation for syncope that occurs in this condition. Increased intramural pressure, stimulating baroreceptors and thereby resulting in reflex bradycardia and vasodilatation, is another mechanism by which syncope can occur. Diastolic dysfunction with inability to increase cardiac output on exercise is an additional mechanism. When the calcification of the aortic valve extends into the upper part of the ventricular septum, complete atrioventricular block can occur and manifests as syncope.

Shortness of breath results from high end-diastolic pressures in the left ventricle and is first apparent on exertion. Shortness of breath,

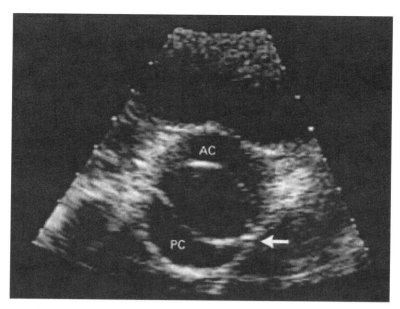

FIG. 24.2. Bicuspid aortic valve (From Bruce CJ, Breen JF. Aortic coarctation and bicuspid aortic valve. *New Engl J Med* 2000;342:249.)

including paroxysmal nocturnal dyspnea, is suggestive of left ventricular dysfunction and portends a poor prognosis. Orthopnea indicates severe left ventricular dysfunction. The left ventricular dysfunction, in aortic stenosis, is diastolic, systolic, or both. Diastolic dysfunction tends to predominate in advanced stages. Diastolic dysfunction is caused by increased left ventricular myocardial thickness, whereas systolic dysfunction is caused by increased dilatation of the left ventricle and decreased myocardial contractility. Severe aortic stenosis can manifest for the first time as congestive heart failure, and affected patients typically have a low volume pulse, an enlarged heart, and a soft murmur. Heart failure is not an uncommon presentation (5), and such patients frequently have normal left ventricular systolic function.

Other modes of presentation include infective endocarditis (see Chapter 20), sudden death, and, occasionally, systemic emboli from the calcified valve (usually resulting in a stroke or amaurosis fugax). About 3% to 5% of patients with aortic stenosis die suddenly without prior symptoms, and the mechanism of death remains unclear, but it has been suggested that it may be a result of ex-

treme intolerance to complete heart block or tachyarrhythmias. Patients with severe aortic stenosis may develop microangiopathic hemolytic anemia as a result of hemolysis at the valve. Infective endocarditis should be considered in patients with aortic stenosis who present with unexplained illness. Arrhythmias and conduction abnormalities have also been described in aortic stenosis. Ventricular arrhythmias are more common than supraventricular arrhythmias, and heart block may occur because of calcification of conducting tissues.

SIGNS

In mild aortic stenosis (when the aortic gradient is less than 50 mm Hg), the pulse is normal. In severe aortic stenosis, the carotid pulse is slow in rising and has diminished volume with a notch on the upstroke—the anacrotic pulse—but it may be normal in elderly patients with noncompliant carotid arteries. With associated aortic regurgitation, a double pulse, or *pulsus bisferiens,* may be felt. The apex beat initially is thrusting and not displaced and reflects the concentric hypertrophy of the left ventricle. A

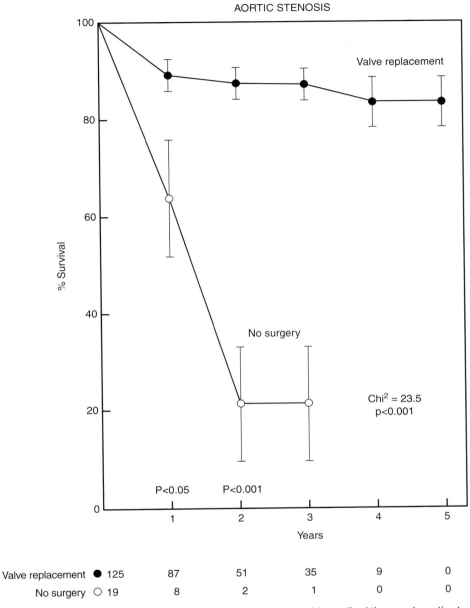

FIG. 24.3A. Survival is better after aortic valve replacement than with medical therapy in patients with severe aortic stenosis. (From Schwarz F, Banmann P, Manthey J, et al. The effect of the aortic valve replacement on survival. *Circulation* 1982;66:1105–1110.) (*Continued*)

displaced apex beat indicates left ventricular dilatation, which suggests that the condition is advanced or that there is associated aortic regurgitation. A systolic thrill may be felt at the base of the heart.

On auscultation there is a midsystolic, crescendo-decrescendo murmur (diamond-shaped murmur), best heard in the second right intercostal space, and the intensity of the murmur increases on expiration. The murmur usually

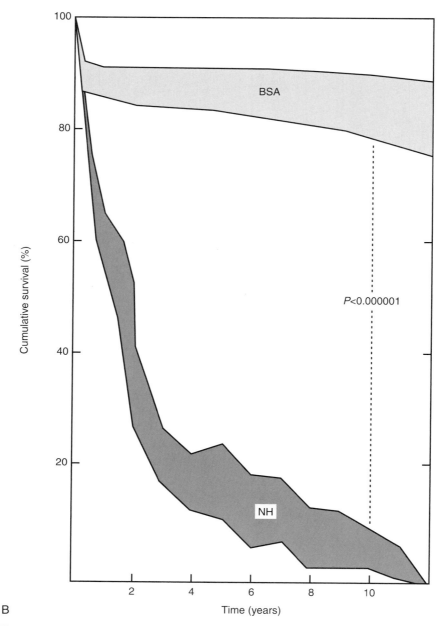

FIG. 24.3B. (*Continued*) Survival is better after aortic valve replacement than with medical therapy in patients with severe aortic stenosis. (From Horstkotte D, Loogen F. The natural history of aortic valve stenosis. *Eur Heart J* 1988;9(Suppl E):57–64.)

radiates to the neck and right clavicle. Clavicular auscultation appears to be more rewarding than the traditional search for transmission of aortic murmurs to the carotid artery (6). In mild aortic stenosis, the peak of the murmur occurs earlier in systole, and as the severity of stenosis progresses, the peak of the murmur occurs later in systole. The decrease in the loudness of the murmur is suggestive of the onset of poor left ventricular function and a low cardiac output. The murmur may display the Gallavardin phenomenon—that is, the selective transmission of the musical component toward the cardiac apex but location of the noisy component (jet noise) to the right of the upper sternum, with transmission toward the carotid arteries. The transmission of these high-frequency components of the murmur to the apex may be mistaken for mitral regurgitation.

The aortic component of the second heart sound is soft or absent when the valves are calcified. A delayed aortic component of the second sound or reverse split is suggestive of severe aortic stenosis. An ejection click may be heard at the apex in bicuspid aortic stenosis, especially in young patients. A third sound implies severe left ventricular dysfunction, whereas a fourth heart sound indicates severe aortic stenosis. Clinical signs of severe aortic stenosis include narrow pulse pressure, soft second heart sound, delayed or reverse split of second heart sound, heaving apex beat, fourth heart sound, and cardiac failure.

HELPFUL TESTS

Electrocardiogram

The electrocardiogram usually shows left ventricular hypertrophy and, occasionally, left axis deviation. In later stages there may be negative P waves in lead V_1 caused by left atrial hypertrophy. First-degree heart block or left bundle branch block is suggestive of calcification of the conducting tissues. The presence of atrial fibrillation is suggestive of associated mitral valve disease or coronary artery disease.

Chest Radiograph

The chest radiograph may show cardiac enlargement, but, typically in the initial stages, the cardiac size may be normal in posteroanterior views. Poststenotic dilatation of the aorta may be seen but can also occur with subvalvular stenosis. Calcification of the aortic valve may be seen in lateral views, particularly in older patients. Signs of pulmonary venous congestion or pulmonary edema may be seen in acute left ventricular failure. When these signs are associated with coarctation of aorta, there may be rib notching.

Echocardiography

Echocardiography may show bicuspid valve (Figs. 24.2 and 24.3), calcified valve, left ventricular hypertrophy, and systolic function (Table 24.2). Women have a much higher incidence of excessive left ventricular hypertrophy, which leads to a supernormal left ventricular ejection fraction (7). Echocardiography is useful in the diagnosis and assessment of severity of aortic stenosis. The degree of aortic stenosis is graded as mild (valve area exceeding 1.5 cm^2), moderate (area exceeding 1.0 to 1.5 cm^2), or severe (area < 1.0 cm^2) (Table 24.3). Echocardiography also helps define the level of obstruction (i.e., valvular, supravalvular, subvalvular). A normal valve appearance excludes significant aortic stenosis in adults. Furthermore, echocardiography allows assessment of left ventricular size, function, and hemodynamics. It is useful in the reevaluation of patients with known aortic stenosis with changing symptoms and signs and in asymptomatic patients with severe aortic stenosis. Doppler imaging allows assessment of the valve gradient. The valve gradient, however, depends on several factors, including left ventricular function, and therefore is not a good indicator of the severity of the disease. For example, a mean valve gradient of less than 50 mm HG may be associated with severe, moderate, or even mild aortic stenosis (8,9). Thus, it is more prudent to use the aortic valve area to determine the severity of aortic stenosis. This may be assessed by the continuity equation.

Exercise Testing

Exercise testing in adults with aortic stenosis has been discouraged largely because of safety issues and is contraindicated in symptomatic patients.

TABLE 24.2. *ACC/AHA recommendations for echocardiography*

Class I: There is evidence and/or general agreement that echocardiography is useful and effective
Diagnosis and assessment of severity of aortic stenosis
Assessment of left ventricular size, function, and hemodynamics
Reevaluation of patients with known aortic stenosis with changing symptoms or signs
Assessment of changes in hemodynamic severity and ventricular function in patients with known aortic stenosis during pregnancy
Reevaluation of asymptomatic patients with severe aortic stenosis
Class II: There is conflicting evidence and/or a divergence of opinion about the usefulness/efficacy of echocardiography
Reevaluation of asymptomatic patients with mild to moderate aortic stenosis and evidence of left ventricular dysfunction or hypertrophy
Class III: There is evidence and/or general agreement that echocardiography is not useful and in some cases may be harmful
Routine reevaluation of asymptomatic adults patients with mild aortic stenosis having stable physical signs and normal left ventricular size and function

ACC/AHA, American College of Cardiology/American Heart Association.
Modified from Bonow RO, Carabello B, de Leon AC Jr, et al. ACC/AHA guidelines for the management of patients with valvular heart disease: executive summary. A report of the American College of Cardiology/American Heart Association Task Force on Practice Guidelines (Committee on Management of Patients with Valvular Heart Disease). *Circulation* 1998;98:1949–1984.

In asymptomatic patients, an abnormal hemodynamic response (e.g., hypotension) is sufficient to consider aortic valve replacement (AVR). Occasionally, in selected patients, it is useful for providing a basis for advice about physical activity.

Cardiac Catheterization

Cardiac catheterization is useful in determining the coronary anatomy and for confirming or clarifying the diagnosis. Cardiac hemodynamic measurement with left- and right-sided heart catheterization is indicated when echocardiography is inadequate. The simultaneous recording of pressures in the left ventricle and in the systemic circulation remains the standard for documenting the presence and severity of aortic stenosis. This requires (a) measurement of transvalvular

flow, (b) determination of transvalvular pressure gradient, (c) calculation of the effective valve area, and (d) determination of the anatomy of the aortic root. A bicuspid aortic valve is often associated with a dominant left circumflex coronary artery and a short main stem.

DIFFERENTIAL DIAGNOSIS

Aortic Sclerosis

Aortic sclerosis can simulate aortic stenosis because, on auscultation, a systolic ejection murmur may be audible. It is commoner in old age and associated with a normal carotid pulse. Echocardiography is necessary to confirm the diagnosis, and typical findings are mild thickening of leaflets without restricted motion or gradient (10).

TABLE 24.3. *Severity of aortic stenosis*

Severity of aortic stenosis	Aortic valve area (cm²)[a]	Aortic valve area index (cm²/m²)[a]	Aortic valve area (cm²)[b]
Normal aortic valve	2–3	—	—
Mild	>1.5	>0.9	≥1.0
Moderate	>1.0–1.5	>0.6–0.9	0.7–1.0
Moderately severe	—	—	0.5–0.7
Severe	>0.8–1.0	≤0.6	<0.5
Critical	0.7	—	—

[a]From Rahimtoola, 1991 SH. Severe aortic stenosis. *Circulation* 1968;38 (Suppl V) : V-61.
[b]From Baim and Grossman

Flow Murmur of Pregnancy; Anemia; and Thyrotoxicosis

These conditions can mimic the murmur of aortic stenosis but are associated with large-volume pulse, a normal echocardiogram, and no gradient.

Mitral Regurgitation

The systolic murmur of mitral regurgitation can be short and therefore be mistaken for aortic stenosis, but these murmurs usually do not radiate to the neck. Echocardiography and Doppler examination may be the only way to confirm the mitral valve abnormality.

Hypertrophic Cardiomyopathy

Hypertrophic cardiomyopathy may also be accompanied by a late systolic murmur, and differentiating features are a jerky pulse, echocardiographic findings of asymmetric septal hypertrophy, and systolic anterior motion of the mitral valve.

Ventricular Septal Defect

Ventricular septal defect is associated with a holosystolic murmur at the left sternal edge with thrill, and Doppler echocardiographic findings of the jet across the septal defect confirm this diagnosis.

THERAPY

Lifestyle

Physical activity is not restricted in asymptomatic patients with mild aortic stenosis. Asymptomatic patients with moderate aortic stenosis should avoid competitive sports that involve high dynamic and static muscular demands; other forms of exercise can be performed safely, but it is advisable to evaluate such patients with an exercise test before they begin an exercise or athletic program. Asymptomatic patients with severe stenosis should limit their activity to relatively low levels.

Pharmacologic Treatment

Drug treatment has no place in the treatment of aortic stenosis in patients who are fit for surgery, but patients should be given antibiotic prophylaxis against infective endocarditis (see Chapter 20 for details). In patients ineligible for surgery because of serious comorbid conditions, medical therapy is used to control symptoms.

Patients with pulmonary edema may benefit from diuretics, digitalis, and angiotensin-converting enzyme inhibitors. Beta blockers and other drugs with negative inotropic effects should be avoided in patients with heart failure caused by aortic stenosis. In patients with angina, cautious use of nitrates and beta blockers may provide relief. Patients with atrial fibrillation should undergo cardioversion; when the latter is unsuccessful, treatment with amiodarone or digitalis may be beneficial.

Aortic Valve Replacement

AVR is mandatory for symptomatic patients because the rate of 5-year survival after the onset of symptoms is 40%. Age alone is not a contraindication. The absolute valve area (or transvalvular pressure gradient) is not usually the primary determinant of the need for AVR. The choice of the prosthetic valve depends on several factors, including the known risks and benefits of each device, the patient's preferences, and individual circumstances of the patient (see Tables 24.4 to 24.6). Symptomatic patients with severe aortic stenosis were shown to have a very high mortality rate without AVR (11–13). AVR results in regression of left ventricular hypertrophy and improves survival, symptomatic state, and impaired left ventricular function (Figs. 24.4, 24.5, and 24.6) (12–14).

The prognosis after surgery depends on age of the patient and comorbid conditions, including left ventricular function and coronary artery disease. A subset of patients with aortic stenosis who had a low mean atrioventricular gradient and severe left ventricular dysfunction (left ventricular ejection fraction less than 0.35) experienced good results when treated with AVR (15). In the same study, another predictor of

TABLE 24.4. *ACC/AHA recommendations for aortic valve replacement*

Class I: There is evidence and/or general agreement that aortic valve replacement is useful and effective
Symptomatic patients with severe aortic stenosis
Patients with severe aortic stenosis undergoing CABG
Patients with severe aortic stenosis undergoing surgery on the aorta or other heart valves
Class IIa: The weight of evidence/opinion is in favor of usefulness/efficacy of AVR
Patients with moderate AS undergoing CABG or surgery of the aortia or heart valves
Asymptomatic patients with severe AS and LV dysfunction
Asymptomatic patients with severe AS and an abnormal response to exercise (e.g., hypotension)
Class IIb: Usefulness/efficacy is less well established by evidence/opinion
Asymptomatic patients with severe AS and ventricular tachycardia
Asymptomatic patients with severe AS and marked or excessive left ventricular hypertrophy (15 mm)
Asymptomatic patients with severe AS and valve area <0.6 cm^2
Class III: There is evidence and/or general agreement that aortic valve replacement is not useful and in some cases may be harmful
Prevention of sudden death in asymptomatic patients with none of the following:
   LV dysfunction, an abnormal response to exercise, ventricular tachycardia, left ventricular hypertrophy, or reduced valve area

---

ACC/AHA, American College of Cardiology/American Heart Association; AVR, aortic valve replacement; AS, atrial stenosis; CABG, coronary artery bypass graft; LV, left ventricular.
   Modified from Bonow RO, Carabello B, de Leon AC Jr, et al. ACC/AHA guidelines for the management of patients with valvular heart disease: executive summary. A report of the American College of Cardiology/American Heart Association Task Force on Practice Guidelines (Committee on Management of Patients with Valvular Heart Disease). *Circulation* 1998;98:1949–1984.

operative mortality was the size of the prosthetic valve: Smaller prostheses (21 mm) were associated with a 47% mortality rate, whereas larger ones (23 mm) were associated with a 15% mortality rate (15). Patients with a small valve annulus that does not permit the use of a 23-mm prosthesis then should be considered for the use of homografts, stentless valves, or enlargement of the aortic root/annulus.

Although asymptomatic patients with aortic stenosis have a normal life span, AVR should be considered in those with severe aortic stenosis (peak-to-peak gradient exceeding 50 mm HG), particularly when any one or more of the

TABLE 24.5. *ACC/AHA recommendations for valve replacement with a mechanical prosthesis*

Class I: There is evidence and/or general agreement that mechanical prosthesis replacement is useful and effective
Patients with expected long life spans
Patients with a mechanical prosthetic valve already in place in a different position than the valve to be replaced
Class II: There is conflicting evidence and/or a divergence of opinion about the usefulness/efficacy of a mechanical prosthesis
Patients in renal failure, on hemodialysis, or with hypercalcemia
Class IIa: The weight of evidence/opinion is in favor of usefulness/efficacy of a mechanical prosthesis
Patients requiring warfarin therapy because of risk factors for thromboembolsim (such as atrial fibrillation, LV dysfunction, previous thromboembolism, hypercoagulable state)
Patients aged 65 years for AVR
Class IIb: Usefulness/efficacy is less well established by evidence/opinion
Valve replacement for thrombosed biologic valve
Class III: There is evidence and/or general agreement that mechanical prosthesis is not useful and in some cases may be harmful
Patients who will not or cannot take warfarin therapy

ACC/AHA, American College of Cardiology/American Heart Association; AVR, aortic valve replacement; LV, left ventricular.
   Modified from Bonow RO, Carabello B, de Leon AC Jr, et al. ACC/AHA guidelines for the management of patients with valvular heart disease: executive summary. A report of the American College of Cardiology/American Heart Association Task Force on Practice Guidelines (Committee on Management of Patients with Valvular Heart Disease). *Circulation* 1998;98:1949–1984.

TABLE 24.6. *ACC/AHA recommendations for valve replacement with a bioprosthesis*

Class I: There is evidence and/or general agreement that bioprosthesis replacement is useful and effective.
Patients who cannot or will not take warfarin therapy
Patients aged 65 years (based on major reduction in rate of valve deterioration after age of 65 years and increased risk of major bleeding in this age group) needing AVR who do not have risk factors for thromboembolism (such as atrial fibrillation, LV dysfunction, previous thromboembolism, hypercoagulable state)
Class IIa: The weight of evidence/opinion is in favor of usefulness/efficacy of a bioprosthesis
Patients considered to have possible compliance problems with warfarin therapy
Class IIb: Usefulness/efficacy is less well established by evidence/opinion
Valve replacement for thrombosed mechanical valve
Patients <65 years
Class III: There is evidence and/or general agreement that mechanical prosthesis is not useful and in some cases may be harmful.
Patients in renal failure, on hemodialysis, or with hypercalcemia
Adolescent patients who are still growing

ACC/AHA, American College of Cardiology/American Heart Association; AVR, aortic valve replacement.
Modified from Bonow RO, Carabello B, de Leon AC Jr, et al. ACC/AHA guidelines for the management of patients with valvular heart disease: executive summary. A report of the American College of Cardiology/American Heart Association Task Force on Practice Guidelines (Committee on Management of Patients with Valvular Heart Disease). *Circulation* 1998;98:1949–1984.

following features are present: left ventricular systolic dysfunction, abnormal response to exercise (e.g., hypotension), ventricular tachycardia, marked excessive left ventricular hypertrophy (15 mm), and valve area less than 0.6 cm². Patients with severe aortic stenosis, with or without symptoms, who are undergoing coronary artery bypass surgery or surgery on the aorta or other heart valves should undergo AVR at the time of surgery. In asymptomatic patients with moderate aortic stenosis, it is generally acceptable to perform AVR in patients who are undergoing mitral valve or aortic root surgery or coronary artery bypass surgery.

One study found that increased left ventricular mass index is associated with increased adverse in-hospital clinical outcomes in patients undergoing AVR (16). The investigators suggested that further studies are needed to address whether outcomes in asymptomatic patients with aortic valve disease could be improved by earlier AVR before a significant increase in left ventricular mass index. Another group of investigators (17), in a prospective study to identify predictors of clinical outcome in adults with severe asymptomatic aortic stenosis, found that an increase in aortic jet velocity of at least 0.3 m per second per year was associated with high risk. Other predictors of severity include a baseline aortic jet velocity

of more than 4.0 m per second and the extent of calcification of the valve. Despite these predictors, the current recommendation for AVR, in patients with severe asymptomatic aortic stenosis, is based on the development of symptoms (18). It is therefore important to educate the patient with aortic stenosis about the expected course of the disease and encourage the patient to seek medical attention as soon as symptoms develop so that valve surgery can be performed promptly.

The Ross procedure with a modified Konno-type enlargement of the aortic annulus is an excellent approach to the treatment of aortic valve disease in neonates and older infants. The procedure can be accomplished with low rates of morbidity and mortality and low rates of reoperation (19). The pulmonary autograft demonstrates durability without development of aortic stenosis, aortic insufficiency, or progressive dilatation. Enlargement of the aortic annulus parallels somatic growth of the neonate or infant (19). The Ross pulmonary autograft procedure has emerged as the operation of choice for young individuals (Fig. 24.7) with aortic valve stenosis and aortic root disease that is not amenable to repair (20). Advantages of this procedure include durability of the pulmonary autograft in the aortic position, freedom from thrombosis and long-term anticoagulation, and the similarity of the

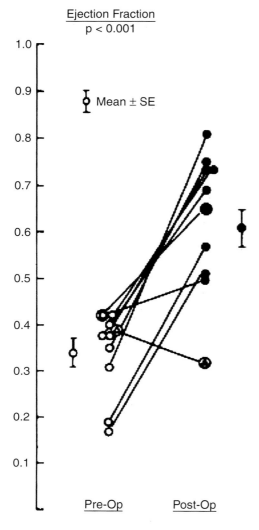

Ejection Fraction
p < 0.001

Mean ± SE

Pre-Op   Post-Op

⬤ Peri-Op MI and late CHB
● Post-Op: Parivalvular Aortic Incompetence

FIG. 24.4. Left ventricular ejection improves and even normalizes after aortic valve replacement in patients with severe aortic stenosis and clinical heart failure. (From Smith N, McAnulty JH, Rahimtoola SH. Severe aortic stenosis with impaired left ventricular function and clinical heart failure: results of valve replacement. *Circulation* 1978;59:255–264.)

pulmonary autograft to the human aortic valve. The indications for the Ross procedure continue to expand; it has been performed in older individuals, the upper limit of patient age being 50 years. Other indications include mechanical or bioprosthetic aortic valve dysfunction, active endocarditis, and, in athletes, the desire to avoid anticoagulation and the extreme physiologic and hemodynamic consequences of their chosen field. Contraindications to the Ross proce-

dure include multivessel coronary artery disease, multiple pathologic processes in which a second valve replacement device is needed, extremes of age, and severely depressed left ventricular function.

Balloon Valvuloplasty

This procedure is useful in infants (in whom the results of surgery are poor) and in children

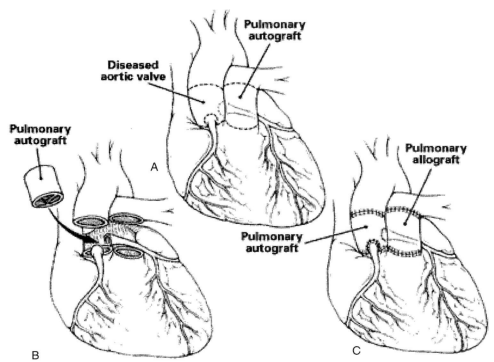

FIG. 24.5. Schematic representation of the Ross operative procedure. First, the aortic valve and the adjacent aorta are excised, leaving buttons of aortic tissue surrounding the coronary arteries (**A**). The pulmonary valve, with a small rim of right ventricular muscle and the main pulmonary artery, is also excised. Next, the pulmonary autograft is sutured to the aortic annulus and to the distal aorta, and the coronary arteries are attached to openings in the pulmonary artery (**B**). A pulmonary-root allograft is then sutured into the right ventricular outflow tract (**C**). (From Kouchoukos NT, Davila-Roman VG, Spray TL. Replacement of the aortic root with a pulmonary autograft in children and young adults with aortic-valve disease. *N Engl J Med* 1994;330:1–6.)

(20,21) and young adults (in whom the valve apparatus is not calcified) (Table 24.7).

Balloon valvuloplasty of aortic stenosis is associated with considerable rates of morbidity and mortality, and it is therefore recommended as a "bridge" to surgery in hemodynamically unstable patients who are at high risk for the need for AVR, as palliation in patients with serious comorbid conditions, and in patients who require urgent noncardiac surgery.

PROGNOSIS AND FOLLOW-UP

In adults, after the onset of symptoms, the 5-year survival rate is 40%. Asymptomatic patients with aortic stenosis have a normal life span (Fig. 24.1).

However, once symptoms develop, the risk of mortality is substantially increased. Of patients in whom the aortic valve is not replaced, about half die within 5 years after angina develops, and half die within 3 years after the onset of syncope; patients with dyspnea or heart failure die only 2 years after these develop (11). Up to 20% of patients with severe congestive aortic stenosis die during childhood, mainly because of progressive heart failure. Patients with mild to moderate aortic stenosis should be monitored for increasing severity.

Patients who have undergone valve replacement should be monitored for failure of the valve prosthesis (particularly biologic valves) and endocarditis.

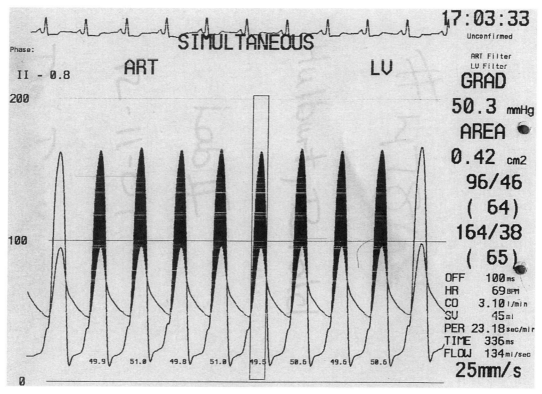

FIG. 24.6. Simultaneous recordings of pressure in the left ventricle and in a peripheral artery show the gradient (difference between the systolic pressures) across the aortic valve.

TABLE 24.7. *ACC/AHA recommendations for aortic balloon valvotomy in adults with aortic stenosis*

Class IIa: The weight of evidence/opinion is in favor of usefulness/efficacy
  A "bridge" to surgery in hemodynamically unstable patients who are at high risk for AVR
Class IIb: Usefulness/efficacy is less well established by evidence/opinion
  Palliation in patients with serious comorbid conditions
  Patients who require urgent noncardiac surgery
Class III: There is evidence and/or general agreement that aortic balloon valvotomy is not useful and in some
    cases may be harmful
  An alternative to AVR

ACC/AHA, American College of Cardiology/American Heart Association; AVR, aortic valve replacement.
Modified from Bonow RO, Carabello B, de Leon AC Jr, et al. ACC/AHA guidelines for the management of patients with valvular heart disease: executive summary. A report of the American College of Cardiology/American Heart Association Task Force on Practice Guidelines (Committee on Management of Patients with Valvular Heart Disease). *Circulation* 1998;98:1949–1984.

PRACTICAL POINTS

- According to the Helsinki Ageing study, almost 3% of the individuals aged between 75 and 86 years have critical aortic stenosis.

- The onset of symptoms is associated with a 2-year survival rate of less than 50%. In contrast, adults with asymptomatic aortic stenosis have an excellent clinical prognosis.

- Clinical signs of severe aortic stenosis include narrow pulse pressure, soft second heart sound, delayed or reverse split of second heart sound, heaving apex beat, fourth heart sound, and cardiac failure.

- The presence of atrial fibrillation is suggestive of associated mitral valve disease or coronary artery disease.

- The valve gradient depends on several factors, including left ventricular function, and is therefore not a good indicator of the severity of the disease. Thus, it is more prudent to use the aortic valve area to determine the severity of aortic stenosis.

- Exercise testing in adults with aortic stenosis has been discouraged largely because of safety concerns and is contraindicated in symptomatic patients. In asymptomatic patients, an abnormal hemodynamic response (e.g., hypotension) is sufficient for considering AVR.

- Asymptomatic patients with severe aortic stenosis should limit their activity to relatively low levels.

- Drug treatment has no place in the treatment of aortic stenosis in patients who are fit for surgery. AVR is mandatory for symptomatic patients because the 5-year rate of survival after the onset of symptoms is 40%.

- Balloon valvuloplasty of aortic stenosis is associated with considerable rates of morbidity and mortality, and it is therefore recommended as a "bridge" to surgery in hemodynamically unstable patients who are at high risk for the need for AVR, as palliation in patients with serious comorbid conditions, and in patients who require urgent noncardiac surgery.

REFERENCES

1. Lindroos M, Kupari M, Heikkila J, et al. Prevalence of aortic valve abnormalities in the elderly: an echocardiographic study of a random population sample. *J Am Coll Cardiol* 1993;21:1220–1225.

2. Subramanian R, Olson LJ, Edwards WD. Surgical pathology of pure aortic stenosis: a study of 374 cases. *Mayo Clin Proc* 1984;59:683–690.

3. Friedman WF. Aortic stenosis. In: Emmanouilides GC, Riemenschneider TA, Allen HD, et al, eds. *Moss and Adams' heart disease in infants, children, and adolescents.* Baltimore: Williams & Wilkins, 1995:1087–1111.

4. Green SJ, Pizzareollo RA, Padmanabhan VT, et al. Relation of angina pectoris to coronary artery disease in aortic valve stenosis. *Am J Cardiol* 1985;55:1063–1065.

5. Murphy ES, Lawson RM, Starr A, et al. Severe aortic stenosis in patients 60 years of age and older: left ventricular function and ten-year survival after valve replacement. *Circulation* 1981;64(Suppl II):II-184–II-188.

6. Spodick DH, Kerigan AT, de la Paz LR, et al. Clavicular auscultation. Preferential clavicular transmission and amplification of aortic valve murmurs. *Chest* 1976;70:337–340.

7. Carroll JD, Carroll EP, Feldman T, et al. Sex-associated differences in left ventricular function in aortic stenosis of the elderly. *Circulation* 1992;86:1099–1107.

8. Griffith MJ, Carey C, Coltart DJ, et al. Inaccuracies of using aortic valve gradients alone to grade severity of aortic stenosis. *Br Heart J* 1989;62:372–378.

9. Rahimtoola SH. Severe aortic stenosis with low systolic gradient. The good and bad news. *Circulation* 2000;101;1892–1894.

10. Otto CM, Lind BK, Kitzman DW, et al. Association of aortic-valve sclerosis with cardiovascular mortality and morbidity in the elderly. *N Engl J Med* 1999;341:142–147.

11. Ross J Jr, Braunwald E. Aortic stenosis. *Circulation* 1968;38(Suppl V):V-61.

12. Horstkotte D, Loogen F. The natural history of aortic valve stenosis. *Eur Heart J* 1988;9(Suppl E):57–64.

13. Schwarz F, Banmann P, Manthey J, et al. The effect of aortic valve replacement on survival. *Circulation* 1982;66:1105–1110.

14. Smith N, McAnulty JH, Rahimtoola SH. Severe aortic stenosis with impaired left ventricular function and clinical heart failure: results of valve replacement. *Circulation* 1978;58:255–264.

15. Connolly HM, Oh JK, Schaff HV, et al. Severe

aortic stenosis with low transvalvular gradient and severe left ventricular dysfunction: result of aortic valve replacement in 52 patients. *Circulation* 2000;1010:1940–1946.

16. Mehta RH, Bruckman D, Das S, et al. Implications of increased left ventricular mass index on in-hospital outcomes in patients undergoing aortic valve surgery. *J Thorac Cardiovasc Surg.* 2001;122:919–928.

17. Rosenhek R, Binder T, Porenta G, et al. Predictors of outcome in severe, asymptomatic aortic stenosis. *N Engl J Med* 2000;343:611–617.

18. Bonow RO, Carabello B, de Leon AC Jr, et al. ACC/AHA guidelines for the management of patients with valvular heart disease: executive summary. A report of the American College of Cardiology/American Heart Association Task Force on Practice Guidelines (Committee on Management of Patients With Valvular Heart Disease). *Circulation.* 1998;98:1949–1984.

19. Ohye RG, Gomez CA, Ohye BJ, et al. The Ross/Konno procedure in neonates and infants: intermediate-term survival and autograft function. *Ann Thorac Surg* 2001;72:823–830.

20. Kouchoukos NT, Davila-Roman VG, Spray TL, et al. Replacement of the aortic root with a pulmonary autograft in children and young adults with aortic-valve disease. *N Engl J Med* 1994;330:1–6.

21. Rocchini AP, Beekman RH, ben Shacher G, et al. Balloon aortic valvuloplasty: results of the valvuloplasty and angioplasty of congenital anomalies registry. *Am J Cardiology* 1990;65:784–789.

25

Tricuspid/Pulmonary Valve Disease

Theodore J. Kolias, Julie A. Kovach, and William F. Armstrong

USUAL CAUSES

Primary tricuspid and pulmonary valve disease occurs less often than disease of the mitral or aortic valve. This may be related to the decreased hemodynamic stress on the valves on the right side of the heart, which are exposed to lower pressures than the left-sided heart valves. Lesions of the right-sided heart valves can be categorized as regurgitant lesions and stenotic lesions.

The most common lesion encountered is tricuspid regurgitation. Minimal tricuspid regurgitation is frequently found in normal patients and should not be considered pathologic in the absence of any other cardiac disease (1). Tricuspid regurgitation can be classified as either functional or organic. Functional tricuspid regurgitation results from dilation or distortion of the tricuspid annulus, whereas organic tricuspid regurgitation occurs as a result of intrinsic disease of the tricuspid valve. Causes of functional tricuspid regurgitation include any conditions that lead to right ventricular dilatation. Examples include left-sided heart diseases such as mitral stenosis or congestive heart failure that lead to pulmonary hypertension and subsequent right ventricular dilatation. Other diseases resulting in pulmonary hypertension, such as pulmonary emboli or primary pulmonary hypertension, may also lead to right ventricular dilatation and subsequent tricuspid regurgitation.

The most common cause of intrinsic tricuspid valve disease that results in tricuspid regurgitation is rheumatic heart disease (2); this is also the most common cause of tricuspid stenosis (3). Rheumatic heart disease most commonly affects the mitral valve (4) and often also involves the aortic valve as well. Isolated tricuspid stenosis or regurgitation secondary to rheumatic disease in the absence of mitral or aortic valve involvement is quite rare.

In adults, the pulmonic valve is the least commonly diseased valve of all the cardiac valves. Pulmonic stenosis is usually congenital in origin. Most frequently, it is caused by congenital fusion of the valve leaflets (5). In contrast, pulmonic regurgitation is usually caused by dilation of the pulmonic valve annulus as a result of pulmonary hypertension or secondary to conditions that dilate the pulmonary artery.

PRESENTING SYMPTOMS AND SIGNS

The presenting symptoms and signs of right-sided heart valve lesions are related to their cause, their effect on venous pressure and right ventricular function, and associated conditions such as mitral stenosis or pulmonary hypertension. Typically, the clinical findings of right-sided heart valve lesions are present only in advanced cases and are commonly overshadowed by left-sided heart disease.

Tricuspid regurgitation, when severe and progressive, typically causes signs and symptoms of right-sided heart failure, such as elevation of the jugular venous pressure, hepatomegaly, abdominal distension with ascites, edema, and congestive hepatopathy, with occasional anasarca in severe advanced cases. Affected patients often experience fatigue and weakness, and they may experience weight loss and cachexia. Examination of their jugular veins frequently reveals a large V wave corresponding to the regurgitant flow from ventricular contraction, as well as a steep Y descent corresponding to brisk early diastolic filling of the right ventricle. These patients often feel throbbing pulsations in their neck, which correspond to the V waves. Auscultation of the heart reveals a holosystolic murmur in the third and fourth intercostal space at the left sternal border. The murmur is accentuated by inspiration, a finding known as the Rivera-Carvallo sign (6). If concomitant right ventricular failure is present, then a right-sided precordial heave may be palpated, and right-sided S3 and S4 may also be heard. If the tricuspid regurgitation is the result of pulmonary hypertension, then an accentuated pulmonic component of S2 may also be heard on auscultation and a diastolic murmur of pulmonic regurgitation may be heard in the second and third intercostal space at the left sternal border (the Graham Steell murmur) (4,7).

Tricuspid stenosis may also manifest with signs and symptoms of right-sided heart failure. Evaluation of the jugular venous pulse reveals a large A wave, known as a cannon A wave, corresponding to atrial contraction against a stenotic orifice. Elevation of the jugular venous pressure is usually present. Auscultation reveals a tricuspid opening snap in diastole, followed by a rumbling diastolic murmur in the third and fourth intercostal space at the left sternal border. If the valve is mobile, then a prominent S1 may also be heard. In contrast to the murmur of mitral stenosis, both the murmur of tricuspid stenosis and the opening snap are increased in intensity with inspiration (the Rivera-Carvallo sign) (6). Because tricuspid stenosis is usually the result of rheumatic heart disease, it is almost always accompanied by rheumatic disease of left-sided heart valves, particularly the mitral valve, and as such, its manifestations may be overshadowed by those of the left-sided lesion.

Isolated disease of the pulmonic valve is quite uncommon and, when it occurs, rarely causes significant symptoms (with the exception of severe congenital pulmonic stenosis). Because pulmonic regurgitation most often occurs as the result of pulmonary hypertension, its manifestations are often overshadowed by those of the pulmonary hypertension. Only rarely does pulmonic regurgitation itself cause clinical manifestations; those that occur are related to right ventricular failure from a right ventricular volume overload. On physical examination, pulmonic regurgitation

is characterized by a diastolic murmur best heard in the second and third intercostal space at the left sternal border. If there is associated pulmonary hypertension, then the intensity of the pulmonic component of S2 may be increased. Signs of right ventricular failure may also be present, such as a prominent right ventricular heave and right-sided S3 and S4 heart sounds (6).

Pulmonic stenosis is characterized by a midsystolic crescendo murmur best heard in the second left intercostal space at the left sternal border. An ejection click often precedes the murmur, and, in contrast to other right-sided cardiac murmurs, the intensity of the ejection click decreases with inspiration (7). Associated findings may include a right-sided S4 and a right ventricular heave. Symptoms typically develop when the stenosis is severe; they include fatigue, dyspnea, exercise intolerance, lightheadedness, syncope, angina, and manifestations of right ventricular failure.

HELPFUL TESTS

The electrocardiogram may be useful in the evaluation of patients with tricuspid or pulmonic valve disease. In patients with pulmonic stenosis, the electrocardiogram often reveals evidence of right ventricular hypertrophy, particularly if the pulmonic stenosis is severe. In patients with isolated tricuspid stenosis, the electrocardiogram may reveal evidence of right atrial enlargement, with a notable absence of right ventricular hypertrophy. If there is concomitant mitral stenosis, then evidence of left atrial enlargement may also be apparent. Atrial fibrillation is also commonly seen.

The electrocardiographic findings in patients with tricuspid or pulmonic regurgitation depend on the cause of the lesion. In cases of regurgitation secondary to pulmonary hypertension, there may be evidence of right ventricular hypertrophy. If right ventricular enlargement has occurred, then a complete or incomplete right bundle branch block may be present. If severe right atrial enlargement has also occurred, then Q waves may be noted in leads V_1 and V_2 that may mimic an anteroseptal myocardial infarction.

The radiographic findings of right-sided heart valve lesions are fairly nonspecific. Tricuspid and pulmonic regurgitation frequently lead to cardiomegaly from right ventricular enlargement. Both tricuspid regurgitation and tricuspid stenosis may lead to right atrial enlargement and prominence of the right border of the cardiac silhouette (4). In the absence of concomitant mitral valve disease, what is most striking is the absence of radiographic signs of pulmonary edema, despite the clinical signs and symptoms of right-sided heart failure.

The mainstay of diagnostic testing in patients with tricuspid or pulmonic valve disease is echocardiography. This method allows direct visualization of the tricuspid and pulmonic valves, thus providing evidence of the cause of the valve lesion. In addition, the mitral and aortic valves can also be evaluated, as can the right atrial and right ventricular size and function. Color Doppler imaging can be used to determine the amount of tricuspid or pulmonic regurgitation (Fig. 25.1), whereas spectral Doppler imaging can be used to measure velocities and determine pressure gradients across the valves, thus allowing for the grading of the severity of tricuspid or pulmonic stenosis. In addition, spectral Doppler imaging can be used to measure the velocity of the tricuspid regurgitation jet; this velocity can then be used to determine the right ventricular systolic pressure (Fig. 25.2). In the absence of pulmonic stenosis, the right ventricular systolic pressure can be used as a surrogate for the pulmonary artery systolic pressure, thus allowing pulmonary hypertension to be diagnosed (1). Finally, echocardiography can also be used to identify other conditions that mimic or cause valvular heart disease, such as atrial tumors or endocarditis.

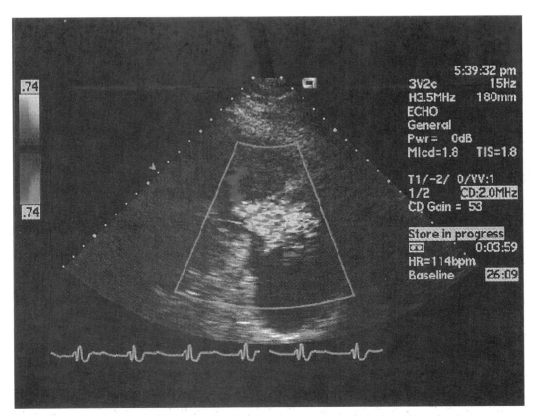

FIG. 25.1. Color Doppler echocardiography demonstrates functional tricuspid regurgitation in a patient with left ventricular failure.

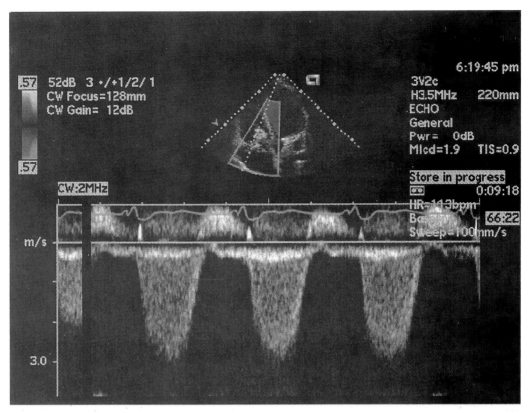

FIG. 25.2. Spectral Doppler echocardiography reveals the tricuspid regurgitation velocity spectrum. The peak velocity can be used to calculate the right ventricular systolic pressure with the modified Bernoulli equation (right ventricular systolic pressure = 4 × peak velocity squared + right atrial pressure).

DIFFERENTIAL DIAGNOSIS

Tricuspid Stenosis

The most common cause of tricuspid stenosis is rheumatic heart disease. In one series evaluating the cause of stenosis in operatively excised stenotic tricuspid valves, rheumatic heart disease accounted for stenosis in 93% of all excised valves (3). As mentioned previously, isolated tricuspid stenosis secondary to rheumatic heart disease is quite uncommon, however, and is usually accompanied by rheumatic mitral disease and, often, aortic disease as well. Other causes of tricuspid stenosis include carcinoid heart disease (8,9), Loeffler's (eosinophilic) endocarditis (6), and prosthetic tricuspid valve malfunction (Table 25.1).

Carcinoid heart disease is caused by a carcinoid tumor, which is a rare malignancy that secretes vasoactive substances, including serotonin, bradykinin, and histamines (6). Patients with carcinoid typically present with flushing, diarrhea, and bronchospasm, and they have elevated urinary levels of the serotonin metabolite 5-hydroxyindoleacetic acid (8). The tumor frequently originates in the appendix, ileum, small

TABLE 25.1. *Causes of tricuspid stenosis*

Rheumatic heart disease
Carcinoid heart disease
Loffler's (eosinophilic) endocarditis
Tricuspid valve endocarditis
Tumor
Prosthetic valve malfunction

intestine, or rectum (6). It is thought that the va-soactive substances secreted by the tumor cause endothelial damage on the right side of the heart, particularly on the right-sided heart valves. The result is fibrosis and thickening of the right-sided heart valves, most commonly the tricuspid valve. Because these vasoactive substances are metab-olized by the lung, left-sided valvular disease is very uncommon and is thought to occur only in the presence of lung metastases or a lesion that allows right-to-left shunting (6).

Loeffler's endocarditis may also cause tricus-pid stenosis through formation of plaques on the right side of the heart, including on the tricuspid valve. The right ventricular plaques seen in this disease are frequently covered with thrombi (6). Other conditions that can mimic tricuspid steno-sis by causing obstruction of flow across the tri-cuspid valve include tumors, such as renal cell carcinoma and right atrial myxoma, and tricus-pid valve endocarditis with very large vegetations that cause obstruction of blood flow.

Tricuspid Regurgitation

Diseases causing tricuspid regurgitation can be divided into two categories: conditions causing organic tricuspid valve disease and conditions causing functional (nonorganic) tricuspid valve disease (Table 25.2). Organic tricuspid valve dis-ease is the less common of the two, and it has numerous causes. These include rheumatic heart disease, carcinoid heart disease, and Loeffler's (eosinophilic) endocarditis, all of which can also cause tricuspid stenosis, as described previously. Other causes include tricuspid valve prolapse, endocarditis, trauma, Marfan's disease (2), radi-ation valve disease (2), prosthetic valve malfunc-tion, and congenital abnormalities, the most com-mon of which is Ebstein's anomaly. Ebstein's anomaly consists of displacement of the sep-tal and posterior leaflets of the tricuspid valve apically into the right ventricle (10). As a re-sult, there is abnormal coaptation of the valve leaflets of the tricuspid valve, resulting in various amounts of tricuspid regurgitation. This abnor-mality is easily detected with echocardiography.

The differential diagnosis of functional tricus-pid valve disease consists of causes of right ven-

TABLE 25.2. *Causes of tricuspid regurgitation*

Organic tricuspid valve disease
Rheumatic heart disease
Carcinoid heart disease
Tricuspid valve endocarditis
Tricuspid valve prolapse
Loffler's (eosinophilic) endocarditis
Ebstein's anomaly
Trauma
Connective tissue disease
Radiation therapy
Prosthetic tricuspid valve malfunction
Functional (nonorganic) tricuspid valve disease
Causes of right ventricular hypertension and dilation
Mitral stenosis
Mitral regurgitation
Left ventricular failure
Primary pulmonary hypertension
Secondary pulmonary hypertension from pulmonary emboli or other causes
Pulmonic stenosis
Causes of right ventricular dilation without right ventricular hypertension
Right ventricular infarction
Right ventricular cardiomyopathy
Atrial septal defect, uncomplicated
Anomalous pulmonary vein

tricular hypertension and causes of right ventric-ular dilation and dysfunction. Any cause of right ventricular hypertension can lead to subsequent dilation of the right ventricle and tricuspid annu-lus, with resultant functional tricuspid regurgita-tion. Common causes include mitral stenosis, left ventricular dysfunction, primary pulmonary hy-pertension, secondary pulmonary hypertension from conditions such as chronic pulmonary em-boli, and pulmonic stenosis. Other causes of right ventricular dilation can also lead to dilation of the tricuspid annulus in the absence of right ven-tricular hypertension. Common causes include coronary artery disease involving the right ventri-cle (11), atrial septal defect, and right ventricular cardiomyopathy.

Distinguishing between functional and or-ganic tricuspid valve regurgitation can be chal-lenging, especially in patients with rheumatic heart disease involving the mitral valve, who may be predisposed to both primary tricuspid valve disease and functional tricuspid regurgi-tation secondary to pulmonary hypertension. In such cases, careful evaluation of the anatomic structure of the valve with echocardiography may be helpful in determining whether there is a

TABLE 25.3. *Causes of pulmonic stenosis*

Congenital pulmonic stenosis
Rheumatic heart disease
Carcinoid heart disease
Infective endocarditis

structural abnormality consistent with rheumatic disease. In addition, estimation of the pulmonary artery systolic pressure with Doppler echocardiography can be helpful; evidence of pulmonary hypertension is suggestive of a functional cause (12).

Pulmonic Stenosis

The most common cause of pulmonic stenosis is congenital pulmonic stenosis, which occurs in between 1 and 7 per 10,000 live births (13). Many patients with congenital pulmonic stenosis survive to adulthood, and they may first come to medical attention as adults (14). Other far rarer causes of pulmonic stenosis include rheumatic heart disease, carcinoid, and infective endocarditis (Table 25.3).

Pulmonic Regurgitation

The differential diagnosis of pulmonic regurgitation can also be divided into two categories: (a) conditions causing dilation of the pulmonic annulus that result in functional pulmonic regurgitation and (b) primary valvular abnormalities (Table 25.4). The predominant causes of dilation of the pulmonic annulus are pulmonary

TABLE 25.4. *Causes of pulmonic regurgitation*

Organic pulmonic valve disease
  Rheumatic heart disease
  Infective endocarditis
  Carcinoid heart disease
  Trauma
  Congenital absence of a pulmonic valve leaflet
  Postsurgical period after repair of congenital heart
    disease
Functional pulmonic regurgitation secondary to
    dilation of the pulmonic annulus
  Pulmonary hypertension
  Connective tissue disease
  Idiopathic dilation of the pulmonary artery

hypertension and connective tissue diseases that cause weakening of the structure of the annulus, such as Marfan's disease (13). Causes of primary valvular problems include rheumatic heart disease (13), carcinoid, and congenital absence of a pulmonic valve leaflet. Infective endocarditis can also cause pulmonic regurgitation, although this valve is the least commonly involved (15). In addition, pulmonic regurgitation has also been seen with the use of a Swan-Ganz pulmonary artery catheter, which, if pulled back inappropriately across the pulmonic valve with the balloon still inflated, may cause trauma to the valve with resultant regurgitation (13). Finally, pulmonic regurgitation may also occur after repair of congenital heart disease, such as repair of tetralogy of Fallot.

COMPLICATIONS

The primary hemodynamic abnormality of tricuspid or pulmonic regurgitation is volume overload of the right ventricle, which is often tolerated for decades. If long-standing, however, especially in the presence of pulmonary hypertension, right ventricular failure may ensue. This is characterized by low cardiac output and elevated systemic venous pressures. Symptoms and signs include fatigue, lethargy, dyspnea with exertion, jugular venous distension, ascites, edema, and, in profound cases, anasarca. Once right ventricular failure occurs, the clinical course may progressively deteriorate.

The other major complication of tricuspid and pulmonic valve disease is endocarditis. Endocarditis of right-sided heart valves occurs most commonly in the setting of intravenous drug abuse. Although underlying tricuspid or pulmonic valve disease can increase the likelihood of endocarditis in this setting, the infection most frequently occurs with normal underlying valves. Other predisposing factors include indwelling catheters and pacemaker wires on the right side of the heart. The tricuspid valve is involved much more frequently than the pulmonic valve (16). The most common pathogen is *Staphylococcus aureus,* accounting for nearly 80% of the cases (16–18). Other pathogens causing right-sided endocarditis include streptococci, enterococci, fungi, and gram-negative organisms; culture-negative infections also occur (16,17). Clinically, right-sided endocarditis typically manifests with fever and a right-sided heart murmur. Evidence of septic pulmonary emboli is often present. Positive blood cultures of the inciting pathogen and echocardiographic evidence of a vegetation on the tricuspid or pulmonic valve may confirm the diagnosis.

THERAPY

Therapy for Pulmonic and Tricuspid Stenosis

The treatment of choice for patients with severe pulmonic stenosis is percutaneous balloon valvuloplasty. Several series have shown excellent short- and long-term results in patients undergoing this procedure (14,19). Patients with only mild disease require no therapy but only periodic monitoring. The indications for intervention in young patients with pulmonic stenosis are outlined in Table 25.5 (5). The treatment for tricuspid stenosis is less well established. There have been reports of percutaneous balloon valvuloplasty for severe tricuspid stenosis (20,21). Because isolated tricuspid stenosis in the absence of tricuspid regurgitation is very uncommon, however, the need for valvuloplasty does not arise often. In patients who have combined tricuspid regurgitation with tricuspid stenosis, an operative

approach is frequently required if intervention is necessary.

Therapy for Tricuspid and Pulmonic Regurgitation

The decision of whether to intervene operatively on the tricuspid valve for tricuspid regurgitation depends on a number of factors. The first factor is whether the tricuspid regurgitation is secondary to an organic abnormality of the valve itself or whether it is functional in origin. If the tricuspid regurgitation is functional, then the cause of dilation of the tricuspid annulus should be ascertained and addressed. If the functional tricuspid regurgitation is secondary to mitral valve disease that necessitates operation, then consideration can be given to repairing the tricuspid valve at the time of mitral valve surgery. In these instances, the degree of tricuspid regurgitation should be determined preoperatively. In patients with severe tricuspid regurgitation and pulmonary hypertension who are undergoing mitral valve repair or replacement, repair of the tricuspid valve with either an annuloplasty ring or a De Vega annuloplasty (22) can be performed at the time of operation. In cases of functional tricuspid regurgitation secondary to other causes of pulmonary hypertension, the therapy of choice is usually treatment of the underlying pulmonary hypertension rather than repair of the valve.

TABLE 25.5. *Recommendations for intervention in the adolescent or young adult with pulmonic stenosis (balloon valvotomy or surgery)*

Indication	ACC/AHA Class[a]
Patients with exertional dyspnea, angina, syncope, or presyncope	I
Asymptomatic patients with normal cardiac output (estimated clinically or determined by catheterization)	
Right ventricular to pulmonary artery peak gradient, >50 mm Hg	I
Right ventricular to pulmonary artery peak gradient, 40 to 49 mm Hg	IIa
Right ventricular to pulmonary artery peak gradient, 30 to 39 mm Hg	IIb
Right ventricular to pulmonary artery peak gradient < 30 mm Hg	III

ACC/AHA, American College of Cardiology/American Heart Association.

[a]Class I: Conditions for which there is evidence and/or general agreement that a given procedure or treatment is useful and effective. Class II: Conditions for which there is conflicting evidence and/or a divergence of opinion about the usefulness/efficacy of a procedure or treatment. (IIa: weight of evidence/opinion is in favor of usefulness/efficacy. IIb: usefulness/efficacy is less well established by evidence/opinion). Class III: Conditions for which there is evidence and/or general agreement that the procedure/treatment is not useful and in some cases may be harmful.

From Bonow RO, Carabello B, de Leon AC Jr, et al., ACC/AHA guidelines for the management of patients with valvular heart disease. *J Am Coll Cardiol* 1998;32:1486–1588.

In patients without pulmonary hypertension in whom organic valve disease causes the tricuspid regurgitation, therapy should be individualized to the patient. Tricuspid regurgitation in this setting is usually well tolerated and usually does not cause symptoms unless or until it is quite severe. Patients who have severe regurgitation and symptoms should be treated with a trial of diuretic therapy. If this therapy fails and signs and symptoms of right-sided heart failure have developed, then tricuspid valve repair or replacement can be considered, although the outcomes are variable (9,23). In cases in which valve replacement is necessary, the options for prosthetic valves include bioprosthetic valves, which do not require anticoagulation, and mechanical prosthetic valves, which require anticoagulation. Because of previously documented problems with thrombosis of mechanical prosthetic valves in the tricuspid position (24), the preferred approach has been a bioprosthetic valve (4), although one study in which newer, lower profile mechanical tilting disc valves were used suggests that the risk of thrombosis may be less than previously reported with other mechanical valves (23).

The treatment of pulmonic regurgitation consists primarily of treating the underlying cause, which most commonly is pulmonary hypertension. Pulmonic regurgitation is usually well tolerated, and the symptoms that patients develop are usually related to the underlying cause. In rare cases in which organic disease of the pulmonic valve causes severe pulmonic regurgitation and right-sided heart failure, pulmonic valve replacement can be performed, typically with a bioprosthetic valve (25).

Therapy for Right-Sided Endocarditis

As with left-sided endocarditis, initial therapy for right-sided endocarditis consists of antibiotics directed against the inciting pathogen. Surgery should be reserved for infection that persists or recurs despite optimal antibiotic therapy or for cases of fungal endocarditis, in which the likelihood of clearing the infection with antibiotics alone is low (16). Patients who develop severe pulmonic or tricuspid regurgitation may ultimately require valve replacement, although this is optimally performed after the infection has been cleared. Complete valvulectomy of the tricuspid valve has also been reported to be successful in helping clear the infection (26,27). Some affected patients may subsequently develop right-sided heart failure and eventually require tricuspid valve replacement (28).

PROGNOSIS AND FOLLOW-UP

The prognosis of tricuspid and pulmonic valve disease depends predominantly on the underlying disease process. For example, the prognosis of patients with rheumatic tricuspid stenosis depends significantly on concomitant mitral and aortic involvement; when these associated valve lesions are treated, the prognosis of these patients is quite good (29). In contrast, the prognosis of patients with carcinoid tricuspid valve disease is much worse, with a 3-year survival rate of only 31% in one series (8).

The prognosis of patients with tricuspid regurgitation also depends on the cause. If the regurgitation is functional, then the cause of pulmonary hypertension may play a significant role in survival. In the absence of pulmonary hypertension, patients with mild or moderate degrees of tricuspid regurgitation generally have a good prognosis. Once right ventricular failure has ensued, however, the prognosis significantly worsens. Patients with Ebstein's anomaly also have limited survival rates, which in one series was 50% at a mean follow-up of approximately 15 years (10). These patients are also at risk for sudden arrhythmic death (30).

The prognosis of patients with congenital pulmonic stenosis is excellent, with a 25-year survival rate that is similar to that of the general population (31). The prognosis of patients with right-sided endocarditis depends on the responsiveness to antibiotics, as well as on the size of the vegetation; vegetations larger than 2 cm are associated with increased rates of mortality (16).

Follow-up of patients with tricuspid or pulmonic valve disease should include periodic history documentation and physical examinations. A baseline echocardiogram with Doppler examination should also be obtained, and follow-up echocardiograms should be obtained in the following situations: in patients with changes in symptoms or signs, patients with severe stenosis or regurgitation, and patients with mild to moderate regurgitation with right ventricular dilatation (32). In addition, all patients with tricuspid regurgitation should undergo an evaluation of the right ventricular systolic pressure, with spectral Doppler imaging of the tricuspid regurgitation signal. Patients who are found to have significantly elevated right ventricular systolic pressure should undergo an evaluation to determine the underlying cause. Finally, antibiotics for prophylaxis against bacterial endocarditis should be prescribed as appropriate.

PRACTICAL POINTS

- Patients suspected of having tricuspid or pulmonic valve disease should undergo two-dimensional echocardiography with Doppler imaging.
- Tricuspid stenosis is usually secondary to rheumatic disease.
- Pulmonic stenosis is usually congenital in origin and is treatable with percutaneous balloon valvuloplasty.
- Tricuspid and pulmonic regurgitation are most often functional rather than due to disease of the valve.
- Functional tricuspid or pulmonic regurgitation is usually best managed by treatment of the underlying cause that leads to dilation of the annulus.
- The major complication of severe tricuspid or pulmonic regurgitation is right ventricular failure, which in some cases may necessitate valve repair or replacement surgery.

REFERENCES

1. Weyman A. *Principles and practice of echocardiography,* 2nd ed. Philadelphia:, Lea and Febiger, 1994.
2. Waller BF, Howard J, Fess S. Pathology of tricuspid valve stenosis and pure tricuspid regurgitation—Part II. *Clin Cardiol* 1995;18:167–174.
3. Waller BF, Howard J, Fess S. Pathology of tricuspid valve stenosis and pure tricuspid regurgitation—Part I. *Clin Cardiol* 1995;18:97–102.
4. Braunwald E. Valvular heart disease. In: Braunwald E, ed. *Heart disease: a textbook of cardiovascular medicine,* 5th ed. Philadelphia: WB Saunders, 1997:1054–1061.
5. Bonow RO, Carabello B, de Leon ACJ, et al. ACC/AHA guidelines for the management of patients with valvular heart disease. A report of the American College of Cardiology/American Heart Association Task Force on Practice Guidelines (Committee on Management of Patients with Valvular Heart Disease). *J Am Coll Cardiol* 1998;32:1486–1588.
6. Cheitlin MD, MacGregor JS. Acquired tricuspid and pulmonary valve disease. In: Rahimtoola SH, Braunwald E, ed. *Atlas of heart diseases. Valvular heart disease.* Philadelphia: Current Medicine, 1997:11.1–11.13.
7. Don Michael TA. *Auscultation of the heart: a cardiophonetic approach.* New York: McGraw-Hill, 1998.
8. Pellikka PA, Tajik AJ, Khandheria BK, et al. Carcinoid heart disease. Clinical and echocardiographic spectrum in 74 patients. *Circulation* 1993;87:1188–1196.
9. Robiolio PA, Rigolin VH, Harrison JK, et al. Predictors of outcome of tricuspid valve replacement in carcinoid heart disease. *Am J Cardiol* 1995;75:485–488.
10. Hong YM, Moller JH. Ebstein's anomaly: a long-term study of survival. *Am Heart J* 1993;125:1419–1424.
11. Vatterott PJ, Nishimura RA, Gersh BJ, et al. Severe isolated tricuspid insufficiency in coronary artery disease. *Int J Cardiol* 1987;14:295–301.
12. Waller BF, Howard J, Fess S. Pathology of tricuspid valve stenosis and pure tricuspid regurgitation—Part III. *Clin Cardiol* 1995;18:225–230.
13. Waller BF, Howard J, Fess S. Pathology of pulmonic valve stenosis and pure regurgitation. *Clin Cardiol* 1995;18:45–50.
14. Chen CR, Cheng TO, Huang T, et al. Percutaneous balloon valvuloplasty for pulmonic stenosis in adolescents and adults. *N Engl J Med* 1996;335:21–25.
15. Ramadan FB, Beanlands DS, Burwash IG. Isolated pulmonic valve endocarditis in healthy hearts: A case report and review of the literature. *Can J Cardiol* 2000;16:1282–1288.
16. Hecht SR, Berger M. Right-sided endocarditis in intravenous drug users. Prognostic features in 102 episodes. *Ann Intern Med* 1992;117:560–566.
17. Robbins MJ, Soeiro R, Frishman WH, et al. Right-sided valvular endocarditis: etiology, diagnosis, and an approach to therapy. *Am Heart J* 1986;111:128–135.
18. Chan P, Ogilby JD, Segal B. Tricuspid valve endocarditis. *Am Heart J* 1989;117:1140–1146.
19. Jarrar M, Betbout F, Farhat MB, et al. Long-term

invasive and noninvasive results of percutaneous balloon pulmonary valvuloplasty in children, adolescents, and adults. *Am Heart J* 1999;138:950–954.

20. Goldenberg IF, Pedersen W, Olson J, et al. Percutaneous double balloon valvuloplasty for severe tricuspid stenosis. *Am Heart J* 1989;118:417–419.

21. Orbe LC, Sobrino N, Arcas R, et al. Initial outcome of percutaneous balloon valvuloplasty in rheumatic tricuspid valve stenosis. *Am J Cardiol* 1993;71:353–354.

22. Holper K, Haehnel JC, Augustin N, et al. Surgery for tricuspid insufficiency: long-term follow-up after De Vega annuloplasty. *Thorac Cardiovasc Surg* 1993;41:1–8.

23. Scully HE, Armstrong CS. Tricuspid valve replacement. Fifteen years of experience with mechanical prostheses and bioprostheses. *J Thorac Cardiovasc Surg* 1995;109:1035–1041.

24. Thorburn CW, Morgan JJ, Shanahan MX, et al. Long-term results of tricuspid valve replacement and the problem of prosthetic valve thrombosis. *Am J Cardiol* 1983;51:1128–1132.

25. Fukada J, Morishita K, Komatsu K, et al. Influence of pulmonic position on durability of bioprosthetic heart valves. *Ann Thorac Surg* 1997;64:1678–1680.

26. Arbulu A, Thoms NW, Wilson RF. Valvulectomy without prosthetic replacement. A lifesaving operation for tricuspid pseudomonas endocarditis. *J Thorac Cardiovasc Surg* 1972;64:103–107.

27. Robin E, Belamaric J, Thoms NW, et al. Consequences of total tricuspid valvulectomy without prosthetic replacement in treatment of *Pseudomonas* endocarditis. *J Thorac Cardiovasc Surg* 1974;68:461–465.

28. Arbulu A, Holmes RJ, Asfaw I. Tricuspid valvulectomy without replacement. Twenty years' experience. *J Thorac Cardiovasc Surg* 1991;102:917–922.

29. Roguin A, Rinkevich D, Milo S, et al. Long-term follow-up of patients with severe rheumatic tricuspid stenosis. *Am Heart J* 1998;136:103–108.

30. Tuzcu EM, Moodie DS, Ghazi F, et al. Ebstein's anomaly: natural and unnatural history. *Cleve Clin J Med* 1989;56:614–618.

31. Hayes CJ, Gersony WM, Driscoll DJ, et al. Second natural history study of congenital heart defects. Results of treatment of patients with pulmonary valvar stenosis. *Circulation* 1993;87:I28–I37.

32. Cheitlin MD, Alpert JS, Armstrong WF, et al. ACC/AHA guidelines for the clinical application of echocardiography: executive summary. A report of the American College of Cardiology/American Heart Association Task Force on Practice Guidelines (Committee on Clinical Application of Echocardiography). Developed in collaboration with the American Society of Echocardiography. *J Am Coll Cardiol* 1997;29:862–879.

26

Acute Pericarditis/Pericardial Effusion

Mani A. Vannan and Mauro Moscucci

ACUTE PERICARDITIS

Definition

Acute pericarditis is a clinical condition characterized by chest pain, typical electrocardiographic (ECG) changes, and a pericardial friction rub. At least two of these features must be present to support the diagnosis.

The pericardium is a double-layered wrapping around the heart that serves many important functions. The outer and inner layers are called the parietal and visceral pericardium, respectively. The potential cavity between these two layers usually contains a small amount (about 15 mL) of pericardial fluid, which serves to lubricate the surfaces. This amount of fluid is not visible by any imaging technique. Clinically relevant disorders of pericardium are acute inflammation (acute pericarditis), pericardial effusion, constrictive pericarditis, congenital absence of the pericardium, and pericardial cysts.

Usual Causes

A wide variety of diseases can affect the pericardium, as listed in Table 26.1. Of these diseases, idiopathic postviral, post–myocardial infarction, drug-induced, and connective tissue disorders and uremia account for most acute pericarditic syndromes seen in the clinical setting. When upper respiratory symptoms precede acute cardiac involvement, the condition is called *postviral pericarditis*. This is because the antecedent infection is usually Coxsackie A or B virus or echovirus (1). The term *acute idiopathic pericarditis* applies when there are no clear-cut antecedent respiratory symptoms. Viral serologic testing is often unhelpful in making the distinction and thus is not a recommended

investigation. Among the entities listed in Table 26.1, the human immunodeficiency virus (HIV) is an increasingly common factor in acute pericarditis (2,3). The condition may be caused by HIV itself or may result from opportunistic infections or neoplasms (such as lymphoma). The presence of pericardial effusion in an HIV syndrome is associated with poor prognosis.

Symptoms

A cardinal symptom of acute pericarditis is *chest pain*. The typical pain of pericardial inflammation is a retrosternal sharp pain radiating to the back near the trapezius edge. It is worse when the patient is in a supine position, and it is either relieved or ameliorated by sitting up. Chest pain may, however, be variable in location, its nature, intensity, and radiation. It could be located retrosternally and radiate to the arm, mimicking ischemic cardiac pain. It may radiate to the epigastrium, mimicking abdominal disease, or worsen on deep inspiration, mimicking pleural pain. Constitutional symptoms are nonspecific and may include dyspnea, general malaise, weakness, hiccups, and cough. A low-grade fever may be present, but occasionally the body temperature may be as high as 40°C.

Signs

Tachycardia and tachypnea are usually nonspecific signs reflecting the general syndrome, although the former may signify significant myocardial inflammation. The hallmark of acute pericarditis is the presence of a pericardial rub. It is a squeaky, high-intensity sound usually heard best at the left lower parasternal edge with the diaphragm of the stethoscope (4). It is also

TABLE 26.1. *Causes of acute pericarditis*

Idiopathic
Infectious
   Bacterial
   Viral
   Mycobacterial
   Fungal
   Protozoal
   AIDS associated
Neoplastic
   Primary
   Secondary (breast, lung, melanoma, lymphoma,
     leukemia)
Immune inflammatory
   Connective tissue diseases (rheumatoid arthritis,
     systemic lupus erythematosus, scleroderma,
     acute rheumatic fever, mixed connective tissue
     disease, Wegener's granulomatosis)
   Arteritis (temporal arteritis, polyarteritis nodosa,
     Takayasu's arteritis)
   Acute myocardial infarction (MI) and post-MI
     (Dressler's syndrome)
   Postcardiotomy
   Posttraumatic
Metabolic
   Nephrogenic
   Aortic dissection
   Myxedema
   Amyloidosis
Iatrogenic
   Radiation injury
   Instrument/device trauma (implantable defibrillator,
     pacemakers catheters)
   Drugs (hydralazine, procainamide, daunorubicin,
     isoniazid, anticoagulants, cyclosporine,
     methysergide, phenytoin, dantrolene, mesalazine)
   Cardiac resuscitation
Traumatic
   Blunt trauma
   Penetrating trauma
   Surgical trauma
Congenital
   Pericardial cysts
   Congential absence of pericardium
   Mulibrey nanism syndrome

AIDS, acquired immunodeficiency syndrome.
(Reproduced with permission from: Restivo J, Hoit B. Manual of Cardiology. Eds. O'Roarke R, et. al. New York, McGraw Hill, pp 585.)

usually heard best during ventricular or atrial systole, and the intensity of the sound may change with position and respiration. Furthermore, it may be evanescent and may be present and absent even within a given day. Occasionally, it may be difficult to differentiate it from a coexistent pleural friction rub. The heart sounds are usually normal, and a third heart sound may be present when there is accompanying significant myocarditis that causes significant valvular re-

gurgitation, which is usually mitral regurgitation. Murmurs are not part of the typical syndrome of acute pericarditis, although the presence of significant valvular regurgitation may be accompanied by specific murmurs.

Helpful Tests

Electrocardiogram

The ECG usually shows normal sinus rhythm except in the case of complicating arrhythmias. There is diffused ST segment elevation and PR segment depression (Fig. 26.1), which then undergoes a typical evolutionary change as listed in Table 26.2. These evolutionary changes in the ECG are pathognomonic of acute pericarditis even in the absence of an audible pericardial friction rub (5,6). ECG changes always reflect a degree of myocardial involvement, inasmuch as the pericardium is electrically inert.

Chest Radiograph

The chest radiograph may be entirely normal or may show evidence of cardiomegaly when there is accompanying significant myocarditis complicated by cardiac enlargement. In the setting of acute left ventricular failure, pulmonary congestion or signs of pulmonary edema may be seen.

Echocardiography

Pericardial effusion of some degree may be seen in up to 60% of cases of acute pericarditis. In acute idiopathic or postviral pericarditis, significant pericardial effusion occurs in only a minority of cases. Echocardiography allows localization, estimation, and comprehensive hemodynamic effects of pericardial effusion. This information is critical if pericardiocentesis is required. Left ventricular dysfunction occurs when there is significant associated myocarditis, and the severity of this dysfunction can be estimated by echocardiography. Furthermore, echocardiography is a tool for follow-up assessment of pericardial effusion, left ventricular dysfunction, and associated functional valvular abnormalities. Pericardial thickening is not reliably assessed by echocardiography. Magnetic resonance imaging

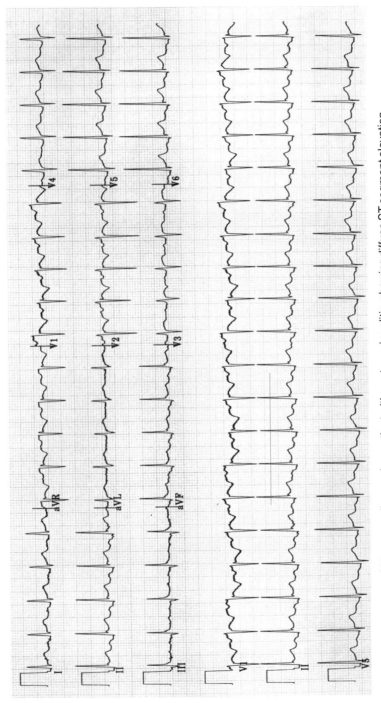

FIG. 26.1. Electrocardiogram in a patient with acute pericarditis, showing diffuse ST segment elevation and PR segment depression.

TABLE 26.2. *Electrocardiographic changes in acute pericarditis*

Stage	Time course	ECG changes
1	ST segment elevation occurs within hours of onset of chest pain and may persist for days	Upward concave ST segment elevations usually not exceeding 5 mm; PR segment depression (except aV$_R$)
2	Hours to days following stage 1	ST segments return to baseline: T waves normal or show loss of amplitude
3	T wave inversions may persist indefinitely (especially when associated with TB, uremia or neoplasm)	T wave inversions
4	Usually completed within 2 weeks, but variability common	ECG normalizes

ECG, electrocardiographic; TB, tuberculosis.
(Reproduced with permission from: Restivo J, Hoit B. Manual of Cardiology. New York, McGraw Hill, pp 587.)

and computed tomography are superior techniques in detecting pericardial thickening (7).

Differential Diagnosis

Myocardial Ischemia

Cardiac ischemia may simulate acute pericarditis, especially if the chest pain is located retrosternally, but lacks other typical characteristics of acute pericarditic pain. In fact, the chest pain may radiate down the arm, which makes it difficult to differentiate cardiac from pericarditic pain. If acute pericarditis is accompanied by significant elevation of myocardial isoenzymes such as troponin I, it becomes even harder to differentiate from myocardial ischemia. Elevation of troponin I level is a marker of myocardial injury, and significant elevation may be seen in younger patients with the postviral syndrome (8). A further confounding factor could be typical changes in ECG in acute pericarditis which may be regional rather than diffused (9). Furthermore, involvement of the PR segment, concave ST segment elevation, lack of simultaneous T wave and ST segment changes, lack of Q wave evolution, and absense of reciprocal ST segment changes all support the diagnosis of acute pericarditis. Echocardiography may help to differentiate the two conditions, in view of the global nature of any wall motion abnormality, which accompanies myocarditis, and the presence of significant pericardial effusion. However, myocarditis may manifest as regional wall motion abnormality, or there may be a regional emphasis on global wall motion abnormality, which may make it difficult to differentiate the two conditions. Ultimately, the clinical picture, especially the prodrome of upper respiratory symptoms, helps confirm the diagnosis of acute pericarditis rather than myocardial ischemia.

Acute Abdomen

Acute pericarditic pain in a lower retrosternal or predominantly epigastric location or radiation to the epigastrium may simulate acute abdomen. The absence of typical ECG changes further complicates the issue of differentiating acute abdomen from acute pericarditis. However, attention to historical details and a helpful echocardiogram may aid in the correct diagnosis.

Acute Pleurisy

Pulmonary infarction or pneumonia may be associated with inflammation of the adjacent pleura, which may mimic chest pain of acute pericarditis. However, the clinical history and ECG changes are unique to these diagnoses and usually help in distinguishing these conditions.

Therapy

Hospital Admission

Most cases of acute pericarditis can be treated on an ambulatory basis. There are specific circumstances in which hospital admission is warranted. If there is persistent, severe chest pain, if the chest pain is accompanied by nondiagnostic ECG changes, or if there is a need to exclude other causes of chest pain, then hospital admission is recommended. Hospital admission is necessary when there is evidence of myocarditis in the form of elevated troponin I levels or elevated jugular venous pulsation accompanied by tachycardia, hypotension, or pulsus paradoxus or a combination of these. The presence of moderate to large pericardial effusion on an echocardiogram usually warrants hospital admission.

Pharmacologic Treatment

Nonsteroidal antiinflammatory drugs (NSAIDs) remain the mainstay for treatment of chest pain. Aspirin and indomethacin are the usual agents used, although indomethacin can potentially reduce coronary blood flow and aggravate myocardial ischemia (10,11). The length of treatment is dictated by symptoms; pain tends to resolve within a week. Steroid therapy is indicated when there is persistent severe pain after 7 to 10 days of NSAID therapy or if the cause of acute pericarditis is uremia or connective tissue disorder. With the latter causes, early use of glucocorticoids helps alleviate pain more effectively and prevents long-term consequences of acute pericarditis. Colchicine is an alternative agent to be used in acute pericarditis when there is persistent, severe pain despite treatment with NSAIDs and steroids (12). Colchicine has also been shown to prevent recurrences effectively and may be the agent of choice to combine with NSAIDs if steroids are contraindicated because of comorbid clinical conditions. Anticoagulants should be avoided in acute pericarditis.

Pericardiocentesis

Therapeutic pericardicentesis is warranted when hemodynamically significant pericardial effusion complicates acute pericarditis. Approximately 15% of patients who develop large pericardial effusions in association with acute pericarditis develop signs of cardiac tamponade. Pericardicentesis is usually effective. Diagnostic pericardiocentesis may be necessary when pericardial effusion complicates acute pericardi-

tis caused by bacterial or fungal infections. In these circumstances, it is also advisable to drain as much of the pericardial fluid as possible, and a catheter may be left in place for further pericardial drainage, because fluid frequently reaccumulates under these conditions.

Pericardiectomy

Pericardiectomy is rarely required in acute pericarditis. Failure of medical treatment and recurrent symptoms of idiopathic or postviral pericarditis are usual indications for pericardiectomy. Pericardiectomy may be required after surgical drainage in bacterial or fungal pericarditis to prevent constrictive pericarditis.

Clinical Course

Most acute pericarditic syndromes resolve within 4 weeks with no long-term sequelae and with complete resolution of symptoms with NSAIDs, steroids, or colchicine or a combination of these. Approximately 25% of patients with acute pericarditis develop refractory or recurrent symptoms, and about 10% show reversible constrictive physiologic characteristics on echocardiographic Doppler examination 4 weeks after the onset of initial symptoms.

PERICARDIAL EFFUSION

Definition

Pericardial effusion is the accumulation of more than the usual amount of fluid in the pericardial sac.

Usual Causes

The causes of acute pericarditis listed in Table 26.1 can be complicated by pericardial effusion. At least 25 mL of pericardial fluid must be present for it to be appreciated by imaging techniques such as echocardiography. The most common causes of large, chronic pericardial effusions are malignancy, idiopathic pericarditis, uremia, infection (including HIV), connective tissue disorder, and radiation therapy (13). Acute large collections of pericardial fluid can occur with cardiac trauma, after cardiac diagnostic or interventional procedures including electrophysiological procedures, after cardiac surgery, after myocardial infarction, and with acute post viral pericarditis.

Symptoms

Clinical manifestations of pericardial effusion vary from absence of any symptoms to life-threatening symptoms consistent with cardiac tamponade. Large, chronic effusions can be entirely asymptomatic, reflecting the ability of the pericardial sac to stretch and adapt to increasing volume. Thus, a rapid accumulation of as little as 200 mL of fluid can produce a hemodynamic impact as significant as that of a 2,000-mL chronic effusion. Symptoms, when they do occur, are nonspecific and often unhelpful. A dull retrosternal ache and dyspnea are the most common symptoms.

Signs

Signs directly caused by effusion are usually insensitive and nonspecific. Cardiac dullness beyond the apex and dullness at the infrascapular region (Ewart's sign) can be confounded by left lower lobe pulmonary disease or left pleural effusion (14). Tachycardia, narrow pulse pressure, and pulsus paradoxus (inspiratory decline in systolic pressure exceeding 12 mm HG) reflect hemodynamically significant pericardial effusion. Pulsus paradoxus may be absent in the presence of significant left ventricular dysfunction. Fever may be present if there is an underlying infectious process.

Helpful Tests

Electrocardiogram

QRS complexes with low voltages as a result of short-circuiting of cardiac potentials by fluid are the characteristic manifestation of pericardial effusion. A low voltage is defined as the total voltage of the QRS complex in all six limb leads of less than 5 mm. Tachycardia reflects hemody-

namic compromise, and electric alternans indicates a swinging heart within a large pericardial effusion.

Chest Radiograph

The chest radiograph may be entirely normal in small to modest-sized effusions. In large effusions, cardiomegaly with loss of usual cardiac contours raises the suspicion of pericardial fluid collection.

Echocardiography

Echocardiography is the definitive test for establishing the presence and the hemodynamic impact of pericardial effusion (Figs. 26.2, 26.3). The range of findings is shown in Table 26.3.

Cardiac Tamponade

Definition

Tamponade is a spectrum of hemodynamic derangements that can be divided into three phases (15). Phase I is characterized by equalization of right atrial and intrapericardial pressures, but not right ventricular or pulmonary capillary wedge pressure (PCWP). In phase II, there is equilibration of right atrial and right ventricular pressures but not PCWP, so that cardiac output is not significantly impacted. Phase III is the clinically evident syndrome of hypotension, tachycardia, tachypnea, and pulsus paradoxus (typically exceeding 20 mm HG). At phase III, intrapericardial pressures have equalized with right atrial and right ventricular pressures and PCWP, and there is significant decrease in cardiac output. Thus, phase III represents the most severe hemodynamic abnormality in the spectrum of pericardial compression and is characterized by pressure and flow abnormalities. Phase II is characterized predominantly by pressure abnormality and a modest degree of flow abnormality (pulsus paradoxus, if present, is usually less than 20 mm HG), whereas phase I consists of only pressure abnormality and is at the mildest end of the spectrum (it may not be clinically evident).

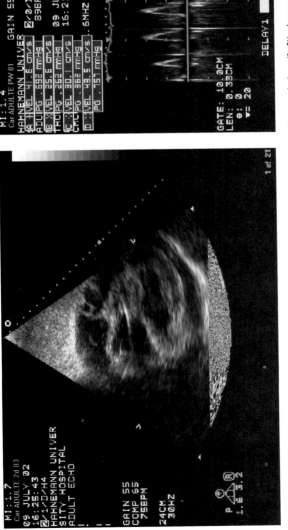
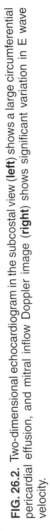

FIG. 26.2. Two-dimensional echocardiogram in the subcostal view (**left**) shows a large circumferential pericardial effusion, and mitral inflow Doppler image (**right**) shows significant variation in E wave velocity.

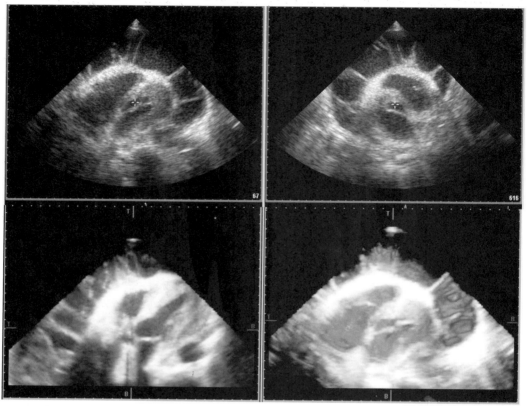

FIG. 26.3. Large circumferential pericardial effusion with fibrinous adhesions. **Top,** Two-dimensional echocardiograms; **bottom,** corresponding three-dimensional echocardiograms.

Echocardiography helps to identify these phases. For example, when there is right-sided heart collapse (phase II), the patient may be mildly symptomatic (tachypnea and tachycardia but no pulsus paradoxus). There may not be a need to perform urgent pericardiocentesis in all such cases. However, when hypotension, pulsus paradoxus, and electrical alternans are present, there is an urgent need to tap the pericardial fluid. Thus, the decision to perform pericardiocentesis should incorporate clinical and echocardiographic findings. Table 26.4 lists the usual indications for urgent pericardiocentesis.

Low-pressure tamponade occurs when the right atrial pressure is less than 10 mm HG, usually because of hypovolemia. In such cases, low intracardiac pressures equilibrate with intrapericardial pressures, compromising cardiac output. Cautious fluid replenishment is usually sufficient, although a subgroup of patients with low-pressure tamponade benefit from pericardiocentesis.

Therapy

Needle Pericardiocentesis

Therapeutic pericardicentesis is warranted in situations listed in Table 26.4. The usual approach is subxiphoid, and monitoring of cardiac rhythm and blood pressure is the minimal requirement for performing a safe procedure. ECG monitoring with electrodes at the needle tip is not essential. Echocardiographic guidance is often useful and is recommended. Hemodynamic monitoring of intracardiac and pericardial pressures is useful

TABLE 26.3. *Echocardiography in pericardial effusion*

Echolucent space between epicardium and pericardium
Visible fluid through diastole and systole indicates at least 25 mL of fluid
First evident anteriorly over the RV free wall and posteriorly behind LV
Typically does not extend beyond the atrium, although large effusions do
Circumferential extent can be determined (determines management)
Loculated effusions cardiac surgery, irradiation, infections
Partial organization and fibrin strands may be identified
RA and RV early diastolic collapse indicates elevated pericardial pressure (elevated RV pressures as in pulmonary hypertension mask this sign)
Right-sided heart collapse is not necessarily tamponade (PPV of 58%, NPV of 92%)
Systolic dominance and expiratory diastolic flow reversal of HV and SVC flows (but difficult to obtain venous Doppler flow signals in over 70% of the patients)
>40% and >25% peak velocity variation in TV and MV Doppler flows (obesity, COPD, LV dysfunction, and large pleural effusions can also cause this)
Posterior loculation (post surgery): LVDC may be the only sign
TEE may be required to identify posterior hematomas

COPD, chronic obstructive pulmonary disease; HV, hepatic vein; LV, left ventricular; LVDC, left ventricular diastolic collapse; MV, mitral valve; NPV, negative predictive valve; PPV, positive predictive valve; RA, right atrial; RV, right ventricular; SVC, superior vena cava; TEE, transesophageal echocardiography; TV, tricuspid valve.

in difficult and borderline cases: for example, when there is suspicion of coexistent restriction or constriction. Removal of all the pericardial fluid is preferred, because it normalizes intracardiac pressures and improves cardiac output. Failure of normalization of right atrial pressure is an indication of *effusive constriction* or myocardial failure or cardiomyopathy, and further testing, including myocardial biopsy, may be required. It is also conventional to leave a pericardial drain with a small multihole catheter, which can also be used to instill sclerosing agents if needed. Pericardial drains can be left in place for several days; at least 48 hours is recommended. Hematocrit, cell count, and glucose level should always be measured in the pericardial fluid and smears, and cultures and cytologic studies should also be done routinely. Needle pericardiocentesis is usually a

TABLE 26.4. *Indications for urgent pericardiocentesis*

Etiologic
  Traumatic (especially hematomas)
  Teratogenic (complication of pacemaker implantation or intracardiac ablation)
  Interventional (e.g., balloon valvotomy, atrial septostomy)
  Neoplasms
Hemodynamic
  Electrical alternans on ECG
  Hypotension (may be absent in hypertension)
  Swinging heart on echocardiogram

ECG, electrocardiogram.

safe procedure, but complications are possible (16–19), as shown in Table 26.5.

Surgical Pericardiocentesis

Surgical drainage may be performed through a subxiphoid incision or a thoracotomy. This is often necessary when there is loculated or posterior effusion, when there are fibrinous adhesions, and when there is need to obtain adequate pericardial tissue for etiologic diagnosis.

Recurrent Pericardial Effusions

Balloon pericardiotomy or a surgical pleuropericardial or peritoneal-pericardial window (the latter window preferred because of larger surface area for fluid absorption) may be necessary to treat recurrent collections as in uremic and malignant pericardial effusions (up to 40%) (20,21). Sclerotherapy with intrapericardial tetracycline, bleomycin, or thiopental are efficient in prevention of recurrences, although chest pain limits tolerance. Surgical pericardiectomy may be required in such cases.

TABLE 26.5. *Complications of needle pericardiocentesis*

Acute RV and LV dysfunction and shock
Pulmonary edema
Myocardial (usually RV), vascular (coronary vein or artery) laceration
Pulmonary laceration
Reflex hypotension
Cardiac arrythymias

LV, left ventricular; RV, right ventricular.

PRACTICAL POINTS

- Diagnosis of acute pericarditis is usually possible on the basis of clinical history, symptoms, and ECG findings.
- ECG findings reflect underlying myocarditis, because the pericardium is electrically inert.
- Absence of audible pericardial rub does not exclude the diagnosis of acute pericarditis.
- Some degree of pericardial effusion is seen on echocardiography in about two thirds of cases.

- Most cases of acute pericarditis resolve completely without long-term sequelae.
- Rapid accumulation of even modest amounts of pericardial fluid can cause hemodynamic compromise.
- Cardiac tamponade is a spectrum of hemodynamic abnormalities and not an all-or-none phenomenon.
- Diagnosis of pericardial tamponade requires incorporation of echocardiographic and clinical data.

REFERENCES

1. Permanyer-Miralda G, Sagrista-Sauleda J, Soler-Soler J. Primary acute pericardial disease: a prospective series of 231 consecutive patients. *Am J Cardiol* 1985;56:623.
2. Steigman CK, Anderson DW, Macher AM, et al. Fatal cardiac tamponade in acquired immunodeficiency syndrome with epicardial Kaposi's sarcoma. *Am Heart J* 1988;116:1105.
3. Heidenreich PA, Eisenberg MJ, Kee LL, et al. Pericardial effusion in AIDS: 4. Incidence and survival. *Circulation* 1995;92:3229.
4. Spodick DH. Pericardial friction. Characteristics of pericardial rubs in fifty consecutive, prospectively studied patients. *N Engl J Med* 1968;278:1204.
5. Spodick DH. Differential characteristics of the electrocardiogram in early repolarization and acute pericarditis. *N Engl J Med* 1976;295:523.
6. Ginzton LE, Laks M. The differential diagnosis of acute pericarditis from the normal variant: new electrocardiographic criteria. *Circulation* 1982;65:1004.
7. Smith WH, Beacock DJ, Goddard AJ, et al. Magnetic resonance evaluation of the pericardium. *Br J Radiol* 2001;74:384.
8. Newby LK, Ohman EM. Troponins in pericarditis: implications for diagnosis and management of chest pain patients. *Eur Heart J* 2000;21:798.
9. Bonnefoy E, Godon P, Kirkorian G, et al. Serum cardiac troponin I and ST-segment elevation in patients with acute pericarditis. *Eur Heart J* 2000;21:832.
10. McGinn JT, Rosati M, McGinn TG. Indomethacin in treatment of pericarditis. *N Y State J Med* 1970;70:1783.
11. Arunasalam S, Siegel RJ. Rapid resolution of symptomatic acute pericarditis with ketorolac tromethamine, a parenteral nonsteroidal antiinflammatory agent. *Am Heart J* 1993;125:1455.
12. Adler Y, Finkelstein Y, Guindo J, et al. Colchicine treatment for recurrent pericarditis. A decade of experience. *Circulation* 1998;97:2183.
13. Corey GR, Campbell PT, van Trigt P, et al. Etiology of large pericardial effusions. *Am J Med* 1993;95:209.
14. Ewart W. Practical aids in the diagnosis of pericardial effusion, in connection with the question as to surgical treatment. *BMJ* 1896;1:717.
15. Reddy PS, Curtiss EI, O'Toole JD, et al. Cardiac tamponade: hemodynamic observations in man. *Circulation* 1978;58:265–272.
16. Tsang TSM, Freeman WK, Sinak LJ, et al. Echocardiographically guided pericardiocentesis: evolution and state-of-the-art technique. *Mayo Clin Proc* 1998;73:647.
17. Armstrong WF, Feigenbaum H, Dillon JC. Acute right ventricular dilation and echocardiographic volume overload following pericardiocentesis for relief of cardiac tamponade. *Am Heart J* 1984;107:1266.
18. Vandyke WH Jr, Cure J, Chakko CS, et al. Pulmonary edema after pericardiocentesis for cardiac tamponade. *N Engl J Med* 1983;309:595.
19. Wolfe MW, Edelman ER. Transient systolic dysfunction after relief of cardiac tamponade. *Ann Intern Med* 1993;119:42.
20. Ziskind AA, Pearce AC, Lemmon CC, et al. Percutaneous balloon pericardiotomy for the treatment of cardiac tamponade and large pericardial effusions: description of technique and report of the first 50 cases. *J Am Coll Cardiol* 1993;21:1.
21. Moriya T, Takiguchi Y, Tabeta H, et al. Controlling malignant pericardial effusion by intrapericardial carboplatin administration in patients with primary non–small-cell lung cancer. *Br J Cancer* 2000;83:858.

27

Pericardial Constriction

Julie A. Kovach and Richard L. Prager

USUAL CAUSES

In pericardial constriction (constrictive pericarditis), a variably thickened layer of visceral or parietal pericardium, or both, surrounds some or all of the cardiac chambers and progressively restricts filling of the ventricles. Because of anatomic pericardial encasement of the heart with resultant marked elevations in atrial pressure, 75% of ventricular filling occurs very rapidly and at high velocity during the first third of diastole, thus causing the characteristic "dip and plateau" or "square root sign" on the left and right ventricular pressure tracings. In most cases, diastolic filling is restricted in both ventricles, which become increasingly interdependent; that is, filling of both ventricles depends on the relative motion of the interventricular septum during diastole, the phenomenon known as ventricular coupling.

Classic "chronic constriction" is conventionally thought of as a process that proceeds over many months to years. However, the clinical spectrum of constrictive pericarditis has changed since the early 1970s in the western hemisphere, primarily because tuberculosis has become relatively infrequent, whereas cardiac surgery has become relatively commonplace. In contrast to the "chronic" variant of constriction, in which symptoms evolve over the course of many months and years and which represents progressive fibrosis of the pericardium, most cases are now "subacute," with constriction evident in the 3- to 12-month period after the pericardial insult (e.g., viral infection of the pericardium or cardiac surgery). The patient with constriction after radiation to the mediastinum for treatment of cancer is the primary exception to this rule, when constriction develops months to years after treatment. Two other variants also exist. In the patient with active pericarditis, the inflamed pericardium can thicken rapidly over a few weeks and produce "acute" symptoms of constriction. Finally, usually after cardiac surgery and at times with acute pericarditis, "transient" constriction develops with elevated jugular venous pressure and clinical signs of constriction. This constrictive pattern resolves after institution of antiinflammatory therapy with nonsteroidal antiinflammatory agents or steroids. Whether these patients go on to develop chronic constriction at a later date is not known.

Knowledge of three other clinical syndromes of constriction that may be acute, subacute, or chronic but are not "classic" is important. In "regional" or local constriction, pericardial thickening is present only over certain chambers of the heart and occurs most frequently shortly after cardiac surgery, when pericardial inflammation and thickening occur over the right side of the heart, or with neoplasm. Affected patients have evidence of pulmonary or systemic venous congestion but usually not both. Effusive-constrictive disease is the variable combination of findings of cardiac tamponade and constriction in some patients. Abnormal pulsus paradoxus is more common in these patients than in patients with constriction. A jugular venous waveform in which the x descent is steeper than the y descent is also suggestive of effusive-constrictive disease, and the presence of Kussmaul's sign in a patient with pericardial effusion is suggestive of effusive-constrictive disease rather than isolated cardiac tamponade. More often than not, the diagnosis is suspected when elevation in jugular venous pressure persists after pericardiocentesis. Finally, latent or "low-volume" constriction should be suspected in the patient with persistent

TABLE 27.1. *Potential causes of pericardial constriction*

Idiopathic
Cardiac surgery
Acute pericarditis (viral)
Mediastinal irradiation
   Hodgkin's lymphoma
   Breast cancer
   Lung cancer
Inflammatory arthritis or vasculitis
   Rheumatoid arthritis
   Systemic lupus erythematosus
   Scleroderma
   Rheumatic fever
Infection
   Tuberculosis
   Fungal
   Bacterial
Trauma
   Blunt trauma
   Penetrating trauma
Hemopericardium
   Traumatic
   Postthrombolytic
   Postsurgical
   Coagulopathy
Neoplasm
   Mesothelioma
   Metastatic cancer
Drugs
   Procainamide
   Hydralazine
   Methysergide
Others
   Whipple's disease
   Amyloidosis
   Sarcoidosis
   Asbestosis

dyspnea, fatigue, and mild lower extremity edema after aggressive diuresis normalizes the central venous pressure. Volume replacement unmasks constrictive hemodynamics.

Before the modern medical and surgical era, pericardial constriction was most commonly caused by tuberculosis or thought to be idiopathic. Of 231 cases of constriction verified by surgery or autopsy at the Mayo Clinic from 1936 to 1982, the causes were idiopathic factors in 73%, pericarditis in 10%, pyogenic infection in 6%, radiation in 5%, and, least frequently, arthritis, post–cardiac surgery, or "other causes" in 2% each (1). In the period from 1985 to 1995, causes in order of incidence were idiopathic in 45 of 135 cases (33%); post–cardiac surgery events (18%); after pericarditis (16%);

after radiation (13%); "other causes," including neoplasm, trauma, and drugs (10%); inflammatory arthritides (7%); and, in rare cases, pyogenic infection (3%). These findings have been confirmed by other investigators (2,3). Other pathologic conditions reported less frequently to cause pericardial constriction include mesothelioma; uremia (chronic, in which affected patients are on dialysis); hemopericardium after trauma or thrombolytic therapy or related to coagulopathies; Dressler's syndrome after myocardial infarction; vasculitis; drugs, including those used for lupus (hydralazine and procainamide) and migraine prophylaxis (methysergide); hypereosinophilia syndromes; amyloidosis; Whipple's disease; and sarcoidosis (Table 27.1).

PRESENTING SYMPTOMS AND SIGNS

The patient with pericardial constriction most often presents with symptoms of venous congestion resembling right-sided heart failure with normal left and right ventricular systolic function. Most common complaints by patients include lower extremity swelling, dyspnea and effort intolerance related to pulmonary venous congestion, and abdominal discomfort from hepatic distension. In the patient with the acute variant of pericarditis with constrictive physiology, chest pain may be the predominant complaint. In advanced cases of constriction, ascites occurs and may be more remarkable than the lower extremity edema, although some patients present with anasarca. Most patients cannot recall any history of antecedent pericarditis. Many of these patients have undergone extensive prior evaluation for hepatic disease with cirrhosis or congestive heart failure before the diagnosis of constriction is suspected. Unsuspected findings on two-dimensional and Doppler echocardiography performed for the diagnosis of congestive heart failure prompted an evaluation for constrictive pericarditis in 40% of patients who underwent pericardiectomy at the Mayo Clinic in the 10 years before 1997 (4).

Most patients with constriction have at least mild tachycardia, especially with even minor exertion. In these patients, stroke volume cannot increase with exercise, and the major compensatory mechanism is an increase in heart rate. Patients with chronic constriction may exhibit atrial fibrillation. Blood pressure is usually normal, but it may be low or even hypertensive. The patient who has undergone aggressive diuresis may have orthostatic hypotension. Abnormal pulsus paradoxus is rare, occurring only if effusive-constrictive disease or chronic obstructive pulmonary disease is present. The patient with severe limitations of cardiac output may manifest peripheral cyanosis with cool extremities. The patient with hepatic failure or cirrhosis from increased hepatic venous pressure may be jaundiced. Funduscopic examination may reveal that retinal veins are engorged. The hallmark of pericardial constriction is elevated jugular venous pressure with rapid and sharp x and y descents, which produce the characteristic W wave on the jugular venous tracing. Often, the jugular venous pressure is so elevated that the veins must be examined with the patient in the sitting position, or even standing, in order to see the top of the venous column. In some patients who have undergone overdiuresis, the jugular venous pressure may not be elevated, but the classic physical findings are unmasked with volume infusion. Kussmaul's sign (the paradoxical increase in jugular venous pressure during inspiration) is present in most patients. A cardiac impulse may not be palpable, leaving the patient with a "quiet precordium," although an early diastolic impulse corresponding to the pericardial "knock" is occasionally detected. The first and second heart sounds are normal. The loud early diastolic S3 or "knock" may be confused with splitting of S1. Hepatomegaly, ascites, and even splenomegaly may be detected on abdominal examination, and lower extremity edema is common. If constriction is regional and restricted to the right side of the heart, systemic venous congestive symptoms may be present, whereas pulmonary congestion may not.

HELPFUL TESTS

The electrocardiogram almost universally displays nonspecific T wave abnormalities. Voltage is usually normal but may be decreased or increased. The chest radiograph shows normal cardiac size but may reveal an enlarged superior vena cava or azygous vein, or both, and often shows bilateral pleural effusions. In the modern era, pericardial calcification is only very rarely identified on chest radiographs.

Transthoracic echocardiography with spectral Doppler imaging may be the first clue to the diagnosis of pericardial constriction. Transthoracic echocardiography is unreliable for the detection of pericardial thickening. Pericardial thickness as measured by transesophageal echocardiography correlates well with measurements by computed tomography ($r > 0.95$, $p < 0.0001$), but this technique has not been widely accepted (5). Two-dimensional echocardiography reveals the restricted motion of the myocardium and the ventricular interdependence with a flat left ventricular posterior wall, absence of diastolic ventricular expansion, and bowing of the interventricular septum toward the left ventricle during inspiration with an abnormal septal "bounce" in early systole. The inferior vena cava is usually dilated, but this can represent elevated central venous pressure from any cause. Doppler echocardiography reveals marked and reciprocal variation in peak mitral and tricuspid inflow velocities with respiration defined as more than a 25% increase in peak mitral E wave velocity in the first beat after the onset of inspiration (6,7). The E wave deceleration time is short and varies excessively with respiration. These Doppler findings detected constriction in 88% of affected patients with in one study (8). Of the remaining patients with constriction documented at surgery, 75% exhibited characteristic respiratory variation after the Doppler examination was repeated in the head-up tilt or sitting position to reduce preload. A pulmonary venous systolic/diastolic flow ratio of more than 0.65 during inspiration and a percentage change in peak pulmonary venous diastolic flow from expiration to inspiration of more than 40% correctly differentiated pericardial constriction from restrictive cardiomyopathy in 86% of patients (9). Measurement of hepatic vein flow with spectral Doppler imaging reveals loss of the normal multiphasic flow pattern. Hepatic venous flow is monophasic and occurs mainly in systole. Doppler tissue imaging is helpful in the differentiation of pericardial constriction from restrictive cardiomyopathy: Longitudinal axis expansion velocities are markedly reduced in restrictive cardiomyopathy and normal in constriction (10).

Gated cine–computed tomography and magnetic resonance imaging are especially useful for the measurement of pericardial thickness (11,12). Pericardial thickness exceeding 3.5 mm suggests the diagnosis of constriction with increase in specificity when pericardial thickness is more than 6 mm (Fig. 27.1). In addition, markedly dilated atria with very small, tube-shaped ventricles may be seen. Also, the distribution of pericardial thickening may assist the surgeon in planning pericardiectomy (Fig. 27.2). Tagged cine–magnetic resonance imaging may be useful for diagnosing local or regional constriction (13).

The combination of Doppler echocardiography in the supine and sitting position and either computed tomography or magnetic resonance imaging confirms the diagnosis of constriction

in 90% to 95% of patients. Cardiac catheterization with hemodynamic measurement is required in the remainder. Coronary angiography should be performed in all patients undergoing catheterization, because the thickened pericardium can cause extrinsic compression with narrowing of coronary arteries that can cause myocardial ischemia under conditions of stress. Typically, the coronary arteries are visualized within the cardiac silhouette, appear to be subepicardial rather than in the usual epicardial location, and have decreased mobility in systole.

Classically, the diastolic pressures in all cardiac chambers are elevated with near equalization (less than 5 mm Hg), unless the patient is volume depleted. The left and right ventricular pressure tracings show the typical "square root sign" with diastolic "dip and plateau," which is also seen in patients with restrictive cardiomyopathy. In constriction, right ventricular and pulmonary artery systolic pressures are only moderately elevated (less than 55 mm Hg), and the

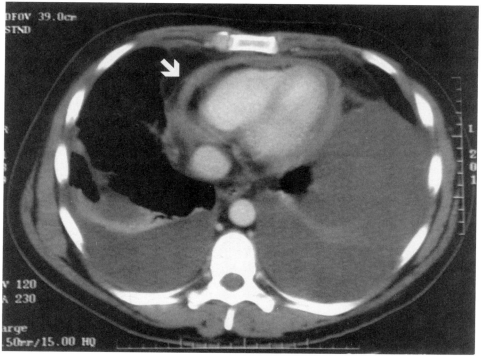

FIG. 27.1. Computed tomographic scan of the heart with pericardium measuring > 10 mm thick (*arrow*).

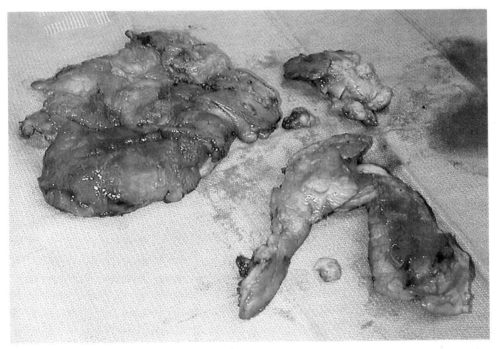

FIG. 27.2. Surgical specimen of extremely thick pericardium from the patient whose computed tomographic scan is shown in Figure 27.1.

right ventricular end-diastolic pressure is approximately one third of systolic pressure. In the patient who does not display these classic findings because of volume depletion, enough volume should be administered intravenously in the catheterization laboratory to raise the central venous pressure, and the measurements should be repeated. In one study in which high-fidelity manometric catheters were used to measure left and right ventricular pressures, discordance between the right and left ventricular pressures during respiration (from ventricular interdependence) accurately separated patients with constriction from those with other causes of heart failure (14). Nevertheless, an occasional patient requires exploratory thoracotomy with inspection and removal of the pericardium or myocardial biopsy to make the diagnosis.

DIFFERENTIAL DIAGNOSIS

The diagnosis of pericardial constriction can be difficult and is often delayed for many months after the onset of symptoms. One study showed little difference in the time from symptom onset to diagnosis in the modern era, despite technical advances in imaging and catheterization. In a cohort of patients with constriction diagnosed from 1936 to 1983, time to diagnosis was 14 months (range, 1 to 348 months), in comparison with 11.7 months (range, 0.1 to 349 months) in patients diagnosed between 1985 and 1995 (1). The differential diagnosis of constrictive pericarditis includes venous obstruction, such as occurs in superior vena cava syndrome from neoplasm; low-protein states, including nephrotic syndrome and cirrhosis; other causes of ascites, including intraabdominal cancers; and diastolic heart failure. Physical examination, imaging techniques, and simple laboratory evaluation can clarify the diagnosis in most patients. Pericardial constriction can be differentiated from restrictive cardiomyopathy in most patients by the combination of Doppler echocardiography and either cine–computed tomography or magnetic resonance imaging. Cardiac catheterization with detailed hemodynamic measurement elucidates the

TABLE 27.2. *Differentiation of pericardial constriction from restrictive cardiomyopathy*

Evaluation method	Constriction	Restrictive cardiomyopathy
Physical examination	Kussmaul's sign usually present Pericardial knock Valve regurgitation rare	Kussmaul's sign may be present Mitral and tricuspid regurgitation common
Doppler echocardiography	> 25% increase in mitral and tricuspid inflow velocity with inspiration	Inspiratory changes absent
CT/MRI	Pericardial thickness > 3.5 mm	Pericardium normal
Cardiac catheterization with hemodynamic measurements	RAP = RVEDP = LEVDP ($\leq$5 mm HG) RVSP < 55 mm RVEDP > 1/3 RVSP Reciprocal changes in RVEDP and LVEDP with inspiration	LVEDP > 5 mm HG higher than RVEDP, although may be equal RVSP may be >55 mm HG RVEDP < 1/3 RVSP No reciprocal changes in RVEDP and LVEDP with inspiration

CT, computed tomography; MRI, magnetic resonance imaging; RAP, right atrial pressure; RVEDP, right ventricular end diastolic pressure; LVEDP, left ventricular end diastolic pressure; RVSP, right ventricular systolic pressure.

diagnosis in the majority of the remainder. In rare cases, exploratory thoracotomy or myocardial biopsy is necessary (Table 27.2).

COMPLICATIONS

Unless constrictive pericarditis is transient and responds to antiinflammatory medications, elevations of central venous pressure are progressive, and cardiac output continues to diminish. Ascites and anasarca may develop with brawny lower extremity edema, hepatic cirrhosis, pulmonary congestion, refractory pleural effusions, renal failure, and death.

THERAPY

Small doses of diuretics may be useful for the management of edema in these patients, but they should be utilized judiciously because hypotension and renal failure may ensue. However, only radical pericardiectomy provides cure for these patients (15). With the earliest reports of pericardial resection for constriction in 1913 by Rehn and Sauerbruch, followed by Churchill's report in 1929 (16,17), the operative approach to "constrictive" limitation of cardiac function began. These early approaches entailed the use of a left anterior lateral thoracotomy, and over the years, various incisions have been used, including left anterior lateral thoracotomy, median sternotomy, and bilateral anterior lateral thoracotomies.

Each of these approaches offers benefits; median sternotomy is favored at our institution. Patients are monitored with arterial lines and pulmonary artery lines and are in the supine position. Upon exploration through the sternotomy, the phrenic nerves are identified, and meticulous dissection is carried out in an area that allows facile identification of a plane between visceral and parietal pericardium or, at a minimum, an adequate plane to begin dissection. Avoiding injury to coronary arteries, the phrenic nerves, and the myocardium is critical, and judicious resection is imperative when calcific deposits invade the myocardium. Once a plane has been achieved, attention is directed to the freeing of the left ventricle first, to prevent right ventricular dilation and failure, which can occur if the right ventricle is freed before the left side (18).

The resection is carried out with wide excision of the pericardium from the left phrenic nerve to the right phrenic nerve and extends from the great arteries on to the inferior diaphragm. The right atrium and superior and inferior vena cava are totally freed, if it is safe to do so. Visceral pericardium or epicardium is removed if involved; if removal is treacherous, the tissue is incised to allow free cardiac expansion. Although the pericardium is not routinely excised posterior to the phrenic nerves, the heart is freed from the pericardium posteriorly using the anterior established plane. Cardiopulmonary bypass is considered only if it is imperative to resect more pericardium or hemodynamic compromise does not allow safe anterior resection.

As pointed out in a review from the Mayo Clinic, etiology of constriction has evolved to include more patients with iatrogenic causes, including previous cardiac surgery as well as postradiation for neoplasia (1). With this trend, three variables were found to be independent predictors of survival after resection: age, preoperative New York Heart Association class, and a postirradiation cause. In the Mayo series, pericardiectomy offered significant relief of symptoms, but it was noted that approximately one third of the patients were found at some point in follow-up to have recurrence of Class III or IV symptoms. Although the mechanism for this may be uncertain and may reflect the primary cause of the constriction and the type of the original procedure, it is imperative that these patients be followed lifelong.

Early studies of pericardiectomy for pericardial constriction demonstrated significant morbidity, including early right ventricular failure, mortality from bleeding, and low cardiac output states. In that era, constriction was generally more chronic, with a considerable incidence of pericardial calcification and fibrosis, which may have increased operative mortality. In a more recent study, operative mortality decreased from 14% in the period 1936 to 1982 to 6% in the modern era (1). Operative mortality rates are lower for patients who underwent surgery earlier in the course of their symptoms; therefore, pericardiectomy should be performed early in the course and should not be delayed until the patient no longer responds to diuretics.

PROGNOSIS AND FOLLOW-UP

As noted previously, patients respond well acutely to pericardiectomy, usually with prompt postoperative diuresis, although a low output state still remains a problem for some patients and resulted in perioperative death in 4% of patients in one series (1). Occasionally, patients have a less dramatic response to surgery, with diuresis over weeks or months. Pericardiectomy is incomplete in some patients because pericardium adherent to the myocardium cannot be removed without risk of myocardial perforation. At 10 years of follow-up, functional class improved markedly from New York Heart Association Class 2.7 ± 0.7 at baseline to 1.5 ± 0.8 at follow-up, and 83% of patients were free of symptoms (1). Late results, however, have not been as promising as might be expected. Diastolic function remains abnormal in 42% of patients late after pericardiectomy and correlates with persistent symptoms (15). Ten-year survival rates are significantly lower for patients who have undergone pericardiectomy than for age and sex-matched controls ($57\% \pm 8\%$ vs. 81%; $p < 0.001$). Late death was predicted by age, functional class, and a postradiation cause of constriction (1). In rare cases, a patient may require repeat surgery if constriction recurs. Because of the risk of late morbidity and mortality, patients who have undergone pericardiectomy require serial long-term follow-up assessments.

PRACTICAL POINTS

- Pericardial constriction should be suspected in patients with symptoms of elevated central venous pressure and normal left ventricular function.
- In the modern era, the most common causes of constrictive pericarditis are postsurgical, postradiation, and the "idiopathic" group, which is probably postviral.
- The combination of physical examination,

Doppler echocardiography, and either computed tomography or magnetic resonance imaging establishes the diagnosis of constriction in more than 90% of patients.
- If the typical Doppler finding of an inspiratory increase in peak mitral inflow E wave velocity of more than 25% is not

(continued)

present, repeating the Doppler examination in the head-up tilt or sitting position increases the detection of constriction.

- If latent or "low-volume" constriction is suspected, administration of

intravenous fluids may assist in the diagnosis.

- Patients who have undergone pericardiectomy for constriction require continued surveillance.

REFERENCES

1. Ling LH, Oh JK, Schaff HV, et al. Constrictive pericarditis in the modern era: evolving clinical spectrum and impact after pericardiectomy. *Circulation* 1999;100:1380–1386.
2. Spodick DH. Constrictive pericarditis. In: Spodick DH, ed. *The pericardium: a comprehensive textbook.* New York: Marcel Dekker, 1997:214–259.
3. Myers RBH, Spodick DH. Constrictive pericarditis: Clinical and pathophysiologic characteristics. *Am Heart J* 1999;138:219–232.
4. Oh JK, Tajik AJ. Doppler features of constrictive pericarditis: response to letter to the editor. *Circulation* 1997;96:3799–3880.
5. Ling LH, Oh JK, Tei C, et al. Pericardial thickness measured with transesophageal echocardiography: feasibility and potential clinical usefulness. *J Am College Cardiol* 1997;29:1317–1323.
6. Hatle LK, Appleton CP, Popp RL. Differentiation of constrictive pericarditis and restrictive cardiomyopathy by Doppler echocardiography. *Circulation* 1989;79:357–370.
7. Oh JK, Hatle LK, Seward JB, et al. Diagnostic role of Doppler echocardiography in constrictive pericarditis. *J Am Coll Cardiol* 1994;23:154–162.
8. Oh JK, Tajik AJ, Appleton CP, et al. Preload reduction to unmask the characteristic Doppler features of constrictive pericarditis: a new observation. *Circulation* 1997;95:796–799.
9. Klein AL, Cohen GI, Pietrolungo JF, et al. Differentiation of constrictive pericarditis from restrictive cardiomyopathy by Doppler transesophageal echocardiographic measurements of respiratory variations in pulmonary venous flow. *J Am Coll Cardiol* 1993;22:1935–1943.
10. Garcia MJ, Rodriguez L, Ares M, et al. Differentiation of constrictive pericarditis from restrictive cardiomyopathy: assessment of left ventricular diastolic velocities in longitudinal axis by Doppler tissue imaging. *J Am Coll Cardiol* 1996;27:108–114.
11. Oren RM, Grover-McKay M, Stanford W, et al. Accurate preoperative diagnosis of pericardial constriction using cine computed tomography. *J Am Coll Cardiol* 1993;22:832–838.
12. Rienmuller R, Gurgan M, Erdmann E, et al. CT and MR evaluation of pericardial constriction. *J Thorac Imag* 1993;8:108–121.
13. Kojima S, Yamada N, Goto Y. Diagnosis of constrictive pericarditis by tagged cine magnetic resonance imaging. *N Engl J Med* 1999;341:373–374.
14. Hurrell DG, Nishimura RA, Higano ST, et al. Value for dynamic respiratory changes in left ventricular and right ventricular pressures for the diagnosis of constrictive pericarditis. *Circulation* 1996;93:2007–2013.
15. Senni M, Redfield MM, Ling LH, et al. Left ventricular systolic and diastolic function after pericardiectomy in patients with constrictive pericarditis: Doppler echocardiographic findings and correlation with clinical status. *J Am Coll Cardiol* 1999;22:1182–1188.
16. Glenn F, Diethelm AG. Surgical treatment of constrictive pericarditis. *Ann Surg* 1962;155:883.
17. Churchill ED. Decortication of the heart delormen for adhesive pericarditis. *Arch Surg* 1929;19:1457.
18. Roberts JR, Kaiser L. Pericardial procedures in mastery of cardiothoracic surgery. In Kaiser L, Kron I, and Spray T, eds. *Mastery of cardiothoracic surgery.* Philadelphia: Lippincott-Raven, 1998:221–229.

28

Abdominal Aortic Aneurysms

Gilbert R. Upchurch, Jr., Thomas W. Wakefield, David M. Williams,
and James C. Stanley

Aortic aneurysms represent a serious vascular disease that is the twelfth most common cause of death in the United States. Abdominal aortic aneurysms (AAAs) develop in 3% to 9% of the population, and rupture of AAAs accounts for nearly 15,000 deaths each year in the United States. The infrarenal aorta is the site of 80% of all aortic aneurysms (1,2). Encounters with this disease will become even more frequent as society ages dramatically during the early decades of the twenty-first century.

USUAL CAUSES

AAAs are characterized by marked inflammation and an imbalance between the production and degradation of structural extracellular matrix proteins (3). Disruption and degradation of medial elastin and collagen are particularly prominent features of AAA formation. In this regard, increased local production of enzymes that degrade elastin and collagen—namely, the matrix metalloproteinases—has been proposed as pivotal in vessel wall degradation and in clinical progression of aneurysmal disease (4–13). Arteriosclerosis, a common finding in AAAs, compromises the structure of the aortic wall but is believed to be a secondary, not a primary, etiologic factor in AAA development. Rarer causes of AAAs include cystic medial necrosis, trauma, dissections, vasculitis, and infection (Table 28.1).

Genetic factors appear important in AAA development; 15% of patients have a first degree relative with an AAA (14). To date, no single gene mutation or protein deficiency has been associated with the common infrarenal AAA. However, a decrease in aortic wall type III collagen has been noted in individuals who have a first-degree relative with an AAA, in comparison with those without this family history of AAAs (15). Increases in the frequency of the Hp 2-1 haptoglobin phenotype, as well as the Kell-positive and MN blood groups, have also been noted in patients with AAAs. In contrast, there is a decrease in the incidence of AAAs in patients with type A Rh-negative blood group (16). In addition, one study suggests that a polymorphic alteration in the human lymphocyte antigen–DR B1 is important in the development of inflammatory AAAs (17). In the next few years, genetic analyses are likely to reveal a number of contributing factors in individuals predisposed to the development of AAAs.

PRESENTING SYMPTOMS AND SIGNS

Most AAAs are asymptomatic. Palpation of the lateral borders of the aorta between the examiner's fingertips on abdominal examination may reveal the existence of an AAA. However, prominent anterior pulsations alone are more likely to be caused by an ectatic, nonaneurysmal aorta. It is often difficult to palpate the infrarenal aorta in the epigastrium above the aortic bifurcation is at the level of the umbilicus. In most patients, physical examination alone is predictably unreliable in detecting AAA. In one series, AAAs were overlooked by physical examination in 62% of patients with known AAAs (18). Physical examination alone as a diagnostic maneuver is clearly not sensitive enough to exclude the diagnosis of an AAA.

Patients with AAAs may also have aneurysms of the femoral or popliteal arteries that are

TABLE 28.1. *Various causes of abdominal aortic aneurysms*

Degenerative
   Abnormal matrix (collagen-elastin) degradation
   Atherosclerosis
Connective tissue disorder
   Cystic medial necrosis
   Marfan's syndrome
   Ehlers-Danlos syndrome
   Pseudoxanthoma elasticum
Trauma
Dissection
Vasculitis
   Takayasu's arteritis
Infection
   Bacterial (salmonella, tuberculosis)
   Syphilis
   Fungal

apparent on physical examination. A study of 251 patients with AAAs from the University of Michigan documented a 14% incidence of aneurysms of the femoral and popliteal arteries, all occurring in male patients (19). The presence of these extremity aneurysms may serve as a clue to the existence of an AAA. It is important to recognize that patients with femoral and popliteal artery aneurysms have an 85% and a 62% chance of having an AAA, respectively (20,21).

In contrast to an intact AAA, a ruptured AAA is always symptomatic. Unfortunately, the classic triad of acute hypotension, back or abdominal pain, and a palpable abdominal mass is an all-too-often inconsistent finding in this setting. A high index of suspicion is mandatory for making a timely diagnosis of these life-threatening lesions. In stable patients, the use of rapid abdominal ultrasonography (US) or computed tomography (CT) has gained popularity in many emergency rooms, because both methods confirm the suspected diagnosis of a ruptured AAA, require no transport time, and are quite sensitive. However, any patient with hypotension and abdominal or back pain with a suspected expanded or ruptured AAA should be transported urgently to the operating room. Symptomatic AAAs represent true surgical emergencies and justify immediate operative intervention, without extensive time-consuming diagnostic studies.

HELPFUL TESTS

Once an AAA is suspected, a logical diagnostic algorithm should be followed to confirm the diagnosis (Fig. 28.1). Plain abdominal or lumbosacral radiographs performed in either the anteroposterior (AP) or lateral projections may suggest the presence of an AAA by demonstrating a rim of calcification in the outer aortic wall. The most useful means of establishing the diagnosis of an AAA is duplex US, a noninvasive, inexpensive test that provides reliable measurements of the aortic diameter (Fig. 28.2). US findings correlate closely with operative measurements of AAA, and interobserver variability of less than 5 mm has been demonstrated in 84% of AP measurements (22). Errors and limitations with US are most often attributed to inexperienced technicians, lack of interpretive skills, or excessive bowel gas.

CT is highly predictive of AAA size. Interobserver variability of less than 5 mm exists in 91% of AP measurements. Of importance is that CT may demonstrate other intraabdominal pathologic processes (22). CT is superior to US in assessing AAA wall integrity, the location and amount of calcification within vessel walls, venous anomalies, retroperitoneal blood, aortic dissection, infection or inflammation, and the proximal and distal extent of the aneurysm (Fig. 28.3). Limitations of CT studies include the need for nephrotoxic iodinated contrast administration, radiation exposure, and cost. Spiral or helical CT, an advance over conventional CT, provides excellent resolution and coronal reconstructions. It has become the study of choice for assessing AAAs before endovascular repair, as well as for identifying postoperative endoleaks in patients treated with endografts (Fig. 28.4).

Magnetic resonance angiography (MRA) with nonnephrotoxic gadolinium and the use of a breath-holding technique, is comparable with CT scanning for AAA measurements (Fig. 28.5). Images are based on T1 relaxation rather than blood flow, which means that slow flow in AAAs does not adversely affect the image. An earlier reported Michigan experience with 43 AAAs revealed that MRA correctly identified maximum

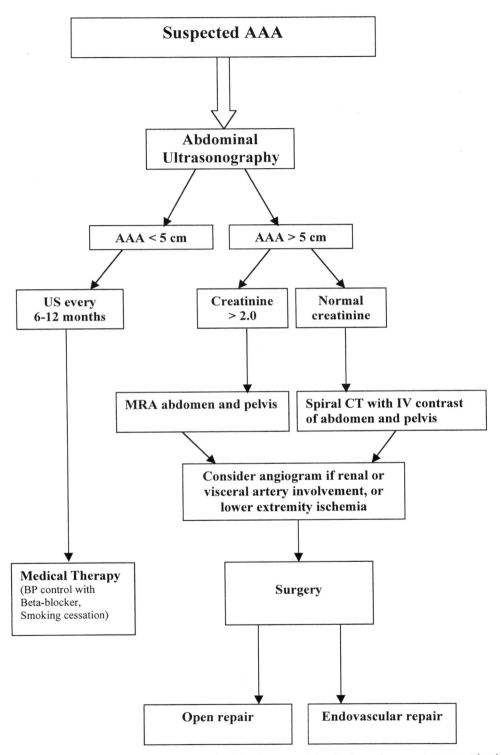

FIG. 28.1. Algorithm for patient suspected of having an abdominal aortic aneurysm on physical examination.

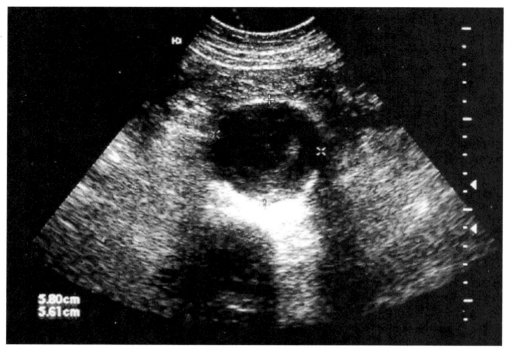

FIG. 28.2. Duplex ultrasonography documenting an abdominal aortic aneurysm.

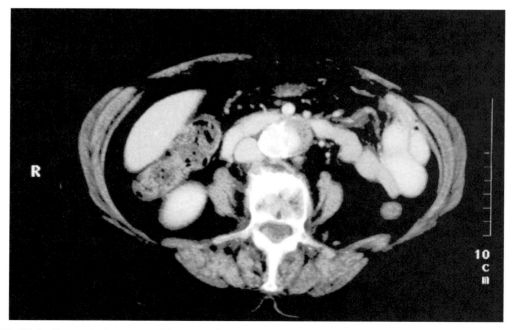

FIG. 28.3. Computed tomographic scan of the abdomen, demonstrating a mycotic abdominal aortic aneurysm.

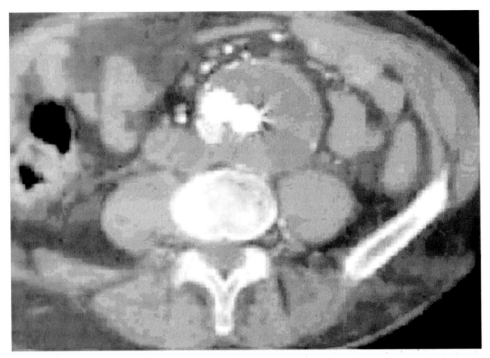

FIG. 28.4. Computed tomographic scan demonstrating the presence of an endoleak after endovascular repair that resolved after a secondary intervention.

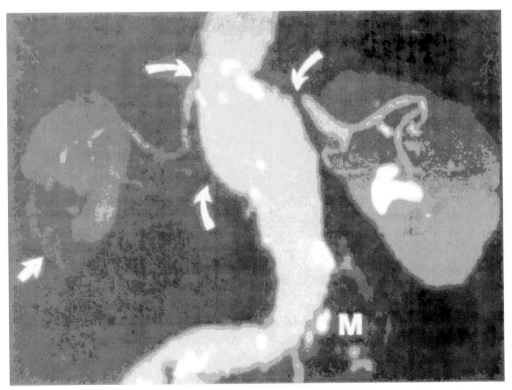

FIG. 28.5. Magnetic resonance angiography documenting renal artery involvement with an abdominal aortic aneurysm.

AAA diameter and had 94% and 98% sensitivity and specificity, respectively, for identifying significant stenoses of the splanchnic, renal, or iliac arteries (23). MRA limitations include the inability to scan patients who have pacemakers, defibrillators, or claustrophobia, and images obscured by artifacts caused by metallic objects, including certain vascular stents. Another disadvantage of MRA is its inability to image calcified plaque, a finding important in endovascular interventions.

Conventional contrast arteriography and digital subtraction angiography are usually obtained when the AAA is suspected to involve the renal or splanchnic vessels or in patients suspected of having moderate or severe lower extremity ischemia (Fig. 28.6). These studies identify the cephalad extent of the AAA, the number and lo-

cation of renal arteries, the state of the splanchnic arteries, and the status of the iliac arteries, as well as the presence of occlusive disease in the lower extremity arteries. Complications of angiography include bleeding or arterial occlusion at the catheterization site, atheroembolism, and impairment of renal function as a result of iodine contrast nephrotoxicity.

DIFFERENTIAL DIAGNOSIS

The patient with the unsuspected AAA may present with presumed exacerbation of chronic back pain or with new onset of abdominal, flank, or back pain, radiating to the groin, secondary to acute AAA expansion or rupture. Without imaging studies or a high index of suspicion, this pain may be confused with that of diverticulitis,

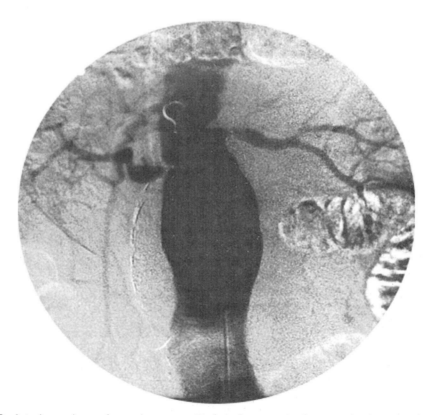

FIG. 28.6. Arteriography performed preoperatively before repair of a complex juxtarenal abdominal aortic aneurysm associated with bilateral high-grade renal artery stenosis.

renal colic, irritable bowel syndrome, inflammatory bowel disease, ovarian torsion, or appendicitis.

COMPLICATIONS

Continued expansion until rupture occurs is the most serious complication of an AAA. It is important to recognize factors contributing to AAA rupture. In accordance with the law of Laplace, a geometric increase in aortic wall pressure occurs with linear increases in AAA size. Thus, an increase in aortic diameter from 2 to 4 cm induces, not a twofold, but a fourfold increase in the pressure/cm^2 on the aortic wall. Rupture is directly proportional to aortic wall pressure. It is also known that aortic elastic tissue loses its integrity with age, and acquired or genetic factors that hasten this process add to the risk of accelerated AAA expansion. Aneurysm expansion greater than 4 mm over a 12-month period suggests that the AAA is unstable and is an indication for early intervention.

An intact asymptomatic AAA with a diameter of 5 cm is generally recognized to carry a risk of rupture of 20% to 30% over 2 to 3 years. The risk of rupture for smaller aneurysms, 3 to 5 cm in size, is less well defined. However, greater AP diameters, chronic obstructive pulmonary disease (COPD), and diastolic hypertension all independently increase the chance of AAA rupture. These factors have been assigned low, medium, and high risk (L, M, H) values as follows: for AP diameter, L is 3 cm, M is 4 cm, and H is 5 cm; for COPD, L is none, M is more than 50% predicted forced expiratory volume in 1 second (FEV$_1$), H is less than 50% predicted FEV$_1$; and for diastolic blood pressure, L is 75 mm HG, M is 90 mm HG, and H is 105 mm HG (24). Thus, the presence of a 5-cm AAA in a patient with severe diastolic hypertension and COPD is a cause for concern, carrying a predicted rupture rate of near 80% in a year, in comparison with a 3-cm AAA in a normotensive patient without COPD, which carries a rupture rate of only a few percent over 5 years (Fig. 28.7).

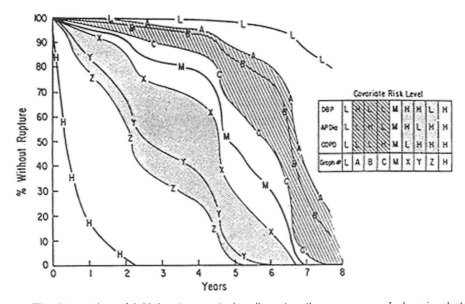

FIG. 28.7. The interaction of initial anteroposterior diameter, the presence of chronic obstructive pulmonary disease, and diastolic blood pressure in contributing to abdominal aortic aneurysm rupture risk. (From Cronenwett JL, Murphy TF, Zelenock GB, et al. Actuarial analysis of variables associated with rupture of small abdominal aortic aneurysms. *Surgery* 1985;98:472–483.)

The risk of death after AAA rupture depends on how quickly an emergency operation can be performed. Unfortunately, nearly 60% of patients with ruptured AAAs die before reaching a hospital, and only 50% of the remainder survive an emergency operation. Thus, AAA rupture carries an 80% rate of mortality (25–28).

SURGICAL THERAPY

Elective operative intervention by an open surgical repair or endovascular graft placement lessens the likelihood of death from AAA rupture. Conventional open operative procedures in elective circumstances in a large population-based study from Michigan carried a 5.6% mortality rate in 1993 (26). Surprisingly, women fared worse than did men after aneurysmectomy for both intact and ruptured aneurysms. The elective mortality rate over an 11-year period in women was 10.7%, in comparison with 6.8% in men in this experience. The explanation for this is not evident, but it suggests both a biologic element and a practice bias exist, which place women at a disadvantage for the operative treatment of AAA.

Conventional Surgical Treatment of Intact Abdominal Aortic Aneurysm

An expeditious operation is important for an open repair of an AAA (29). An aortic operation longer than 5 hours is independently associated with an increase in risk for mortality and significant cardiopulmonary complications (odds ratio, 5.11; 95% confidence interval, 1.69 to 15.52; $p < 0.004$). Other factors associated with poor surgical outcome include operative hypothermia, excessive blood loss, and the need for supraceliac aortic cross clamp. Specific comments about operative technique warrant mention.

Surgical approaches are individualized for each patient, with transperitoneal or retroperitoneal aortic exposure based both on the surgeon's preference and on the aortic disease. The transperitoneal approach is preferred when there is a need to revascularize the right kidney or when the aneurysmal disease extends into the right iliac artery. There are certain anatomic and clinical circumstances in which a retroperitoneal approach may be preferable (30). Relative indications for the retroperitoneal approach include obesity and a history of multiple prior laparotomies, which create hostile adhesions in the abdomen (30). Although the retroperitoneal approach does not significantly decrease mortality or major cardiopulmonary morbidity, it does expedite the return of postoperative bowel function (31,32).

In the past, thrombotic complications of clamping the aorta and renal failure have been important problems. To address these issues, the patients receive systemic anticoagulants with intravenous heparin. Diuresis is established, usually with mannitol administration or, in azotemic patients, loop diuretics. Both anticoagulation and a diuresis are established before the aorta is occluded. The aneurysm is then incised, and any interluminal clot is removed before the aortic graft is sewn in place. The prosthetic grafts currently used are either woven or knitted Dacron or extruded Teflon. After the graft is in place and blood flow is restored to the lower body, it is important that the graft be covered with the aneurysm shell or other retroperitoneal tissue, so as to prevent contact with the intestines. Such contact may lead to later graft-enteric erosion, which is considered a life-threatening complication necessitating graft removal. All patients with aortic grafts should receive antibiotics for invasive procedures, including dental procedures performed at a later date, similar to prophylaxis for bacterial endocarditis in patients with prosthetic cardiac valves.

Conventional Surgical Treatment of Ruptured Abdominal Aortic Aneurysm

The surgical approach to the patient with a ruptured AAA must be focused on saving life. Nearly half these patients subjected to emergency surgery die from complications within the first 30 days after operation (28,33–35). Attention to controlling hemorrhage, restoring aortic blood flow, and avoidance of attempts to reconstruct less diseased vessels, such as asymptomatic stenosis of renal arteries or marginally aneurysmal iliac arteries, becomes very important. A supraceliac aortic cross clamp is often used initially to control continued bleeding, especially in patients with large retroperitoneal hematomas. The proximal aortic cross clamp may then be moved to below the renal arteries once the infrarenal aortic neck has been isolated. Adequate blood replacement and maintenance of normothermia are critical elements in these emergency procedures. After the aortic reconstruction, the adequacy of the blood flow to the colon and lower extremities should be assessed before the patient leaves the operating room. The surgeon should consider delayed abdominal closure after treatment of a ruptured AAA (36). The massive fluid resuscitation and a large retroperitoneal hematoma in these patients may cause the usual abdominal closure to result in a compartment syndrome with decreased perfusion of the splanchnic and renal circulations. Delayed abdominal closure, with the use of a silo similar to that used in pediatric patients with an omphalocele, appears to confer survival benefits in these patients.

Endovascular Surgical Treatment of Intact Abdominal Aortic Aneurysm

By 2000, two endovascular grafts had been approved by the Food and Drug Administration in the United States for treatment of infrarenal AAAs (Fig. 28.8). These grafts differ significantly in design and utility. One device is a modular covered stent graft deployed as a main aortic prosthesis with an ipsilateral iliac artery limb, followed by docking of a contralateral iliac artery graft limb. These endografts are up-sized 10% to 20% in comparison to the native aorta and iliac arteries in order to block flow to the AAA. In contrast, the second device is a unibody graft designed to block flow into the AAA through the use of hooks mounted on Z-stents at the proximal and distal limbs of the graft. These grafts

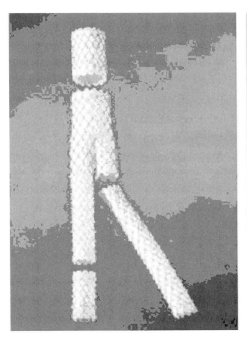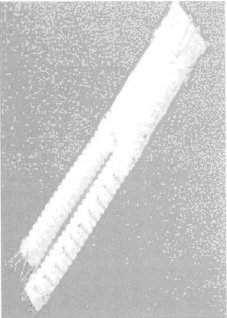

FIG. 28.8. U.S. Food and Drug Administration–approved devices for endovascular treatment of abdominal aortic aneurysms (AneuRx and Ancure grafts).

are then dilated, and the hooks are embedded into the aortic wall. Additional graft designs are being evaluated in a number of clinical trials. Tubular endovascular stent grafts for peripheral and thoracic aortic aneurysms, as well as traumatic arterial disruptions, are also being studied. Most endovascular devices require surgical exposure of the access arteries, usually the proximal common femoral or distal external iliac arteries, although percutaneous endovascular prostheses are in development.

Great care is needed in selecting the length, diameter, and taper of the stent graft to match the aorta and iliac arteries. Many current devices and delivery sheaths are relatively rigid. Therefore, it is important to envision how the prosthesis will sit in the target vessels. Angulation of the proximal and distal infrarenal aortic segments, as well as the iliac arteries, may make graft deployment and fixation impossible. Sizing an artery by angiography alone can be difficult, even with specially constructed calibration catheters or intravascular US. Last, covering the lumbar and inferior mesenteric arteries with the device may lead to graft failure because of continued perfusion of the aneurysm by retrograde blood flow from a branch artery.

PROGNOSIS AND FOLLOW-UP

The current standard for AAA treatment is replacement of the aneurysm with a prosthetic graft by conventional surgical means (Tables 28.2, 28.3). Although endovascular AAA repair may eventually replace open infrarenal AAA repair, the long-term follow-up of endovascular aortic grafts is, to date, limited (Table 28.4). However, it is clear that endovascular repair is equivalent or superior to open repair in terms of decreasing early postoperative morbidity.

Improved preoperative preparation and postoperative care have decreased the rate of mortality after elective AAA repair since the 1960s (26,37). Most mortality after aortic surgery is secondary to myocardial ischemia. Guidelines that establish the need for preoperative cardiac assessment have been formulated. Common risk factors supporting postoperative cardiac event include advanced age, gender, history of diabetes necessitating medication, previous myocardial infarction, and a history of congestive heart failure (38,39). Patients undergoing elective surgery for intact AAAs have fewer postoperative complications and a lower mortality rate than do patients treated on an emergency basis for ruptured AAAs. Coronary artery disease, COPD, and renal insufficiency all increase the hazards of surgery. Increasing complexity of the operation with involvement of the renal and visceral vessels also increases the operative morbidity and mortality. The experience of the surgeon performing the AAA repair also influences outcome.

Operative mortality rates for treating intact AAAs range from 1.4% to 6.5%, with a mean

TABLE 28.2. *Results of open surgical repair of nonruptured abdominal aortic aneurysms*

Study	Year	Study period	Patients	Deaths	Mortality (%)
Crawford	1981	1955–1980	860	41	4.8
McCabe	1981	1972–1977	364	9	2.5
Diehl	1983	1974–1978	350	18	5.1
Hertzer	1984	1978–1981	840	55	6.5
Donaldson	1985	1972–1983	476	24	5.0
Reigel	1987	1980–1985	499	14	2.8
Green	1989	1983–1987	379	8	2.1
Johnston	1989	1986	666	32	4.8
Leather	1989	Not stated	299	11	3.7
Sicard	1989	1983–1988	213	3	1.4
Golden	1990	1973–1989	500	8	1.6
AbuRahma	1991	1983–1987	332	12	3.6
Ernst	1992	1980–1989	710	25	3.5
Total			6,488	260	4.0

Adapted from Ernst CB. Abdominal aortic aneurysm. *N Engl J Med* 1993;328:1167–1173.

TABLE 28.3. *Results of open surgical repair of ruptured abdominal aortic aneurysms*

Study	Year	Study period	Patients	Deaths	Mortality (%)
Crawford	1981	1955–1980	60	14	23
McCabe	1981	1972–1977	73	38	52
Wakefield	1982	1964–1980	116	60	52
Hoffman	1982	1975–1979	152	58	38
Donaldson	1985	1972–1983	81	35	43
Meyer	1986	Not stated	97	45	46
Shackleton	1987	1975–1985	106	43	41
Chang	1990	1983–1989	63	16	25
Ouriel	1990	1979–1988	243	133	55
Sullivan	1990	1978–1989	69	24	35
AbuRahma	1991	1983–1987	73	45	62
Harris	1991	1980–1989	113	72	64
Johansen	1991	1980–1989	180	124	69
Gloviczki	1992	1980–1989	214	97	45
Ernst	1992	1980–1989	91	41	45
Total			1,731	845	49

Adapted from Ernst CB. Abdominal aortic aneurysm. *N Engl J Med* 1993;328:1167–1173.

of 4% (Table 28.2). In contrast, the rate of mortality after ruptured AAA repair nears 50% and has not changed since the 1960s, despite improved preoperative and postoperative care (Table 28.3). Early complications after elective AAA repair include cardiac events (15%), pulmonary insufficiency (8%), renal insufficiency (6%), bleeding (4%), embolization (3%), and wound infection (2%). Late postoperative complications include graft infection and aortoenteric fistula (both 1%). The late complications usually become evident 3 to 5 years after the aortic reconstruction (2).

Several studies have documented the early safety and efficacy of elective endovascular treatment of infrarenal AAAs (40–48) (Table 28.4). Intriguingly, one report has suggested endovascular therapy for ruptured AAAs (49). Twenty-five patients with ruptured aneurysms were treated with endovascular grafts. Five of these patients required conversion to open repair. Two deaths occurred after endograft exclusion of the AAA, which represented a mortality rate of only 10%. It may be concluded that with appropriate preparation and planning, patients with ruptured aneurysms can be treated successfully with endovascular grafts.

The most common complication after endovascular repair of an AAA is an endoleak. An endoleak is defined as persistent blood flow in the aneurysm after the placement of the endovascular graft. Leaks are classified as: (a) graft related, resulting from failure of the hemostatic seal at one end of the endovascular graft or within the fabric of the graft, or (b) graft unrelated, with filling of the aneurysmal sac by back bleeding from

TABLE 28.4. *Results after endovascular repair of abdominal aortic aneurysm*

Series	Patients	Conversion to open repair	30-Day mortality	Persistent endoleak	Other complications
Blum	154	3 (2%)	1 (1%)	9 (6%)	15 (10%)
Moore and Rutherford	46	7 (15%)	0	7 (15%)	27 (rate not stated)
Balm	31	1 (3%)	1 (3%)	3 (10%)	34 in 23 patients
Zarins	190	0 (0%)	5 (2.6%)	17 (9%)	23 (12%)
Beebe	258	5 (2%)	3 (1.2%)	44 (1.6%)	Minor 110 (47%) Severe 10 (3.9%)
Criado	70	5 (7%)	1 (1.4%)	5 (7%)	Not stated

Adapted from May J, White GH, Harris JP. Current designs and results in the treatment of aortic aneurysm. In: Yao JST, Pearce WH, eds. *Modern vascular surgery.* New York: McGraw-Hill, 2000:286–294.

a branch artery. In a large European registry of AAA endovascular grafts, the early endoleak rate was approximately 15% (50). In these cases, the leak sealed spontaneously in 35%, the leak was sealed with the help of a second percutaneous procedure in 18%, and the leak required to open aortic repair in 3%. In this same series, 7% of patients died within 30 days of unrelated causes, 12% had a persistent leak at late follow-up, and 27% were lost to follow-up. An additional 18% of patients developed a late endoleak within the first year of follow-up. It is clear that endoleaks may develop years after placement of the endovascular graft, and their resolution becomes crucial to the success of the endovascular treatment of AAAs.

SUMMARY

AAAs are a major cause of death in the United States, affecting 3% to 9% of the population. Diagnosis of AAA by US is efficient and cost effective, whereas physical examination alone is often unreliable in establishing the presence of an AAA. Large AAAs, greater than 5 cm in diameter, are life-threatening and should be repaired. Small AAAs, 3 to 5 cm in diameter, rupture with unpredictable frequency. Diastolic hypertension and COPD are independent variables contributing to a greater risk of rupture of smaller AAAs. AAAs expanding more than 4 mm in 12 months are more likely to rupture than are AAAs that remain unchanged in size. Elective repair of AAA carries an overall 5.6% mortality rate, and women fare worse than men. Emergency repair of ruptured AAAs carries an operative mortality rate of nearly 50%. The overall rate of mortality from AAA rupture, including patients who die before reaching a hospital, is 80%. The endovascular treatment of selected aneurysms of the abdominal aorta is safe and feasible. Widespread application of endovascular technology must await the maturation of device technology.

PRACTICAL POINTS

- AAAs are the twelfth leading cause of death in the United States and affect 3% to 9% of the population.
- Diagnosis of AAA by US is most efficient and cost effective.
- Large AAAs are greater than 5 cm and are life-threatening.
- Small AAAs, 3 to 5 cm, rupture with unpredictable frequency. Diastolic hypertension and COPD are independent variables contributing to AAA rupture.
- AAA expanding greater than 4 mm over a 12-month period are more likely to rupture than are stable-sized AAAs.
- Elective repair of ruptured AAA carries an overall 5.6% mortality rate. Women fare worse than men do.
- Emergency repair of ruptured AAA carries a mortality rate of nearly 50%. Women fare worse than men do.

- The overall rate of mortality for ruptured AAA, including patients who die before reaching a hospital, is 80%.
- US is best for screening and routine follow-up. MRA or spiral CT is best for preoperative assessment, whereas angiography/DSA may be useful for additional outflow assessment.
- Preoperative planning and attention to technical detail during an expeditious operation are key factors in minimizing blood loss and aortic cross clamp time and thereby in improve overall surgical results after AAA repair.
- Multiple approaches, including transabdominal, retroperitoneal, and thoracoabdominal, should be considered on an individualized basis in operations for aortic disease.

(continued)

- Maintenance of normothermia and avoidance of hypotension are key to preventing poor operative results after repair of a ruptured AAA.
- The endovascular treatment of selected aneurysms of the thoracic and abdominal aorta is safe and feasible.
- In certain patients at high risk and with limited life expectancy, endovascular therapy offers the only reasonable treatment for life-threatening aortic disease.
- Widespread application of endovascular technology to everyday aortic aneurysms must await the maturation of device technology, 5- and 10-year follow-up, and controlled trials of endovascular versus open treatment of aneurysms. In the meantime, patients with endovascular grafts must be monitored indefinitely until the problem of endoleaks is thoroughly understood and resolved.

REFERENCES

1. Cronenwett JL. Arterial aneurysms. In: Rutherford RB, ed. *Vascular surgery.* Philadelphia: WB Saunders, 2000: 1241.
2. Ernst CB. Abdominal aortic aneurysm. *N Engl J Med* 1993;328:1167–1173.
3. Thompson RW, Holmes DR, Mertens RA, et al. Production and localization of 92-kilodalton gelatinase in abdominal aortic aneurysms. An elastolytic metalloproteinase expressed by aneurysm-infiltrating macrophages. *J Clin Invest* 1995;96:318–326.
4. Busuttil RW, Abou-Zamzam AM, Machleder HI. Collagenase activity of the human aorta. A comparison of patients with and without abdominal aortic aneurysm. *Arch Surg* 1980;115:1373–1378.
5. Herron GS, Unemori E, Wong M, et al. Connective tissue proteinases and inhibitors in abdominal aortic aneurysms. Involvement of the vasa vasorum in the pathogenesis of aortic aneurysms. *Arterioscler Thromb* 1991;11:1667–1677.
6. Kohn E, Jacobs W, Kim YS, et al. Calcium influx modulates expression of matrix meralloproteinase-2 (72 kDa type IV collagenase, gelatinase A). *J Biol Chem* 1994;269:21505–21511.
7. Irizarry E, Newman KM, Gandhi RH, et al. Demonstration of interstitial collagenase in abdominal aortic aneurysm disease. *J Surg Res* 1993;54:571–574.
8. Menashi S, Campa JS, Greenhalgh RM, et al. Collagen in abdominal aortic aneurysm: typing, content, and degradation. *J Vasc Surg* 1987;6:578–582.
9. Tamatrina NA, McMillan WD, Shively VP, et al. Expression of matrix metalloproteinases and their inhibitors in aneurysms and normal aorta. *Surgery* 1997;122:264–271.
10. Thompson RW. Basic science of abdominal aortic aneurysms: emerging therapeutic strategies for an unresolved clinical problem. *Curr Opin Cardiol* 1996;11:504–518.
11. Tilson MD, Elefriades J, Brophy CM. Tensile strength and collagen in abdominal aortic aneurysm disease. In: Greenhalgh RM, Mannick JA, Powell JT, eds. *The cause and management of aneurysms.* London: WB Saunders, 1990:97–104.
12. Vine N, Powell J. Metalloproteinases in degenerative aortic disease. *J Clin Sci* 1991;81:233–239.
13. Webster MW, McAuley CE, Steed DL, et al. Collagen stability and collagenolytic activity in the normal and aneurysmal human abdominal aorta. *Am J Surg* 1991;161:635–638.
14. Darling RC 3rd, Brewster DC, Darling RC, et al. Are familial abdominal aortic aneurysms different? *J Vasc Surg* 1989;10:39–43.
15. Powell JM, Greenhalgh RM. Cellular, enzymatic, and genetic factors in the pathogenesis of abdominal aortic aneurysms. *J Vasc Surg* 1989;9:297–304.
16. Webster MW. Genetics of abdominal aortic aneurysm disease. In: Ernst CB, Stanley JC, eds. *Current therapy in vascular surgery,* 4th ed. St. Louis: Mosby, 2001:206–208.
17. Rasmussen TE, Hallett JW Jr, Metzger RLM, et al. Genetic risk factors in inflammatory abdominal aortic aneurysm: polymorphic residue 70 in the HLA-DR B1 gene as a key genetic element. *J Vasc Surg* 1997;25:356–364.
18. Chervu A, Clagett GP, Valentine RJ, et al. Role of physical examination in detection of abdominal aortic aneurysms. *Surgery* 1995;117:454–457.
19. Diwan A, Sarkar R, Stanley JC, et al. Incidence of femoral and popliteal artery aneurysms in patients with abdominal aortic aneurysm. *J Vasc Surg* 2000;31:863–869.
20. Graham LM, Zelenock GB, Whitehouse WM Jr, et al. Clinical significance of arteriosclerotic femoral artery aneurysms. *Arch Surg* 1980;115:502–507.
21. Whitehouse WM Jr, Wakefield TW, Graham LM, et al. Limb-threatening potential of arteriosclerotic popliteal artery aneurysms. *Surgery* 1983;93:694–695.
22. Jaakkola P, Hippelainen M, Farin P, et al. Interobserver variability in measuring the dimensions of the abdominal aorta: comparison of ultrasound and computed tomography. *Eur J Vasc Endovasc Surg* 1996;12:230–237.
23. Prince MR, Narasimham SL, Stanley JC, et al. Gadolinium-enhanced magnetic resonance angiography or abdominal aortic aneurysms. *J Vasc Surg* 1995;21:656–669.
24. Cronenwett JK, Murphy TF, Zelenock GB, et al. Actuarial analysis of variables associated with rupture of small

abdominal aortic aneurysms. *Surgery* 1985;98:472–483.

25. Hannan EL, Kilburn H Jr, O'Donnell JF, et al. A longitudinal analysis of the relationship between in-hospital mortality in New York State and the volume of abdominal aortic aneurysm surgeries performed. *Health Serv Res* 1992;27:517–542.

26. Katz DL, Stanley JC, Zelenock GB. Operative mortality rates for intact and ruptured abdominal aortic aneurysms in Michigan: an eleven-year statewide experience. *J Vasc Surg* 1993;19:804–817.

27. Katz DL, Stanley JC, Zelenock GB. Gender differences in abdominal aortic aneurysm: prevalence, treatment, and outcome. *J Vasc Surg* 1997;25:561–568.

28. Wakefield TW, Whitehouse WM Jr, Wu SC, et al. Abdominal aortic aneurysm rupture: statistical analysis of factors affecting outcome of surgical treatment. *Surgery* 1982;91:586–596.

29. Cambria RP, Brewster DC, Abbott WM, et al. The impact of selective use of dipyridamole thallium scans and surgical factors on the current morbidity of aortic surgery. *J Vasc Surg* 1992;15:43–51.

30. Williams GM, Ricotta J, Zinner M, et al. The extended retroperitoneal approach for treatment of extensive atherosclerosis of the aorta and renal vessels. *Surgery* 1980;88:846–855.

31. Cambria RP, Brewster DC, Abbott WM, et al. Transperitoneal versus retroperitoneal approach for aortic reconstruction: a randomized prospective study. *J Vasc Surg* 1990;11:315–325.

32. Sicard GA, Reilly JM, Rubin BBG, et al. Transabdominal versus retroperitoneal incision for abdominal aortic surgery: report of a prospective randomized trial. *J Vasc Surg* 1995;21:174–183.

33. Gloviczki P, Pairolero PC, Mucha P, et al. Ruptured abdominal aortic aneurysms: repair should not be denied. *J Vasc Surg* 1992;15:851–859.

34. Ouriel K, Geary K, Green RM, et al. Factors determining survival after a ruptured aortic aneurysm: the hospital, the surgeon, and the patient. *J Vasc Surg* 1990;11:493–496.

35. Frank SM, Fleisher LA, Breslo MJ, et al. Perioperative maintenance of normothermia reduces the incidence of morbid cardiac events: a randomized clinical trial. *JAMA* 1997;277:1127–1134.

36. Oelschlager BK, Boyle EM, Johansen K, et al. Delayed abdominal closure in the management of ruptured abdominal aortic aneurysms. *Am J Surg* 1997;172:411–415.

37. Johnston KW. Multicenter prospective study of nonruptured abdominal aortic aneurysms. Part II. Variables predicting morbidity and mortality. *J Vasc Surg* 1989;9:437–447.

38. Eagle KA, Brundage BH, Chaitman BR, et al. Guidelines for perioperative cardiovascular evaluation for noncardiac surgery. A Report of the American College of Cardiology/American Heart Association Task Force of Practice Guidelines (Committee on Perioperative Cardiovascular Evaluation for Noncardiac Surgery). *J Am Coll Cardiol* 1996;27:910–948.

39. Bartels C, Bechtel JRM, Hossmann V, et al. Cardiac risk stratification for high-risk surgery. *Circulation* 1997;95:2473–2475.

40. Blum U, Voshage G, Lammer J, et al. Endoluminal stent-grafts for infrarenal abdominal aortic aneurysms. *N Engl J Med* 1997;336:13–20.

41. Chuter TAM, Wendt G, Hopkinson BR, et al. Transfemoral endovascular insertion of a bifurcated endovascular graft for aortic aneurysm repair: the first 22 patients. *J Cardiovasc Surg* 1995;3:121–128.

42. Moore WS, Rutherford RB. Transfemoral endovascular repair of abdominal aortic aneurysm: result of the North American EVT Phase I Trial. *J Vasc Surg* 1996;23:543–553.

43. Parodi JC, Palmaz JC, Barone HD. Transfemoral intraluminal graft implantation for abdominal aortic aneurysms. *Ann Vasc Surg* 1991;5:491–499.

44. Sternbergh WC, Money SR. Hospital cost of endovascular versus open repair of abdominal aortic aneurysms: a multicenter study. *J Vasc Surg* 2000;31:237–244.

45. Uflacker R, Robison JG, Brothers TE, et al. Abdominal aortic aneurysm treatment: preliminary results with the Talent stent-graft system. *J Vasc Intervent Radiol* 1998;90:51–60.

46. White GH, Yu W, May J, et al. Three-year experience with the White-Yu endovascular GAD graft for transluminal repair of aortic and iliac aneurysms. *J Endovasc Surg* 1997;4:124–136.

47. Woodburn KR, May J, White GH. Endoluminal abdominal aortic aneurysm surgery. *Br J Surg* 1998;85:435–443.

48. Zarins C, White RA, Schwarter S, et al. AneuRx stent-graft versus open repair of abdominal aortic aneurysms. Multicenter prospective clinical trial. *J Vasc Surg* 1999;29:292–305.

49. Ohki T, Veith FJ. Endovascular grafts and other image-guided catheter-based adjuncts to improve the treatment of ruptured aortoiliac aneurysms. *Ann Surg* 2000;232:466–479.

50. Harris PL. The highs and lows of endovascular aneurysm repair: the first two years of the Eurostar Registry. *Ann R Coll Surg Engl* 1999;81:161–165.

29

Nondissecting Thoracic Aneurysms

Sanjay Rajagopalan, Gilbert R. Upchurch, Jr., David M. Williams,
and G. Michael Deeb

"There is no disease more conducive to clinical humility than aneurysms of the aorta."—Sir William Osler

DEFINITION AND HISTORICAL PERSPECTIVE

The term *aneurysm* is derived from the Greek word "aneurysma," which means to widen or dilate. Aneurysms may be either "fusiform," with symmetric oblong dilatation of the aorta, or "saccular," a circular outpouching of the aortic wall. The first descriptive account of an aneurysm was by the Roman physician-philosopher Galen around 160 A.D. Over the past three centuries, a variety of techniques such as simple ligation, wire-induced luminal thrombosis, galvanic current, and periarterial fibrosis were applied, with limited success (1,2). The modern era in the treatment of aneurysmal disease came through the work of Gross, Swan, Lam, and DeBakey, who reported successful treatment of coarctation and aneurysms of the descending thoracic aorta by using resection and replacement (3–6). The first successful aortic arch replacement under cardiopulmonary bypass was performed in 1957 by DeBakey et al. (7). Other advances such as better suture materials, prosthetic grafts, development of anticoagulants, and use of hypothermic circulatory arrest have made it possible to minimize complications on formidable operations, such as aortic arch repair.

ANATOMIC CONSIDERATIONS AND CLASSIFICATION

The thoracic aorta is divided into the ascending, arch, and descending portions. The ascending aorta in turn can be subdivided into the aortic root, which is the part of the aorta that extends from the level of the aortic valve to the sinotubular junction, and the tubular aorta (see Fig. 29.1). Anatomic studies of the aortic root indicate a very consistent relationship among the sizes of the aortic valve leaflets, aortic sinuses, annulus, and sinotubular junction. The aorta at the level of the sinuses is the widest, measuring 3 to 3.3 cm in adults, and is usually 10% to 15% larger than the diameter of the sinotubular junction. The coronary arteries arise at this level. The aortic arch begins at the innominate artery and extends to the origin of the left subclavian artery, where it becomes the descending thoracic aorta. This transition point is the aortic isthmus. The aorta is especially vulnerable to trauma at this site because it is immobilized by the attachment to the thoracic rib cage, pleural reflections, and the left subclavian artery. The abdominal aorta continues from the thoracic aorta and bifurcates at the level of the fourth lumbar vertebra. Aneurysms are classified according to their respective sites of origin as ascending, arch, or descending thoracic aneurysms. Thoracoabdominal aneurysms (TAA), in view of their complexity, are classified according the scheme originally devised by Crawford et al. (8) (Fig. 29.2). This classification is clinically useful in view of implications for both management and incidence of preoperative complications.

MECHANISMS OF ANEURYSM FORMATION

The mechanisms of aneurysm development are complex and probably involve multiple factors, such as abnormalities in matrix (genetic or

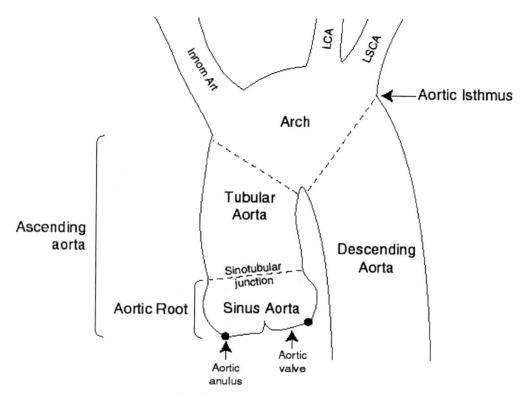

FIG. 29.1. Anatomy of the aorta.

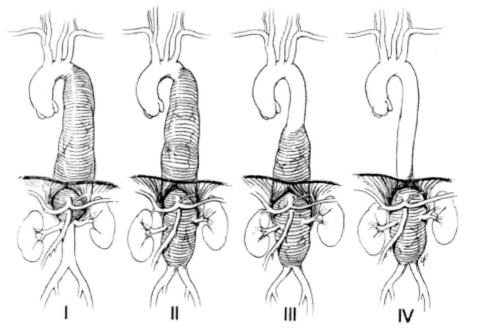

FIG. 29.2. Crawford classification of thoracoabdominal aneurysms.

acquired), excessive activity of matrix degrading enzymes, and hemodynamic factors, that either alone or acting in concert may influence progressive dilation of the aorta.

Abnormalities in Extracellular Matrix

Alterations in matrix structure are fundamental to aneurysm development. A pathologic hallmark of aneurysms, especially those resulting from Marfan's syndrome, is cystic medial necrosis (defined by elastic tissue damage, smooth muscle loss, and the accumulation of basophilic substance in the media). This change occurs to a mild degree as part of the normal aging process and may explain the association between age and the propensity for aneurysms. Marfan's syndrome is an autosomal dominant disorder characterized by mutations in the fibrillin-1 molecule, the main protein component of the microfibril. Microfibrils are extracellular matrix structures displaying a diameter of less than 20 nm and lacking the characteristic 67-nm banding periodicity of interstitial collagen fibers. They form a meshwork in tissues into which elastin is embedded. In the wall of the proximal aorta, the presence of the elastin-associated microfibrillar network gives the aorta added elasticity and compliance. More than 100 mutations have been identified in individuals affected with Marfan's syndrome and other Marfan's syndrome–related "fibrillinopathies," such as MASS (mitral valve prolapse, aortic dilatation, and skin and skeletal manifestations), isolated ectopia lentis, annuloaortic ectasia, and neonatal Marfan's syndrome (9,10). It has been demonstrated that FBN1 mutations can occur in individuals with thoracic aneurysms who otherwise do not meet any criteria for Marfan's syndrome (11). This missense mutation, although rare, is associated with reduced synthesis of fibrillin-1 in dermal fibroblasts. Another disorder, Ehlers-Danlos syndrome type IV, the vascular type, results from mutations in the gene for type III procollagen (COL3A1). Affected patients are at risk for arterial, bowel, and uterine rupture. In this disorder, dissections of the aorta are common, but aneurysmal dilation of the aorta is relatively uncommon (12).

Excessive Activity of Matrix Degrading Enzymes

There is a substantial body of evidence implicating the increased expression and activation of a family of degrading enzymes called matrix metalloproteinases (MMP) in the pathogenesis of abdominal and thoracoabdominal aneurysms. MMP-2, MMP-9, and membrane bound-MMP (MT-MMP) have so far been implicated (13–17). The evidence for a causative role for these enzymes comes from studies in which interruption in the activity of these key enzymes by drugs (18–20) or targeted gene disruption approaches (21) reduces aneurysm development. Correlative human studies have noted an increase in progression of aneurysm size and risk for rupture with an increase in the levels of these enzymes within the aortic wall (22,23). These findings have justified a large multicenter trial for the treatment of small aneurysms with tetracyclines, which are MMP inhibitors (20).

Hemodynamic Factors

With progressive dilation of the aorta, circumferential wall shear stress, as defined by Laplace's law, increases (wall tension and diameter). The pulsatile load (dP/dT) tends to be greatest in the dilated portions (24). Thus, modalities such as beta blockers that reduce dP/dT would be expected to reduce aneurysmal wall stress and the propensity for rupture (25).

ETIOLOGY

Table 29.1 summarizes the causes of thoracic aneurysms. Some of the causes listed, differentially afflict select portions of the aorta. For example, degenerative aneurysms most commonly involve the descending thoracic aorta and the adjacent abdominal aorta, whereas Marfan's syndrome tends to involve the aortic root and tubular ascending aorta. A small percentage of patients develop aneurysms (approximately 1% each type) related to infection (mycotic aneurysm) or previous inflammatory aortitis. Infective aneurysms may involve any location and may arise through the hematogenous seeding of atherosclerotic plaque, with

TABLE 29.1. *Causes of nondissecting thoracic aneurysm*

Degenerative
Hereditary/developmental
Marfan's syndrome
Ehlers-Danlos syndrome (type IV)
Traumatic
Inflammatory
Takayasu's arteritis
Behçet's disease
Polyarteritis nodosa
Kawasaki's disease
Infectious (bacterial, fungal, spirochetal)
Poststenotic

development of focal aortitis and formation of a false aneurysm. Aneurysms associated with blunt trauma most frequently involve the proximal descending aorta in the region of the isthmus. Dilation of the aorta distal to a congenital bicuspid aortic valve or a segment of coarctation may result from hemodynamic flow alterations distal to the stenosis.

Annuloaortic ectasia is a subset of ascending aortic aneurysms that is characterized by progressive dilation of the aortic root, stretching of the leaflets, and functional aortic regurgitation (Fig. 29.3). The valves themselves are structurally normal. In due course, the aortic walls become thin and are prone to dissection. Cystic medial degeneration is the pathologic hallmark of this disorder, which is believed to represent a "fibrillinopathy," akin to Marfan's syndrome. Annuloaortic ectasia is more common in men than in women, typically occurring between the fourth and sixth decades.

INCIDENCE AND CONCOMITANT CONDITIONS

The incidence of thoracic aneurysms in the community (Rochester, Minnesota) is 5 to 10 per 100,000 patient years (26,27). In contrast to abdominal aortic aneurysms (AAAs), which demonstrate a striking predisposition for men

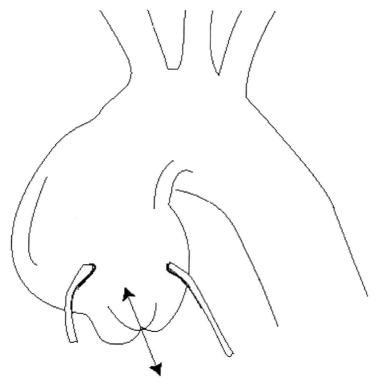

FIG. 29.3. Annuloaortic ectasia. The *arrow* denotes aortic regurgitation.

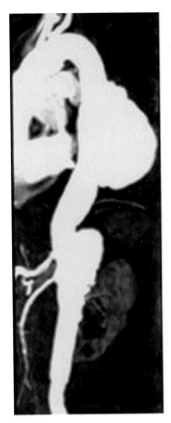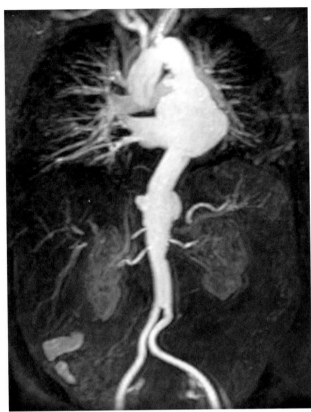

FIG. 29.4. Sagittal and coronal maximum intensity projection images derived from a three-dimensional contrast-enhanced magnetic resonance angiogram that reveal a descending thoracic aneurysm measuring 8.5 cm with an additional aneurysmal segment in the supra-renal portion of the abdominal aorta.

(5:1 male-to-female ratio), thoracic aneurysms afflict men and women equally (27). The presence of a thoracic aneurysm is predictive of a higher likelihood of aneurysms in other locations. Of such affected patients, 25% harbor multiple aneurysms, in contrast to subjects with AAA, of whom only 2% harbor concomitant thoracic aneurysms (28). Figure 29.4 illustrates a large descending thoracic aneurysm in a patient who also has involvement of the suprarenal abdominal aorta. In many instances, the appearance of a thoracic aortic aneurysm postdates that of an AAA, and, indeed, a significant proportion of patients undergoing surgery for thoracic aneurysm have undergone a prior AAA repair. In some patients this represents the *de novo* development

of a new aneurysm; in many other instances, however, this represents the progression of previous diffuse aneurysmal disease (29). Individuals with TAA are often significantly older than patients with ascending aortic aneurysms (especially those associated with Marfan's syndrome) and have concomitant coronary artery disease.

CLINICAL PRESENTATION

The initial manifestation of a thoracic aneurysm is commonly a rupture, in which case it is uniformly fatal (30). Of patients with such aneurysms, 25% are treated on an emergentcy basis; approximately half are treated for frank rupture (31,32). Aneurysm progression in most patients is clinically silent. However, a larger percentage of patients with thoracic aneurysms (approximately 40%) experience symptoms in comparison with patients with AAAs (32,33). This may in part reflect the reluctance to operate on patients in whom the aneurysm is diffuse to begin with, grows even larger, and is therefore much more likely to be symptomatic. The development of abrupt severe chest or abdominal pain may signify aneurysm expansion, rupture, or acute dissection. Thoracic aneurysms may produce localized retrosternal chest pain or back pain related to erosion into the chest wall or spine. The resultant pain may be prominent and may precede the discovery of the aneurysm by several months. Unusual symptoms related to compression of contiguous structures include (a) a new onset of hoarseness, secondary to recurrent laryngeal nerve involvement; (b) cough, secondary to erosion or compression of the tracheobronchial tree; and (c) dysphagia lusoria.

DIAGNOSTIC STUDIES

Chest Radiography

Widening of the mediastinum and unfurling of the ascending aorta on the chest radiograph may be the first clue to the presence of an ascending aortic or aortic arch aneurysm. The chest radiograph may, however, appear completely normal in many cases of ascending aortic aneurysms and in almost all cases of descending thoracic aneurysms and TAAs. Conversely, the presence of mediastinal widening secondary to aneurysmal enlargement cannot always be differentiated from tumors or other enlargements of the mediastinum.

Transesopheageal Echocardiography

Transesophageal echocardiography (TEE) with color-flow Doppler imaging is emerging as an invaluable initial study in the diagnosis and follow-up care of patients with ascending aortic and aortic arch aneurysmal disease, because it simultaneously provides important information on the status of the aortic valve, the aortic arch, and left ventricular function. For suspected dissection of the proximal aorta, a TEE is often the initial di-

agnostic modality of choice in many institutions. Intraoperative monitoring with TEE during ascending aortic repair is helpful in the detection of early prosthetic complications and the adequacy of reparative procedures on the valve. In the follow-up of patients with composite graft replacement of the ascending aorta, TEE is excellent for monitoring the size of the graft and the anastomotic junction, as well as in the simultaneous evaluation of the prosthetic valve. Because patients with an ascending aortic or aortic arch aneurysm are at risk for recurrence of aneurysmal disease in the distal thoracic or abdominal aorta, three-dimensional contrast-enhanced magnetic resonance angiography (MRA) or computed tomographic (CT) scanning should be considered as an periodic surveillance adjunct in addition to TEE (34). For patients with descending thoracic aneurysms, TEE cannot provide complete information, because very often the aneurysm extends beyond the field of view. TEE is therefore not useful in the initial diagnosis or follow-up of patients with descending thoracic and TAA. However, in combination with CT scanning and angiography, it may be of use in monitoring placement of endovascular grafts and in the evaluation of early endoleaks (35).

Computed Tomography

CT techniques are commonly used in the diagnosis of thoracic aortic disease, owing to the widespread availability of CT scanners. They are of particular value in documenting growth rates of aneurysms and in determining timing for surgery, as well as obtaining detailed information on precise extent of the aneurysm (36). Computed tomographic angiography (CTA) combines a rapid bolus intravenous injection with a timed breath-held spiral CT acquisition during peak arterial opacification. Three-dimensional reformatting with maximum intensity projections, curved planar reformations, and shaded surface displays afford excellent visualization of the aorta and major branch vessels. In the patient with a diagnosis of acute rupture, a non–contrast-enhanced CT scan is often the initial diagnostic test of choice, owing to its ready availability (37). Once the rupture is documented, no further studies are indicated, and prompt operative repair should be undertaken. If the rupture is not readily evident, contrast material is administered to more completely delineate the pathologic process and evaluate the possibility of other scenarios, such as dissection, dissecting intramural hematoma, or penetrating aortic ulcer. CTA is often necessary for endovascular planning and is a valuable adjunct in the follow-up of patients after surgery or endovascular graft placement. In the latter case, curved planar reformations are helpful in visualizing the internal anatomy of grafts and stents. The main disadvantage of CTA is its reliance on ionizing radiation and the use of contrast agents with its implications for renal dysfunction.

Magnetic Resonance Imaging

Magnetic resonance (MR) imaging has emerged as a powerful noninvasive tool for the assessment of the thoracic and thoracoabdominal aorta. It obviates the need for iodinated contrast agents and catheter-based arteriography with their associated risks of nephrotoxicity and atheroembolism, respectively. MR protocols used in the systematic evaluation of the thoracic aorta include three-dimensional contrast-enhanced MRA (Fig. 29.4) and T1-weighted spin-echo techniques (black blood) in multiple planes to assess the extent of the aneurysm (Fig. 29.5) and provide information about the involvement of great vessels and their relationship to the aneurysm. Three-dimensional contrast-enhanced MRA data set acquisition is fast (less than 1 minute) and provides detailed images of the thoracic and abdominal aorta. Multiplanar reformations of the image data sets aid in the display of the often complex, tortuous anatomy of aneurysms. The inclusion of post-gadolinium T1-weighted images to the protocol may additionally provide information on inflammatory involvement of the vessel wall in cases of suspected aortitis.

Contrast-Enhanced Aortography

Individuals with ascending aortic aneurysms often need preoperative coronary arteriograms, and an ascending aorta/aortic arch injection may be obtained at that time, very often to delineate origins of aortic arch vessels. Contrast-enhanced

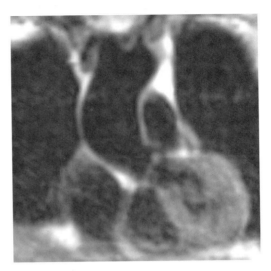

FIG. 29.5. Coronal T1-weighted spin-echo magnetic resonance image revealing a 5-cm ascending aortic aneurysm extending from the sinotubular junction to brachiocephalic artery.

aortography can often be avoided in instances in which detailed information on the extent of the aneurysm and patency of the visceral arteries are provided by MRA and CTA (36). However, if MRA is precluded owing to contraindications (metallic implants or pacemakers) or if MRA or CTA is inadequate in resolving the patency of vessels adjacent to the aneurysm, a contrast-enhanced aortogram may be required. In endovascular planning for descending thoracic aneurysms, in most institutions at this time, it is still the practice to obtain a contrast-enhanced aortogram.

ESTIMATING RISK OF RUPTURE OF A THORACIC ANEURYSM

The risk of rupture of an aneurysm is fundamentally related to its management. Surgical treatment is justified, provided that the risk of short-term rupture is sufficiently high and the risk involved with treatment is lower than that of rupture. The risk of rupture is negligible in thoracic aneurysms smaller than 4 cm; the risk involved with operative intervention is higher than the risk posed by rupture. In the 4- to 5.9-cm range, the risk of rupture rises to 16% at 5 years and is comparable to that involved with surgery.

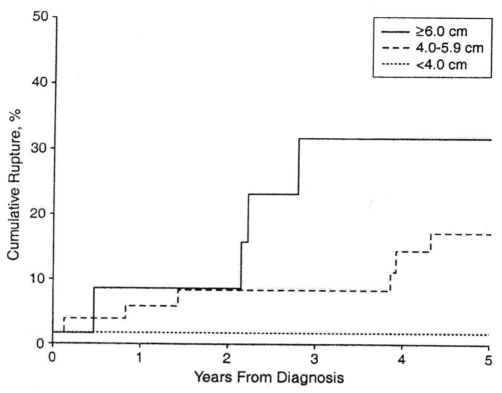

FIG. 29.6. Cumulative probability of rupture of thoracic aortic aneurysms, based on initial diameters.

The risk increases substantially to more than 20% with aneurysms larger than 6 cm (see Fig. 29.6) (27,38). The risk involved in intervention and rupture varies with each patient, depending on underlying medical conditions and other comorbid conditions, and any treatment plan will have to take into account individual variations in susceptibility owing to the concomitant

TABLE 29.2. *Risk factors for nondissecting thoracic aneurysm*

Risk factor	Relative risk
Chronic obstructive pulmonary disease	3.6
Age[a]	2.6
Hypertension	2.6
Presence of symptoms such as pain	2.3
Size[b]	1.7

[a]Risk increases by a factor of 2.6 for each decade of age.
[b]Risk increases by a factor of approximately 2 for each centimeter increase in size.

presence of risk factors that may independently influence risk. For instance, more than 50% of individuals with Marfan's syndrome sustain dissections of ascending aortic aneurysms at diameters much less than 6.0 cm. Therefore, it may be prudent to undertake prophylactic repair of aortic aneurysms in such patients when the diameter of the aorta is far less than that size (39). A number of risk factors have been identified as playing a role in the progression of thoracic aneurysms and TAAs (see Table 29.2). These factors should also be taken in to account in estimating cumulative risk.

MANAGEMENT OF ASCENDING AORTIC AND AORTIC ARCH ANEURYSMS

Medical Management

The medical management of a patient with an aneurysm in any location involves risk factor modification, such as correction of hypertension and cessation of smoking. There is evidence that beta blockade substantially reduces the rate of mortality among individuals with Marfan's syndrome and ascending aortic aneurysms. Shores et al. examined the efficacy of beta blockers (propranolol) in patients with Marfan's syndrome and ascending aortic aneurysm in a randomized, open-label study (40). The presence of aortic regurgitation was a contraindication in the study. The mean dose of propranolol was 212 ± 68 mg, given in four divided doses a day, and the control condition was no beta blocker therapy; patients were then monitored over a 10-year period. The treated group showed a significantly slower rate of aortic dilatation, fewer adverse clinical end points (death, aortic dissection, aortic regurgitation, aortic root aneurysm larger than 6 cm), and a significantly lower mortality rate. The reduction in mortality and in propensity for dissection was so impressive in this study that, on the basis of this alone, most clinicians today believe that control of dP/dT and hypertension is essential in the treatment of all thoracic aneurysms, irrespective of cause or size. In individuals with concomitant aortic regurgitation, the lowering of the heart rate may worsen aortic insufficiency, and the physician may consider the use of other agents devoid of negative chronotropic effects. Even in these patients, a small dose of beta blockers or calcium channel antagonist (diltiazem) may be used cautiously.

Preoperative Evaluation

Patients with ascending aortic and aortic arch aneurysm need to be evaluated thoroughly for the presence of concomitant diseases that may affect their prognosis. A number of these patients may need to undergo routine coronary arteriography to delineate the coronary anatomy and reconfirm the proximal extent and involvement of the sinuses, because this may influence the type of surgery.

Surgical Treatment of Ascending Aortic Aneurysms

Size Thresholds for Recommending Repair and Graft Considerations

Patients with degenerative aneurysms confined to the ascending aorta that exceed 5.5 to 6.0 cm and who have concomitant aortic regurgitation should undergo replacement of the ascending aorta with a synthetic composite graft (see Fig. 29.7) with reimplantation of the coronary arteries. In the event that substantial aortic regurgitation is present with symptoms of heart failure or left-ventricular dysfunction, composite valve and graft replacement may be performed when aneurysms are smaller than the recommended size. In patients with Marfan's syndrome or other inherited collagen disorders, ascending aortic aneurysms exceeding 5.0 cm are enough to warrant prophylactic surgical replacement, in view of a substantially higher risk for rupture (39). Occasionally, patients who have sustained strokes or transient ischemic attacks secondary to severe atherosclerosis involving the ascending aorta and/or aortic arch who have a concomitant degenerative aneurysm smaller than 5.5 cm may undergo repair in combination with valve replacement, coronary artery bypass grafting, or both. Composite homografts may be used in lieu

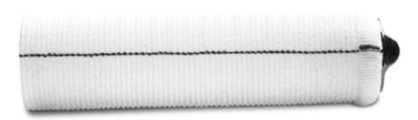

FIG. 29.7. Composite graft (mechanical valve prosthesis within Dacron tube graft).

of synthetic Dacron grafts in the setting of an infective process or when anticoagulation is an issue. The main disadvantages of homografts are their poor long-term durability and lack of ready availability (41). Glutaraldehyde-fixed porcine composite graft is another option for individuals older than 70 years. Although long-term follow-up data on this graft are currently not available, it is believed to be comparable with homografts. This prosthesis is rather short, and so if replacement of the ascending aorta is indicated, a separate Dacron graft must be used to lengthen the aortic root prosthesis.

Composite Graft Replacement of the Aortic Root and Ascending Aorta (Bentall-DeBono Procedure)

This procedure is now synonymous with replacement of the aortic root and the proximal ascending aorta with a composite graft, but in a strict sense it connotes a method of coronary artery implantation in which the coronaries are left attached to the aortic wall and their ostia anastomosed side to side to the graft (42). Important modifications of the original Bentall procedure—such as full-thickness anastomosis of the Dacron graft to the distal ascending aorta and the "button technique," in which the coronary arteries are excised with a collar of tissue around them—have reduced the incidence of anastomotic pseudoaneurysm (41). Some surgeons reinforce the coronary anastomoses with circular collars of Teflon felt ("lifesavers"). Synthetic composite grafts require the same level of anticoagulation as do standard mechanical valves with International Normalized Ratios maintained at recommended levels for the valve.

The Role of Aortic Valve–Sparing Procedures in Ascending Aortic Aneurysm Repair

Valve-sparing procedures are primarily used for patients with ascending aortic aneurysms and anatomically normal valves who do not have Marfan's syndrome. These procedures may be applicable in individuals with aortic regurgitation caused by distortion of leaflet, sinus, and tubular anatomy. Procedures that reestablish this relationship automatically restore cooptation of the leaflets. In individuals with dilation of the tubular aorta and enlargement of the sinotubular junction, simple replacement of the tubular aorta with a consequent reduction of the sinotubular junction diameter to 15% less than the average length of the aortic leaflets, as shown in Fig. 29.8, may be all that is required. Individuals with ascending aortic aneurysms and additional dilation of the sinuses and normal aortic valves may require replacement of the aortic sinuses with remodeling of the aortic root (Fig. 29.9). Several surgeons believe that Marfan's syndrome is a contraindication for valve-sparing surgery, in view of the possibility of dilatation of the aortic annulus after the valve-sparing procedure. However, select groups have demonstrated outstanding long-term results with valve-sparing procedures in patients with obvious manifestations of Marfan's syndrome (43).

Surgical Management of Annuloaortic Ectasia

Surgery is recommended for severe aortic regurgitation or when the aneurysm measures more than 5.0 cm. Replacement of the aortic root with a composite graft is the most commonly performed procedure.

Surgical Treatment of Aortic Arch Aneurysms

Aortic arch aneurysms seldom occur alone and are often associated with aneurysms of the ascending or descending aorta. Operations in the aortic arch are complex, require hypothermic cardiopulmonary bypass, and carry a 5% to 18% risk of focal or diffuse neurologic damage (44,45). In view of this substantial risk, elective surgery for nondissecting aneurysms of the aortic arch is recommended only when the size of the aneurysm exceeds 6 cm (46). The surgical procedure involves separation of the brachiocephalic vessels with a cuff of tissue from the aneurysmal graft, interpositioning of the prosthetic aortic arch, and reimplantation of the vessels into the graft. Retrograde cerebral perfusion via a superior vena cava cannula has been shown to be superior in reducing the neurologic complications of aortic

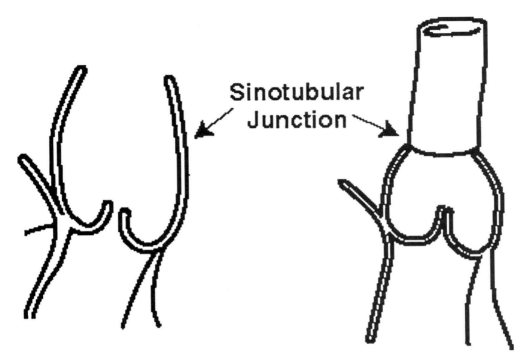

FIG. 29.8. Aortic valve–sparing techniques. Correction of aortic insufficiency by replacing the ascending aorta and adjusting the diameter of the sinotubular junction.

arch replacement (47). The mechanisms underlying better outcome include improvement in the delivery of nutrients to the brain and the ability to flush out air and particulate matter from the cerebral and carotid arteries before establishing antegrade perfusion.

MANAGEMENT OF DESCENDING THORACIC AND THORACOABDOMINAL ANEURYSMS

Medical Management

Control of underlying hypertension and cessation of smoking are cornerstones of medical management. In patients at high risk, this may be the only acceptable intervention. Before elective surgery, it is absolutely critical for patients to discontinue tobacco smoking for a minimum of 1 month. Preoperative optimization of respiratory function with bronchodilator therapy is an important component in the management of patients. Preoperative steroid therapy, however, is controversial because there is anecdotal evidence that this maneuver might precipitate aneurysm rupture (48). There are no data yet on the effects of aggressive lipid lowering and on emerging modalities such as tetracyclines, which seem to work by inhibition of MMP activity (49).

Preoperative Evaluation

As in the management of ascending aortic aneurysms, attention needs to be paid to the presence of concomitant diseases and aneurysms. In view of the high prevalence of coronary disease in this population, preoperative stress testing is often mandated (see Chapter X).

Surgical Treatment of Descending Thoracic and Thoracoabdominal Aneurysms

Size Threshold for Recommending Surgery

The threshold for operative intervention in most degenerative types 1, 2, and 3 TAAs and thoracic

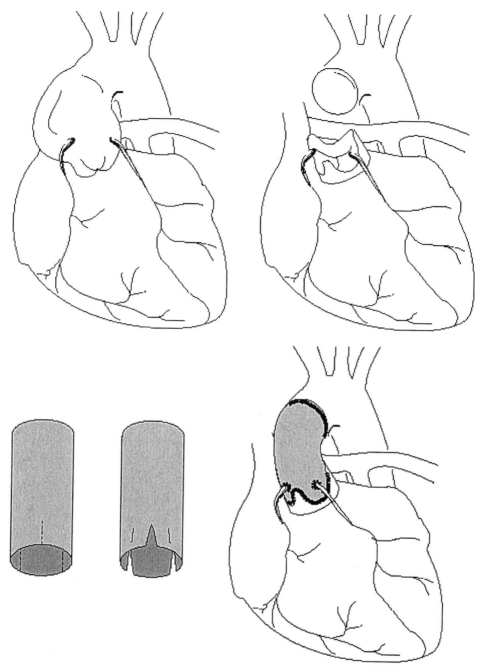

FIG. 29.9. Aortic valve–sparing techniques. Excision of the aortic sinuses and replacement with remodeling of the aortic root and preservation of the aortic valve. (From David TE. Aortic valve sparing operations in patients with ascending aortic aneurysms. *Curr Opin Cardiol* 1997;12:39133–395.)

aneurysms is an aneurysm size of 6 cm, after careful consideration of other comorbid conditions. Because type 4 TAAs really represent AAAs, a threshold of 5 cm or smaller is maintained. The one exception to this rule is in patients with underlying connective tissue disorders such as Marfan's syndrome, for which a number of studies have documented the tendency for such aneurysms to rupture at sizes less than the recommended threshold. In these cases, a 5-cm threshold is probably prudent. Often, the typical degenerative TAA is not uniform in size and presents the additional surgical challenge of the wisdom of extending the resection to subjacent modestly dilated aortic segments.

Surgical graft replacement is the only definite treatment for TAAs. Endovascular treatment (to be discussed) has been applied in the treatment of localized TAAs in the descending aorta.

Repair of Descending Thoracic and Thoracoabdominal Aneurysms (Modified Inclusion Techniques of Crawford)

The two modifications of the Crawford inclusion method currently in vogue are a "clamp-and-sew" technique, often supplemented by adjuncts for organ preservation, and a sequential clamp technique combined with the use of distal aortic perfusion techniques (33,48). Distal aortic perfusion can be provided passively through an indwelling Gott shunt (in which flow is taken from the proximal aorta, the left subclavian artery, or the apex of the left ventricle and channeled to the aorta below the aneurysm or via a retrograde transfemoral approach) or actively through atrial-femoral bypass with the Bio-Medicus pump. Comparable results have been obtained with clamp-and-sew and sequential clamp techniques for the treatment of TAAs. The aortic graft material used in contemporary surgical practice is a Dacron prosthesis. However, in the circumstance of an infected aneurysm, an aortic homograft may be used (50). Polytetrafluoroethylene or Dacron side arm grafts may be used for reconstruction of renal and splanchnic arteries.

Complications Associated with Open Surgical Repair of Descending Thoracic and Thoracoabdominal Aneurysms

The most feared and devastating complication of operative management of descending thoracic aneurysms and TAAs is spinal cord ischemia. The incidence of the complications is partly dependent on the size of the aneurysm (24% in type 2 aneurysms vs. 5% in types 3 and 4 aneurysms, in Crawford's original series of 1,500 cases) and the total duration of the use of the aortic Cross clamp (more than 60 minutes) (51). More contemporary series show a reduction in the overall incidence of these complications to around 12% (31,33,52). Aneurysms in the thoracolumbar region are at most risk for ischemic injury because of the vagaries in arterial supply to the spinal cord in this section (53). Renal failure is another notable complication, occurring in 10% to 15% of individuals. Preexisting renal insufficiency, prolonged aortic Cross clamp time and cholesterol embolization caused by surgical manipulation of the aneurysm all increase risk of postoperative renal failure (51). Respiratory failure necessitating prolonged ventilatory support is also a common complication, occurring in nearly 25% to 45% of patients (32,54).

SURVIVAL AFTER ELECTIVE SURGERY FOR THORACIC ANEURYSMS

Table 29.3 summarizes early mortality and late survival rates for aortic surgery according to the location of the aneurysm. In general, the long-term survival rate among individuals undergoing surgery for TAAs is worse than that among individuals undergoing repair of ascending aortic aneurysms associated with Marfan's syndrome. The majority of the latter patients are young and have no other comorbid conditions. Cardiac events are the most common cause of late mortality among patients with descending thoracic aneurysms and TAAs. In 10% of cases of all thoracic aneurysms, rupture of another aneurysm accounts for death, which argues for periodic surveillance with CT scanning or MRA in every patient with the diagnosis of a thoracic aneurysm.

TABLE 29.3. *Characteristics of nondissecting thoracic aneurysms*

Location	Cause	Early mortality (%)		Late survival (%)		
		Mean	Range	5-Year	10-Year	References
Ascending aorta	Marfan's syndrome	2.5	1–6	78–87	57–73	39,62–65
	Annuloaortic ectasia	3	0–8	65–75	56–75	66–70
	Degenerative	3	0–5	71–75	65	65,66,68,69, 71,72
Aortic arch	Marfan's and degenerative	6	0–19	—	—	44,45,47
Descending aorta	Degenerative	6	3–12	60	—	73–76
Thoracoabdominal aorta	Degenerative	9	7–11	60–65	32–37	32,77,78

ENDOVASCULAR APPROACHES FOR THE MANAGEMENT OF ISOLATED DESCENDING THORACIC ANEURYSMS

Endovascular aneurysm repair involves the transluminal placement of a graft within the aneurysm that excludes the sac from the systemic circulation. The graft is anchored in place by a balloon-expandable or self-expanding externally supported metal stent that supports all or part of the graft and provides a blood-tight seal proximally and distal to the dilated segment of the artery. By avoiding the need for open laparotomy/thoracotomy, application of Cross clamps to the aorta, and the blood loss associated with the opening of the aneurysm sac, this technique has the potential for reducing the rates of morbidity and mortality associated with open aneurysm repair and extends the scope of repair to patients with severe medical comorbid conditions who are not candidates for traditional repair. Despite the obvious advantages, there are three major areas of concern. One is related to the long-term durability of the graft itself, inasmuch as this is currently unknown. Structural failure has been reported in at least one device (55). Second, the ability of the endograft to alter the natural history of progressive expansion of the proximal neck of the aneurysm is currently not known, although data indicate that both the proximal and the distal neck continue to expand, at least with infrarenal AAAs (55). Third, complications that are unique to endovascular repair of aneurysms, such as distal endoleak and embolization, are yet to be resolved.

Endovascular stents are most appropriately placed in patients with a localized aneurysm, restricted to the relatively straight portion of the descending thoracic aorta, anatomically distant from the transverse aortic arch (56–60). In contrast to the endovascular treatment of infrarenal AAAs, there are no natural barriers such as renal arteries that make planning challenging. The primary limitations are restricted to the availability of a prosthesis of sufficiently large diameter to match the aorta adjacent to the graft and the accurate deployment of a large-caliber graft in a high-flow arterial system. Contraindications to the placement of an endovascular graft include the presence of heavy circumferential calcification and excessive mural thrombus.

Complications Associated with Endovascular Treatment of Thoracic Aneurysms

Injuries to Arteries of Access

The passage of large introducer sheaths (7 to 9 mm in size) through diseased, calcific, and tortuous iliac and femoral arteries may result in significant arterial trauma and rupture.

Embolization

Distal embolization caused by manipulation of the endograft within the sac of the aneurysm may result in renal failure, gut infarction, stroke, and lower limb ischemia. The last complication appears to occur more commonly in individuals with luminal thrombus.

Endoleak

An endoleak may be defined as persistent blood flow outside of the lumen of the endograft but within the aneurysm sac or an adjacent arterial segment being treated by the graft. This results in incomplete sealing of the aneurysm sac, continued aneurysm expansion, and eventual rupture. Endoleaks may be classified as graft related (type 1) and non–graft related (type 2).

- Type 1 endoleak results from persistent blood flow caused by inadequate or ineffective seal at the graft ends (proximal or distal).
- Type 2 endoleak results from persistent collateral flow to the aneurysm sac, flowing in a retrograde manner from patent intercostal arteries.

The incidence of endoleaks in a series of patients treated with a self-expanding Z-stent covered by a woven Dacron tube graft was 24%. The majority of endoleaks were type 1 in nature, occurring at the proximal stent graft site adjacent to the left subclavian artery, but in some patients, a type 2 endoleak occurred secondary to persistent collateral arteries (59). The latter was amenable to coil embolization.

Spinal Cord Ischemia

Spinal cord ischemia may still occur (59), although it is relatively rare with current genera-

tion grafts (61). A history of AAA repair once again seems to predispose subjects to this complication, as is this case with open repair.

SUMMARY

Thoracic aortic aneurysms may afflict any portion of the ascending aorta, aortic arch, or descending aorta. The predominant cause of ascending aortic aneurysm is Marfan's syndrome; degenerative aneurysms are common in the thoracoabdominal aorta. The risk of rupture for a thoracic aneurysm increases when the aneurysm exceeds 5 cm in size; intervention is generally recommended when the aneurysm exceeds 6 cm in size. The exception to this rule is patients with Marfan's syndrome, for whom a lower size threshold of 5 to 5.5 cm is currently recommended. TEE, CTA, and three-dimensional contrast-enhanced MRA are valuable for the initial assessment and follow-up of individuals with thoracic aneurysmal disease. Management of underlying hypertension and cessation of smoking are cornerstones of medical management. Surgical graft replacement is the only definitive treatment for ascending aortic and aortic arch aneurysms and TAAs. Spinal cord ischemia is the most feared complication associated with the resection of large thoracic aneurysms and TAAs. Endovascular treatment has been applied in the treatment of localized TAAs in the descending aorta.

PRACTICAL POINTS

- The initial presentation of a thoracic aneurysm is commonly a fatal rupture.
- The chest radiograph appears completely normal in many cases. In suspected dissection of the proximal aorta, TEE is often the initial diagnostic modality of choice. CT and MR imaging techniques are commonly used in the diagnosis of thoracic aortic disease.
- The risk of rupture is negligible in thoracic aneurysms smaller than 4 cm. In the 4- to

  5.9-cm range, the risk rises to 16% at 5 years and to more than 20% with aneurysms larger than 6 cm.
- Patients with degenerative aneurysms confined to the ascending aorta that exceed 5.5 to 6.0 cm in size and who have concomitant aortic regurgitation should undergo replacement of the ascending aort with a synthetic composite graft.
- In patients with Marfan's syndrome

inherited collagen disorders, ascending aortic aneurysms exceeding 5.0 cm in size are enough to warrant prophylactic surgical replacement.

- The threshold for operative intervention in most degenerative types 1, 2, and 3 TAAs and thoracic aneurysms of the descending aorta is 6 cm, after careful consideration of other comorbid conditions.

- Endovascular treatment has been applied in the treatment of localized TAAs in the descending aorta.

REFERENCES

1. Matas R. Surgery of the vascular system. In *Surgery, its principles and practice.* Philadelphia: WB Saunders, 1914.

2. Harrison PW, Chandy J. A subclavian aneurysm cured by cellophane fibrosis. *Ann Surg* 1943;118:478.

3. Gross RE, Bill AHJ, Peirce ECI. Methods for preservation and transplantation of arterial grafts: observations on arterial grafts in dogs: report of transplantation of preserved arterial grafts in 9 human cases. *Surg Gynecol Obstet* 1949;88:689–701.

4. Swan H, Maaske C, Johnson M, et al. Arterial homografts. II. Resection of a thoracic aneurysm using a stored human arterial transplant. *Arch Surg* 1950;61:732–737.

5. Lam CR, Aram HH. Resection of the descending thoracic aorta for aneurysm: a report of the use of a homograft in a case and an experimental study. *Ann Surg* 1951;134:743–752.

6. Debakey ME, Cooley DA. Succesful resection of aneurysm of thoracic aorta and replacement by graft. *JAMA* 1953;152:673–676.

7. Debakey ME, Crawford ES, Cooley DA, et al. Successful resection of fusiform aneurysm of the aortic arch with replacement with homograft. *Surg Gynecol Obstet* 1957;105:657–664.

8. Crawford ES, Crawford JL, Safi H. Thoracoabdominal aortic aneurysms: pre-operative and intraoperative factors determining immediate and long term results. *J Vasc Surg* 1986;3:389–404.

9. Francke U, Furthmayr H. Marfan's syndrome and other disorders of fibrillin. *N Engl J Med* 1994;330:1384–1385.

10. Pereira L, Levran O, Ramirez F, et al. A molecular approach to the stratification of cardiovascular risk in families with Marfan's syndrome. *N Engl J Med* 1994;331:148–153.

11. Milewicz DM, Michael K, Fisher N, et al. Fibrillin-1 (FBN1) mutations in patients with thoracic aortic aneurysms. *Circulation* 1996;94:2708–2711.

12. Pepin M, Schwarze U, Superti-Furga A, et al. Clinical and genetic features of Ehlers-Danlos syndrome type IV, the vascular type. *N Engl J Med* 2000;342:673–680.

13. Goodall S, Crowther M, Hemingway DM, et al. Ubiquitous elevation of matrix metalloproteinase-2 expression in the vasculature of patients with abdominal aneurysms. *Circulation* 2001;104:304–309.

14. Yamashita A, Noma T, Nakazawa A. Enhanced expression of matrix metalloproteinase-9 in abdominal aortic aneurysms. *World J Surg* 2001;25:259–265.

15. Crowther M, Goodall S, Jones JL, et al. Localization of matrix metalloproteinase 2 within the aneurysmal and normal aortic wall. *Br J Surg* 2000;87:1391–1400.

16. Crowther M, Goodall S, Jones JL, et al. Increased matrix metalloproteinase 2 expression in vascular smooth muscle cells cultured from abdominal aortic aneurysms. *J Vasc Surg* 2000;32:575–583.

17. Nollendorfs A, Greiner TC, Nagase H, et al. The expression and localization of membrane type-1 matrix metalloproteinase in human abdominal aortic aneurysms. *J Vasc Surg* 2001;34:316–322.

18. Moore G, Liao S, Curci JA, et al. Suppression of experimental abdominal aortic aneurysms by systemic treatment with a hydroxamate-based matrix metalloproteinase inhibitor (RS 132908). *J Vasc Surg* 1999;29:522–532.

19. Treharne GD, Boyle JR, Goodall S, et al. Marimastat inhibits elastin degradation and matrix metalloproteinase 2 activity in a model of aneurysm disease. *Br J Surg* 1999;86:1053–1058.

20. Thompson RW, Baxter BT. MMP inhibition in abdominal aortic aneurysms. Rationale for a prospective randomized clinical trial. *Ann N Y Acad Sci* 1999;878:159–178.

21. Pyo R, Lee JK, Shipley JM, et al. Targeted gene disruption of matrix metalloproteinase-9 (gelatinase B) suppresses development of experimental abdominal aortic aneurysms. *J Clin Invest* 2000;105:1641–1649.

22. Lindholt JS, Vammen S, Fasting H, et al. The plasma level of matrix metalloproteinase 9 may predict the natural history of small abdominal aortic aneurysms. A preliminary study. *Eur J Vasc Endovasc Surg* 2000;20:281–285.

23. Petersen E, Gineitis A, Wagberg F, et al. Activity of matrix metalloproteinase-2 and -9 in abdominal aortic aneurysms. Relation to size and rupture. *Eur J Vasc Endovasc Surg* 2000;20:457–461.

24. Yin F, Brin K, Ting C, et al. Arterial hemodynamic indexes in Marfan's syndrome. *Circulation* 1989;79:854–862.

25. Prokop EK, Palmer RF, Wheat MW Jr. Hydrodynamic forces in dissecting aneurysms. *In-vitro* studies in a Tygon model and in dog aortas. *Circ Res* 1970;27:121–127.

26. Bickerstaff L, Pairolero P, Hollier L. Thoracic aortic aneurysms: a population based study. *Surgery* 1982;92:1103–1108.

27. Clouse WD, Hallett JW, Schaff HV, et al. Improved prognosis of thoracic aortic aneurysms: a population based study. *JAMA* 1998;280(22):1926–1929.

28. McNamara J, Pressler V. Natural history of arteriosclerotic thoracic aortic aneurysms. *Ann Thorac Surg* 1978;26:468–473.

29. Coselli JS. Thoracoabdominal aneurysms: experience with 372 patients. *J Card Surg.* 1994;9:638–647.

30. Johansson G, Markstrom U, Swedenborg J. Ruptured thoracic aortic aneurysms: a study of incidence and mortality rates. *J Vasc Surg* 1995;21:985–988.

31. Coselli JS, LeMaire SA, Miller CC 3rd, et al. Mortality and paraplegia after thoracoabdominal aortic aneurysm repair: a risk factor analysis. *Ann Thorac Surg* 2000;69:409–414.

32. Svensson LG, Crawford ES, Hess KR. Experience with 1509 patients undergoing thoracoabdominal aortic operations. *J Vasc Surg* 1993;17:357–370.

33. Cambria R, Davison JK, Zannetti S. Thoracoabdominal aneurysm repair: perspectives over a decade with the clamp-and-sew technique. *Ann Surg* 1997;226:294–305.

34. Cesare ED, Giordano AV, Cerone G, et al. Comparative evaluation of TEE, conventional MRI and contrast-enhanced 3D breath-hold MRA in the post-operative follow-up of dissecting aneurysms. *Int J Card Imaging* 2000;16:135–147.

35. Rapezzi C, Rocchi G, Fattori R, et al. Usefulness of transesophageal echocardiographic monitoring to improve the outcome of stent-graft treatment of thoracic aortic aneurysms. *Am J Cardiol* 2001;87:315–319.

36. Jeffrey RB Jr. CT angiography of the abdominal and thoracic aorta. *Semin Ultrasound CT MR* 1998;19:405–412.

37. Coulam CH, Rubin GD. Acute aortic abnormalities. *Semin Roentgenol* 2001;36:148–164.

38. Juvonen T, Ergin M, Galla J. Prospective study of the natural history of thoracic aortic aneurysms. *Ann Thorac Surg* 1997;63:1533–1545.

39. Gott VL, Greene PS, Alejo DE, et al. Replacement of the aortic root in patients with Marfan's syndrome. *N Engl J Med* 1999;340:1307–1313.

40. Shores J, Berger KR, Murphy EA, et al. Progression of aortic dilatation and the benefit of long-term beta-adrenergic blockade in Marfan's syndrome. *N Engl J Med* 1994;330:1335–1341.

41. Safi HJ, Vinnerkvist A, Subramaniam MH, et al. Management of the patient with aortic root disease and aortic insufficiency. *Cardiol Clin* 1998;16:463–75, viii.

42. Bentall H, De Bono A. A technique for complete replacement of the ascending aorta. *Thorax* 1968;23:338–339.

43. David TE. Aortic valve–sparing operations in patients with ascending aortic aneurysms. *Curr Opin Cardiol* 1997;12:391–395.

44. Ergin MA, Galla JD, Lansman SL, et al. Hypothermic circulatory arrest in operations on the thoracic aorta. Determinants of operative mortality and neurologic outcome. *J Thorac Cardiovasc Surg* 1994;107:788–797.

45. Kouchoukos NT. Adjuncts to reduce the incidence of embolic brain injury during operations on the aortic arch. *Ann Thorac Surg* 1994;57:243–245.

46. Kouchoukos NT, Dougenis D. Surgery of the thoracic aorta. *N Engl J Med* 1997;336:1876–1888.

47. Safi HJ, Brien HW, Winter JN, et al. Brain protection via cerebral retrograde perfusion during aortic arch aneurysm repair. *Ann Thorac Surg* 1993;56:270–276.

48. Cambria RP. Thoracoabdominal aneurysms. In: Rutherford R, ed. *Vascular surgery.* Philadelphia: WB Saunders, 2000:1303–1345.

49. Thompson RW, Liao S, Curci JA. Therapeutic potential of tetracycline derivatives to suppress the growth of abdominal aortic aneurysms. *Adv Dent Res* 1998;12:159–165.

50. Coselli JS, Koksoy C, LeMaire SA. Management of thoracic aortic graft infections. *Ann Thorac Surg* 1999;67:1990–1993.

51. Safi HJ, Harlin SA, Miller CC, et al. Predictive factors for acute renal failure in thoracic and thoracoabdominal aortic aneurysm surgery. *J Vasc Surg* 1996;24:338–344.

52. Grabitz K, Sandmann W, Stuhmeier K, et al. The risk of ischemic spinal cord injury in patients undergoing graft replacement for thoracoabdominal aortic aneurysms. *J Vasc Surg* 1996;23:230–240.

53. Savader SJ, Williams GM, Trerotola SO, et al. Preoperative spinal artery localization and its relationship to postoperative neurologic complications. *Radiology* 1993;189:165–171.

54. Svensson LG, Hess KR, Coselli JS, et al. A prospective study of respiratory failure after high-risk surgery on the thoracoabdominal aorta. *J Vasc Surg* 1991;14:271–282.

55. Najibi S, Steinberg J, Katzen BT, et al. Detection of isolated hook fractures 36 months after implantation of the Ancure endograft: a cautionary note. *J Vasc Surg* 2001;34:353–356.

56. Mitchell RS, Dake MD, Sembra CP, et al. Endovascular stent-graft repair of thoracic aortic aneurysms. *J Thorac Cardiovasc Surg* 1996;111:1054–1062.

57. Mitchell RS. Endovascular stent graft repair of thoracic aortic aneurysms. *Semin Thorac Cardiovasc Surg* 1997;9:257–268.

58. Mitchell RS, Miller DC, Dake MD, et al. Thoracic aortic aneurysm repair with an endovascular stent graft: the "first generation." *Ann Thorac Surg* 1999;67:1971–1974.

59. Dake MD, Miller DC, Mitchell RS, et al. The "first generation" of endovascular stent-grafts for patients with aneurysms of the descending thoracic aorta. *J Thorac Cardiovasc Surg* 1998;116:689–703.

60. Bortone AS, Schena S, Mannatrizio G, et al. Endovascular stent-graft treatment for diseases of the descending thoracic aorta. *Eur J Cardiothorac Surg* 2001;20:514–519.

61. Taylor PR, Gaines PA, McGuinness CL, et al. Thoracic aortic stent grafts—early experience from two centres using commercially available devices. *Eur J Vasc Endovasc Surg* 2001;22:70–76.

62. Gott VL, Pyeritz RE, Magovern GJ Jr, et al. Surgical treatment of aneurysms of the ascending aorta in the Marfan syndrome. Results of composite-graft repair in 50 patients. *N Engl J Med* 1986;314:1070–1074.

63. Gott VL, Gillinov AM, Pyeritz RE, et al. Aortic root replacement. Risk factor analysis of a seventeen-year experience with 270 patients. *J Thorac Cardiovasc Sur* 1995;109:536–544.

64. Marsalese DL, Moodie DS, Vacante M, et al. [Mar]fan's syndrome: natural history and long-ter[m] up of cardiovascular involvement. *J Am C* 1989;14:422–428.

65. Svensson LG, Crawford ES, Hess KR

valve graft replacement of the proximal aorta: comparison of techniques in 348 patients. *Ann Thorac Surg* 1992;54:427–437.

66. Cohn LH, Rizzo RJ, Adams DH, et al. Reduced mortality and morbidity for ascending aortic aneurysm resection regardless of cause. *Ann Thorac Surg* 1996;62:463–468.

67. Savunen T, Inberg M, Niinikoski J, et al. Composite graft in annulo-aortic ectasia. Nineteen years' experience without graft inclusion. *Eur J Cardiothorac Surg* 1996;10:428–432.

68. Aoyagi S, Kosuga K, Akashi H, et al. Aortic root replacement with a composite graft: results of 69 operations in 66 patients. *Ann Thorac Surg* 1994;58:1469–1475.

69. Kouchoukos NT, Marshall WG, Wedige-Stecher TA. Eleven-year experience with composite graft replacement of the ascending aorta and aortic valve. *J Thorac Cardiovasc Surg* 1986;92:691–705.

70. Finkbohner R, Johnston D, Crawford ES, et al. Marfan syndrome. Long-term survival and complications after aortic aneurysm repair. *Circulation* 1995;91:728–733.

71. Lewis CT, Cooley DA, Murphy MC, et al. Surgical repair of aortic root aneurysms in 280 patients. *Ann Thorac Surg* 1992;53:38–45.

72. Cabrol C, Pavie A, Mesnildrey P, et al. Long-term results with total replacement of the ascending aorta and reimplantation of the coronary arteries. *J Thorac Cardiovasc Surg* 1986;91:17–25.

73. Verdant A, Cossette R, Page A, et al. Aneurysms of the descending thoracic aorta: three hundred sixty-six consecutive cases resected without paraplegia. *J Vasc Surg* 1995;21:385–390.

74. Borst HG, Jurmann M, Buhner B, et al. Risk of replacement of descending aorta with a standardized left heart bypass technique. *J Thorac Cardiovasc Surg* 1994;107:126–32.

75. Scheinin SA, Cooley DA. Graft replacement of the descending thoracic aorta: results of "open" distal anastomosis. *Ann Thorac Surg* 1994;58:19–22.

76. Kouchoukos NT, Rokkas CK. Descending thoracic and thoracoabdominal aortic surgery for aneurysm or dissection: how do we minimize the risk of spinal cord injury?. *Semin Thorac Cardiovasc Surg* 1993;5:47–54.

77. Hines GL, Busutil S. Thoraco-abdominal aneurysm resection. Determinants of survival in a community hospital. *J Cardiovasc Surg* 1994;35:243–246.

30

Aortic Dissection

Peter G. Hagan, G. Michael Deeb, David S. Williams, and Kim A. Eagle

USUAL CAUSES

Acute aortic dissection is considered the most common acute process involving the aorta that necessitates surgery, even more common than ruptured aortic aneurysm (1,2). Although dissection may develop within an aneurysm and rupture may occur as a complication of dissection, aneurysm and dissection are separate entities that must be clearly distinguished. Dissection of the aorta is classified as type A (proximal) if the ascending aorta is involved or type B (distal) if it occurs beyond the left subclavian artery (3). Separation of the layers of the aortic wall is characteristic and results in the development of a false lumen or channel. Blood enters the intima media space, and further propagation of the dissection may occur in an antegrade or retrograde manner or both. Communication between the true and false lumina may occur via one or more intimal tears. Intramural hematoma (IMH) without an intimal tear is now recognized as a distinct pathologic lesion that is believed to result from hemorrhage of the vasa vasorum and occurs more frequently in the distal aorta (4). IMH may be the initiating event in patients with cystic medial necrosis. Atherosclerotic plaque may ulcerate, which leads to intramural hemorrhage or frank dissection. Typically, penetrating aortic ulcer is a localized lesion of the descending thoracic and abdominal aorta (5). Most patients with aortic dissection have a structural abnormality of the arterial wall, evidence of systemic hypertension, or both (2,6). Several predisposing factors are seen in aortic dissection (Table 30.1). A history of hypertension is documented in the majority of patients and is present in more than 70% of patients with distal dissection (7). Men are more commonly affected than women in a ratio of approximately 2:1, and the incidence of aortic dissection increases with advancing age. Abnormal connective tissue within the aortic wall predisposes patients with Marfan's syndrome and other connective tissue disorders to aneurysm formation and dissection at a much younger age. Dissection should always be suspected in any patient with Marfan's syndrome who has chest, back, or abdominal pain. Similarly, many patients with bicuspid aortic valve have abnormal connective tissue in the aortic wall. As many as one in five patients presenting with acute dissection may have a history of prior or recent cardiac surgery (7). The dissection may result from shared risk factors (advanced age, hypertension, cigarette smoking, vascular disease) and trauma from surgical instrumentation or catheterization of the aorta. Dissection or disruption of the aorta secondary to chest trauma is most often located in the region of the left subclavian artery, where the aorta is relatively fixed by the ligamentum arteriosum (8). Acute aortic dissection has been reported to occur in rare instances during pregnancy, in certain inflammatory disorders, and as a result of cocaine and amphetamine usage.

PRESENTING SYMPTOMS AND SIGNS

Because dissection is a dynamic process that may occur throughout the course of the aorta and because perfusion to any organ system may be compromised, patients present with a broad range of symptoms (Table 30.2). The characteristic feature of acute aortic dissection is the abrupt onset of severe pain, typically in the chest, back, or both. Often the patient can pinpoint the onset of symptoms with "freeze-frame" accuracy. Although a tearing or ripping sensation is an obvious clue, patients are more likely to describe the quality of the pain of aortic dissection as sharp in

TABLE 30.1. *Factors predisposing to aortic dissection*

Advanced age
Hypertension
Male gender
Prior or recent cardiac surgery or aortic catheterization
Trauma
Marfan's syndrome
Connective tissue disorder
Bicuspid aortic valve and/or coarctation of the aorta
Pregnancy
Cocaine or amphetamine use

nature (7). Pain is most often located in the upper back, anterior chest, or upper abdomen.

Migration of pain, another suggestive symptom, appears to be less common than previously thought. Pain may not be part of the presenting symptoms at all, especially in patients presenting with neurologic deficits secondary to stroke. Syncope is a less common but well-described presenting symptom of aortic dissection. Most patients with aortic dissection and syncope have other neurologic or clinical findings, which are useful in suggesting the diagnosis. However, a small percentage of patients present with syncope alone. This implies that aortic dissection should be considered in the differential diagnosis of unexplained syncope, especially in the population at increased risk: the elderly and those with a history of hypertension. Patients may present with clinical features of shock if dissection has resulted in cardiac tamponade or blood loss.

Cardiac failure may be the predominant clinical feature, especially in the presence of aortic regurgitation or myocardial ischemia. Arterial compromise may be caused by direct obstruction by the dissection flap, displacement of the true lumen by the false lumen, or thromboembolic occlusion. This may result in the clinical presentation of gastrointestinal, renal, limb, or spinal cord ischemia. In rare cases, extrinsic compression from the aorta results in hoarseness, dysphagia, or superior vena cava syndrome. Often, pain resolves for a period shortly after the initial presentation, which creates a false sense of the patient's stability. Recurrent pain may herald propagation or extension of dissection.

The physical examination findings are often unremarkable. Classic physical findings such as a pulse deficit or aortic regurgitation murmur are helpful clues but usually absent (7). A pulse deficit is recorded in fewer than 20% of all patients and may be transient if the dissection flap obstructs the arterial ostium intermittently. The murmur of aortic regurgitation is noted in fewer than half of patients with type A dissection (7). The murmur of acute aortic regurgitation may be faint, and other peripheral findings of chronic severe regurgitation, such as wide pulse pressure, are frequently absent. Pleural effusions may be present as a reactive phenomenon or as a result of hemorrhage into the pleural space.

Blood pressure at presentation is highly variable. Hypertension is more common in patients

TABLE 30.2. *Comparison of clinical features between patients with proximal (type A) and distal (type B) acute aortic dissection*

Category	Type A: % present of A	Type B: % present of B	p (A vs. B)
Total patients	289 (62.3%)	175 (37.7%)	—
Mean age (years)	61.2	66.3	<0.0001
Prior history of hypertension	69.3%	76.7%	0.086
Prior cardiac surgery	15.9%	21.1%	0.16
Presenting history			
Anterior chest pain	71.0%	44.1%	<0.001
Back pain	46.6%	63.8%	<0.001
Abdominal pain	21.6%	42.7%	<0.001
Syncope	12.7%	4.1%	0.002
Hypertensive (SBP $\geq$ 150 mm HG)	35.7%	70.1%	<0.001
Mean length of hospital stay (days)	24.1	22.0	0.19

SPB, systolic blood pressure.
Adapted from Hagan PG, Nienaber CA, Isselbacher EM, et al. The International Registry of Acute Aortic Dissection: new insights into an old disease. *JAMA* 2000;283:897–903.

with type B (distal) dissection. Hypotension or shock suggests a serious complication such as rupture or pericardial tamponade and carries a poor prognosis. Presenting features of IMH and penetrating aortic ulcer appear to be similar to those of classic aortic dissection, and progression to classic dissection with intimal tear may occur (5,9).

HELPFUL TESTS

Immediate confirmation of the diagnosis and urgent institution of appropriate therapy are essential (Table 20.3). In addition to being the most frequently encountered acute aortic pathologic process, dissection is important because serious complications develop rapidly. The chest radiograph has traditionally been considered helpful in the initial evaluation of suspected aortic dissection (10). Although a widened mediastinum and an abnormal aortic contour may be suggestive of the diagnosis, they are nonspecific and are absent in more than 10% of patients. With the widespread availability of safe, rapid, and accurate noninvasive imaging techniques, chest radiography should have a limited role in the evaluation of suspected dissection. A normal chest radiograph should not dissuade the clinician from further investigation. Differentiating the pain of aortic dissection from myocardial ischemia is a common clinical dilemma. The presence of a normal ECG in the setting of acute chest pain may lead clinicians away from a diagnosis of myocardial ischemia and toward

TABLE 30.3. *Role of imaging*

Confirmation
    Diagnosis: dissection, IMH, penetrating ulcer
    Location
    Extent
    Intimal tear/communication
Identification
    True lumen
    False lumen thrombosis
    Branch vessel involvement
    Extraaortic extension
    Pericardial effusion
Assessment
    Aortic valve
    LV function

IMH, intramural hematoma; LV, left ventricular.

one of dissection (11,12). However, dissection and myocardial ischemia may occur together, and the electrocardiogram at presentation most often shows nonspecific ST/T wave abnormalities. Thus, the electrocardiogram is frequently unhelpful in the differential diagnosis (7). Laboratory studies are nonspecific and generally unhelpful in the differential diagnosis of aortic dissection. The development of a biochemical assay involving the use of a monoclonal antibody to smooth muscle myosin has been reported to be a rapid and accurate marker in a small number of Japanese patients with acute dissection. Further investigation is under way to determine its role in a larger population (13).

Several accurate imaging modalities are widely available to confirm the presence of aortic dissection. The method of choice in any given center depends on the individual patient, local expertise, and availability. With the advent of multiple noninvasive modalities, the role of aortography has diminished. Previously the gold standard, aortography is performed in fewer than 5% of patients and mainly as a second- or third-line evaluation. Aortography is invasive and time consuming, requires use of potentially nephrotoxic radiocontrast agents, provides limited information regarding cardiac structure and function, and may not detect dissection with false lumen thrombosis or IMH. Advantages of aortography include its ability to assess branch vessel and coronary artery involvement and false lumen hemodynamics, and endovascular therapy with fenestration or stent implantation may be performed during the same procedure. In addition, aortography may be superior to other modalities in detecting localized tears. Overall sensitivity and specificity have been reported at 88% and 94%, respectively (14). Intravascular ultrasonography has been reported to have sensitivity and specificity approaching 100% and is helpful in determining the extent of dissection and branch vessel involvement, and in distinguishing true and false lumina (15). Although intravascular ultrasonography is invasive and its availability may be limited, it is an ideal adjunct to aortography, especially when the clinical suspicion is high and aortography fails to detect an abnormality.

Although the overall sensitivity and specificity of computed tomography (CT), transesophageal echocardiography (TEE), and magnetic resonance imaging (MRI) are excellent, there are advantages and drawbacks to each modality in any given situation; therefore, no technique is uniformly superior to the others. Knowledge of the limitations of each method is important so that the appropriate imaging study may be ordered.

CT is accurate, is widely available, allows visualization of the abdominal aorta, and is the most commonly used initial imaging modality (7,14). With the development of helical CT, its sensitivity appears greater than 95%, and its specificity approaches 100%. Location, extent, and branch vessel involvement can be determined. However, small tears may be missed, and cardiac and aortic valve function cannot be evaluated.

The sensitivity and specificity of TEE are similar to those of CT, and TEE can be performed quickly at the bedside with minimal risk to the patient (16–18). Sensitivity and specificity for multiplane TEE are greater than 90%. Diagnostic difficulty typically occurs in the distal ascending aorta, where there may be a "blind spot" or reverberation artifact that may mimic a dissection flap. M-mode echocardiographic imaging during TEE may be helpful in distinguishing artifact by demonstrating that its motion is parallel to the suspected source and that the image is located at a predictable distance from another structure, such as the aortic or tracheal wall (19). Information regarding the location and extent of dissection, false lumen patency, branch vessel involvement, sites of intimal tear, valvular regurgitation, pericardial hemorrhage, and ventricular function can be obtained in less than a half hour by TEE. Relative cost is low, and risk to the patient is minimal. TEE can also be performed in the operating room to evaluate aortic valve function and assess lumen flow (20). Favorable outcomes in patients who undergo imaging with TEE alone have been reported, and a decision analysis to compare diagnostic techniques concluded that the use of TEE as an initial modality yielded the best outcomes (21,22). We favor TEE because it can be performed quickly in the emergency department with continuous monitoring of

the patient by the physician. A limited transthoracic echocardiogram is helpful in the unstable patient or immediately before TEE to evaluate for the presence of pericardial fluid, left ventricular function, and aortic regurgitation. Occasionally, the dissection flap may be visualized on a transthoracic echocardiogram if the aortic root is involved.

Despite the high sensitivity and specificity of MRI and its superior ability to evaluate arch vessel involvement, it is rarely used (<2%) as an initial diagnostic modality (7,23). Lack of availability, time delay to perform the study, restricted ability to monitor unstable patients during imaging, and incompatibility with metal devices are likely explanations for its limited use. Fast MRI with contrast enhancement enables imaging of the entire aorta in minutes (24). Images may be reformatted in any plane to assess location of intimal tears as well as branch vessel involvement. Because MRI also has excellent sensitivity and specificity, it is likely to become a more popular initial choice, especially in more stable patients.

Most patients undergo more than one imaging study during the evaluation. Frequently, the first study shows aortic abnormalities that are indicative of an acute aortic syndrome but not diagnostic. A second study is thus needed.

DIFFERENTIAL DIAGNOSIS

Because clinical manifestations are diverse and classical signs are often absent, a high clinical index of suspicion is necessary in order to diagnose aortic dissection. The differential diagnosis is extremely broad, and the diagnosis is frequently delayed or missed at presentation. Aortic dissection should be considered in the differential diagnosis of sudden unexplained hypoperfusion to any organ system.

Symptoms may result from several pathophysiologic mechanisms. Separation of the aortic layers typically results in pain that may be felt throughout the chest or abdomen and even to the neck and arms. Some patients develop symptoms of a vasovagal response. Perfusion to any organ may be compromised by hypotension, arterial obstruction by the dissection, or embolization. In rare cases, obstruction or compression of extraaortic structures such as the esophagus or superior vena cava, as outlined previously, may occur. Aortic dissection may mimic a variety of more common and serious conditions such as myocardial ischemia, stroke, pulmonary embolism, and cardiac tamponade. A common clinical dilemma is distinguishing aortic dissection from an acute coronary syndrome. Because appropriate therapy for the latter (thrombolysis/ antiplatelet agents) may be catastrophic in a patient with dissection, accurate diagnosis is essential. Dissection and myocardial infarction may occur together, as the dissection flap obstructs the coronary ostia, more commonly the right coronary artery.

COMPLICATIONS

Because of the diagnostic difficulty and the threat of impending catastrophic complications, aortic dissection is among the most challenging emergencies encountered in clinical practice. Serious complications develop quickly, and the early mortality rate is up to 1% per hour (2). Early death is commonly due to aortic rupture. Rupture may extend into the pericardial sac, causing tamponade, or into the mediastinum or pleural space, resulting in exsanguination. The tear may occlude any of the branches of the aorta at their origins. This may result in coronary ischemia or cerebral malperfusion if the carotid artery is involved. Other vessels may be involved, leading to celiac and mesenteric ischemia, lower extremity ischemia, or renal artery occlusion; less commonly, spinal arteries may be compromised. Multiorgan system failure and aortic rupture are the commonest acute causes of death (7).

THERAPY

Whenever acute aortic dissection is suspected, rapid confirmation of the diagnosis, institution of therapy, and urgent referral for specialist evaluation are essential. Patient preference should be addressed early in the evaluation. Some patients may choose not to pursue further therapy, especially if invasive in nature, because of advanced age and significant comorbidity.

The goal of medical therapy is to control blood pressure and the rate of change of pressure over time (dP/dT) while maintaining peripheral perfusion. A short-acting beta blocker such as esmolol in combination with sodium nitroprusside is typically administered in an intensive care setting. Intraarterial blood pressure monitoring is recommended, and blood pressure should be checked in both arms, to avoid misguided therapy. Endotracheal intubation and mechanical ventilation may be necessary in the unstable patient. Hypotension suggests a serious complication such as cardiac tamponade or rupture. Many patients may suffer, and poorly tolerate, blood loss and intravascular volume depletion. Pericardiocentesis may be harmful in the presence of tamponade caused by type A dissection (25).

Appropriate fluid replacement should be administered in a monitored setting.

Patients with type A dissection should be referred for urgent surgical evaluation. The type of surgery performed depends on the size of the aorta, the condition of the aortic valve, and the presence of coronary artery involvement. Of the International Registry of Acute Aortic Dissection (IRAD) patients with type A dissection, 28% did not undergo surgery, mostly because of advanced age, comorbid medical conditions, patient refusal, IMH, and death before the planned date of surgery (7). Patients who have survived several days after onset of dissection, the initial extremely high-risk period, may undergo semielective surgery (26).

Most stable patients with type B dissection can be successfully treated without surgical intervention. Features that suggest surgical therapy may be warranted for type B dissection include increased aortic diameter (typically, more than 5 cm), organ malperfusion, progression of dissection, subacute rupture or leakage, persistent pain, and persistent hypertension (16).

Currently, the optimal therapy for IMH is unknown. Until the natural history is better understood, it seems reasonable to treat in a manner similar to that for classic dissection.

Percutaneous Therapy

Percutaneous management of acute dissection is being performed more frequently either as an alternative to surgery or as a temporizing measure before operation (27–31).

The objective of endovascular stent graft placement is to stabilize the aorta by sealing the entry tear and promoting thrombosis of the false lumen. Custom-designed endovascular stent placement across the primary entry tear in dissections originating in the descending aorta with or without extension to the ascending aorta has been shown to be technically feasible with promising results in a small number of patients monitored for a relatively short period of time. Stent graft placement is often associated with shrinkage and thrombosis of the false lumen, which may translate into a lower risk of subsequent aneurysm formation, a common long-term complication of dissection. Although the technical support and skills required to implant a custom-made stent are currently limited, endovascular stent placement is a promising alternative to standard therapy.

Fenestration involves perforating the intimal flap that divides the true and false lumina in multiple areas, thereby equalizing pressure and potentially restoring blood flow to arteries being supplied by a compromised lumen. The rate of complications from percutaneous fenestration procedures appears to be low. Many patients show hemodynamic and symptomatic response, which may obviate the need for immediate surgery or improve the clinical status sufficiently to stabilize the patient and reduce the operative risk to an acceptable level. In some cases, a repeat procedure or stent implantation may be necessary for complete relief of obstruction. Fewer than 5% of patients treated at tertiary referral centers currently undergo percutaneous intervention for acute aortic dissection (7). Percutaneous therapy is likely to play a greater role in the management of aortic dissection as materials, technique, and availability improve and as subgroups of patients who benefit from these procedures are identified.

PROGNOSIS

Despite the widespread availability of accurate imaging modalities and advances in surgical and percutaneous therapies, the overall rate of in-hospital mortality from acute aortic dissection remains nearly 30% (Fig. 30.1) (7).

The in-hospital mortality rate among IRAD patients with type A dissection not undergoing surgical therapy was 58%, as opposed to 26% among those undergoing surgical therapy. Death is most often due to aortic rupture and/or multiorgan system failure resulting from malperfusion and cardiac tamponade. Patients with type B dissection who do not require surgical therapy have an in-hospital mortality rate of approximately 10% with effective medical therapy. The mortality rate is approximately 30% among type B patients who require surgery, usually for extension of dissection or organ malperfusion. As in patients with type A dissection, aortic rupture and visceral ischemia are the common causes of death.

FOLLOW-UP

Management of the postacute phase should include stringent blood pressure monitoring and control with a target of less than 120/80 mm HG. Routine follow-up imaging of all patients, typically at 1-, 3-, 6-, and then 12-month intervals, depending on the situation, is recommended because of the risk of recurrence or progression of dissection and aortic enlargement (16). It is generally accepted that patients with uncomplicated type B aortic dissection do well when maximally treated through medical control of blood pressure and heart rate along with close follow-up. However, the optimal long-term management is debated. Most clinicians monitor for symptoms that suggest progression or for enlargement of the aorta by serial imaging. Unfortunately, operation in the chronic phase of dissection is often complicated by extended surgery because of the need to reconstruct vessels and the narrowed true lumen along with frequently encountered adhesions to surrounding tissue. Patients with a maximal aortic diameter of 40 mm or larger and a patent false lumen appear to have a high incidence of aortic enlargement during the chronic phase (32). Surgery or percutaneous stent placement in the early chronic phase may be recommended for these patients. If the aortic diameter is smaller than 40 mm and the false lumen thrombosed,

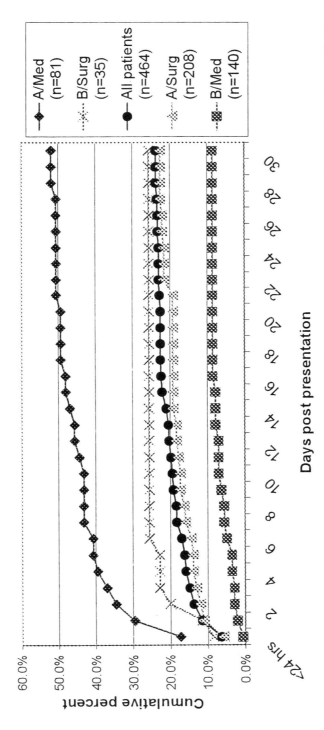

FIG. 30.1. Thirty-day mortality rate among 464 patients with acute aortic dissection by type and management. (Adapted from Hagan PG, Nienaber CA, Isselbacher EM, et al. The International Registry of Acute Aortic Dissection (IRAD): new insights into an old disease. *JAMA* 2000;283:897–903.)

then the risk of enlargement over 10-year follow-up appears to be low. In asymptomatic patients with Marfan's syndrome, prophylactic surgery should be considered when the tubular aorta measures more than 5 cm, especially if there is a family history of dissection or associated significant aortic regurgitation or if a female patient is planning pregnancy (33). Beta blocker therapy has been shown to decrease the rate of aortic enlargement and the incidence of cardiovascular events in Marfan's syndrome (34).

Late death after dissection is often caused by an additional aortic event such as rupture or extension, but it also may result from other associated cardiovascular diseases (35,36). This highlights the need for coronary risk factor assessment and modification in all patients. A multidisciplinary approach is necessary from the time of presentation because comorbidity is common, and the role of medical, surgical, and percutaneous therapy needs to be considered for each patient.

PRACTICAL POINTS

- Presentation is variable; a high clinical index of suspicion is necessary.
- Classic symptoms and signs are often absent.
- The diagnosis should be confirmed and therapy instituted rapidly.

- The majority of patients with type B dissection may be managed medically.
- Strict blood pressure control is necessary during the acute and chronic phases.
- Cardiovascular risk factors must be controlled in all patients.

REFERENCES

1. Pretre R, Von Segesser LK. Aortic dissection. *Lancet* 1997;349:1461–1464.
2. Bickerstaff LK, Pairolero PC, Hollier LH, et al. Thoracic aortic aneurysms: a population-based study. *Surgery* 1982;92:1103–1108.
3. Daily PO, Trueblood HW, Stinson EB, et al. Management of acute aortic dissections. *Ann Thorac Surg* 1970;10:237–247.
4. Nienaber CA, von Kodolitsch Y, Petersen B, et al. Intramural hemorrhage of the thoracic aorta. Diagnostic and therapeutic implications. *Circulation* 1995;92:1465–1472.
5. O'Gara PT, DeSanctis RW. Acute aortic dissection and its variants. Toward a common diagnostic and therapeutic approach. *Circulation* 1995;92:1376–1378.
6. Roberts WC. Aortic dissection: anatomy, consequences and causes. *Am Heart J* 1981;101:195–214.
7. Hagan PG, Nienaber CA, Isselbacher EM, et al. The International Registry of Acute Aortic Dissection (IRAD): new insights into an old disease. *JAMA* 2000;283:897–903.
8. Parmley LF, Mattingly TW, Manion WC, et al. Nonpenetrating traumatic injury of the aorta. *Circulation* 1958;17:1086–1101.
9. Yamada T, Tada S, Harada J. Aortic dissection without intimal rupture: diagnosis with MR imaging and CT. *Radiology* 1988;168:347–352.
10. Earnest F IV, Muhm JR, Sheedy PF II. Roentgenographic findings in thoracic aortic dissection. *Mayo Clin Proc* 1979;54:43–50.
11. Eagle KA, DeSanctis RW. Aortic dissection. *Curr Probl Cardiol* 1989;14:225–278.
12. Slater EE, DeSanctis R. The clinical recognition of dissecting aortic aneurysm. *Am J Med* 1976;60:625–633.
13. Suzuki T, Katoh H, Watanabe M, et al. Novel biochemical diagnostic method for aortic dissection. Results of a prospective study using an immunoassay of smooth muscle myosin heavy chain. *Circulation* 1996;93:1244–1249.
14. Erbel R, Engberding R, Daniel W, et al. Echocardiography in diagnosis of aortic dissection. *Lancet* 1989;1:457–461.
15. Yamada E, Matsumura M, Kyo S, et al. Usefulness of a prototype intravascular ultrasound imaging in evaluation of aortic dissection and comparison with angiographic study, transesophageal echocardiography, computed tomography, and magnetic resonance imaging. *Am J Cardiol* 1995;75:161–165.
16. Diagnosis and management of aortic dissection. Recommendations of the Task Force on Aortic Dissection, European Society of Cardiology. *Eur Heart J* 2001;22:1642–1681.
17. Keren A, Kim CB, Hu BS, et al. Accuracy of biplane

and multiplane transesophageal echocardiography in diagnosis of typical acute aortic dissection and intramural hematoma. *J Am Coll Cardiol* 1996;28:627–636.

18. Sommer T, Fehske W, Holzkuecht N, et al. Aortic dissection: a comparative study of diagnosis with spiral CT, multiplanar transesophageal echocardiography and MR imaging. *Radiology* 1996;199:347–352.

19. Evangelista A, Garcia del Castillo H, Gonzalez-Alujas T, et al. Diagnosis of ascending aortic dissection by transesophageal echocardiography: utility of M-mode in recognizing artifacts. *J Am Coll Cardiol* 1996;27:102–107.

20. Simon P, Owen AN, Havel M, et al. Transesophageal echocardiography in the emergency surgical management of patients with aortic dissection. *J Thorac Cardiovasc Surg* 1992;103:1113–1117.

21. Adachi H, Omoto R, Kyo S, et al. Emergency surgical intervention of acute aortic dissection with rapid diagnosis by transesophageal echocardiography. *Circulation* 1991;84(Suppl III):III-14–III-19.

22. Banning AB, Masani ND, Ikram S, et al. Transesophageal echocardiography as the sole diagnostic investigation in patients with suspected thoracic aortic dissection. *Br Heart J* 1994;72:461–465.

23. Nienaber CA, von Kodolitsch Y, Nicolas V, et al. The diagnosis of thoracic aortic dissection by noninvasive imaging procedures. *N Engl J Med* 1993;328:1–9.

24. Prince MR, Narasimham DL, Jacoby WT, et al. Three-dimensional gadolinium-enhanced MR angiography of the thoracic aorta. *Am J Roentgenol* 1996;166:1387–1397.

25. Isselbacher EM, Cigarroa JE, Eagle KA. Cardiac tamponade complicating proximal aortic dissection. Is pericardiocentesis harmful? *Circulation* 1994;90:2375–2378.

26. Scholl FG, Coady MA, Davies R, et al. Interval or permanent nonoperative management of acute type A dissection. *Arch Surg* 1999;134:402–406.

27. Williams DM, Brothers TE, Messina LM. Relief of mesenteric ischemia in type III aortic dissection with percutaneous fenestration of the aortic septum. *Radiology* 1990;174:450–452.

28. Nienaber CA, Fattori R, Lund G, et al. Nonsurgical reconstruction of thoracic aortic dissection by stent graft placement. *N Engl J Med* 1999;340:1539–1545.

29. Dake MD, Kato N, Mitchell RS, et al. Endovascular stent-graft placement for the treatment of acute aortic dissection. *N Engl J Med* 1999;340:1546–1552.

30. Chavan A, Hausmann D, Dresler C, et al. Intravascular ultrasound-guided percutaneous fenestration of the intimal flap in the dissected aorta. *Circulation* 1997;96:2124–2127.

31. Deeb GM, Williams DM, Bolling SF, et al. Surgical delay for acute type A dissection with malperfusion. *Ann Thorac Surg* 1997;64:1669–1675.

32. Marui A, Takaaki M, Norimasa M, et al. Toward the best treatment for uncomplicated patients with Type B acute aortic dissection: a consideration for sound surgical indication. *Circulation* 1999;100(Suppl II):II-275–II-280.

33. Treasure T. Elective replacement of the aortic root in Marfan's syndrome. *Br Heart J* 1993;69:101–102.

34. Shores J, Berger KR, Murphy EA, et al. Progression of aortic dilatation and the benefit of long-term beta-adrenergic blockade in Marfan's syndrome. *N Engl J Med* 1994;330:1335–1341.

35. DeSanctis RW, Doroghazi RM, Austen WG, et al. Aortic dissection. *N Engl J Med* 1987;317:1060–1066.

36. Glower DD, Fann JI, Speier RH, et al. Comparisons of medical and surgical therapy for uncomplicated descending aortic dissection. *Circulation* 1990;82(Suppl IV):IV-39–IV-46.

31

Cerebrovascular Disease

Susan L. Hickenbottom, Gilbert R. Upchurch, Jr., and James C. Stanley

EPIDEMIOLOGY AND USUAL CAUSES OF CEREBROVASCULAR DISEASE

Stroke is a clinical syndrome characterized by rapidly developing signs or symptoms, or both, of focal neurologic dysfunction with no obvious cause other than vascular origin. Therefore, stroke includes both ischemic and hemorrhagic vascular cerebrovascular events. *Transient ischemic attack* (TIA) is an abrupt, focal loss of neurologic function caused by temporary ischemia, classically defined as lasting less than 24 hours. However, modern imaging techniques have demonstrated that deficits lasting more than a few hours usually result in irreversible cerebral infarction and that most TIAs typically last less than 15 minutes (1). For the same reason, the term *reversible ischemic neurologic deficit* (RIND), referring to symptoms lasting more than 24 hours but less than 7 days, has been abandoned. The colloquial term *cerebrovascular accident* (CVA) is also considered outdated, as it implies a fortuitous origin, while stroke is usually caused by a well-defined etiopathogenic mechanism.

In 1998, the American Heart Association (AHA) estimated that more than 600,000 strokes and 160,000 deaths from stroke occurred in the United States, which makes stroke the third leading killer of Americans and the leading cause of long-term disability among adults (2). More recently, a multiracial study performed in the Cincinnati metropolitan area found that more than 730,000 first-ever and recurrent strokes occur each year in this country (3). Approximately 85% of strokes are ischemic, 10% are caused by parenchymal intracerebral hemorrhage (ICH), and 5% are secondary to subarachnoid hemorrhage (SAH).

Caring for patients with stroke is an expensive undertaking. In 1998, the AHA estimated the to-

tal annual cost for stroke in the United States to be more than $43 billion (2). This estimate included $28.3 billion for direct costs of stroke, such as costs for hospital and acute rehabilitation admission, nursing home care, physician and other health professionals' services, drugs, home health care, and medical durable equipment, and $16 billion for indirect costs, attributable to lost patient wages and productivity.

Stroke is not a single disease process but a heterogeneous group of disorders with similar clinical presentation, and thus stroke can have many different underlying causes. The usual causes of ischemic stroke are outlined in Table 31.1. As with ischemic cardiovascular disease, the most common cause of ischemic cerebrovascular disease is atherosclerosis. Risk factors for ischemic stroke include increasing age, male gender, positive family history of cardiovascular or cerebrovascular disease, hypertension, diabetes, hyperlipidemia, cigarette smoking, atrial fibrillation, carotid artery stenosis, and history of stroke, TIA, or myocardial infarction (4). Other potential risk factors include excessive alcohol intake, sedentary lifestyle, hyperhomocystinemia, hereditary or acquired hypercoagulable states, and obstructive sleep apnea. The usual causes of hemorrhagic stroke (both ICH and SAH) are presented in Table 31.2.

Of course, the most likely cause of stroke in a given patient depends on the patient's age, race, and ethnicity and the spectrum of risk factors. In addition, more than one cause of stroke may be present in the same patient.

PRESENTING SIGNS AND SYMPTOMS

The presenting signs and symptoms of stroke are entirely dependent on the location of brain tissue

TABLE 31.1. *Usual causes of ischemic stroke*

Large-artery atherothromboembolism (~50%)
Thrombosis *in situ*
Artery-to-artery embolism
Small-vessel atherothromboembolism (~15%)
"Lacunar" disease associated with hypertension and
  diabetes
Cardioembolism (~25%)
High risk
  Nonvalvular atrial fibrillation
  Rheumatic heart disease
  Prosthetic cardiac valves
  Infective endocarditis
Moderate risk
  Post–myocardial infarction
  Aortic arch atheroma
  Dilated cardiomyopathy
  Patent foramen ovale/atrial septal aneurysm
Other, less common causes (~10%)
Arterial dissection
Arteritis, including primary angiitis of the central
  nervous system and arteritis associated with
  underlying infectious or immune diseases
Arteropathies, including fibromuscular dysplasia,
  moyamoya disease
Hereditary or acquired hypercoaguable states,
  including polycythemia vera, disseminated
  intravascular coagulation, thrombotic
  thrombocytopenic purpura, dysfibrinogenemia,
  antiphospholipid antibody syndrome, sickle cell
  disease, factor V Leiden mutation, prothrombin
  20210 mutation, protein C/ protein S deficiency,
  antithrombin III deficiency

TABLE 31.2. *Usual causes of hemorrhagic stroke*

Intracerebral hemorrhage (10%)
  Hypertension (>60%)
  Bleeding diathesis (5%–20%)
  Vascular malformation (4%–8%)
  Aneurysm (3%–4%)
  Neoplasm (2%–7%)
  Other causes: cerebral amyloid angiopathy,
    drug-related, cerebral venous occlusive disease,
    hemorrhagic transformation of ischemic arterial
    infarction, arteritis/arteropathies, trauma, after
    carotid endarterectomy or other neurosurgical
    procedures, postmyelography
Subarachnoid hemorrhage (5%)
  Trauma
  Aneurysm (80%–90% of nontraumatic
    subarachnoid hemarrhage)
  Other causes: vascular malformation, arterial
    dissection, drug-related, cerebral venous
    occlusive disease, bleeding diathesis,
    arteritis/arteropathies

involved in the vascular process. Figures 31.1 and 31.2 provide a review of the extracranial and intracranial vascular anatomy involved in cerebrovascular circulation. Figure 31.3 outlines the vascular territories of the cerebral circulation. Stroke syndromes have classically been divided into anterior and posterior circulation distributions, on the basis of presenting signs and symptoms, and furthered subdivided according to the presumed arterial involvement referable to the signs and symptoms. These arterial syndromes and their typical signs and symptoms are outlined in Table 31.3.

Although stroke signs and symptoms are helpful in localizing the stroke to a specific region of the brain or arterial territory, it is important to remember that the clinical presentation typically does not provide any information about stroke etiology. Headache, vomiting, and decreased level of consciousness are somewhat more common with hemorrhagic stroke, but ischemic stroke can present with similar symptoms, especially if the vertebrobasilar arterial system is involved or if a hemispheric stroke is large enough to cause mass effect and increased intracranial pressure. Likewise, thrombotic and embolic strokes cannot be distinguished from each other merely on the basis of presenting signs and symptoms alone.

DIFFERENTIAL DIAGNOSIS AND HELPFUL TESTS FOR THE DIAGNOSIS OF STROKE

Differential Diagnosis of Stroke

The differential diagnosis of stroke includes various other neurologic and medical entities. Keys to distinguishing stroke from other diagnoses include its acute onset (as opposed to subacute onset or chronic progression) and the focality of the presenting neurologic signs and symptoms. In most cases, the correct diagnosis can be established by careful history documentation, physical examination, and diagnostic testing. More recently, however, it has become especially important to be able to diagnose acute ischemic stroke (AIS) rapidly and accurately since the U.S. Food and Drug Administration (FDA) approved the

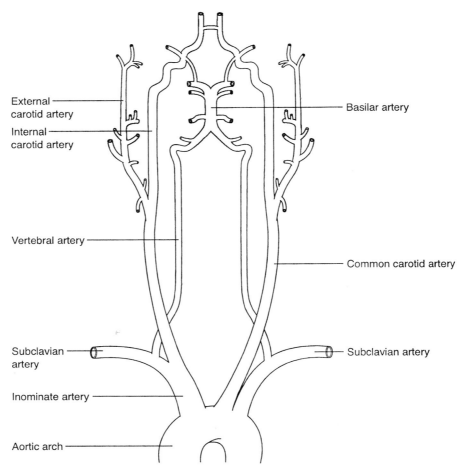

External carotid artery

Internal carotid artery

Basilar artery

Vertebral artery

Common carotid artery

Subclavian artery

Subclavian artery

Inominate artery

Aortic arch

FIG. 31.1. Pictorial representation of the arterial supply to the brain.

use of tissue plasminogen activator (alteplase) for thrombolysis in acute ischemic stroke in 1996 (see Treatment section). Table 31.4 lists the differential diagnoses for acute ischemic stroke and diagnostic tests that can be used to help confirm this diagnosis.

Emergency Diagnostic Evaluation of Acute Stroke

The majority of patients with acute stroke should be initially evaluated in the emergency department. After attention to the issues of oxygenation and hemodynamic stability, a medical history documentation and physical examination should focus on specific stroke risk factors and

causes, followed by clinical localization of the ischemic territory (Table 31.3). Rapid determination of the blood glucose level should be made to rule out hypoglycemia or hyperglycemia as the cause of the neurologic deficit. Laboratory studies, including a complete blood cell count and measurement of electrolytes, glucose, and coagulation parameters, should be obtained. A toxicology screen should be ordered for young patients and any others suspected of illicit drug use. Electrocardiography is needed to assess for evidence of arrhythmia or cardiac ischemia. Emergency computed tomography (CT) is necessary to identify ICH, SAH, or early signs of cerebral ischemia. CT appearances of AIS, ICH, and SAH are demonstrated in Fig. 31.4. It is

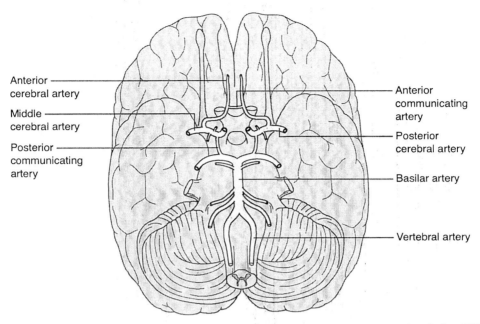

FIG. 31.2. Inferior view of the brain: arterial supply to the brain with attention to the circle of Willis.

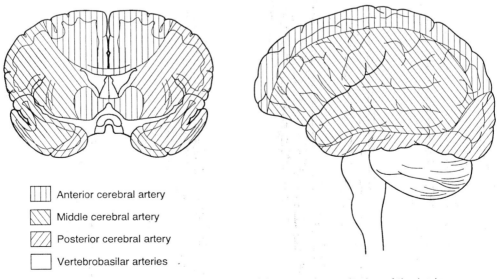

FIG. 31.3. Coronal and lateral views of the vascular territories of the brain.

TABLE 31.3. *Presenting signs and symptoms of stroke by vascular distribution*

Artery	Clinical features
Anterior circulation	
ICA	Ipsilateral monocular vision loss (amaurosis fugax)
	± Contralateral weakness or sensory changes
MCA	Contralateral weakness, sensory changes (more severe in face and arm than in leg)
	± Contralateral visual field deficit
	Aphasia (dominant hemisphere)
	Neglect and other visuospatial difficulties (nondominant hemisphere)
ACA	Contralateral weakness, sensory changes (more severe in leg than in face and arm)
	Personality changes (disinhibition, lack of motivation, disinterest)
Posterior circulation	
PCA	Contralateral visual field deficit ± other visual phenomena
VB	Ipsilateral cranial nerve deficits ± ataxia
	Contralateral or bilateral weakness or sensory changes
	Contralateral or bilateral sensory changes
	Diplopia
	Dysarthria
	Dysequilibrium or vertigo (not in isolation)
	Altered level of consciousness

ACA, anterior cerebral artery; ICA, internal carotid artery; MCA, middle cerebral artery; PCA, posterior cerebral artery; VB, vertebrobasilar system.

important to remember that initial CT scanning in acute ischemic stroke may be normal, or reveal only subtle, early signs of cerebral ischemia. A sample emergency department protocol for the initial evaluation and management of acute stroke is provided in Table 31.5.

Emergency imaging studies may be useful for some treatment decisions. Magnetic reso-

TABLE 31.4. *Differential diagnosis of acute ischemic stroke*

Disorders that mimic acute ischemic stroke	Diagnostic tools
Intracerebral hemorrhage	CT/MRI
Subarachnoid hemorrhage	CT, lumbar puncture, cerebral angiography
Subdural/epidural hematoma	History of trauma, CT/MRI
Structural lesion (e.g., neoplasm)	CT/MRI
Hypoglycemia or hyperglycemia	Fingerstick glucose measurement
Other metabolic derangements	Routine chemistry studies
Seizure	Clinical history, EEG
Complicated migraine	Clinical history
Conversion disorder	Clinical history, psychiatric evaluation

CT, computed tomography; EEG, electroencephalography; MRI, magnetic resonance imaging.

nance imaging (MRI), including diffusion- and perfusion-weighted imaging, may be used to detect early ischemia and identify salvageable penumbral tissue that could be targeted with thrombolytic or neuroprotective therapies. For determination of vascular anatomy, the "gold standard" is conventional catheter angiography, which can demonstrate an acute arterial occlusion or embolus lodged at a vascular bifurcation. Figure 31.5 demonstrates critical stenosis of the carotid artery on conventional angiography. The vasculature can also be evaluated noninvasively with transcranial Doppler ultrasonography, magnetic resonance angiography, or CT angiography, but these techniques may be less accurate than conventional angiography. Furthermore, conventional angiography provides a route for interventional radiologic therapies, such as intraarterial thrombolysis or angioplasty, although these are controversial at present. Discussion of these techniques is beyond the scope of this review; interested readers are referred to a review of diagnostic imaging for stroke (5).

Evaluation of Stroke Etiology

After the hyperacute period of the first few hours after stroke onset, secondary prevention therapy should be initiated for all patients with

TABLE 31.5. *Emergency department protocol for the initial management of presumed acute ischemic stroke*

1. Obtain vital sign measurements, including temperature, pulse, blood pressure, and oxygen saturation; continue to monitor every 15 minutes
2. Begin continuous cardiac and oxygen saturation monitoring
3. Ensure adequate airway/respiratory status
   a. Intubate and initiate mechanical ventilation if necessary
   b. Otherwise, begin oxygen at 2 L per minute via nasal cannula
4. IV access: 0.9 normal saline at 50 mL/hr; saline lock in opposite arm
5. *Stat.* laboratory studies
   a. Serum glucose (may be measured at bedside)
   b. Complete blood cell count with platelet count
   c. Chemistry profile
   d. Coagulation studies (prothrombin time, activated partial thromboplastin time)
   e. Urine pregnancy test for women of childbearing age
   f. Urine toxicology screen
5. Establish patient's weight (measure or estimate)
6. Obtain IV pump for possible infusion therapy
7. Order *stat.* head CT without contrast material
8. No aspirin or other antiplatelet agents, heparin, or warfarin to be given to potential thrombolytic therapy recipients

CT, computed tomography; IV, intravenous.

ischemic stroke. Diagnostic studies are needed to determine the cause of the stroke, because specific treatments are available for specific stroke causes. There is no true "standard" approach to the evaluation of all patients with stroke, and consideration must be given to each patient's medical and neurologic condition, prognosis, and the possible risks and benefits of the interventions being considered.

Brain MRI or CT may be performed in the subacute period to confirm the diagnosis of stroke and to determine the location and extent of ischemic damage, which may help predict outcome from stroke. Other components of the diagnostic workup for ischemic stroke include studies aimed at detecting large-vessel thromboembolism, small-vessel thromboembolism, or cardioembolism. Tests for unusual causes of stroke may also be included if the patient is young (younger than 50 years) or if routine evaluation fails to detect the cause of the stroke. A more detailed discussion of the diagnostic evaluation of stroke is available to interested readers (5).

Large-vessel atherothromboembolism is usually a result of carotid artery stenosis; less commonly, it results from stenosis of the vertebral arteries or the intracranial vessels. Examination of the large vessels should be performed, depending on the localization of the stroke. Patients with anterior circulation strokes (Table 31.3) require evaluation of the carotid arteries, whereas patients with posterior circulation strokes (Table 31.3) require evaluation of the vertebrobasilar system, and both may need evaluation of the intracranial vessels. The extracranial carotid arteries can be evaluated by carotid ultrasonography, whereas both the carotid and vertebral arteries can be reliably imaged with magnetic resonance angiography or CT angiography. The intracranial circulation can be examined by transcranial Doppler ultrasonography, magnetic resonance angiography, or CT angiography. Conventional cerebral angiography is the definitive study, but because this invasive test carries an approximate 1% risk for stroke and significant expense, it is often reserved for situations in which treatment decisions require the additional information.

The diagnosis of small-vessel disease rests on the clinical syndrome, the finding of a small (less than 1.5-cm) deep infarction on CT or MRI, and the absence of an alternative cause (6). The deep small vessels in the internal capsule, corona radiata, thalamus, and pons seem most susceptible to the process of small-vessel occlusive disease. The mechanism of the small-vessel occlusive process is uncertain, but it is most common in patients with long-standing hypertension, diabetes or both.

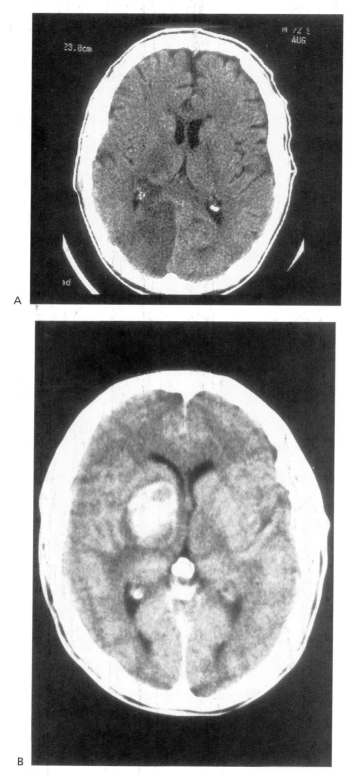

FIG. 31.4. Computed tomographic appearance of acute ischemic stroke (**A**), intracerebral hemorrhage (**B**), and subarachnoid hemorrhage (**C**). Acute ischemic stroke may demonstrate no or only minimal changes on computed tomograms in the acute setting.

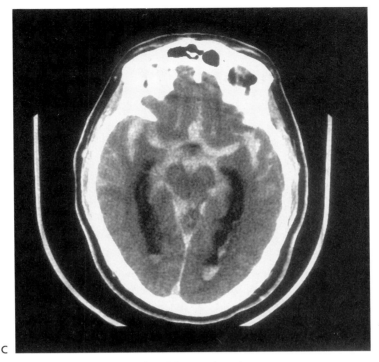

C

FIG. 31.4. *continued*

Cardioembolism should be considered as a possible cause in virtually all patients with ischemic stroke. Embolic events may be multiple and may occur in the territories of any of the major vessels. Cardiac evaluation includes documentation of the clinical cardiac history, clinical examination, an electrocardiogram, and an echocardiogram. Either transthoracic or transesophageal echocardiography may be used as the initial screening test, but transesophageal echocardiography is more sensitive to some abnormalities, including left atrial appendage thrombus and aortic arch atherosclerosis (7). If cardioembolism is suspected but the transthoracic echocardiogram is normal, then transesophageal echocardiography should also be performed.

As with ischemic stroke, diagnostic evaluation of hemorrhagic stroke begins in the emergency department, where emergency imaging with CT is likely to reveal ICH or SAH. Further testing for ICH may include brain MRI or cerebral angiography to try to identify an underlying lesion (e.g., arteriovenous malformation, neoplasm). If

SAH is suspected from the patient's history but initial the CT is normal, lumbar puncture is performed to examine the cerebrospinal fluid for the presence of red blood cells or xanthochromia. Once the diagnosis of SAH has been confirmed, conventional angiography is performed to detect underlying aneurysms or other vascular lesions that necessitate surgical treatment.

THERAPY

This section discusses treatment options for AIS and for secondary prevention of ischemic stroke. A short section on treatment options for hemorrhagic stroke is included, as is a brief discussion of the prevention of stroke complications. Table 31.6 summarizes the medications used for the treatment of AIS and for the secondary prevention of stroke.

Treatment of Acute Ischemic Stroke

Intravenous tissue plasminogen activator (t-PA), specifically alteplase, at a dose of 0.9 mg/kg used

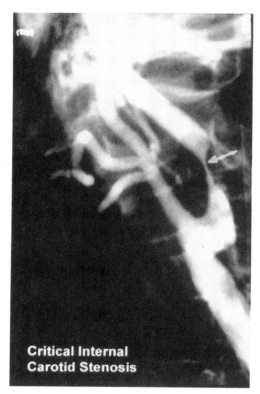

**Critical Internal
Carotid Stenosis**

FIG. 31.5. Demonstration of critical carotid stenosis on conventional angiography.

within 3 hours of symptom onset, is the only FDA-approved treatment for AIS. Its approval arose largely as a result of the National Institute of Neurological Disorders and Stroke (NINDS) rt-PA Stroke Study (8). This study documented an 11% to 13% absolute increase and a 30% to 50% relative increase in favorable outcomes on four different outcome scales at 3 months after stroke. Although there was a statistically significant increase in the rate of symptomatic ICH in the t-PA–treated group (6.4% vs. 0.6% in the placebo group; $p < 0.0001$), there was no significant difference in mortality at 3 months. The European Cooperative Acute Stroke Study I (ECASS-I) found no significant benefit for t-PA therapy in AIS and high rates of treatment-associated ICH but used a longer time window (6 hours) and a higher dose (1.1 mg/kg) than the NINDS t-PA trial, and this trial was also complicated by a very high rate of protocol violations

(involving 109 of 620 patients enrolled) (9). A second European trial, ECASS II, again used a 6-hour time window but used the NINDS dosing regimen of 0.9 mg/kg and required rigorous CT training for its investigators (10). Again, no significant difference in outcome between placebo-treated and t-PA–treated patients was found, but few patients were enrolled within the 0- to 3-hour time window. Symptomatic ICH occurred more frequently in the t-PA–treated group (8.8% vs. 3.4% in the placebo group) but there was no difference in mortality at 3 months. In summary, the trials for intravenous t-PA for AIS demonstrated improved outcome after treatment in selected patients within 3 hours of stroke onset. Although treatment with intravenous t-PA appears to be safe when given up to 6 hours after symptom onset, efficacy has not been proven beyond the 3-hour time window.

Other emergent therapies for AIS (e.g., intraarterial thrombolysis, mechanical reperfusion strategies, defibrinogenating agents) have been evaluated more recently; interested readers are referred elsewhere for general discussion of newer acute stroke therapies (11).

Prevention of Ischemic Stroke

Strategies for secondary prevention of stroke include risk factor modification, pharmacologic treatment with antiplatelet or anticoagulant therapies, and surgical management of carotid artery disease. A more detailed discussion of ischemic stroke prevention, including levels of evidence for the various interventions, can be found in a review article on this topic (12).

Risk Factor Modification

In general, risk factors for ischemic stroke are similar to those for ischemic heart disease; these topics have been discussed extensively in other sections of this text. In addition, nonvalvular atrial fibrillation (NVAF) is one of the strongest risk factors for stroke, and the American Academy of Neurology has issued practice parameters for stroke prevention in NVAF (13). In the general population with NVAF, warfarin with dosing adjusted to yield an International

TABLE 31.6. *Medications used in the treatment of ischemic stroke*

Medication	Standard dosage	Drug interactions	Adverse effects
t-PA (alteplase)	0.9 mg/kg (maximum 90 mg); 10% as IV bolus bolus over 1 minute, then remainder as IV infusion over 1 hour	Anticoagulants, including heparin and warfarin	Systemic and intracranial hemorrhage
Aspirin	50–325 mg q.d.	Other antiplatelet agents, NSAIDs, heparin, warfarin	Dyspepsia, tinnitus, gastrointestinal bleeding
Ticlopidine	250 mg b.i.d.	Aspirin and other antiplatelet agents, NSAIDs, heparin, warfarin, cimetidine, theophylline	Diarrhea, nausea, vomiting, rash, gastrointestinal bleeding, neutropenia, thrombotic thrombocytopenic purpura, aplastic anemia
Clopidogrel	75 mg q.d.	Aspirin and other antiplatelet agents, NSAIDs, heparin, warfarin At high concentrations, may inhibit certain hepatic enzymes and decrease metabolism of various medications	Rash, diarrhea, dyspepsia, gastrointestinal bleeding
Dipyridamole	75–100 mg t.i.d. to q.i.d.; modified-release formulation (200 mg) given in combination with 25 mg aspirin b.i.d.	None	Headache, dizziness, flushing, abdominal distress, diarrhea, vomiting
Warfarin	Individualized according to patient response as measured by international normalized ratio (INR); usual dosages vary from 1 to 10 mg q.d. and are titrated to keep INR between 2.0 and 3.0	Aspirin and other antiplatelet agents, NSAIDs, ticlopidine, clopidogrel, heparin Interacts with multiple other medications through pharmacokinetic mechanisms Consult literature before initiating therapy	Gastrointestinal and other systemic bleeding, warfarin necrosis syndrome, systemic atheromatous embolization ("purple toe" syndrome)

IV, intravenous; NSAID, nonsteroidal antiinflammatory drug; t-PA, tissue plasminogen activator.

Normalized Ratio of 2.0 to 3.0 reduces the risk of stroke by about 70% and is recommended for stroke prophylaxis in patients who can be appropriately monitored. Despite this recommendation, warfarin is generally underused; perhaps only one third to one half of eligible patients with NVAF are managed appropriately (14).

Antiplatelet Therapy

Antiplatelet therapy is often considered the mainstay of secondary prevention of ischemic stroke. This section outlines antiplatelet treatment options that are available for ischemic stroke patients; more detailed discussion of antiplatelet therapy selection can be found elsewhere (15). Aspirin currently remains the standard initial medical treatment for secondary stroke prevention, and numerous trials and metaanalyses have documented an approximate 25% reduction in the odds of stroke recurrence or vascular death in aspirin recipients in comparison with placebo (16). The optimal dose of aspirin for stroke prevention has been controversial in the past, but most authors now agree that low to moderate doses of aspirin (50 to 325 mg) are as effective as high doses and have fewer side effects (15). Several newer antiplatelet agents that have marginal to modest benefit for secondary stroke prevention over aspirin have been introduced: ticlopidine (17); clopidogrel (18); and an extended-release dipyridamole/low-dose aspirin combination (19). The use of ticlopidine for secondary stroke prevention has been curtailed because of its adverse safety profile, including the risk of severe neutropenia and thrombotic thrombocytopenic purpura (20).

Carotid Endarterectomy and Other Surgical Interventions

In addition to pharmacologic agents, surgical intervention with carotid endarterectomy (CEA) may also be appropriate preventive therapy for selected stroke patients. The North American Symptomatic Carotid Endarterectomy Trial (NASCET) and the European Carotid Surgery Trial (ECST) demonstrated marked benefit for CEA over best medical management in symptomatic patients (i.e., those with TIA or nondisabling stroke) with high-grade carotid stenosis, defined as more than 70% in NASCET and more than 80% in ECST (21,22). More recently, NASCET results for symptomatic patients with moderately severe stenosis (50% to 69%) have been published and demonstrate a less robust but still significant benefit from CEA for this population (23). Overall benefit for the two NASCET reports and numbers needed to treat to prevent one stroke are provided in Table 31.7.

Surgical benefits are predicated largely on a low perioperative complication rate. The 30-day rate of stroke and death was 5.8% in the first NASCET report and 7.0% in the ECST. Symptomatic patients should be considered for CEA only if the local complication rate is less than 6%.

CEA for asymptomatic patients is more controversial. Although CEA performed in asymptomatic patients technically is not considered secondary stroke prevention, discussion of this procedure is often grouped with CEA for symptomatic patients for ease of comparison of risks and benefits, as outlined in Table 31.7. The Asymptomatic Carotid Atherosclerosis Study (ACAS) found a modest benefit for prophylactic CEA in carefully selected patients with high-grade (more than 60%) stenosis (24). This benefit occurred in the ideal scenario of combining a select group of patients at low risk (25 patients screened clinically and from ultrasonography laboratories for every 1 patient enrolled in the study) with highly skilled surgeons. Almost one third of the surgeons who applied for credentialing in the trial were rejected or did not complete the certification process (12). Re-creating this ideal scenario in actual clinical practice may not be practical; one study analyzing perioperative mortality in more than 100,000 Medicare beneficiaries found the mortality rate after CEA in average-volume U.S. hospitals to be 1.8%, almost 18 times higher than the surgical mortality rate seen in ACAS (25). Thus, performing prophylactic CEA on asymptomatic patients should be considered on a case-by-case basis, with special attention to the patient's operative risk and the surgeon's perioperative complication rate.

Carotid angioplasty and stent implantation (CAS) has been raised as a possible alternative to CEA for patients with both symptomatic and asymptomatic carotid stenosis. Hospital-based case series have shown that CAS not only is feasible but also may be comparable with CEA for stroke prevention in some patient categories. In a large series on elective stent implantation in the carotid artery in patients considered to be at high risk for surgery, the overall 30-day risk for stroke or death was found to be 6.9%, and the risk for major stroke was 0.7% (26). A randomized prospective trial comparing CAS with CEA for

TABLE 31.7. *Comparison of trials for carotid endarterectomy: NASCET and ACAS*

Trial	Stenosis	Absolute RR	Time	NNT
NASCET	70%–99%	17%	2 years	6
NASCET	50%–69%	6.5%	5 years	15
ACAS	60%–99%	5.9%	5 years	17

ACAS, Asymptomatic Carotid Atherosclerosis Study; NASCET, North American Symptomatic Carotid Endarterectomy Trial; NNT, number needed to treat; RR, risk reduction.

symptomatic patients at high risk is currently underway.

Treatment of Hemorrhagic Stroke

Unfortunately, treatment options for hemorrhagic stroke are limited—only four randomized trials have been performed in ICH (two using dexamethasone, one of glycerol, and one using hemodilution), and none of these trials found a benefit for the therapeutic intervention (27). The benefits of surgical evacuation of the hematoma remain controversial (27–29). The exception is cerebellar ICH, for which surgical evacuation is routinely performed if hemorrhages are larger than 3 cm, especially if the patient has any alteration of level of consciousness (29). Thus, in general, the management of ICH is supportive and includes intensive monitoring of neurologic and cardiovascular status, management of increased intracranial pressure and mass effect, and control of systemic blood pressure. Most authors recommend treatment with intravenous antihypertensive agents to maintain mean arterial pressure at or below 130 mm HG (29).

The management of SAH also includes supportive care, as outlined in the preceding paragraph for ICH (30). However, further interventions aimed at prevention of rebleeding from aneurysmal SAH are usually indicated and include surgical clipping or endovascular coiling of the aneurysm. Appropriate patient selection, surgical techniques, and postprocedure management and prevention of arterial vasospasm are beyond the scope of this text, but several excellent reviews are available (30,31).

Prevention of Complications

Complications of stroke can include aspiration pneumonia, deep venous thrombosis, decubitus ulcers, and limb contractures. Appropriate interventions should begin in the acute treatment phase to prevent these complications.

PROGNOSIS AND FOLLOW-UP

Mortality from ischemic stroke increases progressively with age from about 10% of persons younger than age 65 to 20% of those aged 65 to 74, to 30% among those aged 75 to 84, and to 40% of those aged 85 and older (32). Rates of mortality from hemorrhagic stroke are higher than those for ischemic stroke; case-fatality rates approach 50% for all patients (33). Stroke is far more often disabling than lethal. The AHA estimates that there are over 4 million stroke survivors in this country (2). It is estimated that more than 60% of patients with stroke are left with some residual disability and that fewer than 50% are able to return to work after stroke (34). About one fourth of patients suffer some amount of poststroke depression, which also impedes the ability to perform activities of daily living or return to work.

The major predictor of stroke outcome is initial stroke severity; worse outcomes are seen in patients with more severe deficits (35). The presence of other diseases or medical complications after stroke also appears to worsen outcome (35). Despite these potential prognostic indicators, the variability among individual stroke patients makes prediction of final outcome status after stroke extremely difficult.

PRACTICAL POINTS

- Stroke and other cerebrovascular disorders are the third most common cause of death and the most common cause of long-term disability among Americans.
- More than 50% of strokes could be prevented by identifying and managing stroke risk factors.

- Treatment of acute ischemic stroke with intravenous t-PA (alteplase) is both safe and effective in reducing long-term disability from stroke. There is a 3-hour time window for thrombolysis for acute ischemic stroke.

(continued)

- Thorough evaluation of stroke patients is indicated to identify the cause of the stroke and thus to carry out appropriate secondary prevention through risk factor modification, antiplatelet or anticoagulant therapy, and surgical intervention.

REFERENCES

1. Ay H, Buonanno FS, Rordorf G, et al. Normal diffusion-weighted MRI during stroke-like deficits. *Neurology* 1999;52:1784–1792.
2. American Heart Association. *1998 Heart and stroke statistical update.* Dallas: American Heart Association, 1998.
3. Broderick J, Brott T, Kothari R, et al. The Greater Cincinnati/Northern Kentucky Stroke Study: preliminary first-ever and total incidence rates of stroke among blacks. *Stroke* 1998;29:415–421.
4. Gorelick PB, Sacco RL, Smith DB, et al. Prevention of a first stroke: a review of guidelines and a multidisciplinary consensus statement from the National Stroke Association. *JAMA* 1998;281:1112–1120.
5. Wityk RJ, Beauchamp NJ. Diagnostic evaluation of stroke. *Neurol Clin North Am* 2000;19:357–378.
6. Adams HP, Bendixen BJ, Kapelle LJ, et al. Classification of subtype of acute ischemic stroke. Definitions for use in a multicenter trial. *Stroke* 1993;24:35–41.
7. McNamara RL, Lima JA, Whelton PK, et al. Echocardiographic identification of cardiovascular sources of emboli to guide clinical management of stroke: a cost-effectiveness analysis. *Ann Intern Med* 1997;127:775–787.
8. The National Institute of Neurological Disorders and Stroke rt-PA Stroke Study Group. Tissue plasminogen activator for acute ischemic stroke. *N Engl J Med* 1995;333:1581–1587.
9. Hacke W, Kaste M, Fieschi C, et al., for the ECASS Study Group. Intravenous thrombolysis with recombinant tissue plasminogen activator for acute ischemic stroke: the European Cooperative Acute Stroke Study (ECASS). *JAMA* 1995;274:1017–1025.
10. Hacke W, Kaste M, Fieschi C, et al., for the Second European-Australian Acute Stroke Study Investigators. Randomised double-blind placebo-controlled trial of thrombolytic therapy with intravenous alteplase in acute ischaemic stroke (ECASS II). *Lancet* 1998;352:1245–1251.
11. Hickenbottom SL, Barsan WG. Acute ischemic stroke therapy. *Neurol Clin North Am* 2000;19:379–397.
12. Chaturvedi S, Hickenbottom S, Levine SR. Ischemic stroke prevention. *Curr Treat Options Neurol* 1999;1:113–125.
13. Report of the Quality Standards Subcommittee of the American Academy of Neurology. Practice parameter: stroke prevention in patients with non-valvular atrial fibrillation. *Neurology* 2000;13:57–62.
14. Albers GW, Bittar N, Young L, et al. Clinical characteristics and management of acute stroke in patients with atrial fibrillation admitted to US university hospitals. *Neurology* 1997;48:1598–1604.
15. Albers GW, Easton JD, Sacco RL, et al. Antithrombotic and thrombolytic therapy for ischemic stroke. *Chest* 1998;114:683S–698S.
16. Antiplatelet Trialists' Collaboration. Collaborative overview of randomised trials of antiplatelet therapy. I. Prevention of death, myocardial infarction, and stroke by prolonged antiplatelet therapy in various categories of patients. *BMJ* 1994;308:81–106.
17. Hass WK, Easton JD, Adams HP, et al., for the Ticlopidine Aspirin Stroke Study Group. A randomized trial comparing ticlopidine hydrochloride with aspirin for the prevention of stroke in high-risk patients. *N Engl J Med* 1989;321:501–507.
18. CAPRIE Steering Committee. A randomized, blinded, trial of clopidogrel versus aspirin in patients at risk of ischemic events (CAPRIE). *Lancet* 1998;348:1329–1339.
19. Diener HC, Cuhna L, Forbes C, et al. European Stroke Prevention Study 2. Dipyridamole and acetylsalicylic acid in the secondary prevention of stroke. *J Neurol Sci* 1996;143:1–13.
20. Bennett CL, Weinberg PD, Brozenberg-ben-Dror K, et al. Thrombotic thrombocytopenic purpura associated with ticlopidine. A review of 60 cases. *Ann Intern Med* 1998; 128:541–544.
21. North American Symptomatic Carotid Endarterectomy Trial Collaborators. Beneficial effects of carotid endarterectomy in symptomatic patients with high-grade carotid stenosis. *N Engl J Med* 1991;325:445–453.
22. European Carotid Surgery Trialists' Collaborative Group. Randomised trial of endarterectomy for recently symptomatic carotid stenosis: final results of the MRC European Carotid Surgery Trial (ECST). *Lancet* 1998; 351:1379–1387.
23. Barnett HJM, Taylor DW, Eliasziw MA, et al., for the North American Symptomatic Carotid Endarterectomy Trial Collaborators. Benefit of carotid endarterectomy in patients with symptomatic moderate or severe stenosis. *N Engl J Med* 1998;339:1415–1425.
24. Executive Committee for the Asymptomatic Carotid Atherosclerosis Study. Endarterectomy for asymptomatic carotid artery stenosis. *JAMA* 1995;273:1421–1428.
25. Wennenberg DE, Lucas FL, Birkmeyer JD, et al. Variation in mortality in the Medicare population. *JAMA* 1998;279:1278–1281.
26. Mathur A, Roubin GS, Iyer SS, et al. Predictors of stroke complicating carotid artery stenting. *Circulation* 1998;97:1239–1245.
27. Broderick JP, Brott T, Zuccarello M. Management of intracerebral hemorrhage. In Batjer HH (ed): *Cerebrovascular disease.* Philadelphia: Lippincott-Raven, 1996:417–434.

28. Shah MV, Biller J. Medical and surgical management of intracerebral hemorrhage. *Semin Neurol* 1998;18:513–519.

29. Qureshi AI, Tuhrim S, Broderick JP, et al. Spontaneous intracerebral hemorrhage. *N Engl J Med* 2001;344:1450–1460.

30. Miller J, Diringer M. Management of aneurysmal subarachnoid hemorrhage. *Neurol Clin* 1995;13:451–478.

31. van Gijn J, Rinkel GJ. Subarachnoid hemorrhage: diagnosis, causes and management. *Brain* 2001;124:249–278.

32. Nakayama H, Jorgensen HS, Raaschou HO, et al. The influence of age on stroke outcome. The Copenhagen Stroke Study. *Stroke* 1994;25:808–813.

33. Juvela S. Risk factors for impaired outcome after spontaneous intracerebral hemorrhage. *Arch Neurol* 1995;52:1193–1200.

34. Wozniak MA, Kittner SJ, Price TR, et al. Stroke location is not associated with return to work after first ischemic stroke. *Stroke* 1999;30:2568–2573.

35. Johnston KC, Li JY, Lyden PD, et al. Medical and neurological complications of ischemic stroke: experience from the RANTTAS trial. RANTTAS Investigators. *Stroke* 1998;29:447–453.

32

Deep Venous Thrombosis

Thomas W. Wakefield and William P. Fay

EPIDEMIOLOGY AND USUAL CAUSES OF VENOUS THROMBOSIS

Deep venous thrombosis (DVT) has been estimated to affect more than 250,000 patients per year (1,2). It has also been estimated that DVT and pulmonary embolism (PE) together are responsible for 300,000 to 600,000 hospitalizations and as many as 50,000 deaths per year; other estimates suggest an even higher yearly death rate (3). DVT is responsible for a 21% yearly rate of mortality in the elderly, and the cost of treatment for venous thromboembolism has been estimated to be between $1.0 billion and $2.5 billion per year. Thus, venous thromboembolism remains a significant problem today. Usual risk factors associated with DVT include older age, malignancy, obesity, varicose veins, prior DVT, surgery, vascular injury, immobility, oral contraceptive use, heart failure, and various hypercoagulable states (Table 32.1).

PRESENTING SIGNS AND SYMPTOMS

Lower extremity DVT typically manifests with pain and swelling, particularly in the calf (Table 32.2). However, the abnormal findings associated with DVT are not specific for this diagnosis, and approximately half of all cases are asymptomatic. Therefore, the diagnosis of DVT cannot be reliably established or excluded solely on the basis of the history and physical examination. Depending on the clinical setting, the examiner must maintain a high index of suspicion for DVT, and laboratory testing should be used liberally in the evaluation of patients in whom the diagnosis is suspected.

HELPFUL TESTS FOR DIAGNOSIS OF DEEP VENOUS THROMBOSIS AND PULMONARY EMBOLISM

Tests for the diagnosis of DVT involve indirect tests of historic interest and more current tests that visualize the thrombus. Venous duplex ultrasound imaging is now the standard for DVT diagnosis and has virtually replaced contrast phlebography.

Duplex ultrasound imaging includes analysis of both image and flow. Acute thrombosis is diagnosed from noncompressibility of the vein, vein enlargement, and the lack of collateral veins. Chronic thrombosis is indicated by echogenic thrombi, a small and shrunken vein, and the preference of collateral vessels. Sensitivity, specificity, positive predictive value, and negative predictor value for the diagnosis of acute DVT with color-flow duplex imaging in symptomatic patients are greater than 95% (4). Even for calf vein thrombi, the sensitivity in symptomatic patients is greater than 90%, although the sensitivity in the below-knee position may be much lower in asymptomatic patients being screened.

The excellent specificity of venous duplex imaging allows for therapeutic decisions. Withholding anticoagulation on the basis of a negative scan is safe and reasonable. In a study of 431 negative duplex scans and 66 corresponding phlebograms, only three peroneal thrombi were found on phlebography, whereas more proximal thrombi were not missed (5). Follow-up over 8 months revealed no PE and no recurrent DVT. Some clinicians have also combined clinical characteristics with duplex ultrasound imaging in an attempt to improve upon the results of imaging (6).

TABLE 32.1. *Risk factors for deep venous thrombosis*

Age >40 years
Malignancy
Obesity
Varicose veins
Prior deep venous thrombosis
Surgery
Vascular injury (e.g., catheter-induced)
Immobility
Oral contraceptive use
Heart failure
Hypercoagulable stable
   Antithrombin III deficiency
   Protein C deficiency
   Protein S deficiency
   Factor V Leiden
   Prothrombin 20210A
   Dysfibrinogenemia
   Homocystinemia
   Factor VIII elevations

Thus, venous duplex imaging is now the "gold standard" for the diagnosis of DVT and has replaced contrast phlebography. It is safe, painless, and accurate; requires no contrast material; and can be performed during pregnancy. It is noninvasive and repeatable, it can follow the progression or resolution of DVT, and it detects other abnormalities, such as pseudoaneurysms, venous aneurysms, Baker's cysts, superficial thrombophlebitis, and cellulitis. The incidence of positive studies in a busy vascular laboratory should be approximately 30%.

Magnetic resonance venography (MRV) has demonstrated promise as a diagnostic modality for both DVT and PE. The sensitivity and specificity are 100% and 96% both for DVT (7), and for PE (8). MRV with gadolinium has been found to define thrombus age. During acute DVT, an inflammatory response is found in the vein wall and

TABLE 32.2. *Symptoms and signs of lower extremity deep venous thrombosis*

Pain or tenderness
   (e.g., calf pain elicited by dorsiflexion of foot)
Edema
Skin discoloration
Increased skin temperature
Superficial venous dilatation
Palpable venous cord (superficial thrombophlebitis)

perivenous tissue, and gadolinium extravasates into the inflammation (9). As the DVT organizes and matures, gadolinium enhancement fades as the vein shrinks. In many locations, the inaccessibility of the magnetic resonance imaging machines and the cost limit the use of MRV for DVT diagnosis.

The diagnosis of PE involves ventilation-perfusion (V/Q) scanning or pulmonary angiography; newer techniques include spiral computed tomographic scanning and magnetic resonance imaging. The sensitivity of V/Q scanning is excellent, at 98%, but specificity is low, at 10% (10). However, by combining clinical risk factors with the V/Q scan, sensitivity and specificity greater than 95% have been reported. With a high-probability V/Q scan and two risk factors for PE, the sensitivity for PE diagnosis was 97%; with one risk factor, 84%; and with no risk factors, 82%. Similarly, with a normal V/Q scan, the chance of PE was 0%, no matter what the risk factor status was (11). These results suggest that a normal V/Q scan or a high-probability scan provide good diagnostic information. However, only approximately one third of V/Q scans are in one of these two categories, and so the majority of patients need further testing. Such further testing includes lower extremity venous duplex ultrasound imaging (venous duplex imaging is positive in approximately 10% of cases in these patients) and, more important, pulmonary arteriography. Additional indications for pulmonary arteriography include acute massive PE, inferior vena cava (IVC) interruption, and the planning of pulmonary interventional therapy, such as thrombolysis or pulmonary embolectomy.

Spiral computed tomographic scanning, a relatively new technique for PE diagnosis, has excellent specificity but relatively low sensitivity (50% to 65%), despite promising initial results. However, as the technology has improved, the sensitivity and specificity have also improved, and now emboli at the subsegmental level can be identified (12). Magnetic resonance imaging has demonstrated excellent promise for PE diagnosis.

The use of D-dimer assays has been investigated in the diagnosis of both DVT and PE, and

TABLE 32.3. *Differential diagnosis of lower extremity deep venous thrombosis*

Cellulitis
Superficial thrombophlebitis
Lymphangitis
Arthritis, joint effusion, or hemarthrosis
Hematoma
Ruptured Baker's cyst
Torn gastrocnemius muscle
Achilles tendonitis
Bone fracture
Acute arterial ischemia
Nonthrombotic venous obstruction

sensitivity of 96% to 98% has been reported (13). However, specificity of only 40% to 50% has been found. It is likely that D-dimer testing will supplement other tests such as venous duplex ultrasound imaging and clinical assessment (14).

DIFFERENTIAL DIAGNOSIS

The differential diagnosis of lower extremity DVT is extensive (Table 32.3). In most cases, the correct diagnosis can readily be established by careful history documentation, physical examination, and laboratory testing.

THERAPY

Standard Unfractionated Heparin and Oral Anticoagulation

Treatment for DVT and PE has historically involved anticoagulation with intravenous unfractionated heparin initially, followed by long-term oral anticoagulation. The initial treatment has been revolutionized by the introduction of low molecular weight heparin (LMWH) preparations.

Adequate anticoagulation decreases the risk of recurrent venous thromboembolism by 80%, from a range of 29% to 40% untreated, to a range of 5% to 7% treated (15). During adequate anticoagulant therapy–at least 5 days of heparin and 3 months of oral anticoagulation (International Normalized Ratio, 2.0 to 4.5), LMWH, or adjusted-dose subcutaneous unfractionated heparin—the risk of fatal PE is low: 0.4% and 0.3% during and after treatment for DVT and 1.5% and 0% during and after treat-

ment for PE (16). Anticoagulation with standard heparin must be achieved rapidly, and it has been shown that if therapeutic levels are reached in the first 24 hours, the recurrence rate is lower than if therapeutic levels are not reached in the first 24 hours (level I evidence) (17). Continuous intravenous unfractionated heparin is better than intermittent subcutaneous standard heparin for thromboembolism recurrence (level I evidence).

After standard heparin is begun, what are guidelines for its usage? Heparin administration for 5 days has been compared to that for 10 days, and no difference in recurrent thrombosis has been found (7.1% vs. 7.0%, level I evidence) (18). Oral anticoagulants are begun at maintenance dosing, rather than loading dosing, to decrease the chances of warfarin-induced skin necrosis. Studies (all level I evidence) have evaluated the length of optimal oral anticoagulant therapy. In comparisons of 6 weeks to 6 months of warfarin (Coumadin), the recurrence rate was 18.1% versus 9.5% in favor of longer treatment at 2-year follow-up (19). Another study compared 4 weeks with 3 months of treatment in medical patients; the recurrence rate for 4 weeks was 7.8%, in comparison with 4.0% with 3 months of treatment (20). A third study suggested that oral anticoagulants should be used for longer rather than shorter periods, especially with continuing risk factors (21). The usual recommendation is for a 3- to 6-month period of oral anticoagulation after a first DVT. For example, with reversible or time-limited risk factors and a first thromboembolic event, treatment for 3 to 6 months is recommended, whereas for an idiopathic cause and a first event, treatment for at least 6 months is recommended (22). Natural history studies suggest that after a first DVT, the risk of recurrent thrombosis is 17.5% at 2 years, 25% at 5 years, and 30% at 8 years (23). However, the prognosis after DVT is variable. If DVT is triggered by an isolated event (e.g., trauma or surgery), the risk of recurrence after an adequate course of anticoagulant therapy is low. If DVT occurs in the setting of persistent risk factors, the risk of recurrence is high.

The optimal duration of warfarin therapy after DVT depends on clinical circumstances (Table 32.4). In general, patients with a first

TABLE 32.4. *Duration of anticoagulant therapy after deep venous thrombosis*

Clinical setting	Duration of warfarin therapy
First episode	
Transient cause (e.g., surgery, trauma)	3 months
Idiopathic	3–6 months (or longer)
Persistent risk (e.g., malignancy, hypercoagulable state)	6–12 months (or longer)
First recurrence	6–12 months to indefinite
Second or later recurrence	1 year to indefinite
High risk of recurrent thrombosis	Indefinite

episode of venous thrombosis should receive warfarin for 3 to 6 months. Warfarin therapy for 6 months after a first episode of DVT results in a lower rate of recurrence than does therapy for 6 weeks (24). Patients with a second episode of venous thromboembolism have a significantly lower rate of recurrence if they receive warfarin indefinitely (2.6% risk during 4 years of follow-up) as opposed to 6 months (20.7% risk of recurrence). However, this therapy exposes the patient to a higher risk of bleeding complications (25). Prospective clinical trials addressing the optimal duration of warfarin therapy in patients with a first episode of DVT and an irreversible risk factor considered to place the patient at high risk of recurrence (e.g., malignancy, identifiable thrombophilia such as factor V Leiden) are lacking. Each patient must be considered individually, the duration of therapy depending on the relative bleeding and thrombotic risks.

One study compared a 3-month period of anticoagulant therapy to an additional 24-month period of therapy after a first episode of idiopathic venous thromboembolism. It was concluded that patients should be treated with anticoagulants longer than 3 months (level I evidence) (26). The rate of recurrent venous thromboembolism was 27.4% per patient-year for the shorter course, as opposed to 1.3% per patient-year for the longer course of warfarin, with only minimal increased bleeding. The actual length recommended over and above 3 months is still not determined.

The most important complication of anticoagulation is bleeding. With intravenous unfractionated heparin, the bleeding risk is 11% during the first 5 days. Adding in warfarin and keeping the International Normalized Ratio at 2 to 3 results in an incidence of major bleeding of 6% per year. Specifically for DVT and PE, major bleeding incidences have been reported in 0% to 7% of patients, with fatal bleeding in 0% to 2% (27). Because of the bleeding risks with unfractionated heparin, LMWHs were devised.

Low Molecular Weight Heparin

LMWHs are derived from the lower molecular weight range of heparin by chemical or enzymatic fragmentation. The mean molecular weight of LMWH is 4,000 to 6,500 D, whereas the mean molecular weight of standard unfractionated heparin is 12,000 to 15,000 D. The mean number of saccharide units for LMWH is 13 to 22, whereas that for standard heparin is 40 to 50 (28). Unfractionated heparin is large enough to make a three-way complex between thrombin, antithrombin, and heparin and, as such, inhibits thrombin. This complex usually requires 18 saccharide units. LMWHs are often shorter than 18 saccharide units and, because of this, have less antithrombin activity. For inhibition of factor Xa, such a three-way complex is not required, which allows LMWHs to show more anti–factor Xa activity. Each LMWH has its own ratio of anti–factor Xa to anti–factor IIa activity; most have a ratio between 2:1 to 4:1, in comparison with a 1:1 ratio for standard heparin (28).

The advantages of LMWHs include a decrease in bleeding, less antiplatelet activity, less heparin-induced thrombocytopenia, improved pharmacokinetic profile due to reduced nonspecific plasma protein binding, decreased lipolysis, a half-life that is not dose-dependent, more constant inhibition of anti–factor Xa, less interference with physiologic protein C activation, less complement activation, a lower risk of osteoporosis, less interference with platelet aggregation, and a lower level of fibrin monomer production (29). Because LMWH dosages are based on patient weight, patients do not need to be monitored with blood tests of coagulation. LMWH is administered by subcutaneous injection, and its excretion is renal. The improved bioavailability of LMWHs and the persistence of their anti–factor Xa action are probably key to their efficacy. The action of LMWHs is reversed only partially by protamine sulfate.

Low Molecular Weight Heparin and Deep Venous Thrombosis

LMWHs have been recommended for DVT prophylaxis and treatment of venous thromboembolism. Treatment of DVT is emphasized in this section. Level I studies and metaanalyses comparing LMWHs to standard unfractionated heparin for DVT and PE treatment have demonstrated LMWH to be at least as effective as, if not more effective than, standard heparin (30,31). For DVT, there is a lower risk for major bleeding, recurrent thromboembolic events, and even death (31). One metaanalysis comprising 14 studies and 4,754 patients revealed recurrent venous thrombotic complications of 4.3% for LMWH, in comparison with 5.6% for standard unfractionated heparin (10 studies); a mortality rate of 6.4% for LMWH, in comparison with 8.0% for standard unfractionated heparin (11 studies); major hemorrhage rate of 1.3% for LMWH, in comparison with 2.1% for standard heparin (14 studies); and similar findings when only more proximal DVT was evaluated (32). For proximal (above-knee) thromboses, thrombotic complications were found in 4.8% of patients receiving LMWH, in comparison with 7.8% receiving standard heparin; major hemorrhage in 1.0% versus 8.3%; and mortality in 5.4% versus 8.3% (32).

Low Molecular Weight Heparin and Pulmonary Embolism

For PE, studies have substantiated that LMWH is equivalent to and more convenient than standard unfractionated heparin. Three studies are highlighted in this section. A study of 1,021 patients, 510 given Reviporin sodium (Clivarin, Knoll, Germany) and 511 given standard unfractionated heparin for DVT (73% to 74%) and PE (26% to 27%) found equivalent rates of recurrent venous thromboembolism (5.3% given Riviparin vs. 4.9% given unfractionated heparin), major

bleeding (3.1% vs. 2.3%), mortality (7.1% vs. 7.6%), and fatal PE (0.6% vs. 0.6%). Of importance, the length of hospitalization was only 6.4 days for LMWH, in comparison with 9.4 days for standard heparin (33). A study of 612 patients with clinically suspected PE (70% with DVT) again revealed equivalence between the patients treated with tinzaparin (304) and those treated with standard heparin (308) with regard to combined outcomes of death, bleeding, and recurrent venous thromboembolism (5.9% of those receiving LMWH, 7.1% of those receiving standard heparin) (34). Finally, a study of 200 patients presenting with acute proximal DVT (50% to 60% with asymptomatic PE) found a statistically significant reduction in recurrent venous thromboembolism (0% of those receiving LMWH, 6.8% of those receiving standard heparin), a reduction in mortality (6.2% vs. 8.7%), a reduction in major bleeding (1.0% vs. 1.9%), and a reduction in fatal PE (0% vs. 1.0%) (35).

In summary, LMWH has been found to carry a lower risk for major bleeding, a lower risk for recurrent thromboembolic disease, and a lower mortality rate for DVT and is at least equivalent to standard heparin and certainly more convenient for PE. LMWH dosages are based on patient weight, and patients do not need to be monitored by coagulation tests, except in special circumstances (renal failure). Because of the nonnecessity of monitoring and the use of subcutaneous injections, outpatient treatment at home is a reality and being recommended.

Economic Impact of Low Molecular Weight Heparin

The economic impact of using LMWH rather than standard unfractionated heparin for venous thromboembolism treatment has been investigated. Cost savings have ranged from more than $300,000 for 125 patients (or approximately $2,500 per case) in the United States (36) to approximately $4,000 (U.S. dollars) per case in Canada (37). More than a 60% reduction in cost was found in Europe, Australia, and New Zealand (38), and once-per-day treatment with LMWH resulted in significant cost reductions in Sweden (39). Expanding indications restricting

LMWH only to patients with massive PE, patients with a high risk for major or active bleeding, patients with phlegmasia, and patients already hospitalized for other diseases resulted in more than 80% patient eligibility for home therapy and more than 90% patient satisfaction.

Calf Vein Thrombi

One area of continued controversy involves calf vein thrombi and the need to treat such thrombi. Approximately 20% of calf thrombi extend into the popliteal vein, and extension is associated with a 40% to 50% rate of clinically detectable PE. Isolated calf vein thrombi have been associated with up to a 25% incidence of chronic venous insufficiency 12 months after diagnosis and an approximate 10% incidence of PE at presentation (40). Thus, most authorities today recommend full anticoagulation for calf vein thrombosis, especially for patients with any other risk factors. The ability to use outpatient LMWH will probably end this controversy, inasmuch as all calf-vein thrombi may now be treated with LMWH, and full hospitalization for DVT treatment does not have to be justified.

Patients not Candidates for Low Molecular Weight Heparin Treatment as Outpatients

The use of LMWH thus appears to be possible in 80% to 90% of cases of DVT and PE, with outpatient therapy for many patients. An area of concern is the nondiscriminative use of LMWH for all patients with DVT or PE, regardless of the presenting symptoms and signs. Patients who require more aggressive intervention include those with phlegmasia, young patients with extensive iliofemoral venous thrombosis who may benefit from thrombolysis or thrombectomy, and patients with extensive PE. Others who are not good candidates for outpatient home therapy include patients with active bleeding or significant familial bleeding disorders in which heparin therapy must be closely monitored and may have to be reversed rapidly, those with significant leg edema, those already hospitalized, patients with liver dysfunction or renal insufficiency (creatinine levels of 3.5 mg/dL or less or creatinine clearance of less than 30 mL/minute), pa-

tients with severe obesity (weighing more than 120 kg), and patients who are not able for personal, social, or travel reasons to self-administer LMWH and follow up closely with their physician (41).

Outpatient Treatment Program

The outpatient treatment of venous thromboembolism with LMWH followed by oral anticoagulation requires more than just the writing of a prescription. In order to administer such a program, a physician must take responsibility for the outpatient program, pharmacy services are needed to supply the drug, oral anticoagulation must be monitored and dose-adjusted, visits from nurses must be arranged or follow-up at home established, the patient must be instructed on self-injections, and orthotic services must be provided for the fitting of surgical support stockings (42). It must be remembered that LMWH is only a bridge to longer term oral anticoagulant therapy.

Reimbursement

One area that remains to be fully addressed is reimbursement, inasmuch as Medicare does not pay for the outpatient procurement of LMWH by patients because LMWH is considered a self-injectable drug. This limits the ability to set up a totally outpatient program and protocol. Changes in Medicare reimbursement allow for outpatient coverage if the patient returns to an outpatient facility daily for injections, and Blue Cross/Blue Shield is beginning to pay for some home infusion services. There is little doubt that insurance providers will eventually realize the tremendous cost savings that outpatient LMWH treatment for DVT and PE provides to the health care system. However, until that time, it must be remembered that patients need to know that they may be required to pay for their outpatient therapy out of pocket or that they will need to be initially hospitalized in order for insurance coverage to be provided.

Thrombolysis

The incidence of chronic venous insufficiency after appropriate anticoagulant treatment for DVT has been reported to be 23% after 2 years, 28% after 5 years, and 29% after 8 years (23). Because of this incidence of valvular reflux resulting from DVT, the use of thrombolytic agents to more rapidly clear venous thrombosis has been advocated. Through duplex ultrasonography, it has been found that spontaneous lysis time was 2.3- to 7.3-fold longer in segments with reflux than in segments without reflux (except for the posterior tibial vein; level V evidence) (43). Systemic thrombolysis in two small series (level II evidence) revealed a decrease in the incidence of chronic venous insufficiency with streptokinase, as opposed to systemic standard heparin. However, results depend on complete thrombolysis. Because of this inability to predict complete lysis, combined with the bleeding potential, thrombolysis has fallen out of favor. With the use of intrathrombus urokinase for arterial thrombi, a similar approach with urokinase directly into the venous thrombi was attempted. Initial good results (level V evidence) (44) has led to a national thrombolysis registry (45). In 473 patients, 287 of whom underwent follow-up, 312 urokinase infusions in 303 limbs have been reported. Venous thrombi occurred in the iliofemoral segment in 71% of cases alone, without IVC involvement in 79% and including the IVC in 21% of cases. Two thirds of the patients presented with acute disease, 16% with chronic disease, and 19% with combined acute and chronic disease. Approximately 31% reported prior DVT. The favorite access site for urokinase infusion was the popliteal vein (42% of cases). Complete thrombolysis was achieved in 31% of cases, and partial lysis was achieved in 52% of cases. The mean amount of urokinase needed was 7.8 million units, and the mean time of infusion was 53.4 hours. Predictors of successful lysis included acute DVT and no prior history of DVT. Complications included major bleeding necessitating blood products in 11% and minor bleeding in 16%. The rate of mortality was 0.4%, that of intracranial hemorrhage was 0.2%, and that of subdural hemorrhage was 0.2%. Total lysis was noted in only 31% of the entire series; however, in patients with acute iliofemoral DVT, no previous symptoms, and the use of the popliteal vein access site, total lysis was more frequent. Patency at 12 months was 79% with complete lysis, 58% with more than 50% lysis, and 32% with less than 50% lysis. With complete lysis, absence of valvular reflux was found in 72% of cases, whereas overall valvular reflux was seen in 58% of cases (level V evidence).

Thrombolytic therapy for PE remains controversial. Although agents lyse thrombus effectively, recurrence rates and patient mortality have not been found to be improved (level II evidence). Results are best if patients are young, the embolus is less than 48 hours old, and the embolus is large. Streptokinase, urokinase, and tissue plasminogen activator (46) have all been used (level II evidence). All agents rapidly dissolve clot, but by 7 days, the advantage for all three agents disappears. The benefit of thrombolytic agents for PE thus appears to be greatest in patients who would die as a result of massive PE in the first hour after the PE occurs (up to 10% of cases of PE).

Venous Thrombectomy

Iliofemoral venous thrombectomy has been advocated in the setting of impending venous gangrene. This technique results in mechanical clearing of the venous circulation and may be combined with a temporary arteriovenous fistula to increase patency. Thrombectomy is performed utilizing a Fogarty balloon catheter passed commonly from the femoral level during patient Valsalva maneuvers. The arteriovenous fistula is constructed so that it can be taken down by angiographic, nonsurgical techniques and is made in the groin at the femoral level. Completion venography in the operating room is recommended, because back-bleeding is unreliable for the assessment of complete thrombus clearance. Thrombosis recurrence rates of less than 20% have been reported (level II evidence). The incidence of PE during the first week after thrombectomy is equivalent to the incidence with treatment with anticoagulation only. The frequency of clinical success has been reported to be between 42% and 93% (47). The largest series of 77 legs with a follow-up period of between 5 and 13 years revealed maintenance of patency but a steady decline in valvular competence (level V evidence) (48).

In the only comparative study of iliofemoral venous thrombosis treatment comparing thrombectomy with anticoagulation (31 patients) versus anticoagulation alone (32 patients), the clinical outcome was better at 6 months (40% asymptomatic vs. 7%), iliofemoral vein patency was improved (76% vs. 35%), and femoropopliteal patency was improved with thrombectomy (52% vs. 26%; level II evidence) (47). At 10 years, the number of patients available for follow-up had fallen to 13 in the thrombectomy group and 17 in the anticoagulation-alone group. An improvement in patency in the thrombectomy group was found (83% vs. 41%), and absence of popliteal reflux was found in only 43% of the anticoagulation-alone group, in comparison with 78% in the thrombectomy plus anticoagulation group. Patients with thrombectomy failures included those with chronic iliac vein obstruction creating recurrence of thrombosis and those with prior DVT that resulted in valvular reflux.

Inferior Vena Caval Interruption

IVC interruption for venous thromboembolism is appropriate if traditional anticoagulation fails, if anticoagulant agents are contraindicated, or if there is significant bleeding associated with anticoagulation. Direct IVC ligation, which was initially advocated, resulted in significant lower extremity venous complications and a high rate of recurrent embolism. Thus, initial intraoperative IVC compartmentalization, clip devices, and eventually intravascular venous devices that did not require abdominal operative placement were developed. These devices resulted in a lower rate of venous stasis complications. The most effective device currently available is the Greenfield vena caval filter, a cone-shaped device. This cone shape allows 85% of its length to contain clot and still maintain flow around its periphery, enabling natural fibrinolysis. Indications for IVC filtration include venous thrombosis or PE in a patient with a contraindication to anticoagulation, complication during anticoagulation, recurrent PE in the presence of adequate anticoagulation, or chronic PE with associated pulmonary hypertension and cor pulmonale, and in a patient immediately

after pulmonary embolectomy. Free-floating iliofemoral DVT may be associated with a 60% incidence of PE despite adequate anticoagulation (level V evidence), whereas free-floating IVC thrombi demonstrate a 27% incidence of PE despite adequate anticoagulation (level V evidence) and bilateral free-floating femoral thrombi have a 43% incidence of PE despite adequate anticoagulation (level V evidence), all additional indications for filter placement. In 642 patients reported in the largest experience in the literature with the Greenfield filter, a contraindication to anticoagulation was the most frequent reason for filter insertion, followed by failure of anticoagulation (level V evidence) (49), although more and more devices today are being placed for thromboembolism prophylaxis. Recurrent PE was noted in only 4% of patients over a 20-year follow-up; the long-term IVC patency rate was 96%, independent of anticoagulation; and venous ulceration was noted in only 3% of patients. No patient with suprarenal filter placement (119 cases) was found to have occluded IVC or renal veins over the follow-up period, which suggests that suprarenal filter placement is safe if necessary, such as in pregnant women or women of childbearing potential (50).

Percutaneous insertion versus direct surgical technique offers a number of advantages for the Greenfield filter, including decreased patient discomfort, decreased time of insertion, and decreased cost. With a percutaneous approach with the original 24-French carrier, the incidence of venous thrombosis at the insertion site was reported at 41% (level V evidence). In response to this problem, a titanium Greenfield filter with modified hooks that reduced the carrier size to 12-French in a 14-French sheath was developed. Outcomes for 173 patients with this modified device revealed 97% successful placement, a recurrent PE rate of only 3%, and IVC occlusion in 1% (level V evidence) (51). The venous thrombosis rate at the insertion site was only 2%.

One study compared filter placement with no filter placement in patients with proximal DVT and also compared standard unfractionated heparin with LMWH (level I evidence) (52). A statistically significant advantage was noted in the filter recipients at 12 days with regard to symptomatic or asymptomatic PE, although there were more recurrent DVTs at 2 years in the filter recipients. Unfortunately, filters were not used in this study with the usual indications as mentioned previously. In addition, the association between the filter presence and recurrent DVT is unlikely, unless the filter catches a massive embolus (leading to distal venous hypertension). This has been rare in the 20-year follow-up of the Greenfield filter. Thus, this study has not lessened the benefit of IVC filters in appropriate patients.

Pulmonary Embolectomy

Surgical approaches for PE are indicated for patients with massive embolism with hypotension who require large doses of vasopressors. These are often patients in whom thrombolytic agents have not been successful. Open pulmonary embolectomy as practiced in the past is associated with high rates of morbidity and mortality. Today, open pulmonary embolectomy is limited to patients who require manual cardiac massage for hypotension or those in whom catheter pulmonary embolectomy fails. A catheter for the removal of pulmonary emboli has been developed. Catheter pulmonary embolectomy is performed with local anesthesia by insertion from either the jugular or common femoral vein. This cup catheter is inserted through a transverse venotomy, and the radiopaque catheter is then visualized under fluoroscopic imaging as it is guided into the right side of the heart. The cup is juxtaposed to the embolus, syringe suction is used to aspirate the clot into the cup, and the entire catheter and clot are removed. Multiple retrievals may be necessary to remove enough thrombus to improve pulmonary hemodynamics. In a series of 46 patients treated with this device, emboli were extracted in 76% of cases, and the 30-day survival rate was 70% (level V evidence) (53). Embolectomy was most successful for major PE and massive PE and least helpful for chronic PE; successful embolectomy was predictive of long-term survival. An addition to pulmonary embolectomy is extended support with the use of extracorporeal membrane oxygenation, to allow the lungs time to recover while support is provided.

PRACTICAL POINTS

- DVT and PE remain significant problems today.
- Duplex ultrasound imaging is now the "gold standard" for DVT diagnosis; V/Q scanning, spiral computed tomographic scanning, and pulmonary angiography are the most widely used tests for PE diagnosis.

- Treatment of DVT and PE includes standard unfractionated heparin and LMWH. The use of LMWH allows for outpatient therapy in certain instances. Other treatment alternatives include thrombolysis, venous thrombectomy, IVC interruption, and pulmonary embolectomy.

REFERENCES

1. Coon WW, Willis PW 3d, Keller JB. Venous thromboembolism and other venous disease in the Tecumseh community health study. *Circulation* 1973;48:839–846.
2. Anderson FA, Wheeler HB, Goldberg RJ, et al. A population-based perspective of the hospital incidence and case-fatality rates of deep vein thrombosis and pulmonary embolism. The Worcester DVT Study. *Arch Intern Med* 1991;151:933–938.
3. Peterson KL. Acute pulmonary thromboembolism: has its evolution been redefined? *Circulation* 1999;99:1280–1283.
4. Douglas MG, Sumner DS. Duplex scanning for deep vein thrombosis: has it replaced both phlebography and noninvasive testing? *Semin Vasc Surg* 1996;9:3.
5. Sarpa MS, Messina LM, Villemure P, et al. Significance of a negative duplex scan in patients suspected of having acute deep venous thrombosis of the lower extremity. *Soc Vasc Tech* 1989;13:224.
6. Anand SS, Wells PS, Hunt D, et al. Does this patient have deep vein thrombosis? *JAMA* 1998;279:1094.
7. Carpenter JP, Holland GA, Baum RA, et al. Magnetic resonance venography for the detection of deep venous thrombosis: comparison with contrast

venography and duplex Doppler ultrasonography. *J Vasc Surg* 1993;18:734.

8. Meaney JF, Weg JG, Chenevert TL, et al. Diagnosis of pulmonary embolism with magnetic resonance angiography. *N Engl J Med* 1997;336:1422.

9. Froehlich JB, Prince MR, Greenfield LJ, et al. "Bull's-eye" sign on gadolinium-enhanced magnetic resonance venography determines thrombus presence and age: a preliminary study. *J Vasc Surg* 1997;26:809.

10. Value of the ventilation/perfusion scan in acute pulmonary embolism. Results of the Prospective Investigation Of Pulmonary Embolism Diagnosis (PIOPED). The PIOPED Investigators. *JAMA* 1990;263:2753.

11. Worsley DF, Alavi A. Comprehensive analysis of the results of the PIOPED study. Prospective investigation of pulmonary embolism diagnosis study. *J Nucl Med* 1995;36:2380.

12. Remy-Jardin M, Remy J. Spiral CT angiography of the pulmonary circulation. *Radiology* 1999;212:615–636.

13. Khaira HS, Mann J. Plasma D-dimer measurement in patients with suspected DVT—a means of avoiding unnecessary venography. *Eur J Vasc Endovasc Surg* 1998;15:235.

14. Lennox AF, Delis KT, Serunkuma S, et al. Combination of a clinical risk assessment score and rapid whole blood D-dimer testing in the diagnosis of deep vein thrombosis in symptomatic patients. *J Vasc Surg* 1999;30:794–804.

15. Hirsh J. Heparin. *N Engl J Med* 1991;324:1565–1574.

16. Douketis JD, Kearon C, Bates S, et al. Risk of fatal pulmonary embolism in patients with treated venous thromboembolism. *JAMA* 1998;279:458–462.

17. Hull RD, Raskob GE, Brant RF, et al. Relation between the time to achieve the lower limit of the APTT therapeutic range and recurrent venous thromboembolism during heparin treatment for deep vein thrombosis. *Arch Intern Med* 1997;157:2562–2568.

18. Hull RD, Raskob GE, Rosenbloom D, et al. Heparin for 5 days as compared with 10 days in the initial treatment of proximal venous thrombosis. *N Engl J Med* 1990;322:1260–1264.

19. Schulman S, Rhedin AS, Lindmarker P, et al. A comparison of six weeks with six months of oral anticoagulant therapy after a first episode of venous thromboembolism. *N Engl J Med* 1995;332:1661–1665.

20. Research Committee of the British Thoracic Society. Optimum duration of anticoagulation for deep-vein thrombosis and pulmonary embolism. *Lancet* 1992;340:873–876.

21. Levine MN, Hirsh J, Gent M, et al. Optimal duration of oral anticoagulant therapy: a randomized trial comparing four weeks with three months of warfarin in patients with proximal deep vein thrombosis. *Thromb Haemost* 1995;74:606–611.

22. Hyers TM, Agnelli G, Hull RD, et al. Antithrombotic therapy for venous thromboembolic disease. *Chest* 1998;114:561S–578S.

23. Prandoni P, Lensing AW, Cogo A, et al. The long-term clinical course of acute deep venous thrombosis. *Ann Intern Med* 1996;125:1–7.

24. Deleted in page proofs.

25. Schulman S, Granqvist S, Holmstrom M, et al. The duration of oral anticoagulant therapy after a second episode of venous thromboembolism. The Duration of Anticoagulation Trial Study Group. *N Engl J Med* 1997;336:393–398.

26. Kearon C, Gent M, Hirsh J, et al. A comparison of three months of anticoagulation with extended anticoagulation for a first episode of idiopathic venous thromboembolism. *N Engl J Med* 1999;340:901–907.

27. Levine MN, Raskob G, Landefeld S, et al. Hemorrhagic complications of anticoagulant treatment. *Chest* 1998;114:511S–523S.

28. Ageno W, Turpie AG. Low-molecular-weight heparin in the treatment of pulmonary embolism. *Semin Vasc Surg* 2000;13:189–193.

29. Hirsh J. Low-molecular-weight heparin: A review of the results of recent studies of the treatment of venous thromboembolism and unstable angina. *Circulation* 1998;98:1575–1582.

30. Leizorovicz A. Comparison of the efficacy and safety of low molecular weight heparins and unfractionated heparin in the initial treatment of deep venous thrombosis. An updated meta-analysis. *Drugs* 1996;52:30–37.

31. Lensing AW, Prandoni P, Prins MH, et al. Deep-vein thrombosis. *Lancet* 1999;353:479–485.

32. van den Belt AG, Prins MH, Lensing AW, et al. Fixed dose subcutaneous low molecular weight heparins versus adjusted dose unfractionated heparin for venous thromboembolism. *Cochrane Database Syst Rev* 2000;(2):CD001100.

33. Low-molecular-weight heparin in the treatment of patients with venous thromboembolism. The Columbus Investigators. *N Engl J Med* 1997;337:657–662.

34. Simonneau G, Sors H, Charbonnier B, et al. A comparison of low-molecular-weight heparin with unfractionated heparin for acute pulmonary embolism. The THESEE Study Group. *N Engl J Med* 1997;337:663–669.

35. Hull RD, Raskob GE, Brant RF, et al. Low-molecular-weight heparin vs heparin in the treatment of patients with pulmonary embolism. *Arch Intern Med* 2000;160:229–236.

36. Groce JB 3rd. Patient outcomes and cost analysis associated with an outpatient deep venous thrombosis treatment program. *Pharmacotherapy* 1998;18:175S–180S.

37. Hull RD, Raskob GE, Rosenbloom D, et al. Treatment of proximal vein thrombosis with subcutaneous low-molecular-weight heparin vs intravenous heparin. An economic perspective. *Arch Intern Med* 1997;157:289–294.

38. van den Belt AG, Bossuyt PM, Prins MH, et al. Replacing inpatient care by outpatient care in the treatment of deep venous thrombosis—an economic evaluation. TASMAN Study Group. *Thromb Haemost* 1998;79:259–263.

39. Lindmarker P, Holmstrom M. Use of low molecular weight heparin (dalteparin), once daily, for the treatment of deep vein thrombosis. A feasibility and health economic study in an outpatient setting. Swedish Venous Thrombosis Dalteparin Trial Group. *J Intern Med* 1996;240:395–401.

40. Meissner MH, Caps MT, Bergelin RO, et al. Early outcome after isolated calf vein thrombosis. *J Vasc Surg* 1997;26:749–756.

41. Dunn AS, Coller B. Outpatient treatment of deep vein thrombosis: translating clinical trials into practice. *Am J Med* 1999;106:660–669.

42. Proctor MC, Greenfield LJ, Froehlich JB, et al. *Limitations and value of ambulating treatment of DVT.* Presented at the American Venous Forum, Dana Point, CA, February 1999.

43. Meissner MH, Manzo RA, Bergelin RO, et al. Deep venous insufficiency: the relationship between lysis and subsequent reflux. *J Vasc Surg* 1993;18:596–608.

44. Semba CP, Dake MD. Iliofemoral deep venous thrombosis: aggressive therapy with catheter-directed thrombolysis. *Radiology* 1994;191:487–494.

45. Mewissen MW. Catheter-directed thrombolysis for lower extremity deep vein thrombosis: report of a national multi-center registry. *Radiology* 1999;211:39–49.

46. Turpie AGG. Thrombolytic agents in venous thrombosis. *J Vasc Surg* 1990;12:196–197.

47. Eklof B, Kistner RL. Is there a role for thrombectomy in iliofemoral venous thrombosis? *Semin Vasc Surg* 1996;9:34–45.

48. Juhan CM, Alimi YS, Barthelemy PJ, et al. Late results of iliofemoral venous thrombectomy. *J Vasc Surg* 1997;25:417–422.

49. Greenfield LJ, Proctor MC. Twenty-year clinical experience with the Greenfield filter. *Cardiovasc Surg* 1995;3:199–205.

50. Henke PK, Varma MR, Proctor MC, et al. Suprarenal Greenfield vena caval filter placement. In: *Modern vascular surgery* McGraw-Hill: New York, 2000:427–434.

51. Greenfield LJ, Proctor MC, Cho KJ, et al. Extended evaluation of the titanium Greenfield vena caval filter. *J Vasc Surg* 1994;20:458–465.

52. Decousus H, Leizorovicz A, Parent F, et al. A clinical trial of vena caval filters in the prevention of pulmonary embolism in patients with proximal deep-vein thrombosis. *N Engl J Med* 1998;338:409–415.

53. Greenfield LJ, Proctor MC, Williams DM, et al. Long-term experience with transvenous catheter pulmonary embolectomy. *J Vasc Surg* 1993;18:450–458.

33

Lower Extremity Ischemia

Peter K. Henke, Sanjay Rajagopalan, and Gilbert R. Upchurch, Jr.

EPIDEMIOLOGY AND USUAL CAUSES

Lower extremity limb pain is a common complaint among patients, particularly the elderly. The first step is to define the cause of the lower extremity pain and, in reference to the topic at hand, determine whether ischemic arterial vascular disease is the causal factor. Once other common causes of limb pain such as arthritis, low back pain, and musculoskeletal and neurologic causes are eliminated, the workup for ischemic vascular disease should commence. Peripheral arterial vascular occlusive disease (PAVOD) is by far the most common disease manifestation of systemic atherosclerosis in patients, apart from coronary heart disease, and is estimated to occur in up to 15% of persons older than 55 years. Risk factors for PAVOD are the same as those for atherosclerosis and include increasing age, tobacco use, hypertension, hyperlipidemia, male gender, hyperhomocystinemia, and diabetes. Other, less common causes of lower extremity vascular occlusive disease symptoms include Buerger's disease (primary small-vessel obliterative arteriopathy associated with tobacco use) and systemic arteritides such as Takayasu's arteritis.

The pathophysiologic process of ischemic PAVOD is critical reduction of blood flow secondary to encroachment of the lumen by atherosclerotic plaque. If the vessel lumen cross-sectional area is narrowed by more than 75%, functionally significant stenosis results, as a consequence of the dramatic impact that alterations in diameter can have on flow. This relationship is approximated by Poiseuille's law (1). The degree of vessel stenosis and whether the stenoses or occlusions are in series or parallel are the most important determinants of the severity of the symptoms and presentation. As muscle activity increases (such as with ambulation), tissue

oxygen demand increases, which is compensated for by increased cardiac output, local vasodilation, and increased limb blood flow. In a patient with critical limb ischemia, tissue oxygen demand exceeds delivery even at rest, with anaerobic glycolysis and lactate production, which results in the sensation of pain. The most common anatomic location for infrainguinal atherosclerotic occlusive disease is at the adductor canal (Hunter's canal) in the distal superior femoral artery (SFA)/proximal popliteal artery, followed by iliac artery lesions. Tibial arterial occlusive vascular disease is more common in diabetic patients and often occurs at a younger age, although the basic pathophysiologic process is the same.

PRESENTING SYMPTOMS AND SIGNS

Many asymptomatic patients have underlying PAVOD evident on arteriography. However, because the occlusion/stenoses occur slowly, collateral vessels develop, and muscle units physiologically adapt. Thus, ischemic pain is minimized. In the pelvis and lower extremity, the importance of internal iliac and profunda femoris collateral vessels in maintaining lower limb blood flow cannot be overstated. In general, most patients with cardiovascular disease have PAVOD of the lower extremities, but whether it needs to be addressed beyond general risk factor modification and exercise depends on the signs and symptoms (of which a full spectrum exists). A detailed and useful set of guidelines for reporting the degree of lower extremity ischemia has been published (2).

The most common and least limb-threatening condition is claudication. This is described typically as limb pain, a sensation of heaviness, or numbness that occurs with ambulation, usually for a reproducibly defined distance, and is relieved by rest. It is important to mention the term *disabling claudication,* because this is the most *subjective indication* for an invasive intervention. The decision to perform an intervention should not be done without critical assessment of the patient's symptoms and living situation. The degree of lower extremity ischemic pain that a patient tolerates is individualized and often dependent on age and occupation. Thus, two-block claudication for a sedentary person would not generally warrant intervention. Conversely, a person who ambulates several miles a day for a living may be significantly impaired by the same degree of claudication. The other end of the PAVOD spectrum is rest pain, described as persistent unremitting pain that occurs without any definite preceding lower limb activity. This often occurs at night when the patient is recumbent and the cardiac output is decreased. The pain is usually relieved by limb dependency. Other physical findings with significant ischemic disease include hair loss, muscle atrophy, and marked rubor in the foot. The patient in whom rest pain is diagnosed certainly needs intervention, not only for relief of pain but also to prevent limb loss.

Ulceration is a common manifestation of PAVOD and often accompanies severe claudication and rest pain. It is important to distinguish ischemic ulceration from venous ulcers (usually medial malleolar in the setting of chronic edema and hyperpigmentation) and neuropathic ulcers (secondary to degeneration of sensory nerves with resultant abnormal pressure distribution on the feet with ambulation). These two types of ulcers may coexist within one patient. Isolated ischemic ulcers are painful and usually occur distally on the foot and toes. These ulcers may progress to frank tissue gangrene and necessitate an urgent amputation if infection supervenes. From a therapeutic standpoint, tissue loss is a definite indication for an intervention to improve blood flow. An endovascular or surgical intervention should precede the débridement or amputation to maximize the chances of tissue salvage.

Overall, any intervention must be judged according to whether the risk entailed by the procedure is less than the benefit derived from the intervention and judged against the possible outcome of severe lifestyle disability and limb loss without the intervention.

A clinical scenario that mandates a slightly different workup is the "blue toe syndrome"; in the typical presentation, a single toe or several toes that have a purplish/black appearance, is usually unilateral, and the toes are quite painful. The presumed cause is atheroembolism. It is important to treat the pain with analgesics, to make sure that the patient is taking antiplatelet therapy, and to initiate a workup that defines the embolic source. In general, this includes an echocardiogram (surface or transesophageal); abdominal, femoral, and popliteal ultrasonography to evaluate for aneurysmal disease; and then arch-to-outflow aortography to evaluate for ulcerative atherosclerotic lesions.

Another important differentiation is whether the patient is presenting with chronic or acute lower extremity ischemia. Acute limb-threatening ischemia is a subset of PAVOD that represents a true emergency, in which the physician must determine the magnitude of the ischemia to prevent limb loss. Limb-threatening ischemia is suggested by the "six Ps": limb pulselessness, pain, pallor, paraesthesias, paralysis, and poikilothermia. The acute presentation is usually quite dramatic. The most common cause of acute lower extremity ischemia is a cardiac thromboembolism; the next most common cause is arterial thrombosis *in situ.* For example, a left atrial thromboembolism in a patient with atrial fibrillation and a left ventricular thromboembolism after a myocardial infarction are typical sources of lower extremity emboli. Less common embolic sources are aortic arch plaques or cardiac tumors. The other diagnostic consideration is thrombosis *in situ,* such as in a patient with severe PAVOD with a significant collateral branch occlusion or a popliteal artery occlusion in the setting of an undiagnosed popliteal artery aneurysm. History and physical examination alone can often enable the physician to distinguish these two scenarios, and the therapeutic approach that follows is slightly different, as discussed later.

HELPFUL TESTS

The history and physical examination of any patient with cardiovascular disease should include evaluation for peripheral manifestations of atherosclerotic occlusive vascular disease. Thorough inquiries of claudication, rest pain, stroke, and neurologic and cardiac symptoms should be obtained. On physical examination, particular attention should be paid to all pulses, both in character and in quality. Loss of hair, shiny dry skin, and trophic nail changes should also be looked for and described. Careful evaluation for any evidence of foot ulcers or deep cracks in the skin between the toes should be noted as well. A physician should be able to determine whether the lower extremity arterial occlusive disease is primarily inflow (e.g., aortoiliac, above the inguinal ligament), outflow (e.g., common femoral artery and distally, below the inguinal ligament), or both, primarily on the basis of the presence or absence of femoral pulses.

Once the history and physical examination suggest the presence of PAVOD, the patient's segmental limb pressures/Doppler waveforms and ankle/brachial indices (ABIs) should be measured. The ABI is based on the differential blood pressure between the highest brachial systolic pressure and the best ankle systolic pressure. Much practical and important information is obtained through these simple tests for estimating the anatomic level and magnitude of arterial insufficiency. They also allow serial assessment of the patient for progression of disease. Typical ranges of ABI that correlate with symptoms are shown in Fig. 33.1. Full lower extremity duplex arterial examination is not routinely performed at our institution because it is quite time consuming and has not replaced arteriography as the "gold standard" for determining further intervention,

though some institutions utilize this fully. Again, the most important determinant for intervention is severity of patient's symptoms or the presence of tissue loss in the setting of PAVOD. The absolute ABI values are not to be used solely as a basis for any intervention, and arteriography is discouraged as a screening test. However, patients with an absolute toe pressure of less than 40 mm Hg do have an increased risk of tissue loss and an increased risk of need for a surgical intervention, in comparison with patients with higher pressures but similar claudication symptoms (3). The recommended diagnostic algorithm is shown in Fig. 33.2.

Two situations bear further discussion: noninvasive testing in diabetic patients and in patients with classical ischemic vascular symptoms but nearly normal ABIs. Diabetic patients have a propensity for arterial medial calcification, which results in noncompressible arteries and, thus, invalid ABIs. A toe/brachial index may be a suitable substitute instead, as well as a review of the Doppler waveform pattern. Some surgeons have opted directly for arteriography in diabetic patients with tissue loss and without palpable pulses (F. LoGerfo, personal communication, 4/2000). In patients with suspected significant PAVOD but normal ABIs, exercise ABIs may be useful for unmasking and confirming a significant occlusive lesion A baseline ABI is measured, and the patient is then put on a treadmill for 5 minutes of ambulation. The ABIs are obtained every minute thereafter to determine magnitude of pressure drop and recovery duration. Both of these are proportional to the degree of stenosis and can help clarify an ischemic cause

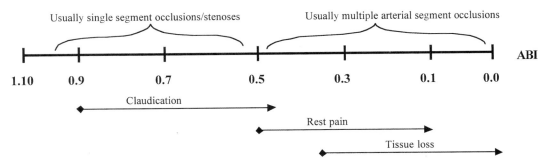

FIG. 33.1. Schematic of generalized ankle/brachial index, symptoms, and anatomic interrelation in patients with peripheral arterial vascular occlusive disease.

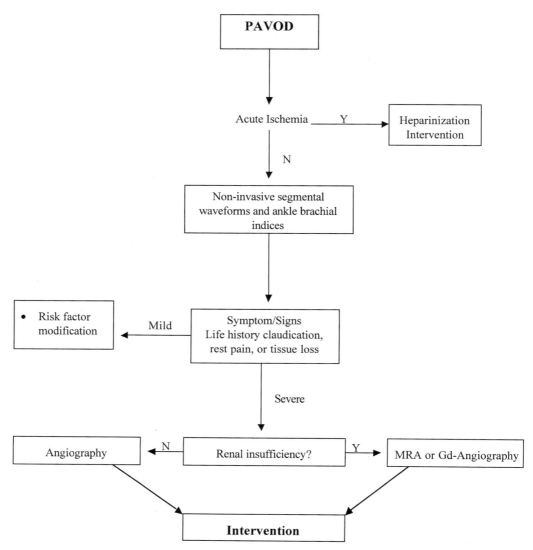

FIG. 33.2. Suggested algorithm for diagnostic evaluation of patients with peripheral arterial vascular occlusive disease.

from other causes of limb pain when the history, physical examination, and resting ABIs do not fully correlate.

Arteriography remains the "gold standard" for determining the anatomic site, severity, and extent of atherosclerotic occlusive disease. It must again be emphasized that patients with stable claudication but without tissue loss should not undergo invasive testing unless interventions are planned because definite risk of complications

exist. The angiographic images are most often performed in the angiography suite with digital subtraction angiographic techniques. These techniques produce high-resolution images and minimize contrast volume. Some institutions have adopted intraoperative angiography, which is immediately followed by an operative procedure if indicated (4). The standard aorta and outflow arteriogram is used to examine the infrarenal aorta, including the renal arteries and oblique views of the pelvis and groin, to define the internal/external iliac and deep/superficial femoral artery bifurcations, respectively. Contrast runoff is performed to assess popliteal and tibial vessels. Foot films are very important for defining suitable targets for a very distal bypass. Of note, in the patient with chronic renal insufficiency in whom contrast-induced nephropathy is a significant risk, gadolinium can be used with good resolution and no impairment of renal function (D. Williams, personal communication, 2/2001). In addition, preprocedural administration of acetylcysteine has been shown to significantly decrease the incidence of nephrotoxicity (5).

Magnetic resonance angiography has emerged as a useful test for arterial anatomy with very good results. In comparison trials with conventional angiography, sensitivity and specificity for MRA was found to be essentially equivalent with arteriography (6,7). Advantages include no contrast-induced nephropathy risk and the noninvasive nature of the procedure. Furthermore, tissue abnormalities can be determined at the same time, and in at least one study, greater sensitivity for very distal run-off vessels was observed (8). However, the specialized magnetic resonance expertise is not widely available at many hospitals and thus has not replaced arteriography as the "gold standard."

THERAPY

All patients with PAVOD require medical and risk factor reduction therapy regardless of whether they will undergo an invasive procedure. Indeed, a comprehensive consensus statement regarding the diagnosis and treatment has been published (9). The overwhelming priority in the treatment of the patient with claudication is the correction of underlying risk factors that not only may contribute to the progression of disease but also may increase the risk of dying from cardiovascular causes. Of equal importance are reassuring the patient that exercise is good for claudication and instituting antiplatelet therapy for overall cardiovascular protection. Only a minority of patients require some intervention, in the form of pharmacotherapy, surgery, or angioplasty.

Risk Factor Modification/Medical Therapy

Exercise Rehabilitation

There is unequivocal evidence that exercise rehabilitation reduces symptom severity and prolongs claudication distance substantially. A metaanalysis of several prospective controlled studies indicates that the maximal walking distance increases by more than 100% (two blocks or more) (10). The predictors of response appear to be supervised training, high levels of claudication pain during the rehabilitation session, and at least 3 months or more of training. Treadmill exercise appears to be far more effective than strength training. Figure 33.3 provides some guidelines for initiation of exercise therapy in the patient with claudication.

Smoking Cessation

All tobacco-using patients with claudication should be referred to a smoking cessation program; for those unable to quit, the use of nicotine replacement therapies in the form of gum, spray, or patch may be considered with intensive counseling. The various nicotine replacement therapies significantly decrease symptoms of the withdrawal syndrome as smokers abruptly stop smoking. The different formulations of these therapies provide alternative methods for delivery and have slightly different onsets of action and durations. In metaanalyses, cessation rates with transdermal nicotine range from 15% to 31%, with a trend toward decreased efficacy in the most highly dependent smokers. Nicotine gum studies demonstrate a similar range of cessation rates; the greatest efficacy is seen with the 4-mg gum in highly dependent smokers. Nasal spray cessation rates range from 26% to 28%, also with greatest efficacy in the most dependent smokers. Limited inhaler studies report cessation rates similar to those for the nasal spray. Bupropion was initially developed and marketed as an antidepressant medication (Wellbutrin), although the mechanism by which bupropion aids in smoking cessation is unknown. The recommended dosage schedule includes a starting dose of 150 mg per day for 3 days, then increasing to twice per day, with an approximately

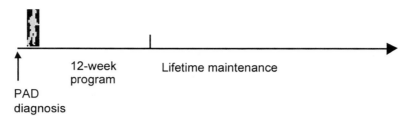

12-week
program

Lifetime maintenance

PAD
diagnosis

- 5 treadmill sessions per week, one hour in duration (3 supervised + 2 unsupervised) for 3-6 months
- Initial workload set by symptom limited Gardner treadmill workload that brings on claudication
- Patient asked to stop and rest when claudication pains of moderate severity (scored 3 or 4 on a 5 point scale)
- Rest periods interspersed with periods of treadmill walking
- In return visits if patient can walk for >10 minutes at the lower work load then speed increased till patient at 3 mph then grade increased

FIG. 33.3. A prescription for exercise. PAD, peripheral arterial disease.

25% efficacy rate for tobacco use cessation. In one published clinical trial (11), "treatment with sustained-release bupropion alone or in combination with a nicotine patch resulted in significantly higher long-term rates of smoking cessation than use of either the nicotine patch alone or placebo." Abstinence rates were higher with combination therapy than with bupropion alone, but the difference was not statistically significant.

Weight Loss

It is generally believed that obesity may contribute to reduction in claudication distance, and weight loss may alleviate this reduction. All obese patients with symptomatic claudication should be encouraged to lose weight.

Glycemic Control

There is a strong correlation between duration of diabetes and risk of claudication and chronic critical limb ischemia. However, the data on strict diabetes control and amelioration of symptoms of claudication are conflicting. The United Kingdom Prospective Diabetes Study (UKPDS) examined a variety of end points, including peripheral vascular complications with aggressive glycemic control, using a variety of measures including insulin, sulfonylureas, and metformin in patients with type II diabetes. Tight glycemic control in the study was not associated with improvement in risk for macrovascular events, including peripheral vascular events (12). Because patients with peripheral vascular disease are at risk for the development of foot complications, they should be advised to inspect their feet regularly, avoid pressure points with specially designed footwear, and pay immediate attention to minor cracks and fissures in the skin.

Treatment of Hyperlipidemic States

For the patient with peripheral arterial disease (PAD), the National Cholesterol Education Program guidelines for the patient with established coronary artery disease are applicable. To this effect, low-density lipoprotein cholesterol levels above 125 mg/dL should be treated aggressively with statins. Data from the Veterans Affairs High-Density Lipoprotein Cholesterol Intervention Trial (VA-HIT) are especially relevant to the diabetic patient population, whose metabolic profile often comprises low levels of high-density lipoprotein and elevated triglyceride levels (13). These patients would benefit from fibrate therapy.

Hypertension Control

Although there are no data linking blood pressure control to the natural history of PAD, the overall cardiovascular protective effects are so overwhelming that hypertension control is of great importance. Due consideration should also be given to secondary causes of hypertension, especially renal artery stenosis. According to the UKPDS data and the Hypertension Optimal Treatment (HOT) study results, control of blood pressure appears to be far more important than tight glycemic control in diabetic patients (12,14). The choices for antihypertensive therapies should be guided by Joint National Committee VI guidelines (15). In this regard, it must be emphasized that there is no evidence that beta blockers adversely affect mild to moderate claudication, and they should be considered strongly, especially for the patient with concomitant coronary artery disease. For diabetic hypertensive patients, angiotensin-converting enzyme inhibitors ought to be first choice. On the basis of the benefit of angiotensin-converting enzyme inhibitors in patients with established atherosclerosis, these drugs may be preferred over calcium channel blockers in the initial therapy of uncomplicated hypertension in the patient with PAD.

Correction of Hyperhomocystinemia

Although hyperhomocystinemia is a strong risk factor for PAD but whether the correction of elevated homocysteine levels with B vitamins and folic acid results in lowering of vascular related end points is unknown. However, it is recommended that patients be screened for hyperhomocystinemia and treated if their levels were found to be high.

Pharmacotherapy for Claudication

Pharmacotherapy for claudication is not meant to replace risk factor modification or exercise rehabilitation but rather to complement it. The drugs that are currently in use are mentioned as follows.

Cilostazol

Cilostazol is a type III phosphodiesterase inhibitor that is both a vasodilator and an antiplatelet agent. It also has favorable effects on the lipoprotein profile, including a 15% reduction in triglyceride levels and a 10% increase in high-density lipoprotein levels. A large phase III clinical trial that was composed of eight separate double-blinded trials involving more than 2,000 patients confirmed the efficacy of cilostazol in improving treadmill walking time and quality of life. Initial benefit may not be seen for up to 3 months after initiation of the drug, and the drug effect wanes within a month of discontinuation. Cilostazol is metabolized to a large extent by the CYP3A4 pathway but has no effect on the activity of this enzyme system. Drugs that inhibit these pathways may result in an increase in drug levels (see Table 33.1). Because of concerns about the use of phosphodiesterase inhibitors in patients with depressed left ventricular systolic function, the use of cilostazol is contraindicated in patients with congestive heart failure and a left ventricular ejection fraction of less than 40%.

Pentoxifylline

Pentoxifylline is a substituted xanthine derivative that, unlike theophylline, has hemorheologic properties (i.e., it is an agent that alters blood viscosity). In early clinical trials, pentoxifylline was shown to improve initial claudication distance and peak walking time, but subsequent studies have failed to demonstrate any improvement in these parameters.

Beraprost

Beraprost sodium is a new, stable, orally active prostaglandin I_2 analogue with antiplatelet and vasodilating properties. In a single-blinded phase III study involving more than 500 patients with moderate claudication, beraprost at a dosage of 40 μg three times a day was shown to improve pain-free claudication distance as well as peak walking time (16). Secondary end points included incidence of critical cardiovascular events (death, myocardial infarction, peripheral or

TABLE 33.1. *Drugs used in treatment of claudication*

Drug	Dosage	Strength of evidence in trials[a]	Side effects	Interactions
Cilostazol	50–100 mg b.i.d.	Class I	Headache, diarrhea, palpitations, and dizziness	Substances that inhibit CYPA4 or CYP2C19, including macrolide antibiotics, ketoconazole, grapefruit juice, and omeprazole,
Pentoxifylline	400 mg t.i.d.	Class II	Nausea, bloating, and dizziness	Theophylline (increases levels)
Beraprost	40 μg t.i.d.	Class II	Headache, flushing	—

[a]Class I: General agreement that the therapy is efficacious. Class II: Conflicting/diverging opinions on efficacy. Class III: Not useful/harmful.

coronary percutaneous transluminal angioplasty or bypass surgery, transient ischemic attack, stroke, and critical limb ischemia) and beraprost appeared to have a favorable reduction in these events. This drug is not yet available in the United States. On a more recent trial in the U.S., this agent did not demonstrate efficacy.

Agents under Investigation

Carnitine

Metabolic abnormalities in the lower extremity muscles have been demonstrated in patients with PAD. There has been a direct correlation between metabolic intermediates of carnitine metabolism and impaired exercise performance, and therefore studies have investigated the role of supplementing L-carnitine or its potent analogue, propionyl-L-carnitine. Two phase II double-blinded placebo-controlled trials have demonstrated improvements in peak walking times with propionyl-L-carnitine in comparison with placebo in select subgroups of patients who have more severe symptoms at baseline (17,18). To achieve a benefit, the drug must to be taken at doses of 1 g twice a day for a duration of 1 year.

L-*Arginine*

L-Arginine, the precursor for nitric oxide synthesis has been demonstrated to have favorable effects in improving peak walking time and pain-free claudication time in small trials (19). The precise mechanism may be more complex than

a simple restoration of L-arginine stores in the body. The dose of this drug, which is consumed as a bar, is 1 g orally twice a day.

Angiogenic Growth Factors

Angiogenic growth factors are proteins that have been shown to stimulate the growth of capillary blood vessels *in vitro* and *in vivo* in simple animal models of hind limb ischemia. Various growth factors have been implicated, including vascular endothelial growth factor (VEGF), fibroblast growth factor, and platelet-derived growth factor. In addition, potent transcription factors such as hypoxia inducible factor alpha (HIF1-α) that are important for the regulation of VEGF levels are also being tested in early phase I and phase II trials. Whether the administration of these factors by themselves or in combination result in a meaningful improvement in claudication symptoms remains to be seen.

Surgical and Endovascular Therapy

Surgical and interventional options are available for patients in whom medical/exercise therapy has failed and those with an acutely ischemic limb [classified as threatened limb, category IIa or IIb (2)] (Fig. 33.4). If limb-threatening ischemia exists, the first order the physician should convey is full heparinization (100 to 150 U/kg, intravenous bolus). The history and physical examination are crucial in determining the next step: namely, whether to proceed directly to the operating room or the angiography suite (Table 33.2).

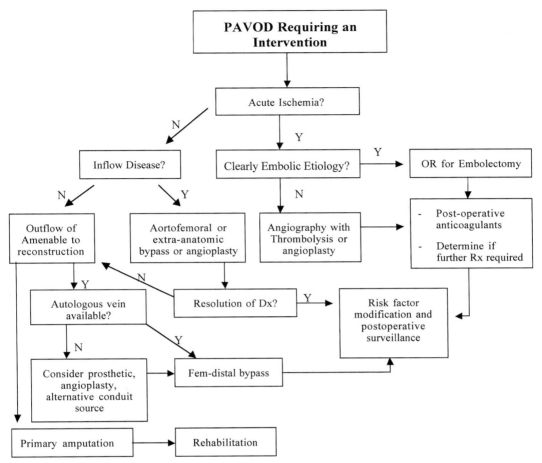

FIG. 33.4. Suggested algorithm for therapeutic approach to patients with peripheral arterial vascular occlusive disease deemed suitable for an intervention.

If evidence suggests that the process is embolic in the setting of nonsignificant underlying PAVOD, the patient should proceed directly to the operating room for open embolectomy. Conversely, if there is any question of whether the process is embolic or thrombotic, angiography with the option for thrombolysis is the best course. In two well-controlled trials comparing thrombolysis with direct surgery (20,21), the outcomes of 6-month amputation and death rate were not significantly different, although major bleeding complications were more numerous in patients receiving thrombolytics. Furthermore, long-term revascularization durability after thrombolysis is also not as good in comparison with surgical therapy (21). Thus, thrombolysis can be recommended for semiacute ischemia (less than 14 days) with reasonable results, although often as a prelude to a surgical bypass.

Endovascular therapies are becoming more commonplace with the availability of stents and catheter devices and as the number of practitioners willing to perform this type of intervention increases. At present, lesser symptoms, such as modest claudication, do not warrant this less invasive approach (with the endovascular techniques described), because they have not proved to be more efficacious than exercise and risk factor modification alone (22). The endovascular

TABLE 33.2. *Comparison of operative embolectomy with angiography and lysis for acute lower extremity ischemia*

Presumed diagnosis	Thromboembolism	Thromboses *in situ*
Procedure	Operative embolectomy	Angioplasty with lysis
Pertinent history and physical examination findings	Acute onset of symptoms	Slower onset of symptoms
	No prior PAVOD diagnosis	History of PAVOD
	Recent cardiac event	No cardiac history
	Timing well documented	Older patient
	Normal findings on contralateral limb examination	Abnormal findings on contralateral limb examination
Anatomic conditions	Aortic bifurcation	May be diffuse/occlusive or distal arteries
	Femoral bifurcation	
	Popliteal artery disease	
Advantages	Rapid restoration of blood flow	Define anatomy for bypass
	Simple	Lyse small artery thrombi
	Minimal hemorrhagic risk	No anesthesia risk
	Possible lower cost	
Disadvantages	Anesthetic	Hemorrhagic risk
	Wound infection potential	Failed lysis
		Contrast risk
		Slower restoration of blood flow

PAVOD, peripheral arterial vascular occlusive disease.

approach is appealing, because it is less invasive, is less physiologically stressful, offers decreased hospital length of stay, and possibly reduces cost in comparison with open operative therapy. The arterial lesions best treated with angioplasty, stent implantation, or both are those in larger arteries such as the aorta or common iliac artery with short concentric stenotic lesions and unobstructed runoff, for which 5-year patency rates are nearly equivalent to those after surgical repair (23) (Fig. 33.5). Restenosis rates with iliac intervention tend to be low, and stent implantation in conjunction with angioplasty in this situation has not been shown to decrease recurrent stenosis or increase patency rates (24,25). Longer segment external iliac, SFA, and popliteal or distal lesions can, technically, be successfully repaired by angioplasty; however, long-term patency rates are lower than at other sites and significantly lower than those for open operative bypass (26). Recanalization of short occlusions in the iliac artery or SFA is also being more commonly pursued with the endovascular route, with reasonable patency rates (Fig. 33.6). However, morbidity and mortality rates are not significantly lower than those with open repair, as documented in one study (25,27).

The disadvantages of endovascular techniques for infrainguinal disease primarily concern the durability and long-term patency, as well as the increased need for further interventions that often increase cost and patient discomfort. At the current time, the authors recommend primary use of angioplasty for focal aortic, iliac, or short SFA stenotic lesions (less than 3 cm) with adequate runoff and in infrainguinal arteries in patients with prohibitive operative risks. In younger patients with long segment iliac or femoral artery disease, operative bypass provides better long-term durability with low morbidity and mortality rates. However, all physicians who treat peripheral vascular disease must individualize these options and tools.

The surgical options for bypass are briefly reviewed as follows. It is imperative that inflow disease be addressed first. Oftentimes, in combined inflow and outflow disease, improving inflow alone suffices in relieving most of the patients' symptoms, and more distal arterial disease necessitates no further intervention. In general, inflow or aortoiliac disease is treated with an aortobifemoral prosthetic bypass. Inflow reconstruction yields a good result before further infrainguinal reconstructions (28). In patients in whom this

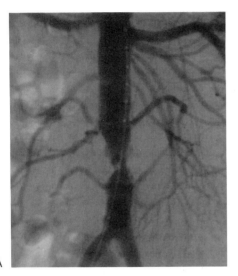
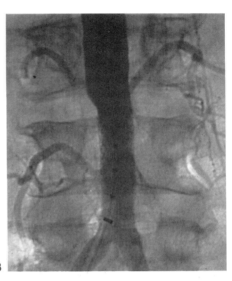

A   B

FIG. 33.5. Angiograms of a patient who had a history of lifestyle-limiting claudication and a high-grade aortic focal stenosis. Although his resting ankle/brachial indices (ABIs) were approximately 0.8, his exercise ABIs dropped dramatically to 0.4. A high-grade focal infrarenal aortic stenosis (more than 80%) **(A)** is seen with a 45–mm HG pressure gradient **(B).** A balloon angioplasty and stent implantation procedure was done; the resultant postprocedural angiogram showed an excellent technical result. No appreciable pressure gradient was measured after the procedure. The postoperatively, his pedal pulses were palpable and he had full relief of his symptoms.

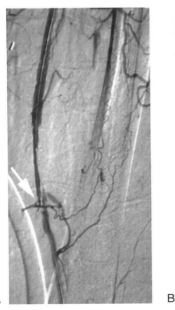
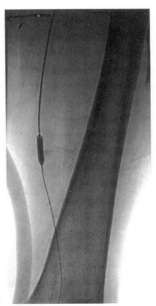
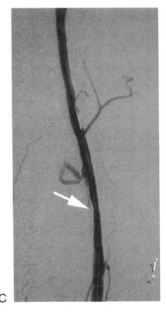

A   B   C

FIG. 33.6. Views in a patient with severe claudication and no available autologous conduit. **A,** A short segment superior femoral artery (SFA)occlusion was the main anatomic finding (*arrow*). **B,** The balloon has followed the wire across the occluded segment, probably in the subintimal plane. **C,** Recanalization of the SFA was successful, with a good angiographic result (*arrow*). After the procedure, the patient experienced full relief of his symptoms.

procedure is not feasible (e.g., those with hostile conditions in the abdomen), an axillofemoral or thoracobifemoral bypass may be performed. Infrainguinal or outflow disease presents more options and more controversy. The proximal artery is most often the common femoral artery, and the distal artery is that which arteriographically provides the best anatomic target for outflow to and across the foot. For example, a patient with a nonhealing ulcer on the great toe with an SFA occlusion, a diseased popliteal artery, and a patent anterior tibial artery should undergo a femoral-to-anterior tibial bypass (Fig. 33.7).

The options for bypass conduit are an autologous vein (usually the ipsilateral greater saphenous vein), prosthetic material, the umbilical vein, or a cryopreserved vein. The latter two options are much less commonly used and are not discussed here. Several large trials have detailed the comparative efficacy between prosthetic and autologous tissue as an infrainguinal bypass conduit (29,30). These studies suggest the following: (a) In any below-knee bypass in which a vein is available (arm or leg), an autologous conduit should be used, and (b) an above-knee bypass should be performed with the ipsilateral greater saphenous vein, if available; however, the use of prosthetic material as an initial conduit is not unreasonable, inasmuch as long-term patency results are not appreciably different over 2 to

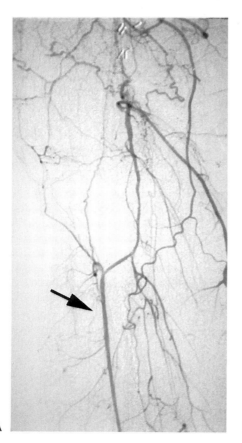 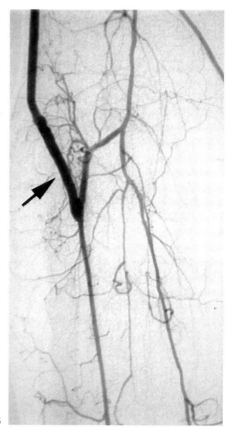

A   B

FIG. 33.7. Example of peripheral arterial vascular occlusive disease affecting the popliteal-tibial arteries, with rest pain and a nonhealing ulcer. The patient had an adequate ipsilateral autologous conduit and underwent a femoral–to–dorsalis pedis bypass with reversed GSV (greater saphenous vein). **A,** The preoperative angiogram shows an adequate anterior tibial artery target (*arrow*). **B,** The postoperative angiogram shows a patent graft (*arrow*) with no evidence of any technical defects.

3 years of follow-up between these two conduit types. Our current practice is to use an autologous vein if available and a prosthetic as a second choice. In the patient in whom no autologous vein is available and the patient's limb is in jeopardy, good efficacy has been reported with the use of a prosthetic conduit with a distal vein patch in limited series (31). The debate between *in situ,* reversed, and nonreverse translocated vein bypasses can be summarized as saying that current studies suggest clinical equipoise and should be based on the surgeon's own preference and best outcomes (32–34).

Postoperatively, patients who receive an endovascular stent or angioplasty are usually prescribed a combined antiplatelet regimen of aspirin and clopidogrel for six weeks, on the empirical basis of coronary stent trials (35). Aspirin is recommended in all patients to decrease graft occlusion, as well as for its cardiac protective effects. A study comparing infrainguinal autologous bypass with and without adjunctive ticlopidine has shown superior graft patency rates in those receiving this antiplatelet agent, but further trials are needed to fully evaluate this adjunct (36). It is also probably beneficial for patients to receive anticoagulation with a vitamin K antagonist, such as warfarin (Coumadin), in high-risk grafts prone to thrombosis, such as those with prosthetic below-knee and composite grafts (31).

PROGNOSIS/OUTCOMES

Medical therapy with risk factor modification and an exercise program has been shown to very effective in increasing walking distance for patients who are compliant with the regimen. This has already been emphasized. Overall, 5-year assisted patency rates in infrainguinal bypass grafts and 10-year rates in aortoiliac grafts approach 80%, and the limb salvage rate is even higher (28–31,33,34). Endovascular therapeutic outcomes are more dependent on the anatomic location and runoff beyond the occlusive lesion; for example, in one large prospective trial, common iliac angioplasty was associated with a 5-year patency rate of 60%, whereas that for femoral/popliteal angioplasty was only 40% (23). In other smaller studies, the 2-year assisted patency rate for iliac

angioplasty was between 45% and 90%, depending on anatomic factors (24,26), whereas that for SFA angioplasty at 1 year was 46% patency (25). Perioperative mortality rates are in the range of 1% to 3% (28–31). The presence of PAVOD itself is the harbinger of severe generalized atherosclerotic disease, and approximately 30% to 50% of these patients die over a 5-year span after their intervention (37). In fact, patients with multivessel coronary artery disease have a fivefold greater mortality rate if coexistent PAVOD is present (38).

Early operative failure (within 30 days), such as stent or bypass occlusion, does occur in a minority of patients (less than 10%). These patients usually require an aggressive revascularization attempt, whether it is with thrombolytic agents, angioplasty, and stent implantation or with graft thrombectomy and correction of the technical problem (or repeat grafting). Late angioplasty failures may be treated with repeat angioplasty or conversion to open operation, and late bypass graft failures should usually be treated with a new bypass, preferable avoiding the previously operated fields.

Overall, an aggressive approach to limb salvage with surgical and endovascular approaches results in decreased amputation rates, increased survival rates, and an improved quality of life (39,40). Only about 5% of patients have no distal outflow artery target and are candidates for primary amputation if rest pain or tissue loss persists. Amputation is associated with decreased long-term survival, particularly in patients with end-stage renal disease (41).

FOLLOW-UP

Several long-term care issues of PAVOD patients need to be emphasized. First, once the bypass or intervention has been completed successfully, these patients may require further surgery for limb infection or amputation. Occasionally, a patient with a functioning bypass may require an amputation for persistent infection. This scenario is more common in diabetic and renal failure patients. More commonly, chronic limb pain and swelling with decreased mobility plagues a certain number of these patients. Postoperative

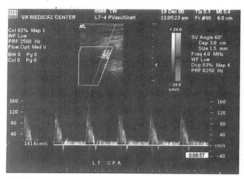
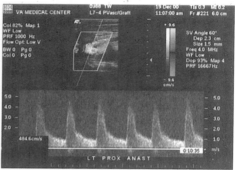

A

HISTORY:
      THIS IS A FOLLOW-UP EVALUATION POST GRAFT PLACEMENT.
PERIPHERAL ARTERIAL DUPLEX SCAN.

LEFT:

COMMON FEMORAL ARTERY: 141   CM/SEC

PROXIMAL ANASTAMOSIS: 484   CM/SEC

PROXIMAL GRAFT: 162   CM/SEC

DISTAL GRAFT: 76   CM/SEC

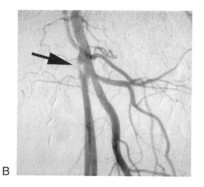

B

FIG. 33.8. A, Example of 3-month graft surveillance duplex scans of left femoral–to–below-knee popliteal bypass, showing a high-grade focal lesion at the proximal vein graft anastomosis. Velocities are as shown with a PSV ratio of 3.4. **B,** A confirmatory angiogram reveals a high-grade focal stenosis (*arrow*). The patient underwent a successful vein patch angioplasty with intraoperative normalization of graft flows and more than a 0.15 increase in the ankle/brachial index. The likely pathophysiologic process was neointimal hyperplasia, as judged at surgery.

physical therapy, with structured exercise programs and compression stockings to reduce edema that inevitably occurs after most bypasses, is useful. The cause of postoperative edema has not been fully defined but is probably a combination of lymphatic disruption, reperfusion injury, and, in some instances, venous insufficiency (42). An important study by Abou-Zamzam et al. showed that preoperative ambulatory functional status was the best predictor of postoperative ambulatory status and that mortality was due mostly to comorbid diseases, not to the surgery itself (43). Because a majority of operative patients require further procedures related to PAVOD, the decision for intervention is not to be taken lightly; it should be discussed with the patient and the patient's family, to affirm realistic outcome expectations (44). These outcome issues are now

prominent in studies examining the functional patient outcome rather than just technical aspects (43, 45).

Another important issue in follow-up is that after the intervention, whether percutaneous or operative, these patients need to be monitored for their lifetime by a vascular specialist. As part of the follow-up in patients after angioplasty, especially for infrainguinal lesions, high-risk lesions (e.g., those in the long segment of the external iliac artery) or individuals at high risk (those who continue to smoke), it is recommended that ABIs be obtained every 3 months for 1 year and every 6 months thereafter. In patients with an infrainguinal autologous vein bypass, duplex graft surveillance has proven efficacy for prolonging graft patency and limb salvage and is cost effective (46–48).

Intraoperatively, a duplex scan is performed along the whole graft, and abnormalities and flow velocity are noted and corrected (49). Graft abnormalities tend to occur at the proximal and distal anastomotic sites in reversed grafts and at sites of retained valves or injury in the *in situ* grafts. The detection of significant graft stenoses before thrombosis (for which later graft salvage is nearly impossible) is imperative. For example, a peak systolic velocity ratio of greater than 3.5 (at the point of stenosis in comparison with the proximal flow) and a mean graft velocity of less than 50 cm/second are the currently recommended criteria for critical stenosis that should be operatively corrected (50) (Fig. 33.8). Our protocol is an intraoperative

scan (with or without angiogram), followed by scans every 3 months for 1 year and then every 6 months for the next year, and then yearly throughout life of the graft, although the most cost-effective algorithm has not yet been fully determined. Last, development of significant symptoms of PAVOD in the contralateral limb occurs in approximately 25% of patients. Again, risk factor modification and exercise can often stave off the need for any further interventional treatment on the contralateral limb and should be the goals. The setting of an operative or endovascular intervention is a prime time to emphasize the lifestyle changes that are critical in these patients to ensure a longer life.

PRACTICAL POINTS

- Peripheral arterial occlusive disease is prevalent in patients with coronary heart disease and should be actively identified from the history and physical examination.
- Noninvasive testing should be an extension of the physical examination and allows quantification of arterial ischemia.
- Risk factor reduction, establishment of an exercise program, and cessation of tobacco use are top management priorities, whether

an invasive procedure is performed or not.
- Endovascular angioplasty/stent implantation therapy has the best outcomes in short, focal large-artery stenoses.
- Surgical therapy for PAVOD is durable, with excellent long-term patency.
- PAVOD is a marker of severe generalized atherosclerosis, and the 5-year mortality rate is significant.
- Patients with PAVOD need lifelong care.

REFERENCES

1. Barnes RW. Hemodynamics for the vascular surgeon. *Arch Surg* 1980;115:216–223.
2. Rutherford RN, Baker JD, Ernst C, et al. Recommended standards for reports dealing with lower extremity ischemia: revised version. *J Vasc Surg* 1997;26:517–538.
3. Bowers BL, Valentine RJ, Myers SI, et al. The natural history of patients with claudication with toe pressures of 40 mmHg or less. *J Vasc Surg* 1993;18:506–511.
4. Melliere D, Cron J, Allaire E, et al. Indications and benefits of simultaneous endoluminal balloon angioplasty and open surgery during elective lower limb revascularization. *Cardiovasc Surg* 1999;7:242–246.
5. Tepel M, van der Giet M, Schwarzfeld C, et al. Prevention of radiographic-contrast-agent-induced reductions in renal function by acetylcysteine. *N Engl J Med* 2000;343:180–184.
6. Baum RA, Rutter CM, Sunshine JH, et al. Multicen-

ter trial to evaluate vascular magnetic resonance angiography of the lower extremity. *JAMA* 1995;274:875–880.
7. Owen RS, Carpenter JP, Baum RA, et al. Magnetic resonance imaging of angiographically occult runoff vessel in peripheral arterial occlusive disease. *N Engl J Med* 1992;326:1577–1581.
8. Meaney JFM, Ridgway JP, Chakraverty S, et al. Stepping-table gadolinium enhanced digital subtraction MR angiography of the aorta and lower extremity arteries: preliminary experience. *Radiology* 1999;211:59–67.
9. Weitz JI, Byrne J, Clagett GP, et al. Diagnosis and treatment of chronic arterial insufficiency of the lower extremities: a critical review. *Circulation* 1996;94:3026–3049.
10. Gardner AW, Poehlman ET. Exercise rehabilitation programs for the treatment of claudication pain. A meta-analysis. *JAMA* 1995;274:975–980.

11. Jorenby DE, Leischow SJ, Nides MA, et al. A controlled trial of sustained-release bupropion, a nicotine patch, or both for smoking cessation. *N Engl J Med* 1999;340:685–691.

12. Intensive blood-glucose control with sulfonylureas or insulin compared with conventional treatment and risk of complications in patients with type 2 diabetes (UKPDS 33). UK Prospective Diabetes Study (UKPDS) Group. *Lancet* 1998;352:837–853.

13. Rubins HB, Robins SJ, Collins D, et al. Gemfibrozil for the secondary prevention of coronary heart disease in men with low levels of high-density lipoprotein cholesterol. Veterans Affairs High-Density Lipoprotein Cholesterol Intervention Trial Study Group. *N Engl J Med* 1999;341:410–418.

14. Hansson L, Zanchetti A, Carruthers SG, et al. Effects of intensive blood-pressure lowering and low-dose aspirin in patients with hypertension: principal results of the Hypertension Optimal Treatment (HOT) randomised trial. HOT Study Group. *Lancet* 1998;351:1755–1762.

15. The sixth report of the Joint National Committee on prevention, detection, evaluation, and treatment of high blood pressure. *Arch Intern Med* 1997;157:2413–2446.

16. Lievre M, Morand S, Besse B, et al. Oral beraprost sodium, a prostaglandin I2 analogue, for intermittent claudication : A double-blind, randomized, multicenter controlled trial. *Circulation* 2000;102:426–431.

17. Brevetti G, Diehm C, Lambert D. European multicenter study on propionyl-L-carnitine in intermittent claudication. *J Am Coll Card* 1999;34:1618–1624.

18. Brevetti G, Perna S, Sabba C, et al. Propionyl-L-carnitine in intermittent claudication: double-blind, placebo-controlled, dose titration, multicenter study. *J Am Coll Cardiol* 1995;26:1411–1416.

19. Maxwell AJ, Anderson BE, Cooke JP. Nutritional therapy for peripheral arterial disease: a double-blind, placebo-controlled, randomized trial of HeartBar. *Vasc Med* 2000;5:11–19.

20. Ouriel K, Veith FJ, Sasahara AA. A comparison of recombinant urokinase with vascular surgery as initial treatment for acute arterial occlusion of the legs. *N Engl J Med* 1998;338:1105–1111.

21. Weaver F, Comerota AJ, Youngblood M, et al. Surgical revascularization versus thrombolysis for nonembolic lower extremity native artery occlusions: results of a prospective randomized trial. *J Vasc Surg* 1996;24:513–523.

22. Leng GC, Davis M, Baker D. Bypass surgery for chronic lower limb ischaemia. *Cochrane Database Syst Rev* 2000;(3):CD002000.

23. Johnston KW, Rae M, Hogg-Johnston SA, et al. 5-year results of a prospective study of percutaneous transluminal angioplasty. *Ann Surg* 1987;206:403–413.

24. Tetteroo E, van dr Graaf Y, Bosch JL, et al. Randomised comparison of primary stent placement versus primary angioplasty followed by selective stent placement in patients with iliac-artery occlusive disease. *Lancet* 1998;351:1153–1159.

25. Gray BH, Sullivan TM, Childs MB, et al. High incidence of restenosis/reocclusion of stents in the percutaneous treatment of long-segment superficial femoral artery disease after suboptimal angioplasty. *J Vasc Surg* 1997;25:74–83.

26. Powell RJ, Fillinger M, Walsh DB, et al. Predicting outcome of angioplasty and selective stenting of multisegment iliac artery occlusive disease. *J Vasc Surg* 2000;32:564–569.

27. Matsi PJ, Manninen HI. Complications of lower limits percutaneous transluminal angioplasty: a prospective analysis of 410 procedures on 295 consecutive patients. *Cardiovasc Intervent Radiol* 1998;21:361–366.

28. Eagleton MJ, Illig KA, Green RM, et al. Impact of inflow reconstruction on infrainguinal bypass. *J Vasc Surg* 1997;26:928–938.

29. Veterans Administration Cooperative Study Group 141. Comparative evaluation of prosthetic, reversed, and *in situ* vein bypass grafts in distal popliteal and tibial-peroneal revascularization. *Arch Surg* 1988;123:434–438.

30. Veith FJ, Gupta SK, Ascer E, et al. Six-year prospective multicenter randomized comparison of autologous saphenous vein and expanded polytetrafluorethylene grafts in infrainguinal arterial reconstructions. *J Vasc Surg* 1986;3:104–114.

31. Neville RF, Tempesta B, Sidawy AN. Tibial bypass for limb salvage using polytetrafluoroethylene with a distal vein patch. *J Vasc Surg* 2001;33:266–272.

32. Harris PL, Veith FJ, Shanik GD, et al. Prospective randomized comparison of *in situ* and reversed infrapopliteal vein grafts. *Br J Surg* 1993;80:173–176.

33. Taylor LM Jr, Edwards JM, Porter JM. Present status of reversed vein bypass grafting: Five-year results of a modern series. *J Vasc Surg* 1990;11:193–206.

34. Donaldson MC, Whittemore AD, Mannick JA. Further experience with an all-autogenous tissue policy for infrainguinal reconstruction. *J Vasc Surg* 1993;18:41–48.

35. Tangelder MJD, Lawson JA, Algra A, et al. Systematic review of randomized controlled trials of aspirin and oral anticoagulants in the prevention of graft occlusion and ischemia events after infrainguinal bypass surgery. *J Vasc Surg* 1999;30:701–709.

36. Becquemin J. Effect of ticlopidine on the long-term patency of saphenous-vein bypass grafts in the legs. *N Engl J Med* 1997;337:1726–1731.

37. Cheng WK, Ting ACW, Lau H, et al. Survival in patients with chronic lower extremity ischemia: a risk factor analysis. *Ann Vasc Surg* 2000;14:158–165.

38. Burek KA, Sutton-Tyrell K, Brooks MM, et al. Prognostic importance of lower extremity arterial disease in patients undergoing coronary revascularization investigation. *J Am Coll Cardiol* 1999;34:716–721.

39. Kalra M, Gloviczki P, Bower TC, et al. Limb salvage after successful pedal bypass grafting is associated with improved long-term survival. *J Vasc Surg* 2000;33:6–16.

40. Hallett JW Jr, Byrne J, Gayari MM, et al. Impact of arterial surgery and balloon angioplasty on amputation: a population-based study of 1155 procedures between 1973 and 1992. *J Vasc Surg* 1997;25:29–38.

41. Dossa CD, Shepard AD, Amos AM, et al. Results of lower extremity amputations in patients with end-stage renal disease. *J Vasc Surg* 1994;20:14–19.

42. AbuRahma AF, Woodruff BA, Lucente FC. Edema after femoropopliteal bypass surgery: lymphatic and venous theories of causation. *J Vasc Surg* 1990;11:461–467.

43. Abou-Zamzam AM Jr, Lee RW, Moneta Gl, et al. Functional outcome after infrainguinal bypass for limb salvage. *J Vasc Surg* 1997;25:287–297.

44. Nicoloff AD, Taylor LM Jr, McLafferty RB, et al. Patient recovery after infrainguinal bypass grafting for limb salvage. *J Vasc Surg* 1998;27:256–266.

45. Dawson I, van Bockel JH. Outcome measures after lower extremity bypass surgery: there is more than just patency. *Br J Surg* 1999;86:1105–1106.

46. Calligaro KD, Musser DJ, Chen AY, et al. Duplex ultrasonography to diagnose failing arterial prosthetic grafts. *Surgery* 1996;120:455–459.

47. Visser K, Idu MM, Buth J, et al. Duplex scan surveillance during the first year after infrainguinal autologous vein bypass grafting surgery: costs and clinical outcomes compared with other surveillance programs. *J Vasc Surg* 2000;33:123–130.

48. Lundell A, Lindblad B, Bergquist D, et al. Femoropopliteal-crural graft patency is improved by an intensive surveillance program: a prospective randomized study. *J Vasc Surg* 1995;21:26–34.

49. Bandyk DF, Johnson BL, Gupta AK, et al. Nature and management of duplex abnormalities encountered during infrainguinal vein bypass grafting. *J Vasc Surg* 1996;24:430–438.

50. Gibson KD, Caps MT, Gillen D, et al. Identification of factors predictive of lower extremity vein graft stenosis. *J Vasc Surg* 2001;33:24–31.

34

Pulmonary Embolism

John G. Weg, Melvyn Rubenfire, and Lazar J. Greenfield

EPIDEMIOLOGY AND USUAL CAUSES

Pulmonary embolism (PE) and deep venous thrombosis (DVT) are two manifestations of one disease, venous thromboembolism (VTE). DVT is confirmed by venography in more than 80% of patient with PE that is proven by angiography (1). However, on average, only 35% to 45% of patients with PE demonstrate DVT by ultrasonography or impedance plethysmography (2), and even fewer (about 15%) show clinical evidence of DVT (3).

The incidence of PE in the United States is estimated to be about 600,000 per year (4). This may well be an underestimate because PEs are not clinically diagnosed in a majority of patients with PE at autopsy (5). Furthermore, in a study to determine the accuracy of detecting PE at autopsy, careful dissection identified PE in 52% of right lungs but only 12% in the left lungs evaluated by routine techniques (6).

VTE occurs in the milieu of stasis of blood flow, damage to the vascular wall, and activation of the clotting system, particularly in the presence of acquired or inherited thrombophilic factors. Approximately 80% to 90% of PEs originate in the veins of the lower extremity, the initial thrombi originating in the calf veins. They may, however, originate in more proximal sites, particularly in patients undergoing gynecologic surgery, parturition, and prostate surgery. Upper extremity DVTs are an increasing cause of PE, associated with the placement of central venous catheters (often with sepsis), malignancy, thrombophilic states, prior leg vein thrombosis, and malignancy (7).

Recognition of the predisposing factors ("causes") of VTE form the cornerstone of diagnosis. Surgery within the previous 3 months and immobilization interactive factors are identified in more than half of patients with VTE. Other common risk factors include congestive heart failure, obesity, malignancy, lower extremity trauma, therapeutic estrogen, cerebral vascular accidents, pregnancy and the puerperium, venous varicosity/insufficiency, history of thrombophlebitis, and travel lasting 4 hours or more (the "economy class syndrome") (3,8–11).

The annual incidence of idiopathic VTE is about 0.04% in the general population and increases to 0.1% to 0.4% in family members of symptomatic carriers of prothrombotic mutations. One or more markers of hypercoagulability can be identified in more than 60% of patients with VTE, particularly when it is idiopathic. The most common are factor V Leiden and activated protein C resistance (APCR), which are found in 11% to 21% of VTE and are present in 5% of white people but are rare in black and Asian populations; APCR may be acquired (Table 34.1). The estimated risk of DVT is sevenfold in factor V Leiden carriers and increased further by pregnancy and the use of birth control pills. Although the reason is not clear, paradoxically, the prevalence of factor V Leiden or APCR in patients with isolated PE seems to be about half of that in patients with isolated DVT (without symptoms of PE). DVT and PE are about equally prevalent in the prothrombin mutation G to A at point 20210, which carries a three- to fourfold risk of VTE. There is a 15-fold relative risk of VTE during pregnancy with this mutation, and when the mutation is combined with factor V-Leiden, the risk is greater than 100-fold. Hyperhomocysteinemia is the second most common factor associated with VTE and is found in about 25% of patients with idiopathic VTE. A plasma homocysteine level above the ninety-fifth percentile (more than

TABLE 34.1. *Heritable and acquired thrombophilia and venous thromboembolus*

Genetic trait	Prevalence in population	Prevalence in VTE subjects	Relative risk of VTE	Relative risk of recurrent VTE[a]
Homocysteinemia (above 17 μmol/L)	5%	25%	2–3	3
Factor V Leiden	5% of white people 2% of Hispanics 0.3% of Asians <1% of blacks	11%–21% Not known for others	Heterozygous: 7 Homozygous: 80	0–4
Prothrombin 20210	2%	<5%		0
Factor V Leiden and prothrombin 20210	0.1%	3%	3–4 ~20	~4
Homocysteine and factor V Leiden (men only)	0.3%	2.7%	10 for any VTE 20 for idiopathic VTE	Unknown

VTE, venous thromboembolus.
[a]After anticoagulants are discontinued.

17 μmol/L) increases the risk of DVT by two- to threefold and is associated with a nearly threefold risk of recurrence (Table 34.1). The relative contribution of lower levels of homocysteine is not established. However, in men with hyperhomocysteinemia and factor V-Leiden, there is a 20-fold increase in VTE. High levels of factor XI are also a risk factor for DVT; the risk doubles at high levels, which are present in 10% of the population. Other, less common genetic causes of hypercoagulability that increase the risk for VTE include elevated factor VIII levels, deficiencies of antithrombin III, deficiencies of proteins C and S, and abnormal plasminogen levels. Antiphospholipid antibodies, including anticardiolipin, associated with the lupus anticoagulant and ovarian stimulation for *in vitro* fertilization are acquired risk factors. It is reasonable to initially search for APCR, homocysteinemia, and the prothrombin mutation G20210 in a patient with idiopathic VTE (no obvious identifiable risk factor), VTE in a patient younger than 45 years, a patient with recurrent VTE, or a patient with a family history of VTE if oral contraceptives or pregnancy are being considered (11,12).

PRESENTING SIGNS AND SYMPTOMS

Combinations of clinical findings in patients with PE are both extremely sensitive and extremely nonspecific. Dyspnea or tachypnea (respiratory rate, more than 20 breaths/minute) occurred in 90% of patients with PE in the Prospective Inves-

tigation of Pulmonary Embolism Diagnosis (PIOPED) study; dyspnea or tachypnea or signs of DVT (despite their inaccuracy) occurred in 91%; dyspnea or tachypnea or pleuritic pain occurred in 97%; and dyspnea or tachypnea or pleuritic pain, or radiographic evidence of atelectasis or parenchymal abnormality, occurred in 98%. The frequency of individual findings in PIOPED and the urokinase/streptokinase studies are shown in Table 34.2 (3,8,9). In PIOPED, in patients without prior cardiopulmonary diseases, only tachypnea (70%), dyspnea (73%), chest pain (66%), and crackles were found in the majority of patients with PE, and only crackles showed a statistical difference from the findings in the patients without PE. These signs and symptoms are found in many diseases, are very common in sick patients, and are almost uniformly present in patients in intensive care units.

HELPFUL TESTING FOR THE DIAGNOSIS OF VENOUS THROMBOEMBOLISM

The diagnosis of VTE requires objective testing: namely, an imaging study.

Ventilation/Perfusion Lung Scanning

This has been the usual initial imaging study for PE. However, lower extremity, noninvasive imaging studies are a satisfactory alternative. The only ventilation/perfusion (V/Q) results that

TABLE 34.2. *Signs and symptoms in pulmonary embolism*

Sign/symptom	PIOPED (no prior cardiopulmonary disease)		UK/SK trials: PE (N = 327) (%)
	PE (N = 117) (%)	No PE (N = 248) (%)	
In majority			
Respirations (>16/min)	—	—	92
Respirations (>20/min)	70	68	—
Dyspnea	73	72	84
Chest pain	66	59	88
Pleuritic pain	—	—	74
Apprehension	—	—	59
Crackles	51	40[a]	58
Cough	37	36	53
S2P	23	13[a]	53
Frequent			
Hemoptysis	13	8	30
Pulse >100	30	24	44
Sweats	11	8	27
Syncope	—	—	13
Leg pain	26	24	—
Temperature (>37.8°C)	7	12	43
Diaphoresis	—	—	36
S4 Gallop	24	14[a]	34
Phlebitis	—	—	32
Edema	—	—	24
Murmur	—	—	23
Cyanosis	—	—	19
Uncommon			
Palpitations	10	18	—
Holman's sign	4	2	—
Wheezing	9	11	—
Angina-like pain	4	6	—
Right ventricular lift	4	2	—
Pleural friction rub	3	2	—
S3 Gallop	3	4	—

PE, pulmonary embolism; PIOPED, Prospective Investigation of Pulmonary Embolism Diagnosis; SK, streptokinase; UK, urokinase.

[a] $p < 0.001$.

Adapted from Weg JG. Venous thromboembolism: pulmonary embolism and deep venous thrombosis. In: Irwin R, Cerra F, Tippe J. eds. *Intensive care medicine,* 4th ed. New York: Lippincott-Raven, 1999:650–672.

permit definitive, rational clinical decision making are those indicating high probability (more than one segmental or larger perfusion defect with normal ventilation—a mismatch) and those that are normal (no significant defects). In PIOPED, a high-probability V/Q scan had a positive predictive value of PE in 87% of patients, and the likelihood of PE was greater than 96% if the clinical suspicion was high. However, PE was found in only 74% of patients with this reading who had a history of prior PE. PE was present in 4% of those with a normal or near normal V/Q scan. Only 27% of patients had high (13%) and normal (14%) readings. Intermediate- and low-probability V/Q scans should be reported as nondiagnostic. PE was found in 33% of patients with intermediate-probability scans and 14% of patients with low-probability scans, an incidence too high to abandon the diagnosis of PE and too low to initiate treatment (13). Of patients with substantial chronic obstructive pulmonary disease, only 5% had high-probability scans, and they had PE. There were no normal scans; lung scans are also of little value in patients with acute respiratory failure (14,15).

Pulmonary Angiography

Pulmonary angiography is the "gold standard" for the diagnosis or exclusion of PE. In the 1,111 angiograms in PIOPED, the correct diagnosis was made in 96% of the patients on the basis of a 1-year outcome study; 4% of studies were nondiagnostic or incomplete. There were five deaths among patients with unstable severe cardiopulmonary disease. In comparison, one patient died after a ventilation scan. Major complications occurred in an additional nine patients, and less severe complications occurred in 60 patients. Complications did not correlate with pulmonary artery pressure but were more common in patients in a medical intensive care unit (16).

Lower Extremity Studies

Noninvasive studies have all but replaced venography in the diagnosis of DVT. A positive study is sufficient to diagnose VTE, because there is no difference in the need for anticoagulation. However, because approximately 20% or more of patients with PE have nondiagnostic lower extremity studies, these studies are insufficient to exclude the diagnosis of PE. Real-time B-mode compression color (color duplex) ultrasonography is preferred and should include imaging of the calf and external iliac veins (see Chapter 32 for additional information).

Contrast-Enhanced Spiral Computed Tomography

There has been no prospective validation of this technique in a sufficiently large study. Its sensitivity is approximately 70% [95% confidence interval (CI), 58% to 80%], and its specificity is 88% (95% CI, 81% to 93%), with a positive predictive value of 76% (95% CI, 64% to 85%). For main and segmental vessels, the sensitivity was reported to be 94% (95% CI, 86% to 98%) and the specificity, 94% (95% CI, 68% to 96%) (17). A larger review reported sensitivities of 53% to 100% and specificities of 81% to 100% (18). The identification of subsegmental clots has been less than 30%, but about 6% to 36% of PEs have been limited to subsegmental vessels, and 17% of PIOPED patients with low-probability V/Q scans had only subsegmental clots (19). In 115 patients who had ultrasonography, 15 had positive results on both ultrasonography and CTs, and the CT alone was positive in an

additional four patients (20). A small study comparing a dual-detector helical CT with pulmonary angiography revealed a sensitivity of 90% and a specificity of 94% for CT (21).

Finally, in a prospective study of 259 patients, the sensitivity of CT angiography was only 70% (95% CI 62–78) and specificity 91% (95% CI 86–95%). The likelihood ratio for a negative CT was 0.3—close to that of a low probability scan in PIOPED. The false negative rate was reduced from 30 to 20%, if ultrasonography was negative and to 5% if the lung scan was also nondiagnostic. The false positive rate was 15% in lobar arteries and 38% in segmental arteries. (21a)

Thus, enhanced spiral CT cannot be recommended at this time as a screening test for PE. It is satisfactory for central clots, but if it is negative, pulmonary angiography or a positive lower extremity study is required. The sensitivity and specificity, especially with the new generation of multislice rapid-acquisition dual scanners with thin collimation (1 to 1.25 mm), and thus the role of enhanced spiral CT in the diagnosis of VTE await the results of PIOPED-II, a National Heart, Lung, and Blood Institute, National Institutes of Health study, which is in progress.

Magnetic Resonance Imaging

The sensitivity and specificity of magnetic resonance angiography with contrast enhancement shares with helical contrast enhanced CT the attributes of being minimally invasive and permits the interpretation at a work station which improves results. In small prospective studies, it has shown promise. In one study it had a sensitivity of 100% and a specificity of 87%, but all the clots were in main or segmental vessels (22). In another small study, the sensitivity was 85% and the specificity was 96%; however it missed four subsegmental emboli (23). Magnetic resonance venography is exceptionally accurate in upper and lower extremity iliac and pelvic (including ovarian) veins (24).

D-Dimer Assays

The currently available D-dimer (a specific fibrin degradation product) assays appear to be useful in excluding the diagnosis of VTE *in association with other testing.* In studies using a variety of D-dimer assays, the reported negative predictive values were 94% to 100% (25). However, in a study of 1,171 patients among whom the prevalence of PE was only 17%, the need for additional testing was evident:- With a negative D-dimer and a normal V/Q scan, the posttest probability of PE was 0.4% (95% CI, 0.0% to 2.3%); if the V/Q was nondiagnostic, the posttest probability of PE was 2.8% (95% CI, 1.4% to 4.8%); and if the V/Q was high probability, the posttest probability of PE was 65.4% (95% CI, 44.3% to 82.8%). In 930 consecutive patients evaluated by one of 43 emergency department physicians using a combination of a negative whole blood D-dimer agglutination test and a low probability from a clinical prediction model, PE was excluded in 437 (46.9%) patients. The negative predictive value was 99.5% based on no VTE in a three month follow-up. (27c) False-positive D-dimer tests are more common in patients with cancer and in postoperative patients. They are likely to be increased in patients with sepsis and similar conditions. The most prudent use of a D-dimer test is still unclear. It is more likely to be helpful where the likelihood of PE is low when combined with other data. (27b)

Echocardiography

Transthoracic echocardiography may identify right ventricular dysfunction and substantial pulmonary hypertension. These findings are nonspecific; they are not markers for PE and were found in only 56% of patients with PE in a prospective study (28). Transesophageal echocardiography has identified main pulmonary artery and intracardiac emboli in 12 of 24 patients in shock with neck vein distention (29). In several small studies of patients with cor pulmonale, transesophageal echocardiography has had sensitivities of only 58% to 65% in identifying emboli (30).

Nonspecific Tests

In PIOPED, some nonspecific abnormality was present in 80% of chest roentgenograms: atelectasis or consolidation in 65% and pleural effusion in 48%. The so-called classic findings of wedge-shaped infiltrates, prominent central pulmonary arteries and pulmonary artery cutoffs, and decreased peripheral vascularity occurred in less than 25% of those studies; these findings are particularly difficult to see on portable anterior-posterior chest roentgenograms. Similarly nonspecific electrocardiographic findings were seen in 70%: Tachycardia and nonspecific ST-T wave changes were common; again, the so-called classic but nonspecific findings of S_1, S_2, S_3, complete right bundle branch block; and S_1, Q_3, T_3 patterns were seen in only about 10%. Left-axis deviation was more common than right-axis deviation. The nonspecific findings of hypoxemia, an increased alveolar-to-arterial oxygen [$P(A-a)O_2$] gradient, and hypocarbia were equally present in patients with and without PE. The absence of findings in these nonspecific tests lowers the likelihood of PE but does not exclude PE; their presence does not confirm PE. However, these studies may identify other conditions that simulate PE (3).

RECOMMENDED DIAGNOSTIC ALGORITHMS

The two algorithms in Figs. 34.1 and 34.2 provide a rational approach to the diagnosis of VTE–PE and DVT, because the requirement for anticoagulation is the same. Fitted compression stockings worn for 3 months to prevent the postphlebitic syndrome are recommended for patients with symptomatic proximal DVT (31). If there is clinical evidence of DVT or pregnancy, the lower extremity studies are favored; availability will also influence the choice of study (11). Anticoagulation is required if the V/Q reading is of high probability, unless there is a history of PE or a low clinical suspicion. With the latter two, confirmation of VTE via noninvasive studies or pulmonary angiogram should be obtained. If the V/Q reading is normal, anticoagulants should not be given. If ultrasonography, including the calf or impedance plethysmography (less sensitive), yields positive results, anticoagulation is required. If the V/Q reading is nondiagnostic and the lower extremity noninvasive studies are negative, a pulmonary angiogram should be obtained. These recommendations are based on large, randomized,

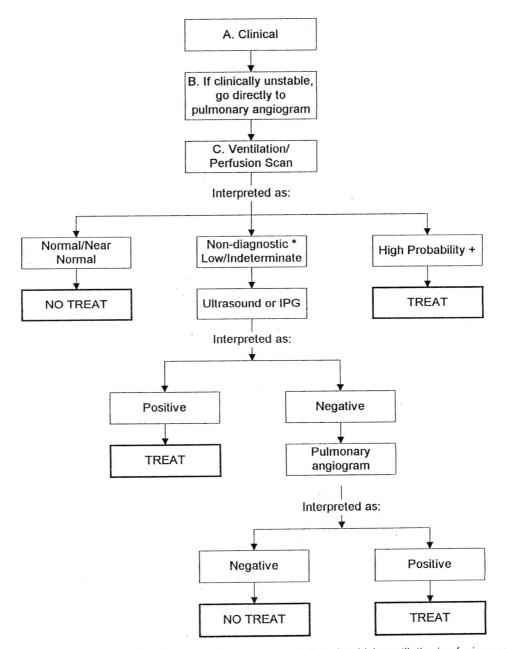

FIG. 34.1. An algorithm for the diagnosis of pulmonary embolism, in which ventilation/perfusion scanning is the initial imaging study. *If clinical suspicion is *very* low, some will not proceed. †If clinical suspicion is low or if there is a history of pulmonary embolism, obtain a pulmonary angiogram. (Adapted from Weg JG. Venous thromboembolism: pulmonary embolism and deep venous thrombosis. In: Irwin R, Cerra F, Tippe J, eds. *Intensive care medicine,* 4th ed. New York: Lippincott-Raven, 1999:650–672.)

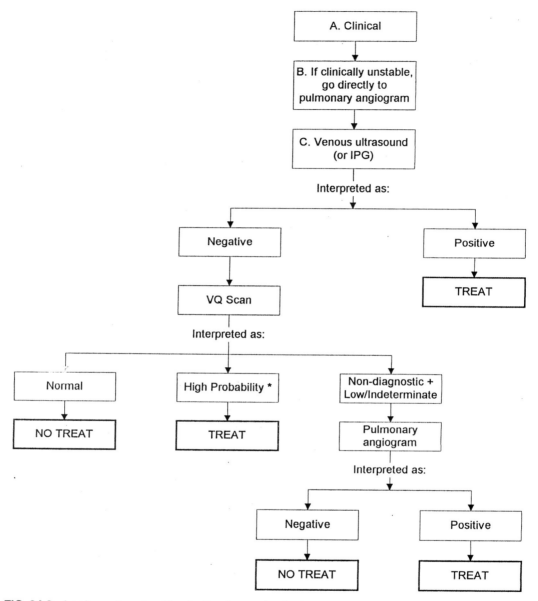

FIG. 34.2. An alternative algorithm for the diagnosis of pulmonary embolism, involving lower extremity noninvasive studies: compression ultrasonography (preferred) or impedance plethysmography. *If clinical suspicion is low or if there is a history of pulmonary embolism, obtain a pulmonary angiogram. †If clinical suspicion is *very* low, some will not proceed. (From Weg JG. Current diagnostic techniques for pulmonary embolism. *Semin Vasc Surg* 2000;13:182–188.)

prospective, consistent multicenter studies that use objective validation criteria, outcome, or both; this is a 1A recommendation (1, benefit/risk clear; A, methods strong).

DIFFERENTIAL DIAGNOSIS

The alternative diagnoses in patients with PE are extensive. Signs, symptoms, chest roentgenograms, electrocardiograms, and arterial blood gas measurements cannot differentiate the patient with PE from one with the other diagnostic possibilities in Table 34.3. Many of these entities may also occur concomitantly with PE.

THERAPY

The current preferred treatment for acute proven VTE with PE and DVT is low molecular weight heparin (LMWH), subcutaneously for 5 to 7 days, and an inhibitor of the synthesis of vitamin K–dependent coagulation factors, such as

TABLE 34.3. *The differential diagnosis of pulmonary embolism*

Cardiovascular
  Acute myocardial infarction
  Dissecting thoracic aortic aneurysm
  Congestive heart failure
Pulmonary
  Intrathoracic malignancy
  Pneumonia
  Exacerbation of chronic obstructive pulmonary
    disease
  Exacerbation of diffuse infiltrative disease (e.g.,
    idiopathic pulmonary fibrosis, sarcoidosis)
  Atelectasis
  Respiratory failure
  Hypoxemia (etiology undetermined)
  Pleuritis
Infectious
  Sepsis
  Urinary tract infection (chest, flank, back pain)
  Extrapulmonary abscess
  Peritonitis
Neurologic
  Cerebral vascular accident
Others
  Collagen vascular disease
  Transplant rejection
  Pancreatitis
  Musculoskeletal pain
  Hyperventilation
  Sighing respiration

warfarin, for more than 3 months. These recommendations are based on large, randomized, prospective, consistent multicenter studies that used objective validation, outcome, or both; this is a 1A recommendation (1, benefit/risk clear; A, methods strong) (32,33). LMWH is preferred throughout pregnancy, but warfarin should not be used during pregnancy for VTE (11). Patients with proximal DVT should also wear fitted compression stockings for at least 3 months to reduce the incidence of the postphlebitic syndrome (31). An appropriate anticoagulation regimen reduces the rate of mortality caused by PE to less than 2.5%, in contrast to a mortality rate of 25% to 35% in historical controls (34,35). If PE is strongly suspected, 5,000 to 10,000 IU of unfractionated heparin (UFH) should be given immediately intravenously unless there is a high risk or contraindication to anticoagulation.

Low Molecular Weight Heparin

LMWH has been shown to be at least as effective as UFH in preventing recurrence of thrombotic events, reducing mortality rates, and minimizing bleeding. In some studies and meta-analyses, it has been superior to UFH in these areas (36). Its first major advantage is accurate, effective dosing by body weight–anti-Xa U/kg, without laboratory monitoring for the anticoagulant effect, whereas it is necessary with UFH. However, the physician should consider monitoring plasma anti–factor Xa activity in patients who are pregnant, have a creatinine clearance of less than 30 mL/minute, or are very obese (32). Second, it facilitates outpatient treatment of many patients with DVT and the early outpatient treatment of PE in the *stable* patient once a system is in place for outpatient care, including (a) administration of LMWH; (b) monitoring the patient for recurrence and complications of bleeding; and (c) monitoring warfarin therapy. The minimal patient criteria for outpatient treatment include stable status, *normal* vital signs (pulse, respiration, blood pressure, and temperature), a low bleeding risk, absence of severe renal disease, and good control of other disease processes. Early discharge results in improved quality of life. The third major advantage is a substantial

TABLE 34.4. *Guidelines for low-molecular-weight heparins approved for use in the United States and Canada*

Drug	Dose	Approved
Dalteparin sodium	200 IU/kg/d anti–factor Xa Should not exceed 18,000 IU/dose	Canada
Enoxaparin sodium	1 mg/kg q12 h SC *or* 1.5 mg/kg/d SC Single daily dose should not exceed 180 mg	United States and Canada
Nadroparin calcium	86 IU/kg anti–factor Xa b.i.d. SC × 10 d *or* 171 IU/kg/d SC anti–factor Xa Should not exceed 17,100 IU/dose	Canada
Tinzaparin sodium	175 IU/kg/d SC anti–factor Xa	United States and Canada

reduction in costs (37,38). Cost reduction results from decreased hospital stays, decreased costs of laboratory monitoring, and decreased rates of recurrence of VTE that would occur in patients who undergo inadequately anticoagulation with UFH in the first 24 hours. Table 34.4 provides guidelines for LMWH that are currently approved in the United States or Canada or both.

Unfractionated Heparin

UFH intravenously is an effective alternative to LMWH; UFH may also be given subcutaneously but in larger doses. UFH requires initial monitoring every 4 to 6 hours until a stable therapeutic level is obtained, along with prompt and vigorous dose adjustment (Table 34.5). The activated partial thromboplastin time (aPTT) is in general use. However, variations in reagents and clot detection systems require titration with protamine sulfate or an amidolytic assay to ensure that the aPTT of 1.5 to 2.0 time control levels represents the therapeutic range of 0.2 to 0.4 heparin units (32). The thrombin clotting time (TCT) is the preferred measurement. The target is 0.2 to 0.4 heparin units. The TCT is linear over a range of 0.2 to 0.6 heparin units (in contrast to the alinear aPTT, with its frequent reports of more than 100 times control levels). The TCT has better correlation with predicted heparin units and is less altered by warfarin. If the aPTT is less than 1.5 times control levels or if the TCT is less than 0.2 heparin units, the risk of recurrence increases. UFH in a dose of 1,300 IU/hour or more than 30,000 U/24 hours (18U × 70 kg × 24 hours = 30,240 IU) is necessary to achieve and maintain a therapeutic range. If venous access is poor or absent, subcutaneous heparin can be considered;

TABLE 34.5. *Body weight–based dosing of intravenous unfractionated heparin[a]*

aPTT seconds[b]	Dose change (U/kg/hr)	Addition action	Next aPTT (hours)
<35 (<1.2 × mean normal)	+4	Bolus with 80 IU/kg	6
35–45 (1.2–1.5 × mean normal)	+2	Bolus with 40 IU/kg	6
46–70[c] (1.5–2.3 × mean normal)	0	0	6[d]
71–90 (2.3–3.0 × mean normal)	−2	0	6
>90 (>3 × mean normal)	−3	Stop infusion 1 hr	6

aPTT, activated partial thromboplastin time.

[a]Initial dosing; loading 80 IU/kg; maintenance infusion; 18 IU/kg/h (aPTT in 6 hr).

[b]The therapeutic range in seconds should correspond to a plasma heparin level of 0.2 to 0.4 IU/mL by protamine sulfate or 0.3 to 0.6 IU/mL by amidolytic assay. When aPTT is stable at 6 hr or longer, steady-state kinetics can be assumed.

[c]Heparin, 25,000 IU in 250 μL of 5% dextrose in water (D_5W). Infuse at rate dictated by body weight through an infusion apparatus calibrated for low flow rates.

[d]During the first 24 hr, repeat aPTT every 6 hr. Thereafter, monitor aPTT once every morning unless it is outside the therapeutic range.

Adapted from Weg JG. Venous thromboembolism: past, present, and future. *Semin Respir Crit Care Med* 2000;21:575–588; and from Raschke RA, Reilly BM, Guidry JR, et al. The weight-based heparin dosing nomogram compared with a "standard care" nomogram. A randomized controlled trial. *Ann Intern Med* 1993;119:874–881.

the usual subcutaneous dose of UFH is about 50,000/24hours.

Oral Anticoagulants

Oral anticoagulation should be started with warfarin, 5 mg/day, in the evening of the first day and adjusted to obtain an international normalized ratio (INR) of 2 to 3. Warfarin should be continued to maintain this range for 3 to 6 months for the first VTE with a recognized cause. If the first VTE is idiopathic (no recognized cause), warfarin should be continued for more than 6 months. If there is a recurrence of VTE or if there are risk factors such as unresolved cancer, unresolved anticardiolipin antibody, or antithrombin III deficiency, anticoagulation is maintained for 12 months to a lifetime. The appropriate duration of anticoagulation is not established for patients with a first VTE associated with factor V Leiden, prothrombin 20210, hyperhomocystinemia, deficiency of factor C or S, multiple thrombophilias, and recurrent VTEs caused by concomitant risk factors (32,33). The duration of warfarin therapy for preventing recurrent VTE has generally been 3–12 months to a target INR of 2.0 to 3.0. Longer duration of therapy reduces recurrent events, but at the expense of an increase in major bleeding. In a recent controlled trial of 508 patients with idiopathic VTE, long term low intensity warfarin, targeting INR to 1.5 to 2, was shown to be a low risk and effective strategy in patients with or without hypercoagulable factors. After 4.3 years of treatment (mean 2.1 years), recurrent VTE occurred in 7.2 per 100 person years on placebo and only 2.6 per 100 person years on low intensity warfarin. Death occurred in 8 patients on placebo and 4 allocated to warfarin and major hemorrhage occurred in 2 patients on placebo and 5 allocated to low-intensity warfarin. (33a) Patients with the antiphospholipid antibody syndrome appear to require an INR of more than 3.

If the INR is elevated and bleeding is severe, fresh-frozen plasma can be used to reverse the effect of warfarin; with minor bleeding, oral vitamin K is effective; and with INR elevations without bleeding, the warfarin can be stopped for 1 to 3 days (31).

Other Agents

Recombinant hirudin (lepirudin and argatroban) is approved in the United States for treatment of heparin-induced thrombocytopenia. They have been at least as effective as heparin in clinical trials.

Thrombolytic Agents

The role of thrombolytic agents (urokinase, streptokinase, tissue plasminogen activator, alteplase, and reteplase) is not well established. Despite multiple randomized controlled studies of over 1,000 patients since 1970, no clinically important reduction in morbidity, including objectively proven recurrent VTE, or in mortality rates has been demonstrated (8,9,39). Over the first 2 to 24 hours, thrombolytics produce a greater reduction in pulmonary vascular pressures, pulmonary vascular resistance, V/Q scan findings, and angiographically evident extent of clot than does heparin alone. However, there is no difference in lung scans at 1, 5 to 7, and 14 to 30 days (8,9,39). Thrombolytic therapy carries an 8% risk of major hemorrhage in some studies; fatal hemorrhage occurred in slightly more than 2% of patients and intracranial bleeding in a similar percentage. The risk is fourfold in patients older than 70 years. It also carries morbidity-related costs of about $1,160 (streptokinase) to $2,750 (recombinant tissue plasminogen activator), in addition to the costs of heparin, warfarin, and complications.

In a recent randomized trial of 256 patients with PE and pulmonary hypertension or right ventricular dysfunction, there was no reduction in hospital mortality between those receiving altepase plus heparin (3.4%) vs. haparin alone (2.2%) (39b).

Most clinicians reserve thrombolytic therapy for patients with proven massive PE with hemodynamic instability (shock) despite heparin and resuscitative efforts with fluids and vasopressors (32,33,39,40). Although reduction in mortality rates among such patients has not been documented in a randomized trial, this group does represent patients with a mortality rate of 20% to 30%. Some physicians also give thrombolytics for patients with PE and severe hypoxemia or echocardiographic evidence of right ventricular dysfunction, citing nonrandomized trials with all their biases. However, because right ventricular dysfunction has been reported in 40% to 80% of patients with PE, and because the rate of mortality due to PE is only about 2%, such extensive use does not appear to be warranted (41)

Inferior Vena Caval Interruption

Inferior vena caval interruption is recommended for (a) a contraindication to or complications (e.g., major bleeding) of anticoagulant therapy in a patient with or at high risk of VTE; (b) documented recurrent VTE despite adequate anticoagulation; (c) chronic or recurrent PE with pulmonary hypertension; (d) transvenous extraction of PE; (e) pulmonary embolectomy; and (f) pulmonary thromboendartectomy of major central PE (32,33,40). It has also been used in patients with massive PE and upper extremity PE. The largest experience is with the Greenfield filters; they have a 20-year efficacy rate of 95% and a patency rate of about 96% (42). One randomized study of 106 patients in which inferior vena caval filters with anticoagulation were compared with anticoagulation alone in patients with proximal DVT (not with the recommended indications cited previously) showed a reduction in PE at 12 days but an increased recurrence of DVTs at 2 years (43). However, the filters were of various unrecorded types and were inserted by different individuals at multiple sites. The bird's nest filter is also effective but is associated with a higher rate of vena caval occlusion (44). Filters have also been used for primary prophylaxis in patients with a high risk of bleeding, such as those with visceral cancer, those who have sustained extensive trauma, and those undergoing hip or knee surgery (45,46).

Pulmonary Embolectomy and Transvenous Catheter Extraction

These procedures are reserved for patients in shock despite heparin and resuscitative efforts with fluids and vasopressors, who also usually have a contraindication to thrombolytic therapy (33). The rate of operative mortality has been reported as 10% to 75% in retrospective case series. Transvenous catheter pulmonary embolec-

tomy has been reported to carry a 70% rate of 30-day survival.

Designer Drugs

In addition to the previously described lepirudin and argatroban, new anticoagulants developed by design in the laboratory are undergoing clinical trials. They include the indirect thrombin inhibitor danaparoid (Orgaran 10172), an oral agent; the direct thrombin inhibitors napsagatran and melagatran, an oral agent; the indirect factor Xa inhibitors; synthetic pentasaccharides; the direct factor Xa inhibitors Dx 9065a SK549, SF303, and YM60828; inhibitors of the factor XIIa/tissue factor pathway SR90107/ORG 31540; and nematode anticoagulant proteins (NAPC2). They hold the promise of being just as effective as or more effective than heparin/warfarin, providing a reliable, reproducible effect, not requiring monitoring, carrying a decreased risk of bleeding and ease of administration. A critical issue will be the cost/benefit ratio (47,48).

PREVENTION OF VENOUS THROMBOEMBOLISM

Primary prophylaxis of VTE should be a major focus of every physician who cares for patients at risk. The many risk factors for VTE and the efficacy of prevention are well established (49). The risk factors include hip fractures, total hip and knee replacement, major open urologic surgery, gynecologic surgery and neurosurgery, multiple trauma, spinal cord injury, lower extremity fractures, acute myocardial infarction and ischemic stroke, and patients in intensive care units in whom the signs and symptoms of PE are ubiquitous (15).

Important reductions in VTE can be achieved with the use of LMWH, minidose UFH (5,000 IU every 8 or 12 hours), adjusted-dose UFH, and low-dose warfarin; elastic graduated compression stockings; intermittent pneumatic compression devices; or various combinations of these. Specific recommendations are available (49). There exists a serious gap between published guidelines for prevention of VTE and clinical practice (50).

PRACTICAL POINTS

- A consideration of VTE must include the predisposing causes, both acquired (e.g., stasis, surgery, trauma) and inherited (prothrombotic factors), and the signs and symptoms.

- The definitive diagnosis of VTE requires imaging; PE is documented by a high-probability V/Q scan (no history of PE), a positive result of a noninvasive study, a positive pulmonary angiogram, a positive spiral contrast-enhanced CT (segmental or larger vessels), a positive venogram. PE is excluded by a normal V/Q scan or a negative pulmonary angiogram.

- Standard treatment includes LMWH subcutaneously for 4 to 5 days and warfarin for ≥3 months, starting on the first day.

- Thrombolytic therapy is indicated if there is hemodynamic instability (shock) despite resuscistative efforts with fluids and vasopressors.

- Inferior vena caval interruption is indicated when there are (a) contraindications to or complications (e.g. major bleeding) of anticoagulants in patient with or at high risk of VTE; (b) documented recurrent VTE despite adequate anticoagulation; and (c) chronic or recurrent PE with pulmonary hypertension. It is also indicated for patients undergoing transvenous extraction, pulmonary embolectomy, or thromboembolectomy.

- Pulmonary embolectomy or transvenous extraction is indicated for patients in shock despite resuscitation, usually with contraindication to thrombolytic therapy.

- **Primary prophylaxis is the most efficient treatment of VTE.**

REFERENCES

1. Girard P, Musset D, Parent F, et al. High prevalence of detectable deep venous thrombosis in patients with acute pulmonary embolism. *Chest* 1999;116:903–908.
2. van Rossum AB, van Houwelingen HC, Kieft GJ, et al. Prevalence of deep vein thrombosis in suspected and proven pulmonary embolism: a meta-analysis. *Br J Radiol* 1998;71:1260–1265.
3. Stein PD, Terrin ML, Hales CA, et al. Clinical, laboratory, roentgenographic, and electrocardiographic findings in patients with acute pulmonary embolism and no pre-existing cardiac or pulmonary disease. *Chest* 1991;100:598–603.
4. NIH Consensus Development. Prevention of venous thrombosis and pulmonary embolism. *JAMA* 1986;256:744–749.
5. Stein PD, Henry JW. Prevalence of acute pulmonary embolism among patients in a general hospital at autopsy. *Chest* 1995;108:978–981.
6. Morrell MT, Dunhill MS. The post-mortem incidence of pulmonary embolism in a hospital population. *Br J Surg* 1986;55:347–352.
7. Prandoni P, Polistena P, Bernardi E, et al. Upper-extremity deep vein thrombosis. Risk factors, diagnosis, and complications. *Arch Intern Med* 1997;157:57–62.
8. The Urokinase Pulmonary Embolism Trial: a national cooperative study. *Circulation* 1973;47(Suppl):1–108.
9. Urokinase Streptokinase Pulmonary Embolism Trial. Phase II results. *JAMA* 1974;229:1606–1613.
10. Ferrari E, Chevallier T, Chapelier A, et al. Travel as a risk factor for venous thromboembolic disease: a case-control study. *Chest* 1999;115:440–444.
11. Weg JG. Venous thromboembolism in pregnancy. *Semin Respir Crit Care Med* 1998;19:231–241.
12. Kyrle PA, Minar E, Hirscl M, et al. High plasma levels of factor VIII and the risk of recurrent venous thromboembolism. *N Engl J Med* 2000;343:457–462.
13. The PIOPED Investigators. Value of the ventilation/perfusion scan in acute pulmonary embolism: result of the prospective investigators of pulmonary embolism diagnosis (PIOPED). *JAMA* 1990;263:2753–2759.
14. Lesser BA, Leeper KV Jr, Stein PD, et al. The diagnosis of acute pulmonary embolism in patients with chronic obstructive pulmonary disease. *Chest* 1992;102:17–22.
15. Neuhaus A, Bentz RR, Weg JG. Pulmonary embolism in respiratory failure. *Chest* 1978;73:460–465.
16. Stein PD, Athanasoulis C, Alavi A, et al. Complications and validity of pulmonary angiography in acute pulmonary embolism. *Circulation* 1992;85:462–468.
17. Mullins MD, Becker DM, Hagspiel KD, et al. The role of spiral volumetric computed tomography in the diagnosis of pulmonary embolism. *Arch Intern Med* 2000;160:293–298.
18. Rathbun SW, Raskob GE, Whisett TL. Sensitivity and specificity of helical computed tomography in the diagnosis of pulmonary embolism: a systematic review. *Ann Intern Med* 2000;132:227–232.
19. Stein PD, Henry JW. Prevalence of acute pulmonary embolism in central and subsegmental pulmonary arteries and relation to probability interpretation of ventilation-perfusion lung scans. *Chest* 1997;111:1246–1248.
20. Cham MD, Yankelvitz DF, Shaham D, et al. Deep venous thrombosis: detection by using indirect CT venography. *Radiology* 2000;216:744–751.

21. Qanadli SD, Hajjam ME, Mesurolle B, et al. Pulmonary embolism detection: prospective evaluation of dual-section helical CT versus selective pulmonary arteriography in 157 patients. *Radiology* 2000;217:447–455.

21a. Perrier A, Howarth N, Didier D, et al. Performance of helical computed tomography in unselected outpatients with suspected pulmonary embolism. *Ann Int Med* 2001;135:88–97.

22. Meaney JF, Weg JG, Chenevert TL, et al. Diagnosis of pulmonary embolism with magnetic resonance angiography. *N Engl J Med* 1997;336:1422–1427.

23. Gupta A, Frazer CK, Ferguson JM, et al. Acute pulmonary embolism: diagnosis with MR angiography. *Radiology* 1999;210:353–359.

24. Moody AR, Pollock JG, O'Connor AR, et al. Lower-limb deep venous thrombosis: direct MR imaging of the thrombus. *Radiology* 1998;209:349–355.

25. Quinn DA, Fogel RB, Smith CD, et al. D-Dimers in the diagnosis of pulmonary embolism. *Am J Respir Crit Care Med* 1999;159:1445–1449.

26. Ginsberg JS, Wells PS, Kearon C, et al. Sensitivity and specificity of a rapid whole-blood assay for D-dimer in the diagnosis of pulmonary embolism. *Ann Intern Med* 1998;129:1006–1011.

27. Farrell S, Hayes T, Shaw M. A negative SimpliRED D-dimer assay result does not exclude the diagnosis of deep vein thrombosis or pulmonary embolus in emergency department patients. *Ann Emerg Med* 2000;35:121–125.

27b. ten Wolde M, Kraaijenhagen RA, Prins MH, et al. The clinical usefulness of D-dimer testing in cancer patients with suspected deep venous thrombosis. *Arch Int Med* 2002;162:1880–1884.

27c. Wells PS, Anderson DR, Rodger M, et al. Excluding pulmonary embolism presenting to the emergency department by using simple clinical model and D-dimer. *Ann Int Med* 2001;135:98–107.

28. Miniati M, Monti S, Pratali L, et al. Value of transthoracic echocardiography in the diagnosis of pulmonary embolism: results of a prospective study in unselected patients. *Am J Med* 2001;110:528–535.

29. Krivec B, Voga G, Zuran I, et al. Diagnosis and treatment of shock due to massive pulmonary embolism. *Chest* 1997;112:1310–1316.

30. Pruszczyk P, Torbicki A, Pacho R, et al. Noninvasive diagnosis of suspected severe pulmonary embolism. *Chest* 1997;112:722–728.

31. Brandjes DP, Buller HR, Heijboer H, et al. Randomized trial of effect of compression stockings in patients with symptomatic proximal-vein thrombosis. *Lancet* 1997;349:759–762.

32. Hyers TM, Agnelli G, Hull RD, et al. Sixth ACCP consensus conference on antithrombotic therapy: antithrombotic therapy for venous thromboembolic disease. *Chest* 2001;119:176S–193S.

33. Weg JG. Venous thromboembolism: past, present, and future. *Semin Respir Crit Care Med* 2000;21:575–588.

33a. Ridker PM, Goldhaber SZ, Danielson E. Rosenberg Y, et al. Long-term, Low-Intensity Warfarin for the Prevention of Recurrent Venous Thromboembolism: A Randomized, Double-Blind, Placebo-Controlled Trial. *N Engl J Med.* In press, 2003.

34. Carson JL, Kelley MA, Duff A, et al. The clinical course of pulmonary embolism. *N Engl J Med* 1992;326:1240–1245.

35. Douketis JD, Kearon C, Bates S, et al. Risk of fatal pulmonary embolism in patients with treated venous thromboembolism. *JAMA* 1998;279:458–462.

36. Dolovich LR, Ginsberg JS, Douketis JD, et al. A meta-analysis comparing low-molecular-weight heparins with unfractionated heparin in the treatment of venous thromboembolism: examining some unanswered questions regarding location of treatment, product type, and dosing frequency. *Arch Intern Med* 2000;160:181–188.

37. Levine M, Gent M, Hirsh J, et al. A comparison of low-molecular-weight heparin administered primarily at home with unfractionated heparin administered in the hospital for proximal deep-vein thrombosis. *N Engl J Med* 1996;334:677–681.

38. O'Brien BO, Levine M, Willan A, et al. Economic evaluation of outpatient treatment with low-molecular-weight heparin for proximal vein thrombosis. *Arch Intern Med* 1999;159:2298–2304.

39. Dalen JE, Alpert JS, Hirsh J. Thrombolytic therapy for pulmonary embolism: is it effective? Is it safe? When is it indicated?. *Arch Intern Med* 1997;157:2550–2556.

39b. Konstantinides S, Geibel A, Heusel G, et al. Heparin plus alteplase compared with heparin alone in patients with submassive pulmonary embolism. *N Engl J Med* 2002;347:1143–1150.

40. ACCP Consensus Committee on Pulmonary Embolism. Opinions regarding the diagnosis and management of venous thromboembolic disease. *Chest* 1996;109:233–237.

41. Goldhaber SZ, Visani L, DeRosa M. Acute pulmonary embolism: clinical outcomes in the International Cooperative Pulmonary Embolism Registry (ICOPER). *Lancet* 1999;353:1386–1389.

42. Greenfield LJ, Proctor MC. Recurrent thromboembolism in patients with vena cava filters. *J Vasc Surg* 2001;33:510–514.

43. Decousus H, Leizorovicz A, Parent F, et al. A clinical trial of vena caval filters in the prevention of pulmonary embolism in patients with proximal deep-vein thrombosis. Prevention du Risque d'Embolie Pulmonaire par Interruption Cave Study Group. *N Engl J Med* 1998;338:409–415.

44. Dorfman GS. Percutaneous inferior vena caval filters. *Radiology* 1990;174:987–992.

45. Emerson RH, Cross R, Head WC. Prophylactic and early therapeutic use of Greenfield filter in hip and knee joint arthroplasty. *J Arthroplasty* 1991;6:129–135.

46. Greenfield LJ, Proctor MC, Michaels AJ, et al. Prophylactic vena caval filters in trauma: the rest of the story. *J Vasc Surg* 2000;32:490–497.

47. Agnelli G, Sonaglia F. Clinical status of direct thrombin inhibitors. *Crit Rev Oncol Hematol* 1999;31:97–117.

48. Weitz JI, Hirsh J. New anticoagulant drugs. *Chest* 2001;119:95S–107S.

49. Geerts WH, Heit JA, Claggett GP, et al. Prevention of venous thromboembolism. *Chest* 2001;119:132S–175S.

50. Stratton MA, Anderson FA, Bussey HI, et al. Prevention of venous thromboembolism: adherence to the 1995 American College of Chest Physicians consensus guidelines for surgical patients. *Arch Intern Med* 2000;160:334–340.

35

Pulmonary Hypertension and Cor Pulmonale

Diagnosis and Management

Melvyn Rubenfire

The majority of patients with chronic heart and lung diseases associated with dyspnea and fatigue have some degree of pulmonary hypertension. The diagnosis, assessment of severity and prognosis, and treatment strategies for pulmonary hypertension can be made with a relatively high degree of certainty by experienced practitioners.

Pulmonary hypertension is defined by Doppler echocardiography as a tricuspid valve regurgitant velocity exceeding 3.0 to 3.5 m/second, corresponding to a right ventricular systolic pressure (RVSP) of 40 mm HG or higher and a mean pulmonary artery pressure higher than 20 mm HG (1). This chapter focuses on chronic pulmonary hypertension that is not attributable to the left-sided heart disease and valvular disease.

USUAL CAUSES AND WORLD HEALTH ORGANIZATION CLINICAL CLASSIFICATION OF PULMONARY HYPERTENSION AND ASSOCIATED TRIGGERS

The World Health Organization (WHO) classification of pulmonary hypertension (PH), an expanded differential diagnosis, and definite and possible triggers for PH are summarized in Table 35.1 (1). It is helpful to think of the differential diagnosis as precapillary and postcapillary PH. The most common causes of PH and right-sided heart failure are postcapillary, such as left-sided heart failure and aortic and mitral valvular disease characterized by pulmonary venous hypertension and resistance to drainage. Because of therapeutic implications, pulmonary emboli, both central and peripheral, must always be the first consideration in precapillary PH. The term *secondary pulmonary hypertension* has been abandoned in the revised WHO classification, which categorizes PH by a shared pathologic process and treatment options (Table 35.1):

1. Pulmonary arterial hypertension (PAH).
2. Pulmonary venous hypertension.
3. Disorders of the respiratory system and or hypoxemia.
4. Chronic thrombotic or embolic disease.
5. Disorder directly affecting the pulmonary vasculature.

Because pulmonary arterial hypertension (PAH) is insidious in onset but often rapidly progressive, it is important to have a high index of suspicion for persons at risk because of associated diseases and exposures. Patients at high risk include those with scleroderma-related disorders and lupus, congenital heart disease, sleep apnea, cirrhosis and portal hypertension, human immunodeficiency virus (HIV) infection, and a family history of primary pulmonary hypertension (PPH); chronic cocaine users; and those using anorexigens (2). There is also an increased prevalence of PAH in patients with anemia, including thalassemia and sickle cell disease; those with hyperthyroidism; and those who are obese. Each of these conditions is associated with a marked increase pulmonary blood flow that could be a trigger, but the association is not clear.

TABLE 35.1. *Classification, diseases, and triggers associated with pulmonary hypertension as modified from the WHO classification*

1. **Pulmonary arterial hypertension**
   1.1 Primary Pulmonary hypertension
      a. Sporadic
      b. Familial
   1.2 Related to:
      a. Collagen vascular diseases: scleroderma-related disorders, lupus, mixed connective tissue diseases, and less common Takayasu's giant cell, ulcerative colitis, Wegener's granulomatosis, rheumatoid arthritis, and juvenile rheumatoid arthritis
      b. Congenital systemic-to-pulmonary shunts: high pressure or flow, left to right at atrial, ventricular, or pulmonary artery level
      c. Portal hypertension (portopulmonary hypertension)
      d. HIV infection
      e. Drugs/toxins (L-tryptophan, toxic rapeseed oil, cocaine, heroin)
      f. Anorexigens (amphetamines, fenfluramine, dexfenfluramine)
      g. POEMS syndrome (myeloma variant)
      h. Other possible triggers: obesity, anemia (Thalassemia), hyperthyroidism
   1.3 Persistent pulmonary hypertension of the newborn
2. **Pulmonary venous hypertension with resistance to drainage**
   2.1 Left atrial and left ventricular disease (LV failure, diastolic dysfunction, atrial myxoma)
   2.2 Left-sided valvular disease (mitral stenosis or insufficiency)
   2.3 Extrinsic compression of pulmonary veins by fibrosing mediastinitis, lymph nodes, invasive tumors (breast, lung, lymphoma)
   2.4 Pulmonary venoocclusive disease: primary PVOD, lupus, radiation, chemotherapeutic drugs (bleomycin, mitomycin C, cyclophosphamide, etoposide), tumor infiltration
3. **Pulmonary hypertension associated with disorders of the respiratory system and/or hypoxemia**
   3.1 Chronic obstructive lung disease
   3.2 Interstitial lung diseases
   3.3 Sleep apnea, obstructive or primary hypoventilation
   3.4 Chronic high altitude: "chronic mountain sickness"
   3.5 Alveolar-capillary dysplasia
   3.6 Lymphangioleiomyomatosis
   3.7 Disorders of respiratory excursion: marked obesity, severe kyphoscoliosis, neuromuscular disorders
4. **Pulmonary hypertension due to chronic thromboembolic or thrombotic disease**
   4.1 Thromboembolic obstruction of proximal or central pulmonary arteries
   4.2 Obstruction of distal pulmonary arteries
      a. Pulmonary embolism (thromboemboli, tumor, ova and/or parasites, foreign body)
      b. *In situ* thrombosis
      c. Sickle cell disease
5. **Pulmonary hypertension due to disorders directly affecting the pulmonary vasculature**
   5.1 Inflammatory
      a. Schistosomiasis
      b. Sarcoidosis
      c. Other
   5.2 Pulmonary capillary hemangiomatosis

HIV, human immunodeficiency virus; LV, left ventricular; POEMS, polyneuropathy, organomegaly, endocrinopathy, M protein, skin changes; WHO, World Health Organization.

From Rich S, ed. *Executive summary.* From the World Symposium on Primary Pulmonary Hypertension, Evian, September 6–10, 1998. Cosponsored by the World Health Organization (http://www.who.int/ncd/cvd/pph.html).

COMMON SIGNS AND SYMPTOMS IN PULMONARY HYPERTENSION

The signs and symptoms associated with PH are summarized in Table 35.2. Mild PH (pulmonary artery systolic pressure less than 40 to 45 mm HG, or mean pulmonary artery pressure of 20 to 25 mm HG) is generally not associated with symptoms, except in active persons (who participate in, e.g., aerobic sport, dancing), who experience decreased energy and endurance. The WHO PH functional assessment classification (Table 35.3) is very useful for describing and risk-stratifying patients (1).

Symptoms attributable to PH are similar to those in left-sided heart failure, valvular disease, and lung disease. PH should be suspected as the cause in the setting of risk factors, triggers, and associated diseases. The symptoms depend on the functional limitation and the degree of hemodynamic impairment.

Each of the symptoms has one or more hemodynamic correlates:

1. Dyspnea and fatigue are correlated with decrease in rest and exercise stroke volume, cardiac output, and oxygen transport.

2. Angina-like chest pains on exertion are correlated with increased right ventricular (RV) myocardial oxygen demand and pulmonary artery pressures in excess of aortic pressure.

3. Presyncope and syncope and postural, tussive, and exercise systemic hypotension are correlated with decreased RV filling, decreased left ventricular (LV) filling, and LV compression by the right ventricle.

4. Abdominal pain, anorexia, edema, and ascites are correlated with gastric distention, increasing venous pressure, tricuspid insufficiency, and RV diastolic dysfunction.

5. Raynaud's phenomenon is characteristically found in patients with scleroderma-related disorders and in 10% of patients with PPH.

Physical findings depend on the cause and severity of PH. Most patients with a Doppler echocardiographic RVSP of more than 60 mm HG or a pulmonary artery systolic pressure of more than 50 mm HG obtained invasively have one or more cardiac findings. Patients with lung disease severe enough to cause more than moderate PH can be identified by decreased breath sounds, chest deformities, rales consistent with interstitial lung disease, abnormal jugular venous

TABLE 35.2. *Common presenting symptoms and signs in pulmonary hypertension, depending on related disease*

Symptoms
General: fatigue, weakness, Raynaud's phenomenon, generalized swelling
Cardiac: chest pain consistent with angina, atypical chest pains, palpitations
Pulmonary: dyspnea, orthopnea, and hemoptysis (rare in PAH)
Gastrointestinal: nausea, anorexia, abdominal bloating and fullness, occasionally severe abdominal pains
Neurologic: lightheadedness with positional change: presyncope and syncope with effort, cough, and at rest
Signs
General: anxiety, depression
Blood pressure: normal to low (occasionally hypertension)
Jugular venous pulse: distension with prominent a and V waves, estimated RA pressure > 5–20 mmHG, giant V waves with tricuspid regurgitation,
Carotid pulse: normal or low amplitude
Lungs: usually normal, rales with parenchymal disease
Cardiac: left parasternal RV lift, palpable pulmonic closure sound, increased split of S2 with increased P2 (heard at the apex); systolic murmur at left fourth ICS increasing with inspiration (tricuspid insufficiency), soft diastolic decrescendo murmur of pulmonic regurgitation in left third ICS, systolic ejection murmur at left second or third ICS, RV S4 and/or RV S3 gallop at lower left and/or right sternal border
Abdomen: pulsatile and enlarged liver, ascites, splenomegaly with portopulmonary hypertension and severe right-sided heart failure, distension
Extremities: peripheral edema, clubbing, Raynaud's phenomenon, sclerodactyly, loss of digital pulp (scleroderma related disorders)
Skin: pallor, plethora, cyanosis, telangectasias, livedo reticularis

ICS, intercostal space; PAH, pulmonary arterial hypertension; RA, right atrial; right ventricular.

TABLE 35.3. *World Health Organization pulmonary hypertension functional assessment classification*

Class I: Ordinary physical activity does not cause undue dyspnea or fatigue, chest pain, or near syncope
Class II: Slight limitation of physical activity; ordinary physical activity causes undue dyspnea or fatigue, chest pain, or near syncope
Class III: Marked limitation of physical activity; comfortable at rest, but less-than-ordinary activity causes undue dyspnea or fatigue, chest pain, or near syncope; signs of right-sided heart failure may be present
Class IV: Inability to carry out any physical activity without symptoms; dyspnea and/or fatigue may even be present at rest; discomfort is increased by any physical activity; signs of right-sided heart failure are usually present

wave or pressure, a murmur of tricuspid insufficiency, and often clubbing of the fingers and toes and cyanosis.

Long-standing Eisenmenger's syndrome (severe PH associated with congenital intracardiac shunt at the atrial, ventricular, or pulmonary artery level) with predominant right-to-left shunting is characterized by cyanosis at rest or with exercise, clubbing of the fingers and toes, and often murmurs of tricuspid insufficiency and pulmonic insufficiency. Because the right ventricle hypertrophies over a period of years, patients

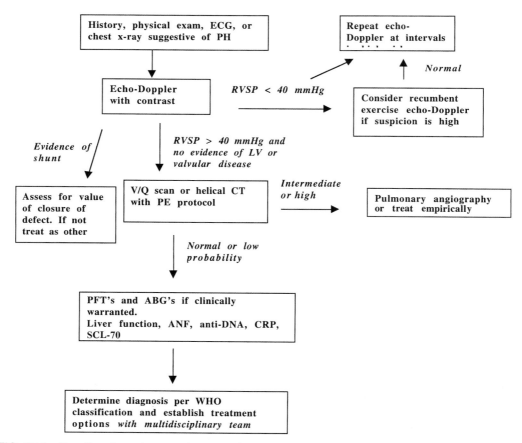

FIG. 35.1. Algorithm for pulmonary hypertension assessment in symptomatic individuals or those at high risk.

are often only mildly symptomatic until very late in the course. Patients with atrial septal defects and anomalous pulmonary venous drainage (about 2%) can rapidly develop severe PH that resembles PPH and manifests without clubbing of the fingers and toes or without cyanosis. Cyanosis can be due to intracardiac right-to-left shunting or to low cardiac output and decreased alveolar-capillary diffusion.

CLINICAL ALGORITHM FOR ASSESSMENT OF PULMONARY HYPERTENSION AND DIFFERENTIAL DIAGNOSIS

Figure 35.1 provides an algorithm for the assessment of PH. The algorithm provides a logical sequence in which to consider cost and therapeutic implications at each decision point that should be influenced by medical history and physical examination: for example, venous disease or pulmonary embolus, cirrhosis, evidence of sclerodactyly, telangiectasias, obesity or use of anorexigens, Raynaud's phenomenon, and cyanosis. The clinical presentations of diseases associated with precapillary PH overlap. Diagnosis and management require a multidisciplinary approach and liberal referral to physicians experienced in evaluating and treating PH.

HELPFUL TESTS IN THE ASSESSMENT OF PULMONARY HYPERTENSION

Electrocardiogram

The electrocardiogram (ECG) has a high degree of sensitivity (more than 75% to 80%) for detecting right ventricular hypertrophy in symptomatic patients with severe PH. The sensitivity is less than 40% when the ECG is read without clinical information or when the ECG is unedited and computerized. Frequent misdiagnoses include inferior, anterior, and septal infarction; inferior and anterior ischemia; and left posterior fascicular block. The ECG is not an effective screening tool in asymptomatic or mildly symptomatic persons. The most common ECG patterns in PH include a right axis deviation of the QRS interval of more than 90 degrees, a qR in

V_1, a right axis deviation, and increased voltage (more than 2.5 mm) of the p wave in lead II. The increased voltage is associated with a fourfold increase in mortality rate (3). Atrial premature beats are occur frequently, but atrial fibrillation, atrial flutter, and serious ventricular arrhythmias are not common. The upper ECG tracing in Fig. 35.2 demonstrates the typical ECG findings in PPH. It was obtained in a 37-year-old woman with WHO Class IV PPH. Her pretreatment mean pulmonary artery pressure (mPA) was 75 mm HG, and her pulmonary vascular resistance (PVR) was 24 Wood units. The lower ECG tracing is after 2 years of treatment with intravenous epoprostenol, at which point her disease was WHO Class I, her mPA was 30 mm HG, and her PVR was 6 Wood units. After treatment, there is less QRS right axis deviation (120 degrees vs. 90 degrees), lower R wave voltage in V_1 to V_3, and persistent but less ST segment abnormality of RV strain or ischemia.

Chest Radiograph

The magnitude of lung disease (emphysema, fibrosis, masses, and skeletal deformity) needed to induce significant PH is usually detectable on the chest radiograph. Chest radiographic indicators of PH include enlargement of the right ventricle, the right atrium, the superior vena cava, and the main pulmonary artery and its major branches. The criteria for PH is found in 95% of patients with PPH and only 4% of controls matched for age, gender, and body surface area. Figure 35.3 demonstrates the baseline and on-treatment chest radiograph in the 37-year-old woman with PPH described previously.

Doppler Echocardiography

Doppler echocardiography is an effective screening tool for detecting PH and for monitoring progression. The tricuspid regurgitant velocity (TRV) is proportional to the gradient between the RV and RA and is used to calculate the RVSP with Bernoulli's equation:

$$RVSP = 4 \times TRV^2 + \text{estimated RA pressure}$$

$$\text{in millimeters of mercury.}$$

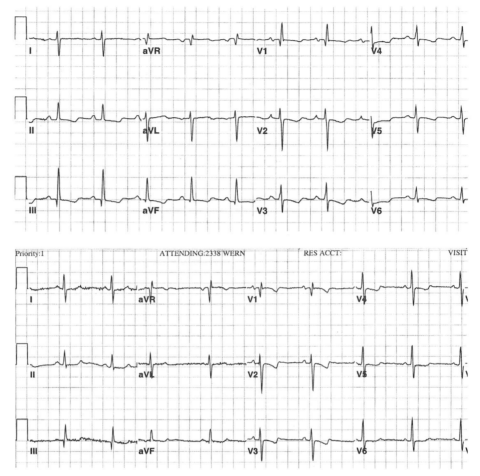

FIG. 35.2. Electrocardiographic tracings in a 37-year-old woman with primary pulmonary hypertension. **Top,** Tracing shows right ventricular hypertrophy and right ventricular strain, a qR in lead V_1, peaked enlarged p wave in lead II, and a right axis deviation of 120 degrees. **Bottom,** Tracing obtained after 2 years of treatment with intravenous epoprostenol.

Some authorities estimate the RA pressure from the size of the inferior vena cava and its response to respiration, and others use a fixed value (range, 10 to 14 mm HG). The TRV (in meters per second) should be provided to allow the clinician to add an estimate of the RA. Doppler echocardiography is sensitive for PH, but the TRV should be viewed in the context of clinical parameters, the size of the right atrium, and the size and function of the right ventricle (e.g., a mild increase in RVSP with dilated right atrium and right ventricle should prompt further studies). Agitated saline contrast material should be used to facilitate the measure of the TRV, particularly when the clinical estimate is mild PH, and to identify intracardiac shunts and a patent foramen ovale. A patent foramen ovale can be the explanation for rest and exercise arterial desaturation. The common anatomic findings in severe PH include dilated right atrium and right ventricle, flattened or D-shaped septum, and often a small, compressed left ventricle (4). Pericardial effusions are not common but may be predictive of a poor outcome. Doppler findings include significant

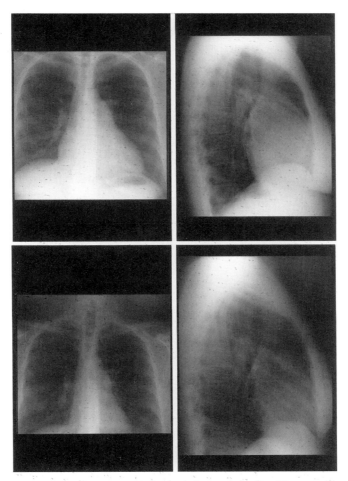

FIG. 35.3. Top, Posteroanterior and lateral chest radiograph in the 37-year-old woman with World Health Organization Class IV pulmonary artery hypertension with shortness of breath, demonstrating enlarged pulmonary artery and major branches, enlarged right atrium and right ventricle, and decreased pulmonary vascularity. **Bottom,** Film taken after 1 year of treatment with intravenous epoprostenol.

tricuspid and pulmonic regurgitation, from which the RVSP and pulmonary artery diastolic pressures can be calculated.

The WHO recommendations for Doppler echocardiography in persons at risk for PH are presented in Table 35.4 (1). The RVSP on screening Doppler echocardiography is often normal or mildly increased; a TRV of 3.0 to 3.5 m/second on Doppler echocardiography corresponds to an RVSP of 40 to 50 mm HG. Under these circum-

stances, patients at high risk (first-degree relatives of patients with sporadic or familial PPH patients, those with scleroderma-related disorders) or with portal hypertension should be considered for a right-sided heart catheterization supplemented by exercise if the resting study is inconclusive. Although it is a very effective screening tool and is useful for detecting response to therapy in moderately severe PH, Doppler echocardiography is less useful in monitoring progress

TABLE 35.4. *Recommended schedule for Doppler echocardiography for the detection of pulmonary hypertension in persons at high-risk*

Conditions present	Schedule
High risk	
Familial PPH: all first-degree relatives	When symptoms appear or at 3–5 year intervals if asymptomatic
Sporadic PPH: all first-degree relatives	When symptoms appear
Scleroderma spectrum of diseases	Annually with or without symptoms
Intermediate and low risk	
Liver disease/portal hypertension	When symptoms appear or at time of liver transplant listing
Murmur or congenital heart disease	At least once; repeat if symptoms or signs of PH appear
HIV infection	When symptoms appear
History of cocaine or anorexigen use	When symptoms appear

HIV, human immunodeficiency virus; PH, pulmonary hypertension; PPH, primary pulmonary hypertension.

and prognosis in severe PH, for which it adds little to clinical parameters.

Computed Tomography and the Ventilation/Perfusion Lung Scan

The ventilation/perfusion (V/Q) lung scan is the "gold standard" for the diagnosis of acute pulmonary embolus, and a normal or low-probability V/Q scan can be used to exclude chronic thromboemboli when the PH is moderate to severe. However, the best tool for assessing chronic thromboembolic PH is helical computed tomographic (CT) contrast-enhanced pulmonary angiography. The advantage of helical CT is the ability to screen for chronic central pulmonary thromboemboli that may be amenable to thromboendarterectomy (5). When PH is moderate or more severe and the helical CT pulmonary angiogram is "normal" or indicates low probability, the V/Q scan is needed to exclude third- and fourth-order pulmonary branch pulmonary embolus. When the V/Q scan is normal or indicates low probability, the algorithm shown in Fig. 35.1 is continued. In severe PH, it may be necessary to confidently exclude central thromboemboli by performing pulmonary angiography.

With mild to moderate PH, the differential diagnosis includes hypoxic/parenchymal, thromboembolic, and intrinsic vascular occlusive disease (scleroderma-related disorders, vasculitis, PPH). Depending on the clinical findings, chest radiograph, and probability of parenchymal lung disease, a high-resolution CT scan (1-mm cuts) may be obtained first or at the time of a helical

CT pulmonary angiogram. A high-resolution CT scan is recommended for patients with PH associated with collagen vascular disease, to detect interstitial fibrosis, inflammatory pneumonitis, and alveolitis that may be amenable to immunosuppressive therapy. The CT scan can detect PH in parenchymal lung disease. A main pulmonary artery diameter larger than 29 mm has a sensitivity of 87%, a specificity of 89%, and a positive predictive value of 0.97 for identifying patients with an mPA of more than 20 mm HG (6).

Magnetic Resonance Angiography

Magnetic resonance studies can be used to characterize both anatomy and physiology in PH (7,8). Estimates of RVSP and mPA can be obtained from flow velocities with the Bernoulli equation, as with Doppler echocardiography. Magnetic resonance imaging and magnetic resonance angiography can be used to assess RV and LV chamber volume and ejection fraction, detect intracardiac shunts, and image both acute and chronic central and peripheral pulmonary emboli (9). The resources for these studies, particularly software, are, however, not widely available.

Serologic and Hepatic Function Studies

After excluding hypoxemia, parenchymal lung disease, systemic to pulmonary shunts, and pulmonary emboli, the remaining differential diagnosis (Fig. 35.1) consists of entities associated with PAH or intrinsic pulmonary vascular occlusive disease (Table 35.1). Serologic studies are necessary to screen for the collagen vascular diseases: sedimentation rate, C-reactive protein, antinuclear antibody, and SCL-70 antibody. Distinguishing the scleroderma-related disorders and other collagen vascular disease from PPH has clinical implications and often requires specialty consultation.

Portopulmonary hypertension, found in nearly 1% of patients with chronic liver disease and 10% of those referred for liver transplantation, can be excluded in the absence of a history of alcohol abuse, blood transfusions, or hepatitis and in the presence of normal liver function. Because of the clinical implications, HIV screening should be considered in PAH. Hepatitis C is a suspected trigger for PAH, but because of its frequency in the population, the relationship is unclear.

Pulmonary Function Studies and Arterial Blood Gas Measurements

Pulmonary function testing are useful in the assessment of dyspnea but are not indicated in severe PH unless there is clinical evidence for structural lung disease on examination or chest radiograph. The usual pattern in severe PH without lung disease is a moderate decrease in diffusion capacity, mild reduction in ventilatory capacity, and no significant obstructive or restrictive physiologic processes (10). In scleroderma-related disorders with PH, pulmonary fibrosis, and hypoxemia, there is often a marked reduction in diffusion capacity and a restrictive ventilation pattern.

Functional Assessment with Exercise

Assessment of exercise capacity in patients with mild to severe forms of PH is recommended for risk stratification, for selection of a treatment strategy, to measure the response to therapy, and to assist in determining eligibility for more aggressive therapies. The two most useful measures are a standardized 6-minute walk test with continuous measurement of cutaneous oxygen saturation and a submaximal or symptom-limited bicycle or treadmill exercise test with or without direct measurement of oxygen consumption. Because symptom-limited stress testing is poorly tolerated in patients with worse PH than WHO Class II, our institution prefers the 6-minute walk. The walk is easily tolerated, and results correlate highly with PH class and prognosis. The inability to walk at least 300 m and a decrease in oxygen saturation by 10 or more units are associated with a marked increase in mortality rate and can be used to select patients for lung transplantation (10).

Cardiopulmonary exercise testing with gas exchange measurements can be obtained safely in patients with moderate to severe PH, and they correlate with clinical severity, but their clinical utility is not established (11).

Right-Sided Heart Catheterization and Assessment of Pulmonary Vasodilator Reserve

Right-sided heart catheterization is necessary in the majority of patients with precapillary pulmonary artery hypertension to verify the diagnosis and exclude pulmonary venous hypertension, assess prognosis, assist in selecting the best treatment option, and measure the pulmonary vasodilator reserve (12) (Fig. 35.1). A similar approach is recommended for patients with thromboembolic PH not amenable to thromboendarterectomy, in whom intravenous epoprostenol or the subcutaneous prostacyclin analogue treprostinil (Remodulin) may be used. At this time, there is little clinical value in performing a vasodilator trial in patients with PH associated with lung disease and hypoxemia.

PULMONARY HYPERTENSION ASSOCIATED WITH CHRONIC LUNG DISEASE

Of the patients with chronic obstructive pulmonary disease (COPD) that is complicated by cor pulmonale, about 50% die within 7 years of diagnosis, but without cor pulmonale, survival averages 13.5 years (13,14). The signs of PH in COPD are occult and can be precipitous. Patients with COPD or pulmonary fibrosis and PH often exhibit relatively sudden (weeks to months) "unexplained" deterioration in cardiac function with minimal change in lung function that can be attributed to cor pulmonale. Acute infections are often blamed for the rapid deterioration, and worsening hypoxemia can be due to reversal of flow through an unrecognized patent foramen ovale.

Severe PH is rare, but has important consequences, in COPD. In a series of patients with chronic lung disease referred to a transplantation center, PH was generally mild to moderate (15). The mPA averaged 25 ± 6 mm HG, and the pulmonary vascular resistance index was mildly elevated at 4.4 ± 1.7 Wood units/m². However, a reduced RV ejection fraction (less than 45%) was present in 59% of patients with COPD and in 66% with cystic fibrosis (15). LV ejection fraction was less than 45% in nearly 20% of patients with PH, was less than 4% in those without PH, and was not related to coronary disease. Simple ECG criteria for cor pulmonale (frontal plane P axis of +90 degrees or more, and S1, S2, S3 QRS pattern) during an acute exacerbation of COPD are associated with a 50% increase in mortality rate (16).

CHRONIC THROMBOEMBOLIC PULMONARY HYPERTENSION

Chronic thromboembolic pulmonary hypertension (CTEPH) results from incomplete lysis of large, organized thrombi in the main pulmonary artery or large secondary branches. Although important to exclude, pulmonary embolus is not a common cause of chronic PH (17). Recurrent and multiple small pulmonary emboli can lead to severe PH that resembles PPH, possibly because of genetic susceptibility. Symptoms in CTEPH overlap with those of coronary disease, asthma, congestive heart failure, cirrhosis, COPD, and deconditioning (18). Signs and symptoms of PH (Table 35.3) in patients with pulmonary embolus, deep venous thrombosis, and hypoxemia should prompt an assessment for central pulmonary emboli with helical CT angiography. The goal is not simply to detect evidence of pulmonary emboli but also to identify patients with central pulmonary emboli that are amenable to thromboendarterectomy (19). If the helical CT with contrast material or the V/Q scan is consistent with chronic pulmonary emboli or inconclusive in patients with a history of deep venous thrombo-

sis, pulmonary angiography is necessary to detect central (surgically remedial) disease.

An inferior vena caval filter should be inserted in all patients with evidence of central or peripheral CTEPH with PH. Lifelong anticoagulation with warfarin, unless absolutely contraindicated, is necessary to prevent *in situ* thrombi, recurrent deep venous thrombosis, and thromboemboli that can bypass the filter via the left ovarian or testicular vein draining to the left renal vein.

The prognosis of patients with severe PH attributable to pulmonary emboli is poor. In a series of 49 patients treated with anticoagulants and monitored for an average of 18.7 months (range, 6 to 72 months), the mortality rate was 33%; most deaths were from progressive right-sided heart failure (20). Risk for death was related to the degree of hypoxemia, mPA, exercise capacity, and association with COPD. In properly selected patients, pulmonary thromboendarterectomy can be lifesaving, can reduce the PH, and can improve right-sided heart function and well-being (19). Figure 35.4 demonstrates the fibrous material successfully removed from two patients undergoing a pulmonary thromboendarterectomy. Surgery is generally indicated in WHO PH Class III and Class IV with a PVR greater than 3 Wood units. Obtaining good surgical results requires a highly experienced team. The mortality rates ranges from 2% to 25% depending on risk factors and experience. Markedly impaired RV function and tricuspid insufficiency increase the risk but do not preclude surgery. Right-sided heart failure and transient mental status changes can complicate the postoperative course. More than 90% of survivors recover to the level of New York Heart Association Class I or II (19). Patients with CTEPH should be screened for hypercoagulability.

PULMONARY ARTERIAL HYPERTENSION

There are an estimated 200 thousand persons in the United States with PAH, the WHO category that encompasses the more severe forms of diseases of the pulmonary vasculature (Table 35.1) (1). PAH encompasses PPH (sporadic and familial) and PH related to the following triggers or associated diseases: scleroderma-related disorders

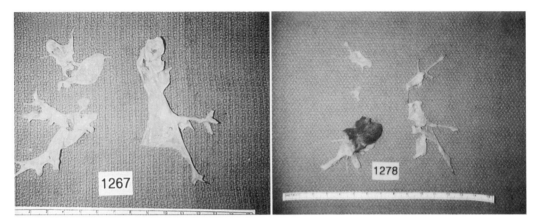

FIG. 35.4. Example of the fibrinous and fibrous material removed during successful pulmonary thromboendarterectomies in two patients with severe chronic thromboembolic pulmonary hypertension.

(estimated frequency, 0.1% to 10%), atrial septal defect (2% to 4%), Eisenmenger's reaction, portal hypertension (10% of transplant-eligible patients), HIV (0.5%), and drugs and toxins such as the anorexigens (1/16,000) (3).

Severe PH with the characteristic and unusual pulmonary arteriolar plexiform lesions found in PPH was attributed to aminorex fumarate, a popular anorexigen used for obesity in Europe in the 1960s (12). The risk of developing PH in persons who use the modern anorexigens dexfenfluramine and fenfluramine with or without phentermine (formulations with phentermine are commonly known as "fen-phen") is estimated at 28 cases per million person-years of exposure (21). There is a probability that these agents can increase the frequency of severe PH in patients with other disorders, including collagen-vascular diseases, hypoxia/sleep apnea, and COPD. Other recognized triggers of plexogenic arteriopathy include toxic rapeseed oil, cocaine, and L-tryptophane, which was available over the counter in the United States as a diet supplement and used for restless sleep (1). A relationship among triggers, genetic susceptibility, and severe PH is highly likely (Fig. 35.5). The germ line mutation associated with familial PPH has been demonstrated in the sporadic form (22).

The majority of cases of PPH are sporadic, but in 6% to 10% of cases, there is one or more affected family member (12). The onset of symptoms occurs earlier in familial PPH (genetic anticipation), and asymptomatic relatives of patients with PPH who are genetic carriers have an abnormal pulmonary artery pressure response to exercise (23). The disease is transmitted as an autosomal dominant trait with incomplete penetrance. Varying degrees of abnormality in bone morphogenic peptide (BMPR2) and related peptides may explain the incomplete penetrance in familial PPH and may contribute as well to the genetic susceptibility to triggers (22).

PPH occurs more commonly in women (about threefold), but the gender difference is not seen in children (12). Because of the frequent peripartum presentation, the association with oral contraceptives (possibly coincidental because of age and gender), and the known prothrombotic effects of estrogens, there is poorly confirmed speculation that estrogens play a role in the initiation or progression of PPH. The classic presentation in PPH and triggered PAH is a healthy-appearing young to middle-aged woman complaining of dyspnea and fatigue and often atypical chest pains that are ignored or considered anxiety until months later when accompanied by edema, syncope, or both. It is uncommon (but must be considered) for patients with collagen vascular diseases to present with PH as the first manifestation of disease, but PPH may resemble scleroderma and lupus. About 10% of PPH patients have Raynaud's phenomenon, and levels of antinuclear antibodies are often elevated.

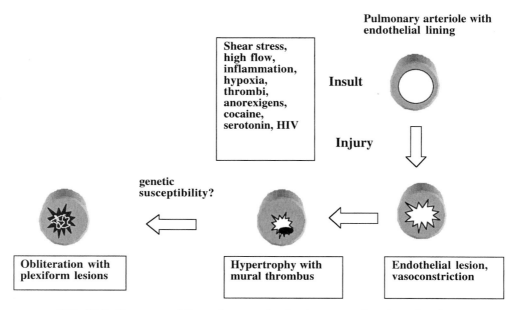

FIG. 35.5. Summary of the pathogenesis of pulmonary artery hypertension.

Long-term survival with PPH has improved markedly with the use of calcium channel blockers, anticoagulants, and epoprostenol (12). The median length of survival now exceeds 5 years. Independent predictors of mortality include baseline portal hypertension more severe than Class II, p wave in lead II over 2.5 mm, distance walked of less than 300 m and desaturation of more than 9 units on a pretreatment 6-minute walk test, and the PVR (3,10,24). After treatment with epoprostenol, predictors of a poor outcome include (a) failure to improve by at least one functional class, (b) a 6-minute walk distance of less than 300 m, (c) a high RA pressure, (d) a mixed venous oxygen saturation of less than 60%, and (e) a failure of the cardiac output to increase and the PVR to decrease significantly (approximately 25%) (24–27).

Algorithm for the Differential Diagnosis in Pulmonary Artery Hypertension

The diagnostic algorithm for patients with a clinical presentation consistent with PAH is fairly constant in experienced centers (Fig. 35.1). Serologic studies are necessary to exclude rheumato-logic diseases but may be inconclusive. An antinuclear antibody level higher than 1/320 or an elevated C-reactive protein should prompt the investigation of collagen vascular disease. Patients with severe PH can have an isolated elevation of the antinuclear antibody level in a speckled pattern, a positive SCL-70 antibody measurement, or anticardiolipin antibodies and no other manifestations of scleroderma or lupus. Experience is limited, but immunosuppressive therapy has been effective in some forms of PAH, such as lupus-related vasculitis. Patients with an established diagnosis of PPH should be assessed continually for collagen vascular disorders.

Pulmonary angiography is not necessary in the evaluation of severe PAH when the V/Q scan is of low probability and when clinical probability is not high. The pulmonary angiogram in PPH resembles that of CTEPH (with the exception of webs, filling defects, and cutoffs). The primary and secondary branches are symmetrically enlarged, and there is pruning or loss of branching from tertiary vessels. Relatively large central insite thrombi have been reported in PPH.

Pulmonary venoocclusive disease (PVOD), which was once classified as a form of PPH, can

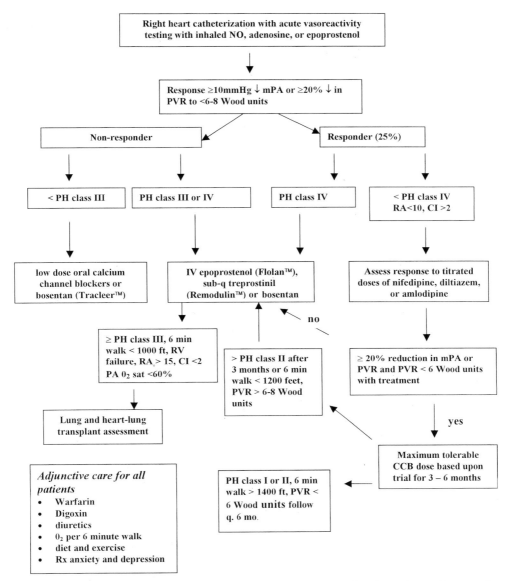

FIG. 35.6. Algorithm for management of pulmonary artery hypertension, based on pulmonary hypertension class and vasoreactivity.

be present with moderate to severe PH. PVOD may be idiopathic or associated with collagen diseases and cancer chemotherapy. The presentation is similar to that of PAH, but the chest radiograph demonstrates pulmonary venous hypertension, pleural effusions, or congestive heart failure in the setting of normal LV systolic and diastolic function. PVOD can result in a high-probability

V/Q scan and be misdiagnosed as thromboembolic PH. The pulmonary angiogram in PVOD shows no evidence of intraluminal thrombi, and the pulmonary capillary wedge (PCW) pressure is generally (but not always) elevated in one or more sites (28). The confirmation of PVOD requires a lung biopsy, and treatment is lung transplantation.

Right-Sided Heart Catheterization and Pulmonary Vasodilator Reserve in Pulmonary Artery Hypertension

Right-sided heart catheterization should be performed in patients with PAH to confirm the diagnosis and exclude PVOD, and a pulmonary vasodilator trial should be performed to determine therapeutic options and prognosis (Fig. 35.6). Such studies should be performed in centers with experience with PH.

Experience is necessary in performing and interpreting the results. A mean pulmonary artery pressure of 30 mm HG or RVSP of 60 mm HG has serious implications in patients with COPD, thromboemboli, and postcapillary PH, but it is compatible with a relatively good prognosis in patients with Eisenmenger's syndrome, scleroderma-related disorders, and PPH. Pressure has little meaning without a determination of cardiac output (CO) and a calculation of resistance. The impedance to emptying of the right ventricle is the major determinant of RV failure and compensatory hypertrophy and dilatation. RV impedance is proportional to the total pulmonary vascular resistance (TPVR):

$$TPVR = mPA / CO,$$

which includes the contribution of the pulmonary venous pressures. More important in precapillary PH is the PVR, also known as the *pulmonary arteriolar resistance,* which is the portion of resistance that is precapillary:

$$PVR = (mPA - PCW) / CO.$$

Resistance can be expressed in Wood units, the direct result of the equation, or multiplied by 80 to convert to dyne-cm per second^{-5} (1 Wood unit = 80 dyne-cm/sec^{-5}). Resistance is often expressed, corrected for the body surface area in children, by using the cardiac index rather than cardiac output, or pulmonary vascular resistance index.

Use of a four-lumen balloon flotation catheter with thermodilution (additional lumen for stiffening wire) facilitates entering the pulmonary artery and obtaining satisfactory pulmonary artery occlusive pressure (PAOP), PCW pressure, and cardiac output. The PAOP obtained with or without balloon inflation can be inaccurate in severe PH. The hypertrophied or occluded arteriole is not capable of transmitting the true left atrial pressure. To calculate the PVR when an accurate PAOP or PCW cannot be obtained (about 5%), the PCW is estimated at 12 mm HG if the RA pressure is lower than 12 mm HG and at 15 mm HG if the RA pressure is higher than 12 mm HG. The latter is based on the common finding of an elevated LV diastolic pressure from RV compression in severe PH. Simultaneous PCW and LV diastolic pressure recordings are necessary when an increase in pulmonary venous pressure is possible.

Inhaled nitric oxide (iNO), intravenous adenosine, or intravenous epoprostenol can be used to assess pulmonary vasodilator reserve (12,29). Each is safe in properly selected patients. Empirical use or a hemodynamic trial of calcium channel blockers without a trial of short-acting agents should be avoided (30). A positive response to these agents (defined as more than a 20% reduction in mPA or PVR or a decrease in mPA by 10 mm HG) correlates with the likelihood of a similar response to calcium channel blocker therapy (29). In a small study comparing iNO and adenosine for predicting the response to nifedipine in PPH, Ricciardi et al. (31) found iNO to be better tolerated (patients experienced chest pain and hypotension with intravenous adenosine) and considerably higher positive and negative predictive value. Other advantages of iNO are that the onset of action is rapid, the half-life is less than 60 seconds, the test requires only 5 to 7 minutes, and, because iNO has no effect on systemic pressures, it is extremely safe. My colleagues and I have conducted more than 450 trials in PH with iNO without adverse events. There is no established value or safety in testing vasodilator reserve in precapillary PHH with intravenous nitroglycerin or nitroprusside.

Lung Biopsy

Lung biopsy is not necessary for confirming the diagnosis in most patients with PAH. There is a significant risk of morbidity and mortality from major bleeding from lung biopsies in severe PH.

In centers with a multidisciplinary team that includes an experienced thoracic surgeon and a pathologist interested in lung disease, open-lung biopsy may be conducted in patients with mild to moderate pulmonary hypertension to diagnose active vasculitis, pulmonary venoocclusive disease, pulmonary capillary hemangiomatosis, and the rare overlap syndromes, and interstitial lung disease. Knowledge of each of these findings would have an impact on therapeutic strategies.

Therapeutic Strategies for Pulmonary Artery Hypertension

"Because PPH is a rare disease whose complexity poses tremendous challenges to the treating physician, it is recommended that patients be referred to a center with experience in the management of this disease. The referring physician must, nevertheless, play a major role in the day to day care of these patients" (32). This consensus statement, published in 1993, applies to all forms of PAH. The therapeutic approaches to PPH, PAH, and related disorders listed in Table 35.1 are fundamentally equivalent. Inoperable PH attributable to pulmonary thromboemboli is considered in the same category by some authorities.

The drugs available to improve effort tolerance, increase cardiac output, and decrease pulmonary artery pressure and resistance in PH are listed in Table 35.5. Figure 35.6 is a treatment decision tree for pharmacologic therapy for PAH. In patients with evidence of pulmonary artery vasodilator reserve, approximately 25%, the oral calcium channel blockers nifedipine, diltiazem, and amlodipine may reduce symptoms and prolong life (33). Because of an increased risk, a trial of oral calcium channel blockers should not be performed regardless of the response to iNO or intravenous epoprostenol in patients with WHO Class IV PH, overt right-sided heart failure, mRA of higher than 12 mm HG, cardiac index of less than 2 L/minute/m^2, or systemic pressure less than 95 to 100 mm HG. Even the initial administration of a small dose (10 to 20 mg) of nifedipine can result in severe systemic hypotension and death.

Patients with PH that is more severe than WHO Class II who do not respond to calcium channel blockers or have a contraindication to

TABLE 35.5. *Treatment options with vasodilator drugs in pulmonary hypertension*

Drug	Dosage	Indications and exclusions
Calcium channel blockers	Nifedipine, 30–240 mg extended-release, given q12h if dose exceeds 30 mg Diltiazem, 60–480 mg extended-release, given q12h if dose exceeds 60 mg Amlodipine, 2.5–20 mg, given q12 h	Classes II and III[a] with pulmonary vasodilator reserve Avoid in patients with Class IV[a] and RV failure
Endothelin antagonists	Bosentan (Tracleer), 62.5 mg q12h, titrated to 125 mg q12h	PAH in patients with Classes II, III, and possibly IV[a] Do not use in patients with liver disease, persons infected with HIV, women with potential for pregnancy
Prostacyclin derivatives	Treprostinil (Remodulin): continuous subcutaneous infusion at rate of 10–100 μ/kg/min (avg. 20–40 μg/kg/min) Epoprostenol (Flolan): continuous intravenous infusion at rate of 4–150 μg/kg/min (avg. 20–40 μg/kg/min)	PAH and CTEPH in patients with Classes III and IV[a] PAH and CTEPH in patients with high-risk Class III and all Class IV[a]

CTEPH, chronic thromboembolic pulmonary hypertension; HIV, human immunodeficiency virus; PAH; pulmonary arterial hypertension; RV, right ventricular.
[a]World Health Organization pulmonary hypertension Functional assessment classification.

a calcium channel blocker trial are candidates for the new endothelin antagonist bosentan (Tracleer), subcutaneous treprostinil (Remodulin), or intravenous epoprostenol (Flolan).

Endothelin Antagonists

Bosentan is a novel dual endothelin-receptor antagonist that has been shown to be effective in PAH (34,35). Endothelin-1 is an endogenous vasoconstrictor that promotes smooth muscle proliferation and appears to play a role in the pathogenesis and natural history of PH. Levels of endothelin-1 are elevated in the lungs of patients with PH (36). In two placebo-controlled trials, bosentan improved exercise tolerance, increased time to clinical worsening, increased CO, and reduced PVR in patients with PAH (PPH and connective tissue disease) (34,35). Nonfatal hepatotoxicity has occurred with bosentan, which is metabolized in the liver and interacts significantly with drugs through the P-450 system. It is approved by the U.S. Food and Drug Administration for PAH, but prescription privilege is limited to experienced physicians who are assisted by a regional distribution system that send a month's supply after receiving report of normal liver function. The cost of bosentan is about $2,500 per month. Although considerably easier to take and less expensive than intravenous epoprostenol, its long-term safety, effect on survival, and safety in combination with other drugs remain to be seen. Contraindications to bosentan include liver disease, portopulmonary hypertension, HIV infection, and, in women, lack of a high level of protection from pregnancy.

Prostacyclin

The prostacyclin analogue epoprostenol has markedly improved the quality of life and changed the natural history of PPH, portopulmonary hypertension, Eisenmenger's syndrome, the scleroderma spectrum of diseases, and thromboembolic hypertension (37–40). It is the drug of choice for patients with PAH who have WHO Class IV PH and patients with Class III PH with poor prognostic features. Epoprostenol is administered by continuous intravenous infusion through an indwelling Hickman catheter and an infusion pump the size of a portable radio. It is a short-acting (3- to 5-minute half-life) analogue of prostaglandin I_2, the naturally occurring vasodilator prostacyclin. It may acutely decrease mPA and PVR and increase CO and oxygen transport, but the absence of an initial response is not predictive of the subsequent clinical or hemodynamic outcome. The long-term hemodynamic benefits are associated with pulmonary arteriole remodeling, gradual improvement in RV function, and antiplatelet/antithrombotic effects (41). The dose of epoprostenol is increased gradually by an experienced nurse or physician according to symptoms and tolerance of side effects. Most patients tolerate side effects, which include rash, flushing, jaw claudication, and diarrhea. Thrombocytopenia (platelet count range, 25 to 75,000 mL^3) occurs in about 10% to 20% of patients. The mechanism is obscure but may be exaggerated by hypersplenism in portal hypertension and possibly by hyperperfusion of the spleen from excessive dosages and a high CO. A local skin infection, bacteremia, and septicemia occur in about 5% to 10% of patients taking intravenous epoprostenol. Despite the potential problems, patients are tolerant because of the improvement in well-being that occurs in more than 75%, which is accompanied by a marked reduction in mortality rate.

Treprostinil, an analogue of epoprostenol with a longer half-life, is administered as a continuous subcutaneous infusion and is approved by the U.S. Food and Drug Administration for similar indications. In comparison with placebo, treprostinil has similar but less powerful effects on hemodynamic parameters than does epoprostenol. It increases the distance on the 6-minute walk, reduces dyspnea, and improves quality of life (42). A major limitation of treprostinil is an annoying pain at the infusion site, resulting in intolerance in about 10% of patients.

Evolving Drug Therapies for Pulmonary Artery Hypertension

Several new treatment options are in various stages of clinical development in the management of PAH, including iNO, selective subtype A endothelin receptor antagonists, oral and inhaled prostacyclin analogues, and the phosphodiesterase-5 inhibitors exemplarized by sildenafil (43). It is highly likely that small doses of combinations of each of these agents will prove to be highly effective and complementary. The pathophysiologic process of PAH is related to abnormal synthesis of endothelium-derived nitric oxide and prostacyclin and excessive levels of endothelin, the endothelium-derived potent vasoconstrictor and mitogen. Clinical trials are under way with oral (beraprost) and inhaled (aerosolized iloprost) analogues of prostacyclin, which may be effective in persons not requiring high dosages and in patients with PH associated with lung disease (44,45). Cyclic guanidine monophosphate increases in response to sildenafil, the phosphodiesterase-5 inhibitor, and to L-arginine, the nitrate donor in the synthesis of endothelium-derived relaxing factor (nitric oxide). Each has possible therapeutic value in PAH both alone and in combination with other strategies (46,47).

Treatment of Refractory Pulmonary Artery Hypertension

Long-term survival rates are poor in patients at high risk with PAH and PPH (less than 12 to 18 months after diagnosis) (12). In patients in whom epoprostenol treatment fails, high-risk options include atrial septostomy and lung or heart-lung transplantation. Atrial balloon septostomy is primarily a bridge to transplantation. It should not be performed in patients with end-of-life indicators or in extremis. Initial experience with blade septostomy was relatively poor, but balloon septostomy is performed safely by experienced teams using intraatrial ultrasound guidance (48,49). By creating a right-to-left intra-atrial shunt that results in arterial oxygen saturation percentage in the mid-80s, balloon septostomy increases LV filling and stroke volume and "unloads" the right side of the heart.

Single- or double-lung transplantation is considered in PAH patients whose condition remains WHO Class III or IV after treatment with epoprostenol for longer than 3 months and earlier in some centers (50). Other indicators of a poor prognosis that can be used for referral and listing for transplantation include baseline RA pressure higher than 12 to 15 mm HG, mPA higher than 55 mm HG, cardiac index less than 2 L/minute/m^2, a 6-minute walk distance of less than 300 m, and exercise desaturation greater than 9 units (10,12,26,27). International guidelines for the selection of patients for lung transplantation in severe PAH have been published, but practice patterns vary considerably in the United States and Europe (50,51). Single- or double-lung transplantation is the preferred procedure in the United States, and heart-lung transplantation is preferred in the majority of European centers. The rate of operative survival after lung transplantation for PPH is over 90%. However, the 1- and 5-year survival rates are relatively poor, at 85% and 50%. Most transplantation survivors improve to New York Heart Association Class I or II.

GENERAL TREATMENT MEASURES IN PULMONARY ARTERY HYPERTENSION AND COR PULMONALE ASSOCIATED WITH LUNG DISEASE

The general approach to moderate to severe forms of PH and cor pulmonale, defined as right-sided heart failure associated with chronic lung disease, is similar to treatment of all forms of heart failure. Critical to success is a good social support system, comprehensive patient and family education, and attention to lifestyle measures that promote wellness. Depression and anxiety should be assessed and treated with the assistance of social workers or psychologists working as part of a team who are aware of the diseases and clinical issues, including prognosis. There is no contraindication to the use of nonsedating anxiolytics and, in particular, antidepressants in these patients.

Cachexia and associated muscle wasting and weakness in cor pulmonale contribute significantly to the symptoms and functional limitation. The cardiac workload and cost of work of breathing at any given external workload (e.g., carrying packages) is proportional to the effort required. Nutrient supplements and exercise to maintain and increase muscle tone, strength, and aerobic capacity, preferably in a pulmonary rehabilitation program, should be considered. Obesity is common in patients with PPH. Body fat, regardless of the degree of obesity, increases cardiopulmonary work. Weight loss to an ideal body weight should be encouraged, with specific recommendations and goals and use of nutrition counseling.

Continuous use of nasal oxygen to maintain an arterial saturation of at least 90% increases exercise performance, can eliminate episodic nocturnal and exertional hypoxemia, and may reduce the rate of progression of PH and mortality even in the presence of progressive loss of pulmonary function (52). Oxygen requirements should be determined during exercise with monitoring of cutaneous oxygen saturation.

In contrast to PAH, there is no apparent benefit, and there is possibly harm, from vasodilator therapy in PH associated with respiratory diseases and hypoxemia (53,54). Amlodipine is safe for treating systemic hypertension in COPD with PH. Diltiazem, verapamil, and beta blockers should be used with caution because of negative inotropic effects on the right ventricle. The concern that vasodilator drugs will worsen oxygen delivery by increasing perfusion in poorly ventilated lungs has not been observed in most controlled trials. Angiotensin-converting enzyme inhibitors and angiotensin receptor blockers can be used alone and in combination with other drugs.

Digoxin increases the CO in PH with normal LV function and is generally indicated in patients with PH and cor pulmonale (55,56). However, digitalis toxicity is more common in patients with COPD and cor pulmonale. The target drug level is about 1 ng/mL.

Diets should be high in protein and complex carbohydrates, low in fat, and low in salt (2 g or less of sodium per day). Both the loop and potassium-sparing diuretics are effective. Caution is necessary to avoid dehydration and orthostatic hypotension, which can be a reflection of underfilling of the left or right ventricle and not of a decrease in total body water. Spironolactone (25 to 200 mg/day) is particularly effective when the liver is congested and can be used effectively in conjunction with loop diuretics.

There is consensus that long-term anticoagulation with warfarin reduces the rate of mortality in severe forms of pulmonary artery hypertension, but no controlled trials have been reported regarding the use of warfarin in other causes of cor pulmonale (57,58).

PRACTICAL POINTS

- The WHO classification of PH includes (a) PAH, (b) pulmonary venous hypertension, (c) disorders of the respiratory system and or hypoxemia, and (d) chronic thrombotic or embolic disease.
- Pulmonary artery hypertension (PAH) is insidious in onset but often rapidly progressive. Patients at high risk include those with scleroderma-related disorders, congenital heart disease, sleep apnea, portal hypertension, HIV infection, and a family history of PPH; those who use cocaine; and those who use anorexigens.
- PH should be considered in any patient with dyspnea, peripheral edema, angina,

  presyncope, and syncope. Doppler echocardiography is the most useful tool for screening for PH in patients at risk or with symptoms.
- When PH is considered to be precapillary according to the Doppler echocardiogram, the diagnostic algorithm should include a V/Q scan, serologic studies, and pulmonary function tests in selected patients.
- Right-sided heart catheterization and testing for pulmonary artery vasodilator reserve are very helpful for assessing prognosis and determining therapeutic choices in PAH.

(continued)

- PH associated with chronic pulmonary embolus should be considered for an inferior vena caval filter and pulmonary thromboendarterectomy.
- Hypoxic PH can be reversible with oxygen and treatment of sleep apnea.
- Treatment of right-sided heart failure due to PH should include diuretics, digoxin, warfarin, diet, exercise, and oxygen as needed, all based on the results of a 6-minute hall walk.
- Specific treatment for PAH includes calcium channel blockers, endothelin antagonists, subcutaneous and intravenous prostacyclin derivatives, atrial septostomy, and lung transplantation.

REFERENCES

1. Rich S, ed. *Executive summary.* From the World Symposium on Primary Pulmonary Hypertension, Evian, France, September 6–10, 1998, cosponsored by The World Health Organization (*http://www.who.int/ncd/cvd/pph.html*).
2. Galie N, Manes A, Uguccioni L, et al. Primary pulmonary hypertension. Insights into the pathogenesis from epidemiology. *Chest* 1998;114:184S–194S.
3. Bossone E, Paciocco G, Iarussi D, et al. The prognostic role of the ECG in primary pulmonary hypertension. *Chest* 2002;121:513–518.
4. Bossone E, Duong-Wagner TH, Paciocco G, et al. Echocardiographic features of primary pulmonary hypertension. *J Am Soc Echocardiogr* 1999;12:655–662.
5. Auger WR, Channick RN, Kerr KM, et al. Evaluation of patients with suspected chronic thromboembolic pulmonary hypertension. *Semin Thorac Cardiovasc Surg* 1999;11:179–190.
6. Tan RT, Kuzo R, Goodman LR, et al. Utility of CT scan evaluation for predicting pulmonary hypertension in patients with parenchymal lung disease. *Chest* 1998;113:1250–1256.
7. Boxt LM, Katz J. Magnetic resonance imaging for quantification of RV volume in patients with pulmonary hypertension. *J Thorac Imaging* 1993;8:92–97.
8. Kondo C, Caputo GR, Mansu T, et al. Pulmonary hypertension: pulmonary flow quantification and flow profile analysis with velocity encoded cine MR imaging. *Radiology* 1992;183:751–758.
9. Kreitner KF, Mayer E, Voigtlaender T, et al. Three-dimensional contrast-enhanced magnetic resonance angiography in a patient with chronic thromboembolic pulmonary hypertension before and after thromboendarterectomy. *Circulation* 1999;99:1101.
10. Paciocco G, Martinez F, Bossone E, et al. Oxygen desaturation on the six-minute walk test and mortality in untreated primary pulmonary hypertension. *Eur Respir J* 2001;17:647–652.
11. Sun X-G, Hansen JE, Oudiz RJ, et al. Exercise pathophysiology in patients with primary pulmonary hypertension. *Circulation* 2001;104:429–435.
12. Rubin LJ. Primary pulmonary hypertension. *N Engl J Med* 1997;336:111–117.
13. Bishop JM, Cross KW. Physiologic variables and mortality in patients with various categories of chronic respiratory disease. *Bull Eur Physiopathol Respir* 1984;20:495–500.
14. Traver GA, Cline MG, Burrows B. Predictors of mortality in chronic obstructive pulmonary disease. *Am Rev Respir Dis* 1979;119;895–902.
15. Vizza CD, Lynch JP, Ochoa LL, et al. Right and left ventricular dysfunction in patients with severe pulmonary disease *Chest* 1998;113:576–583.
16. Inclan RA, Fuso L, De Rosa M, et al. Electrocardiographic signs of chronic cor pulmonale: a negative prognostic finding in chronic obstructive pulmonary disease. *Circulation* 1999;99:1600–1605.
17. Egermayer P, Peacock AJ. Is pulmonary embolism a common cause of chronic pulmonary hypertension? Limitations of the embolic hypothesis. *Eur Respir J* 2000;15:440–448.
18. Moses KM, Auger WR, Fedullo PF. Chronic major-vessel thromboembolic pulmonary hypertension. *Circulation* 1990;81:1735–1743.
19. Jamieson SW. Experience and results with 150 pulmonary thromboendarterectomy operations over a 29-month period. *J Thorac Cardiovasc Surg* 1993;106:116–127.
20. Lewczuk J, Piszko P, Jagas J, et al. Prognostic factors in medically treated patients with chronic pulmonary embolism. *Chest* 2001;119:818–823.
21. Abenhaim L, Moride Y, Brenot F, et al. Appetite-suppressant drugs and risk of primary pulmonary hypertension. *N Engl J Med* 1996;335:609–616.
22. Thomson JR, Machado RD, Pauciulo MW, et al. Sporadic primary pulmonary hypertension is associated with germline mutations of the gene encoding BMPR-II, a receptor member of the TGF-beta family. *J Med Genet* 2000;37:741–745.
23. Grunig E, Janssen B, Mereles D, et al. Abnormal pulmonary artery pressure response in asymptomatic carriers of primary pulmonary hypertension gene. *Circulation* 2000;102:1145–1150.
24. Ewert R, Wensel R, Opitz C, et al. , for the Pulmonary Hypertension Group. Prognosis in patients with primary pulmonary hypertension awaiting lung transplantation. *Transplant Proc* 2001;33:3574–3575.
25. Miyamoto S, Nagaya N, Satoh T, et al. Clinical correlation and prognostic significance of the six minute walk test in patients with primary pulmonary hypertension. *Am J Respir Crit Care Med* 2000;161:487–492.
26. Shapiro SM, Oudiz R, Cao T, et al. Primary pulmonary hypertension: improved long-term effects and survival with continuous intravenous epoprostenol infusion. *J Am Coll Cardiol* 1997;30:343–349.
27. Higenbottam T, Butt AYK, McMahon A, et al. Long

term intravenous prostacyclin (epoprostenol or iloprost) for treatment of severe pulmonary hypertension. *Heart* 1998;80:151–155.

28. Bailey CL, Channick RN, Auger WR, et al. "High probability" perfusion lung scans in pulmonary venoocclusive disease. *Am J Respir Crit Care Med* 2000;162:1974–1978.

29. Ricciardi MJ, Knight BP, Martinez FJ, et al. Inhaled nitric oxide in primary pulmonary hypertension: a safe and effective agent for predicting response to nifedipine. *J Am Coll Cardiol* 1998;32:1068–1073.

30. Ricciardi MJ, Bossone E, Bach DS, et al. Echocardiographic predictors of an adverse response to a nifedipine trial in primary pulmonary hypertension: diminished left ventricular size and leftward ventricular septal bowing. *Chest* 1999;116:1218–1223.

31. Ricciardi MJ, Knight BP, Rubenfire M. Safety and efficacy of nitric oxide and adenosine in predicting nifedipine response in primary pulmonary hypertension. *J Am Coll Cardiol* 1997;29:58A.

32. Rubin LJ. Primary pulmonary hypertension. ACCP consensus report. *Chest* 1993;104:236–250.

33. Rich S, Kaufmann E, Levy PS. The effect of high doses of calcium-channel blockers on survival in primary pulmonary hypertension. *N Engl J Med* 1992;327:76–81.

34. Channick RN, Simonneau G, Sitbon O, et al. Effects of the dual endothelin-receptor antagonist bosentan in patients with pulmonary hypertension: a randomised placebo controlled study. *Lancet* 2001;358:1119–1123.

35. Rubin LJ, Badesch DB, Barst RJ, et al. Bosentan therapy for pulmonary artery hypertension. *N Engl J Med* 2002;346:896–903.

36. Giaid A, Yanagisawa M, Langleben D, et al. Expression of endothelin-1 in the lungs of patients with pulmonary hypertension. *N Engl J Med* 1993;328:1732–1739.

37. Barst RJ, Rubin LJ, Long WA, et al. A comparison of continuous intravenous epoprostenol (prostacyclin) with conventional therapy for primary pulmonary hypertension. *N Engl J Med* 1996;334:296–301.

38. Plotkin JS, Kuo PC, Rubin LJ, et al. Successful use of chronic epoprostenol as a bridge to liver transplantation in severe portopulmonary hypertension. *Transplantation* 1998;65:457–459.

39. Badesch DB, Tapson VF, McGoon MD, et al. Continuous intravenous epoprostenol for pulmonary hypertension due to the scleroderma spectrum of disease. A randomized, controlled trial. *Ann Intern Med* 2000;132:425–434.

40. McLaughlin VV, Genthner DE, Panella MM, et al. Compassionate use of continuous prostacyclin in the management of secondary pulmonary hypertension. A case series. *Ann Intern Med* 1999;130:740–743.

41. McLaughlin VV, Genthner DE, Panella MM, et al. Reduction in pulmonary vascular resistance with long-term epoprostenol (prostacyclin) therapy in pulmonary hypertension. *N Engl J Med* 1998;338:273–277.

42. Simmoneau G, Barst RJ, Galie N, et al. Continuous subcutaneous infusion of treprostinil, a prostacyclin analogue, in patients with pulmonary arterial hypertension. *Am J Respir Crit Care Med* 2002;165:800–804.

43. Bailey CL, Channick RN, Rubin LJ. A new era in the treatment of primary pulmonary hypertension. *Heart* 2001;85:251–252.

44. Hoeper MM, Schwarze M, Ehlerding S, et al. Long-term treatment of primary pulmonary hypertension with aerosolized iloprost, a prostacyclin analogue. *N Engl J Med* 2000;342:1866–1870.

45. Nagaya N, Uematsu M, Okano Y, et al. Effect of orally active prostacyclin analogue on survival of outpatients with primary pulmonary hypertension. *J Am Coll Cardiol* 1999;34:1188–1192.

46. Wilkens H, Guth A, Konig J, et al. Effect of inhaled iloprost plus oral sildenafil in patients with primary pulmonary hypertension. *Circulation* 2001;104:1218–1222.

47. Nagaya N, Uematsu M, Oya H, et al. Short-term oral administration of L-arginine improves hemodynamics and exercise capacity in patients with precapillary pulmonary hypertension. *Am J Respir Crit Care Med* 2001;163:887–891.

48. Sandoval J, Gasper J, Pulido T, et al. Graded balloon dilation atrial septostomy in severe pulmonary hypertension. *J Am Coll Cardiol* 1998;32:297–304.

49. Moscucci M, Dairywala IT, Chetcuti S, et al. Balloon atrial septostomy in end-stage pulmonary hypertension guided by a novel intracardiac echocardiographic transducer. *Catheter Cardiovasc Interv* 2001;52:530–534.

50. Pielsticker EJ, Martinez FJ, Rubenfire M. Lung and heart-lung transplant practice patterns in pulmonary hypertension centers. *J Heart Lung Transplant* 2001;20:1297–1304.

51. Maurer JR, Frost AE, Estenne M, et al. International guidelines for the selection of lung transplant candidates. *Heart Lung* 1998;27:223–229.

52. Zielinski J, Tobiasz M, Hawrylkiewicz I, et al. Effects of long term oxygen on pulmonary hemodynamics in COPD patients: a 6-year prospective study. *Chest* 1998;113:65–70.

53. Packer M, Medina N, Yushak M. Adverse hemodynamic and clinical effects of calcium channel blockade in pulmonary hypertension secondary to obliterative pulmonary vascular disease. *J Am Coll Cardiol* 1984;4:890–895.

54. Melot C, Hallemans R, Naeije R, et al. Deleterious effect of nifedipine on pulmonary gas exchange in chronic obstructive pulmonary disease. *Am Rev Respir Dis* 1984;130:612–618.

55. Rich S, Seidlitz M, Dodin E, et al. The short-term effects of digoxin in patients with right ventricular dysfunction from pulmonary hypertension. *Chest* 1998;114:787–792.

56. Mathur PN, Powles ACP, Pugsley SO, et al. Effect of digoxin on right ventricular function in severe chronic airflow obstruction: a controlled clinical trial. *Ann Intern Med* 1981;95:283–288.

57. Cohen M, Edwards WD, Fuster V. Regression in thromboembolic type of primary pulmonary hypertension during 2.5 years of antithrombotic therapy. *J Am Coll Cardiol* 1986;7:172–175.

58. Frank H, Mlczoch J, Huber K, et al. The effect of anticoagulant therapy in primary and anorectic drug-induced pulmonary hypertension. *Chest* 1997;112:714–721.

36

Congenital Heart Disease in Adults

Julie A. Kovach, Albert P. Rocchini, and Edward L. Bove

More than 1 million adults in the United States currently have congenital heart disease. Many have undergone surgery for repair or palliation of their heart defects and are cared for in their communities (1). Because of advances in surgical and medical care over the past several decades, an additional 20,000 patients per year with congenital heart disease reach adulthood. This chapter reviews the clinical characteristics of five of the most common cardiac lesions with expected survival to adulthood: atrial septal defect, ventricular septal defect, coarctation of the aorta, patent ductus arteriosus, and tetralogy of Fallot.

ATRIAL SEPTAL DEFECT

Atrial septal defects (ASDs) are the most common of the congenital cardiac defects first diagnosed in adulthood, totaling approximately 30% of cases of congenital heart disease diagnosed in adults. Ostium secundum ASDs, which are defects in the region of the fossa ovalis, are most frequent and represent 75% of all ASDs. The ostium primum defect, which is absence of the lower part of the interatrial septum at the crux, occurs in 15% of patients, is typically associated with a cleft mitral valve, and is most often diagnosed in childhood. Sinus venosus defects, 10% of all ASDs, usually occur in the interatrial septum just inferior to the orifice of the superior vena cava and are associated with anomalous drainage of a pulmonary vein or veins from the right lung. In rare cases, the sinus venosus defect is of the inferior vena cava type visible below the fossa ovalis and immediately superior to the orifice of the inferior vena cava. Even more rare is the coronary sinus defect, which results from absence of part of the roof of the coronary sinus with left-to-right shunting (Fig. 36.1). Infrequently,

ASD may present as part of a genetic disorder, such as Holt-Oram syndrome, also known as "heart-hand" syndrome, which is characterized by ASD, usually secundum in type, and distinctive abnormalities of the bones of the forearms, hands, and upper limbs. In regions of the world with high prevalence of rheumatic fever, affected patients may present with both secundum ASD and rheumatic mitral stenosis, the combination of which is the Lutembacher complex. In these individuals, the severity of the mitral stenosis may be underestimated because of the coexisting left-to-right shunt.

A patent foramen ovale is defined as a persistent flaplike opening between the atrial septum primum and secundum at the region of the fossa ovalis, caused by incomplete sealing off after birth. Patent foramen ovale is present in up to 25% adults, is not due to embryologic absence of septal tissue, and should not be confused with the ASD. The patent foramen ovale may become significant if paradoxical embolization occurs through the opening.

Presenting Symptoms and Signs

The physiologic hallmark of ASD is shunting of blood from the left atrium to the right atrium during late systole and early diastole. If significant, shunting produces volume overload of the right ventricle in diastole and increased flow through the pulmonary vascular bed. The magnitude of left-to-right shunting depends not only on the size of the defect but also on the relative stiffness of the left versus the right ventricles and the proportional resistances of the pulmonary and the systemic vasculature. In an aging adult with decreased ventricular compliance due to systemic hypertension or increased left ventricular

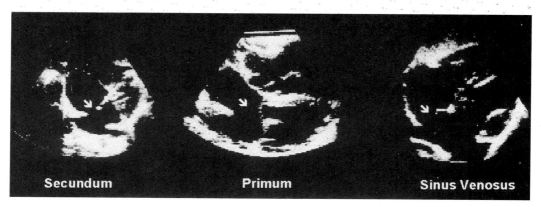

FIG. 36.1. Subcostal echocardiographic views of ostium secundum, ostium primum, and sinus venosus atrial septal defect. The defect is noted by the *arrow.*

diastolic pressure from cardiomyopathy or ischemia, a previously small left-to-right shunt may increase in size and cause new symptoms. In the patient with a very large ASD, fixed pulmonary hypertension (Eisenmenger's physiology) may supervene, and the shunt may reverse, becoming bidirectional or predominantly right to left. Most patients with ASD are asymptomatic until the third or fourth decade of life, unless the defect is quite large. Dyspnea on exertion manifests in 30% of patients by the third decade and in 75% by the fifth decade of life. Effort intolerance and fatigue are common. By 40 years of age, the patient frequently experiences palpitations from atrial fibrillation or flutter; less frequently, sick sinus syndrome may be present in patients with sinus venosus defects. Symptoms of systemic venous congestion and right-sided heart failure (e.g., edema, ascites) may occur in 10% of affected 40-year-olds. The patient with ostium primum ASD may present with fatigue due to bradycardia from complete atrioventricular block. Symptoms of pulmonary congestion from uncorrected mitral regurgitation may be prominent in these patients. In rare cases, the adult with a small ASD may suffer a cerebrovascular event or peripheral emboli as a result of paradoxical embolization through the defect. Finally, the adult with Eisenmenger's syndrome may be cyanotic at rest or develop cyanosis with exertion.

In the patient with a large left-to-right shunt, the jugular veins may be distended with "left atri-alization" of the pressure waveform (a wave = V wave). A dynamic right ventricular impulse may be palpated at the left sternal border, and a prominent pulmonary artery pulsation may be noted at the upper left sternal margin. The first heart sound is normal. The second heart sound is, as a rule, widely split with loss of respiratory variation. Respiratory changes in systemic venous return to the right atrium are offset by reciprocal changes in the volume of the left-to-right shunt, thus ameliorating the respiratory changes in stroke volumes of the right and left ventricles that cause physiologic splitting (2). If there is pulmonary hypertension, the pulmonic component of S2 may be loud and even palpable in the second left intercostal space. Because of increased pulmonary flow, a pulmonic systolic ejection murmur is present and often incorrectly assumed to represent an "innocent" murmur. Although common in children, a tricuspid diastolic flow rumble is rarely appreciated in adults. No murmur is produced by flow directly across the ASD because the interatrial pressure difference is small and velocity of flow is low (Table 36.1).

Helpful Tests

On electrocardiogram (ECG), most affected adults display normal sinus rhythm. In one study of adults with a first diagnosis of ASD, atrial fibrillation or flutter was found in 8%, complete

TABLE 36.1. *Clinical symptoms, signs, and evaluation of the adult with congenital heart disease*

	ASD	VSD	Coarctation of the aorta	PDA	TOF
Common presenting symptoms	Dyspnea Fatigue Atrial fibrillation	Asymptomatic murmur Cyanosis if Eisenmenger's syndrome present	Hypertension	Asymptomatic murmur	Uncorrected: dyspnea and cyanosis Corrected: dyspnea
Characteristic physical examination finding	Fixed split S2	Holosystolic murmur	Blood pressure differential between upper and lower extremities	Continuous murmur Differential cyanosis if Eisenmenger's syndrome present	Uncorrected: single P2 pulmonic flow murmur Corrected: murmurs of pulmonic insufficiency, VSD, aortic insufficiency
ECG findings	Secundum ASD: IRBBB with RAD Primum ASD: IRBBB with LAD	RAD, RVH if Eisenmenger's syndrome present	LVH	Normal RVH if Eisenmenger's syndrome present	Uncorrected: RVH Corrected: RBBB with wide QRS
Chest radiograph findings	Cardiomegaly with shunt vascularity	Cardiomegaly with shunt vascularity	"3" sign Rib notching	Normal	Uncorrected: RVH with decreased pulmonary vessels Corrected: depends on sequelae of operation
Other helpful tests	Echocardiography, cardiac catheterization	Echocardiography, cardiac catheterization	MRI or spiral CT	Echocardiography	Echocardiography, cardiac catheterization

ASD, atrial septal defect; CT, computed tomographic scanning; ECG, electrocardiographic; IRBBB, incomplete right bundle branch block; LAD, left axis deviation; LVH, left ventricular hypertrophy; MRI, magnetic resonance imaging; PDA, patent ductus arteriosus; RAD, right axis deviation; RBBB, right bundle branch block; RVH, right ventricular hypertrophy; TOF, tetralogy of Fallot; VSD, ventricular septal defect.

heart block (presumably in patients with ostium primum ASD) in 1%, and complete right bundle branch block in 8% (3). A junctional or low atrial rhythm with inverted P waves in the inferior leads may be present in patients with sinus venosus ASD that is caused by disruption of the sinus node. Classically, the ECG shows an incomplete right bundle branch block with right axis deviation in secundum ASD and left axis deviation in primum ASD. Patients with Eisenmenger's physiology may manifest right atrial and/or right ventricular hypertrophy with widening of the QRS interval (Fig. 36.2). On chest radiograph, more than 80% of affected adults older than 40 years display moderate to severe cardiomegaly, especially of the right atrium and ventricle. The proximal pulmonary arteries may be prominent. More than 30% of affected patients demonstrate "shunt vascularity," with prominent small pulmonary arteries in the periphery of the lung fields (Fig. 36.3). The peripheral pulmonary arteries may be diminutive with "pruning" if fixed pulmonary vascular obstruction exists (4).

Echocardiography is the most practical and cost-effective technique for the demonstration and characterization of the anatomy and physiologic consequences of most types of ASD. Transthoracic echocardiography may demonstrate right atrial and ventricular enlargement and paradoxical septal motion consistent with volume overload of the right ventricle, and it is helpful for assessing right and left ventricular function (Fig. 36.4). The ostium primum ASD is particularly well seen on transthoracic echocardiography. "Echo dropout" of the midportion of the interatrial septum on two-dimensional echocardiography characterizes the secundum ASD, but this finding may represent a

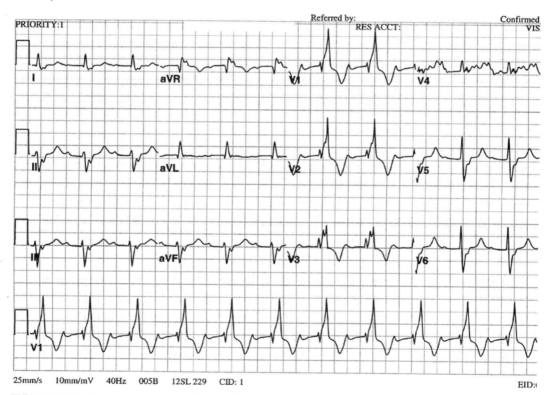

FIG. 36.2. Electrocardiogram of patient with very large secundum atrial septal defect, which demonstrates normal sinus rhythm with first-degree atrioventricular conduction delay, right bundle branch block with right ventricular enlargement, and left axis deviation.

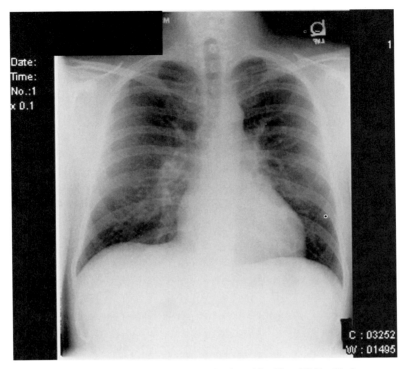

FIG. 36.3. Chest radiograph of the same patient depicted in Fig. 36.2 with large secundum atrial septal defect, which demonstrates right ventricular enlargement and prominent peripheral pulmonary arteries, consistent with "shunt vascularity."

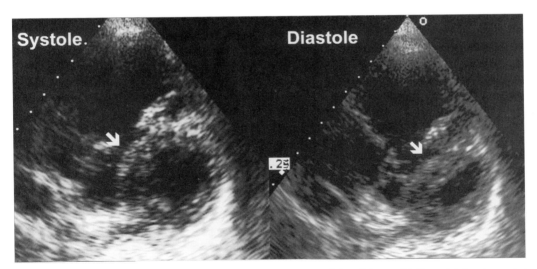

FIG. 36.4. Parasternal short-axis echocardiographic views of the right and left ventricles in systole and diastole, showing the septal motion typical of right ventricular volume overload in large ASD. The right ventricle is markedly dilated. In systole, the interventricular septum is normally positioned, and the left ventricle is round, which suggests that the left ventricular pressure exceeds the right ventricular pressure in systole. In diastole, the interventricular septum is bowed into the left ventricle consistent with elevated right ventricular diastolic pressure.

false-positive sign that is due to the relative "thinness" of the fossa ovalis in comparison to the surrounding septal tissue, especially in the four-chamber view. Color and spectral Doppler echocardiography may demonstrate flow across the defect, especially in the subcostal view, in which ASD flow is parallel to the ultrasound beam. In some patients, the secundum ASD may be visualized only after intravenous injection of agitated saline microbubbles, which are seen passing from the right atrium into the left atrium. Conversely, a "negative contrast effect," or clear space in the bubble-filled right atrium, may be seen when unopacified blood shunts from left to right across the defect. Transesophageal echocardiography more clearly reveals the defect

at the fossa ovalis in secundum defect and is superior to transthoracic echocardiography for the diagnosis of sinus venosus defects in adults (Fig. 36.5) (5,6). In addition, Doppler echocardiography demonstrates the direction of shunting, allows quantitation of the left-to-right shunt, and permits estimation of the right ventricular systolic pressure. Phase-contrast cine magnetic resonance imaging and cine computed tomography can accurately depict the morphologic features of all types of ASD and are not as invasive as transesophageal echocardiography, but they are more expensive and are not available in most practice settings (7).

Cardiac catheterization is recommended in most adults older than 40 years for

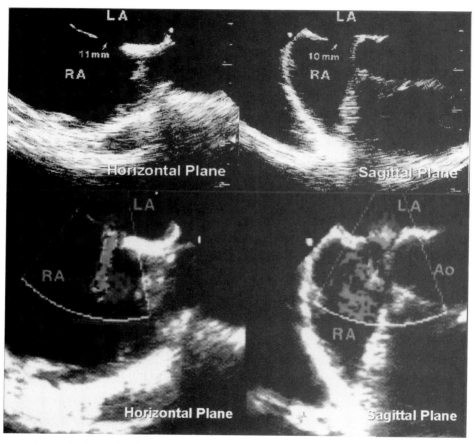

FIG. 36.5. Transesophageal echocardiography of secundum atrial septal defect in the horizontal and sagittal planes. On color Doppler echocardiography, a left-to-right shunt was demonstrated.

characterization of coronary artery anatomy, and it is required in younger adults if fixed pulmonary vascular obstruction is suspected. In these patients, reversibility of pulmonary vascular disease should be evaluated at the time of catheterization with the use of appropriate pulmonary vasodilators, because this may influence the decision for repair.

Differential Diagnosis

ASD should be suspected in all adults who present with effort intolerance, dyspnea, or palpitations, especially those with right-sided heart enlargement on chest radiograph, echocardiography, or ECG or with typical physical examination findings such as a fixed, widely split second heart sound. In the differential diagnosis, the physician might consider other causes of right-sided heart enlargement, including primary tricuspid or pulmonic valve disease, arrhythmogenic right ventricular dysplasia, primary pulmonary hypertension, and other intracardiac and extracardiac shunts. Transthoracic echocardiography with intravenous saline contrast should be performed with careful attention to the superior interatrial septum to assess for unexpected sinus venosus defects. If an explanation for the right-sided heart enlargement is not found on surface echocardiography, transesophageal echocardiography should be performed. If sinus venosus ASD is detected, the drainage of the pulmonary veins should be carefully sought.

Complications

Most patients with unrepaired ASD survive to adulthood, but life expectancy is not normal, although not as dire as was estimated in early natural history studies. The mortality rate has been estimated at 6% per year after 40 years of age (8). In general, young women with ASD who become pregnant successfully deliver healthy infants without maternal or fetal complications, provided that pulmonary hypertension is not present. However, supraventricular arrhythmias occur more commonly during pregnancy and can complicate the care of these patients (9). Atrial arrhythmias, especially atrial fibrillation,

are common in these adults, occurring in 10% of 40 year olds with unrepaired ASD, and increase the risk of paradoxical embolization. Operation, especially when performed in patients older than 40, may not prevent the later development of atrial fibrillation, perhaps because of scar formation at the atrial incision site (10). In one study, moderate pulmonary hypertension (systolic pulmonary artery pressure, 40 to 60 mm HG) developed in 26% of patients. Severe pulmonary hypertension (pulmonary systolic pressure, higher than 60 mm HG) develops only rarely and was present in only 7% of adults, although it may manifest at a very young age even in patients with small defects (11). In these patients, it is possible that unrelated pulmonary vascular disease (e.g., primary pulmonary hypertension) may coexist with the ASD or may be triggered by relatively small increases in pulmonary blood flow. Interestingly, development of pulmonary hypertension may occur more frequently in patients with sinus venosus ASD than in those with ostium secundum ASD (26% vs. 9%, respectively) (12). In infants with large ASD, the tendency for recurrent upper and lower respiratory tract infections is well documented. Although it is less well documented in adults, one study of medical management versus surgical closure of ASD in adults suggested that recurrent pulmonary infections were more common in the group whose ASD was not closed (13). In older patients with significant unrepaired ASD (left-to-right shunt blood flow ratio at least 1.5:1), right-sided heart failure may develop with peripheral edema and even ascites. Endocarditis is uncommon in patients with secundum ASD but is more common in patients with primum ASD and cleft mitral valve (Table 36.2).

Therapy

Regardless of the patient's age, closure of the secundum ASD improves symptoms and exercise tolerance and prevents the later development of congestive heart failure in symptomatic patients with a pulmonary-to-systemic blood flow ratio (Qp/Qs) of 1.5:1 or higher. Closure of the defect prolongs survival if performed before the age of 40 (10,11,14,15). ASD closure at an

TABLE 36.2. *Treatment, complications, and follow-up of adults with congenital heart disease*

Condition	Recommendations for repair	Common complications	Follow-up	Endocarditis prophylaxis
ASD	All primum ASD and sinus venosus if symptomatic and Qp/Qs $\geq$ 1.5:1 *or* Secundum ASD if asymptomatic with big RV	CHF Atrial fibrillation	Every 2–5 years after repair	No for secundum ASD and sinus venosus Yes before and after repair for primum ASD
VSD	Qp/Qs $\geq$ 1.5:1 and symptoms Qp/Qs $\geq$ 2.0:1 without symptoms	CHF Endocarditis Eisenmenger's syndrome	Every 2–5 years after repair	Yes before repair No 6 months after repair
Coarctation of the aorta	Upper extremity hypertension and gradient $\geq$ 20 mm HG	Stroke Aortic aneurysm Aortic valve disease Endocarditis and endarteritis	Yearly with MRI or CT of aorta every 2–5 years	Yes
PDA	Audible murmur	Rare Eisenmenger's syndrome Rare endarteritis	Periodically	Yes if audible No 6 months after closure
TOF	All affect adults without Eisenmenger's syndrome who have not previously undergone repair As needed for sequelae of operation	Pulmonary insufficiency RV failure Atrial and ventricular dysrhythmias	Yearly	Yes

ASD, atrial septal defect; CHF, congestive heart failure; CT, computed tomography; MRI, magnetic resonance imaging; PDA, patent ductus arterious; Qp/Qs, ratio of pulmonary blood flow to systemic blood flow; RV, right ventricle; TOF, tetralogy of Fallot; VSD, ventricular septal defect.

earlier age may prevent later occurrence of atrial fibrillation to some degree. However, atrial fibrillation is still frequent after repair and is associated with late stroke (10). Whether simultaneous performance of the Maze procedure for atrial fibrillation in the older patient with ASD prevents later arrhythmias is unknown. ASD closure is also recommended for asymptomatic patients younger than 40 years with a Qp/Qs of 1.5:1 or higher if right-sided heart enlargement is present, primarily for the prevention of right-sided heart failure. Closure of ASDs in asymptomatic older adults is more controversial. In one large study, 521 patients older than 40 years with secundum ASD were randomly assigned to undergo surgical closure or receive medical therapy and were monitored for more than 7 years (15). The risk of the combined end point (death, pulmonary embolism, major arrhythmic event, cerebrovascu-

lar embolic event, recurrent pulmonary infection, functional class deterioration, or development of heart failure) was higher in the medically managed group than in the surgical group (hazard ratio of 1.99, $p < 0.01$). Although there was no difference in mortality rate between medical and surgical groups during this period of follow-up, the authors propose surgical closure in all patients older than 40 with secundum ASD with a Qp/Qs of 1.7:1 or higher who do not have fixed pulmonary hypertension. Some patients with small secundum ASD and a history of paradoxical embolization may benefit from closure.

Indications for closure of sinus venosus and ostium primum ASD are less well defined. The higher incidence of mitral valve abnormalities in patients with ostium primum ASD and the higher risk of the development of pulmonary hypertension in patients with sinus venosus ASD suggest that most of these defects should be closed.

All studies of long-term outcomes after ASD repair have involved patients who underwent surgical closure through the standard surgical approach. Excellent short- and intermediate-term outcomes of percutaneous closure of ASDs with various devices have been reported (16–18). There are currently two transcatheter atrial septal devices that have been improved for clinical use in the United States (the CardioSEAL device, NMT Corporation, Boston, Massachusetts, and the AMPLATZER Septal Occluder, AGA Medical Corporation, Golden Valley, Minnesota). The CardioSEAL device is approved for closing the patent foramen ovale in individuals who have documented cerebral vascular accidents or other proven embolic events that are refractory to medical therapy, and the AMPLATZER Septal Occluder is approved for the closure of secundum ASD.

Individuals must have a secundum ASD or patent foramen ovale to be a candidate for device closure. Neither sinus venosus or primum ASDs can be closed with any of these devices. Patients with defects with circumferential septal rims are the best candidates for closure. A patient is considered a candidate for device closure if the diameter of the ASD is less than 28 to 30 mm by transthoracic echocardiogram and if the diameter is less than 34 mm when stretched by a balloon catheter at the time of catheterization. In addition, the ASD must have a rim that is more than 4 mm away from all other cardiac structures, including the superior and inferior vena cavae, pulmonary veins, and the atrioventricular valves. Defects with multiple fenestrations can occasionally be closed with a single device, but multiple widely spaced defects are more difficult, and sometimes impossible, to close.

There have been a number of articles that established the safety and efficacy of the AMPLATZER device. One study reviewed the records of 89 patients who underwent either surgical closure ($n = 44$) or AMPLATZER device closure ($n = 45$) of an ASD performed between March 1998 and May 2000 (19). These investigators demonstrated that transcatheter closure with the AMPLATZER Septal Occluder carries the advantages of fewer complications, avoidance of cardioplegia and cardiopulmonary bypass, shorter hospitalization, reduced need for blood products, and less patient discomfort. However, as with any other comparison between a surgical procedure and a transcatheter intervention, these authors acknowledged that the surgeon's ability to close any ASD regardless of anatomy remains an important advantage of surgery. Similar results were reported in a multicenter nonrandomized study (20).

The experience from 13 European centers using the CardioSEAL double-umbrella devices to close interatrial communications in 334 patients has been reviewed (21). The investigators concluded that this device produced excellent results when used to close defects of small to moderate size. However, results are less optimal and complications occurred when attempts were made to close very large defects. In summary, the AMPLATZER Septal Occluder and the CardioSEAL umbrella work equally well for closing small to medium-sized defects (less than 20-mm stretched diameter); however, for defects larger than 20 mm, the AMPLATZER Septal Occluder had a significantly better closure rate and a lower incidence of complications.

Percutaneous closure of ASDs eliminates scarring at the atrial suture line from surgery and, theoretically, may prevent atrial arrhythmias if performed at an early age. Also, minimally invasive, direct-access surgical techniques for ASD closure have been reported with no operative or late mortality and rare complications (22). Percutaneous treatment or minimally invasive surgery may be feasible for ASD closure in many patients.

Bacterial endocarditis prophylaxis is not necessary for the preoperative patient with secundum or sinus venosus ASD. Six months after secundum or venosus ASD repair, endocarditis prophylaxis may be discontinued. Prophylaxis should be given to all patients with primum ASD before and after surgery.

Prognosis and Follow-up

In all adults with congenital heart disease, the physician must consider the complications of the lesion that has not been repaired (the natural history of the unrepaired defect), potential residua of incomplete repair, and sequelae of the operation. Patients with ASD who have undergone surgical closure in childhood, with either primary suture or patch closure, do well. El-Najdawi et al described long-term outcomes in 334 patients who underwent repair of primum ASD (partial atrioventricular septal defect) with or without mitral valve repair (23). Ten-, 20-, and 40-year survival rates were 93%, 87%, and 76%, respectively. Reoperation was required in 11% of patients, usually for mitral valve regurgitation or stenosis. When secundum ASD is repaired in childhood, operative mortality rates are less than 2%, and long-term survival is almost normal (24). In patients undergoing operation after 40 years of age, the operative mortality rate is slightly higher (5.8%) but still considered reasonable, and cardiovascular events may be less frequent than in medically treated patients (11.1% vs. 20.7%; hazard ratio, 2.0; $p = 0.004$) (15). Late atrial fibrillation is common and is associated with cerebrovascular events but is perhaps less frequent in patients undergoing operation before 40 years of age (10). Therefore, patients with ASD closed either in childhood or adulthood should not be considered "cured" but should be monitored for later development of arrhythmias and given anticoagulants if necessary.

VENTRICULAR SEPTAL DEFECT

Although ventricular septal defect (VSD) is the most common congenital heart defect diagnosed in childhood, it represents the third most common congenital cardiac anomaly in adults after ASD and patent ductus arteriosus (PDA) and accounts for 10% of congenital heart disease in adults. Spontaneous closure of small VSDs before adolescence (as occurs in approximately 60% of patients) (25), patient attrition due to congestive heart failure or arrhythmias in patients with large VSD, and prior surgery are the reasons for the decreased incidence of VSD in adults. Locations of defects in the interventricular septum include perimembranous (beneath the crista supraventricularis when viewed from the right ventricle and in the outflow tract of the left ventricle be-

neath the aortic valve when viewed from the left ventricle) in 70%, muscular (either single or multiple in the muscular portion of the septum) in 20%, supracristal or subpulmonic (beneath the pulmonary valve undermining the aortic valve annulus and associated with aortic valve prolapse and insufficiency) in 5%, and inlet, or "atrioventricular canal," defects (beneath the septal leaflet of the tricuspid valve) in 5% to 8%.

Presenting Symptoms and Signs

The presentation of the adult with VSD is usually related to one of two extremes of very small or very large-sized defects, inasmuch as most moderate or larger defects are diagnosed and surgically corrected in childhood. With small or "restrictive" VSDs, first described by Henri-Louis Roger in 1879 and given the moniker "maladie de Roger," a large pressure difference exists between the left and right ventricle with a small left-to-right shunt and low pulmonary artery pressure. The affected adult patient is asymptomatic but reports that a loud murmur was detected in childhood, perhaps during a sports physical examination. In rare cases, adults may present with fever, septic emboli, and peripheral manifestations of endocarditis that result from infection of the "jet" lesion on the right ventricular free wall, most commonly after a dental procedure. The first and second heart sounds are normal. Typically, a loud, harsh Grade IV/VI holosystolic murmur is auscultated in the third or fourth intercostal space at the left sternal margin associated with a palpable thrill. The murmur of the muscular VSD is very loud and harsh but may terminate abruptly in mid- to late systole as the defect is closed by myocardial contraction during systole. In some adults with supracristal VSD, a high-pitched diastolic blowing murmur of aortic insufficiency may be heard.

By adulthood, patients with large or "nonrestrictive" VSDs invariably progress to Eisenmenger's syndrome with equilibration of right and left ventricular systolic pressures or development of suprasystemic pulmonary artery pressure with shunt reversal. Dyspnea is usually prominent, and exertional syncope is common. Occasionally, a patient may present with a cerebrovascular event caused by paradoxical embolization or brain abscess from septic embolization. The patient may have cyanosis at rest or with exercise and usually exhibits clubbing of the fingers and toes. The jugular venous pressure is elevated. A right ventricular heave may be palpated at the left sternal border, and a prominent pulmonary artery impulse may be detected with or without a palpable pulmonic component of the second heart sound. A very loud P2 and right-sided S4 or S3 or both are common. Because shunting across the VSD is now minimal, the typical VSD murmur is absent. A holosystolic murmur of tricuspid regurgitation or a diastolic blowing murmur of pulmonary insufficiency that is augmented with inspiration may be heard.

Occasionally, a moderate-sized VSD is first recognized in adults. In these patients, with defects usually less than half the size of the aortic orifice and a Qp/Qs of 2:1 or higher, symptoms include dyspnea, effort intolerance, and fatigue. If there is a history of a very loud murmur that has diminished or disappeared over the years, development of Eisenmenger's physiology should be suspected. If aortic insufficiency has progressed, the diastolic murmur may be loudest and physical findings of left-sided heart failure may be prominent with a displaced left ventricular impulse and a left-sided S3. In these patients, the holosystolic murmur of the VSD is generally softer than in patients with small VSDs. If aortic insufficiency accompanies the VSD, the combined pansystolic and diastolic murmurs may be interpreted as a continuous murmur.

Helpful Tests

In patients with restrictive VSD, the ECG and chest radiograph are normal. The ECG is generally normal in the patient with moderate-sized VSDs, although it may reveal right axis deviation. The chest radiograph in these patients may show cardiomegaly with enlarged left atrium and left ventricle (from the increased flow that returns from the lungs to the left side of the heart) and prominent central pulmonary arteries with "shunt vascularity." In the patient with shunt reversal due to Eisenmenger's physiology, the ECG shows prominent right axis shift with right atrial and right ventricular hypertrophy and possible right ventricular "strain" repolarization abnormality with QRS widening. Frequently, premature ventricular contractions are captured on routine ECG or ambulatory ECG monitoring. On chest radiograph, right-sided heart enlargement is notable with dilated, sometimes calcified central pulmonary arteries and tapering or "pruning" of the pulmonary vessels in the periphery. On transthoracic color and spectral Doppler echocardiography, the hallmark of VSD is usually high-velocity flow from the left ventricle to the right ventricle at the site of the defect in the interventricular septum (Fig. 36.6). In some patients, a ventricular septal aneurysm forms as a result of partial or complete closure of a perimembranous

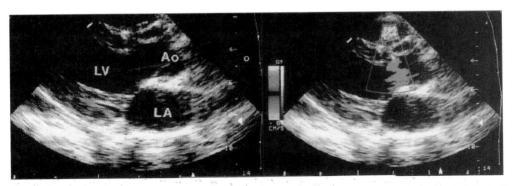

FIG. 36.6. Transthoracic echocardiogram of a small perimembranous ventricular septal defect. Turbulence in the right ventricle, seen at the site of the defect on the color Doppler echocardiogram, resulted from the high-velocity left-to-right shunt.

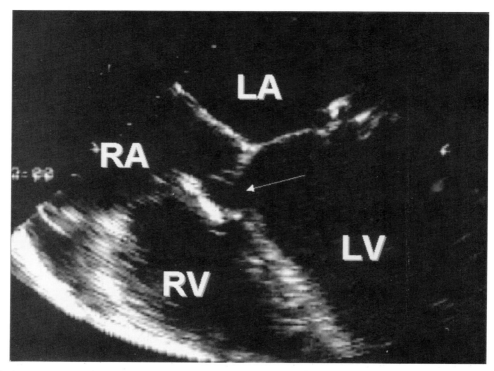

FIG. 36.7. Transesophageal echocardiogram of a ventricular septal aneurysm formed when the septal leaflet of the tricuspid valve became adherent to the perimembranous ventricular septal defect. No left-to-right shunt was visible on the color Doppler echocardiogram.

VSD by portions of the septal leaflet of the tricuspid valve (Fig. 36.7). The sonographer must carefully interrogate all regions of the septum from multiple views with color and spectral Doppler imaging in order not to miss small defects. Nevertheless, very small muscular VSDs with characteristic murmurs, especially if multiple, may not be visualized on transthoracic or even the more sensitive transesophageal echocardiogram. Intravenous injection of agitated saline microbubbles is not usually helpful in the diagnosis of small VSD, because the shunt is left to right. Adults with very large VSD and Eisenmenger's physiology may have no shunt whatsoever or a small right-to-left shunt demonstrated by color or spectral Doppler imaging at the defect site. Echocardiography is also instrumental for the evaluation of additional cardiac lesions, including aortic valve prolapse and insufficiency and subpulmonic obstruction, which may develop in late adolescence or adulthood as

a result of hypertrophy of the crista supraventricularis. Cine magnetic resonance imaging and computed tomography may elegantly display all types of VSD but are not generally available.

In adults in whom closure of a moderate-sized VSD is under consideration, right- and left-sided heart catheterization may be necessary. Knowledge of pulmonary artery pressure and pulmonary vascular resistance is mandatory for making the decision for or against closure. In individuals with pulmonary arteriolar resistance that is two-thirds the systemic arteriolar resistance or more, lack of pulmonary vascular reactivity in response to pulmonary vasodilators such as oxygen or nitric oxide at the time of cardiac catheterization is predictive of high operative mortality risk. In rare cases, patients require open-lung biopsy to examine the pulmonary vessels for evidence of irreversible pulmonary vascular obstruction.

Differential Diagnosis

In the patient with restrictive VSD, the differential diagnosis includes other lesions that may produce a holosystolic murmur. Although the murmurs of mitral and tricuspid regurgitation are pansystolic, their locations (cardiac apex or lower left sternal border) and respiratory changes (augmentation of the tricuspid murmur with inspiration) help differentiate them from the murmur of VSD. Only rarely is the murmur of tricuspid or mitral regurgitation (e.g., with a flail leaflet) as harsh as that of VSD and associated with a palpable thrill. In patients with VSD and aortic insufficiency, the additive systolic and diastolic murmurs may be confused with the continuous murmur of the patent duct, ruptured sinus of Valsalva aneurysm, coronary artery fistula, or systemic–to–pulmonary artery collateral vessels such as those that occur with pulmonary atresia.

Complications

Until the mid-1990s, bacterial endocarditis was thought to be the only significant potential complication of the restrictive VSD, with incidences of 1.9 per 1,000 patient years in unrepaired simple VSD and 3.5 per 1,000 patient years if aortic regurgitation coexisted with the VSD (26). The incidence of endocarditis after closure of the VSD decreases to 0.75 per 1,000 patient years. However, in a study of 188 adults (aged 17 to 72) with small unrepaired VSD, 26.6% of whom had additional cardiac lesions such as bicuspid aortic valve and coarctation of the aorta, complications occurred in 53% of patients (27). Of note, spontaneous closure of the VSD occurred in 19 patients (10%, all between the ages of 17 and 45; mean age, 27 years). Serious complications occurred in 46 patients (25%): infective endocarditis in 11%, progressive aortic insufficiency in 5%, and symptomatic arrhythmias, most commonly atrial fibrillation, in 8.5%. Irreversible pulmonary vascular obstruction (Eisenmenger's syndrome) inexorably develops before adulthood in the patient with a large, nonrestrictive VSD and carries the potential for complications such as endocarditis; right-sided heart failure; hemoptysis;

erythrocytosis with the attendant risks of hyperviscosity, hyperuricemia, and gout; renal insufficiency; cholelithiasis; and sudden cardiac death. Maternal and fetal mortality rates among pregnant women with Eisenmenger's syndrome exceed 50% and are higher in women with pulmonary hypertension due to VSD than with that due to ASD (28). Aortic insufficiency develops in 2% to 7% of patients with VSD over time, occurs more commonly in adults older than 20 years, and is classically associated with the supracristal or subpulmonic type of defect, although it may occur in perimembranous VSD (29). In 25% of these patients in one study, the severity of aortic insufficiency remained stable over time. Aortic insufficiency is much more common in the Asian population with subarterial VSD, developing in 64% of 139 asymptomatic patients in one study (30). The authors of this study found that aortic prolapse and insufficiency developed only in patients with a VSD diameter larger than 5 mm and recommended closure in these patients.

Therapy

Currently, the only recommended therapy for patients with restrictive VSD is bacterial endocarditis prophylaxis for dental and other procedures. With future advances in the technique of percutaneous closure of VSDs, it is possible that the risk accompanying the procedure will one day be lower than the risk of complications in these patients and closure may eventually be recommended.

Surgical closure is recommended for adults with a Qp/Qs of 1.5:1 or higher with symptoms, evidence of left ventricular enlargement or dysfunction, and pulmonary hypertension that is not severe. If pulmonary vascular resistance is normal, closure of defects with a Qp/Qs of 2:1 or higher in the asymptomatic patient is probably warranted to prevent the progression to pulmonary hypertension, because the risk of death is four times higher in these patients (31). Patients with severe pulmonary hypertension (pulmonary-to-systemic vascular resistance ratio higher than 2:3) who have a net left-to-right shunt flow ratio of 1.5 or higher may safely undergo repair only if reversibility of pulmonary resistance can be demonstrated at catheterization or by lack of permanent vascular obstruction on lung biopsy. Because aortic insufficiency is progressive in patients with supracristal VSD, closure seems warranted if insufficiency is more than mild or is shown on serial echocardiography to be progressive. A history of endocarditis, especially if recurrent, may also be an indication for closure.

Studies of percutaneous transcatheter closure of VSDs have, to this time, included a limited number of patients with fairly brief follow-up (32,33). Device deployment is currently limited to muscular VSD and was successful in approximately 85% of patients, with a residual shunt present in 30%. Major complications or death occurred in 4 of 55 patients in the two studies. Thus, this procedure should be considered experimental. As with ASDs, a minimally invasive surgical approach to closure of VSD is used at some centers (34).

Patients with fixed pulmonary vascular obstruction have a very high mortality rate with repair and should not undergo operation. At this time, there is no curative therapy for patients with Eisenmenger's syndrome. Pregnancy should be strongly discouraged and sterilization of the patient or, preferably, the sexual partner offered, because even minor noncardiac surgery conveys significant risk in these patients. Pregnancy termination may be considered for certain patients. Continuous intravenous prostacyclin may improve hemodynamics and quality of life in symptomatic patients with pulmonary hypertension and congenital heart disease (35). In 20 such patients on chronic prostacyclin therapy, mean pulmonary artery pressure decreased by 21%, cardiac index improved from 3.5 ± 2.0 L/minute/m^2 to 5.9 ± 2.7 L/minute/m^2, and New York Heart Association functional class improved from 3.2 ± 0.7 to 2.0 ± 0.9 ($p < 0.0001$). Surgical treatment of patients with Eisenmenger's syndrome either with heart-lung transplantation or with single- or double-lung transplantation and concomitant intracardiac repair has been performed in a limited number of patients, with a disappointing one-year survival rate of less than 60% (36,37).

All patients with unrepaired VSD should receive endocarditis prophylaxis, although this may be discontinued 6 months after surgical closure if no associated valvular abnormalities such as aortic insufficiency are present.

Prognosis and Follow-up

As noted previously, the course of unrepaired patients with small VSD may not be as uneventful as originally thought; 25% of patients eventually experience endocarditis, progressive aortic regurgitation, left ventricular dysfunction, or atrial arrhythmias. However, there was no significant difference in survival from the normal population in the study (27). In patients with unrepaired VSD and Eisenmenger's syndrome, survival rate is 77% at 15 years of age but only 42% at 25 years of age. Death occurs suddenly in 30% of patients and is due to congestive heart failure in 25%, hemoptysis in 15%, and pregnancy, noncardiac surgery, and endocarditis in the remainder (38).

The life expectancy of patients with VSD and normal pulmonary vascular resistance repaired in childhood is nearly normal. Of 296 patients who underwent surgical closure during the early operative era of 1954 to 1961, the survival rate was 80% at a mean of 26.8 years of follow-up (39). Mortality rates were higher in patients who underwent operation after the age of 5 years, in those with elevated pulmonary vascular resistance higher than 7 Woods units, and in those with transient or permanent complete heart block. Complete heart block infrequently occurs late after VSD repair and is not less frequent after atriotomy than after a ventricular incision (40). Atrial fibrillation occurs in approximately 8% of patients after repair, and the frequency increases at older ages (27). Ventricular arrhythmias are common but generally benign; however, a higher incidence of sudden death has been reported in patients with surgically managed VSDs than in those with medically managed VSDs, presumably from ventricular arrhythmias (31).

Patients with small, nonrestrictive VSDs and those who have had VSD closure should be monitored periodically with auscultation, ECG, chest radiography, and echocardiography for potential progression of aortic insufficiency, new development of subpulmonic stenosis, deterioration of left and right ventricular function, and arrhythmias.

COARCTATION OF THE AORTA

Approximately 20% of all cases of coarctation of the aorta are diagnosed in adolescence and adulthood. In the adult, coarctation of the aorta is characterized by a narrowing of the descending thoracic aorta distal to the left subclavian artery at the site of the ligamentum arteriosum (postductal coarctation); the narrowing is composed of a discrete ridge of tissue extending into the aortic lumen (Fig. 36.8). In rare cases, the patient may have hypoplasia of the aorta proximal to the subclavian artery (preductal), which may extend distally. Coarctation is two to five times more common in boys and men than in girls and women, but it is the most common congenital cardiac anomaly in patients with the female chromosomal XO abnormality (Turner's syndrome). A bicuspid aortic valve is present in 50% to 85% of adults with coarctation. Other noncardiac

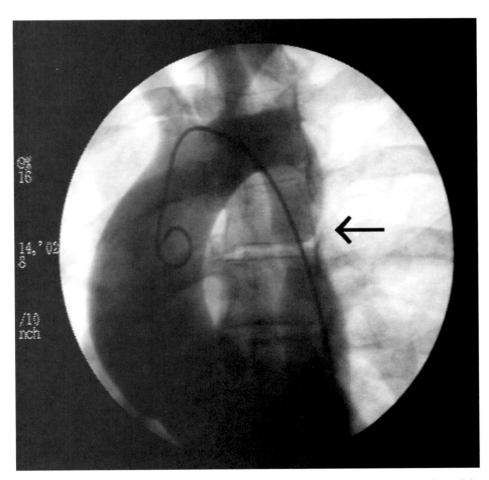

FIG. 36.8. Angiogram of the aorta from the posteroanterior projection. A discrete ridge of tissue is noted distal to the ostium of the left subclavian artery at the *arrow.*

abnormalities associated with coarctation include berry aneurysms of the circle of Willis in 10% of patients and aneurysm of the ascending aorta with or without dissection (most often in conjunction with bicuspid aortic valve).

Presenting Symptoms and Signs

Before the second or third decade of life, most adults are asymptomatic. Coarctation of the aorta is suspected when hypertension is detected on routine physical examination in the upper extremities (in patients with a discrete ridge distal to the left subclavian artery) or only in the right upper extremity (in patients with hypoplasia of the transverse portion of the arch). If hypertension is severe, the patient may experience headache, dizziness, epistaxis, or pulmonary congestion from congestive heart failure. If the coarctation is severe and collateral vessels are few, the patient may experience lower extremity fatigue or claudication. The adult with severe coarctation and few collateral vessels may also exhibit more muscularity and better development of the upper torso than of the lower body. Regrettably, the presenting symptom of untreated coarctation in the adult is too often cataclysmic, with aortic dissection or rupture, subarachnoid hemorrhage, myocardial infarction from premature coronary artery disease, or infective endocarditis or endarteritis. On physical examination, the patient usually has mild or moderate systolic hypertension in the right or both arms. The systolic pressure of the legs is diminished, although the diastolic pressures in upper and lower extremities are similar, which results in a widened pulse pressure in the arms. Femoral arterial pulses are diminished or absent, and there is a delay between the brachial and femoral pulse upstrokes when palpated simultaneously. Of note, however, is that femoral pulses may be fairly normal and the systolic pressure gradient between the arms and the legs may not be excessive if extensive collateral vessels have developed. If prestenotic dilation of the aorta is marked, a pulsatile aorta may be palpated in the suprasternal notch with a systolic thrill. On cardiac examination, the left ventricular impulse may be hyperdynamic. An ejection click from the bicuspid aortic valve can

be heard with an aortic ejection murmur or diastolic murmur if aortic stenosis or insufficiency, respectively, is present. An S4 is usually present on auscultation. A harsh, late systolic murmur from the coarctation is usually audible at the left sternal border and is loudest in the interscapular region of the back at the site of the aortic narrowing. A crescendo-decrescendo systolic murmur may be heard widely throughout the back and chest from intercostal collateral artery formation.

Helpful Tests

The ECG may be normal or display left atrial enlargement or left ventricular hypertrophy, whether hypertension is severe or not. The pathognomonic chest radiographic abnormality is the "3 sign" on the posteroanterior view: the upper limb of the "3" is caused by prestenotic dilation of the aorta or the left subclavian artery, followed by the indentation of the coarctation and poststenotic dilation of the aorta, which forms the lower limb of the "3." Resorption of bone from increased flow through intercostal arteries causes the characteristic notching of the posterior of ribs three through eight bilaterally. If the left subclavian artery arises below the coarctation, rib notching may occur only on the right side. Because the anterior intercostal arteries do not travel in the costal grooves, anterior rib notching does not occur.

The sensitivity for visualization of the coarctation site is 87% by transthoracic echocardiography from the suprasternal notch view, a view not usually part of the standard adult echocardiographic examination. Turbulence at the site of narrowing will be evident on color-flow Doppler echocardiograms. Persistent flow in the descending or abdominal aorta throughout diastole on spectral Doppler echocardiography is consistent with the diagnosis. A gradient across the coarctation may be measured by continuous-wave Doppler imaging. However, Doppler imaging may underestimate the "true" gradient across the narrowing because of the presence of collateral vessels. Finally, the status of the aortic valve, left ventricular mass and function, and ascending aorta can be ascertained by echocardiography.

Magnetic resonance angiography or spiral computed tomographic scanning are imperative for visualizing the entire aorta, to assess for aneurysm and abnormalities of branch vessels. Aortography with hemodynamic measurements of the gradient at rest and possibly with exercise, evaluation of branch vessels, and identification of collateral arteries should be performed before intervention. In most adults, coronary angiography should be performed before surgery because premature coronary artery disease is prevalent.

Differential Diagnosis

Although the differential diagnosis of hypertension in the young adult includes essential hypertension and other secondary causes of hypertension, coarctation of the aorta is suspected when differential blood pressures and pulses are detected in the upper and lower extremities. In rare cases, a coarctation of the aorta may be confused with a "pseudocoarctation" caused by tortuosity and "buckling" of the descending thoracic aorta without true narrowing or a gradient. Aortography with pressure measurements across the "coarctation" clarifies the diagnosis in these patients.

Complications

Untreated coarctation of the aorta is associated with very high mortality rate: 75% at age 50 years and 90% by age 60 (41). Before the age of 30, coarctation-related death usually results from aortic rupture, infective endocarditis of the bicuspid aortic valve or endarteritis at the coarctation site, or cerebral hemorrhage from ruptured berry aneurysm. After 30 years of age, congestive heart failure is common, and two-thirds (2/3) of affected adults older than 40 years have symptoms of heart failure (42). Hypertension with possible secondary organ system involvement is universal in older adults with untreated coarctation. Aortic dissection at the coarctation site or the noncoarcted proximal ascending aorta is common and can occur more often in women during pregnancy. Approximately 10% of patients,

whether they undergo coarctation repair or not, require later aortic valve replacement. Premature coronary artery disease may lead to myocardial infarction in affected young men in the second or third decade of life. The risk of hemorrhagic stroke persists even after repair.

Therapy

Although the absolute upper-to-lower extremity gradient considered to be "significant" is not clearly established, most authors recommend repair for all patients with coarctation of the aorta who have upper extremity hypertension and an upper-to-lower extremity gradient or directly measured gradient of at least 20 mm HG across the coarctation. In most adults, the preferred method for treatment of coarctation is either the use of balloon-expandable stents or surgical repair, because the coarctation is more fibrotic and less distensible than in children and is thus less responsive to balloon angioplasty alone. Surgical repair is associated with low mortality rate (less than 1%) and, rarely, with paraplegia from spinal cord ischemia (0.4%), a more common complication in patients with poorly developed collateral vessels (43).

Percutaneous balloon dilatation of native aortic coarctation has been performed in adults. In one study of 27 adults, the procedure was successful initially in 23 patients (44). Recoarctation is not uncommon after balloon angioplasty of native coarctation, developing in 22.8% of patients in one study (45). Late aneurysm formation has also been reported. The implementation of endovascular stent implantation for coarctation has resulted in excellent immediate and intermediate outcomes with little restenosis at 1 year and few immediate complications, which have included stent migration, aortic disruption, pseudoaneurysm of the femoral artery access site, and stroke (46,47).

Currently, surgical repair of most adults with coarctation of the aorta is recommended, except in centers with considerable experience in the use of endovascular stents for this purpose. Percutaneous balloon angioplasty alone does not result in good long-term outcomes in most adults. Endocarditis prophylaxis is required for all adults with coarctation of the aorta before and after repair.

Prognosis and Follow-up

Survival after surgical repair of aortic coarctation is influenced by the presence or absence of recoarctation or aneurysm formation at the repair site. Late survival also depends on associated lesions, including aortic valve disease, aneurysm of the ascending aorta, and cerebral aneurysm and is related to age at time of repair. Of patients who undergo repair of coarctation in childhood, 83% survive 25 years, in comparison with a 25-year survival rate of 75% among those who undergo repair between the ages of 20 and 40 and a 15-year survival rate of 50% among patients who undergo repair after 40 years of age (48). In one study of adults with coarctation who underwent repair at a mean age of 16 years, average age at death was 38 years; the 30-year actuarial survival rate was 72%. Of the late deaths, 37% were from coronary artery disease, 12% were sudden from unknown cause, 9% were from heart failure, 7% were from ruptured aortic aneurysm, and 7% were from stroke (49).

Although hypertension resolves or lessens in severity in many patients after repair, blood pressure response is dependent on age at the time of surgery. Among patients who undergo coarctation repair during childhood, the incidences of normotension are 90% at 5 years, 50% at 20 years, and 25% at 25 years after surgery. Of patients who do not undergo repair until after age 40, 50% have persistent hypertension, and most others have a hypertensive response to exercise, although the need for antihypertensive medication is reduced (48,50). Recoarctation after surgical repair of various types (e.g., end-to-end anastomosis, subclavian flap, Dacron patch aortoplasty, interposition graft) is generally infrequent, averaging 3% to 10% in most studies, but was reported in 22 (26.2%) of 84 adults in one series, 73% of whom had undergone an end-to-end type repair (51). In one study of 891 patients who underwent surgical repair and were monitored for up to 24 years, aneurysms formed at the site of repair in 48 patients (5.4%) (52). The majority of individuals who developed aneurysms had a synthetic patch as part of the coarctation repair.

Of these, 30 patients underwent reoperation, and there were four deaths. All 18 patients who did not undergo aneurysm repair died of aneurysm rupture.

Therefore, all adults with coarctation of the aorta should be monitored yearly for complications or sequelae of the repair; for the development of other cardiovascular complications, including aortic valve stenosis or insufficiency, cerebral aneurysm rupture, and aneurysm of the ascending aorta; and for aggressive treatment of hypertension and modification of other risk factors for coronary atherosclerosis. Women with coarctation who wish to become pregnant should undergo coarctation repair before conception because of the risk of aortic dissection and rupture. One research group proposed that the combination of magnetic resonance imaging of the aorta and a routine clinic visit with physical examination is the most cost-effective way to monitor these patients (51). Periodic echocardiography may be required for the assessment of progression of aortic valve disease. All patients with aneurysm formation at the site of prior coarctation surgery should be monitored carefully with consideration for reoperation with aneurysm repair.

PATENT DUCTUS ARTERIOSUS

The ductus arteriosus is an embryologic structure that permits pulmonary blood flow to bypass the lungs *in utero* by connecting the main pulmonary artery at the bifurcation to the descending aorta. At birth, pulmonary arterial pressure drops, and the ductus usually closes. In certain infants, especially premature neonates, infants with low birth weight, infants born at high altitude, and those with maternal rubella exposure, the ductus arteriosus remains patent, and blood flow direction reverses to left to right. Indeed, if the duct does not close spontaneously by 2 months of age, it is typically destined to remain patent unless closed by interventional methods.

Presenting Symptoms and Signs

In many adults, a very small PDA may be "silent" and found serendipitously on echocardiography performed for other reasons. Most adults with small PDAs are asymptomatic, with the rare exception of patients with infective endarteritis of the duct. If the duct is of moderate size and was not closed in childhood, the patient presents with symptoms of left ventricular volume overload from the left-to-right shunt, including dyspnea, effort intolerance, fatigue, palpitations, and left-sided heart failure. The adult with very large PDA and irreversible pulmonary hypertension presents with symptoms of right-sided heart failure and Eisenmenger's syndrome, as described in the section on VSD.

In patients with small PDAs, jugular venous pressure is normal. The first and second heart sounds are usually normal. A continuous murmur is heard in the second left intercostal space, with a crescendo beginning immediately after S1, peaking at or shortly after S2, and with a decrescendo throughout diastole. In the patient with a moderate to large shunt and low pulmonary vascular resistance, peripheral pulses are bounding and the pulse pressure is widened. The left ventricular impulse may become hyperdynamic, and the continuous murmur, known as the Gibson's murmur, is louder with a "machinery" quality. With a large left-to-right shunt, an aortic flow murmur and a diastolic rumble of increased mitral flow may be heard. As irreversible pulmonary hypertension supervenes and pulmonary and systemic pressures equalize, the continuous murmur diminishes and may be heard only in systole. The murmur eventually disappears. When the shunt direction reverses and becomes predominantly right to left, the classic "differential cyanosis" appears, and clubbing develops in the toes but not the fingers. Other physical findings of severe pulmonary hypertension ensue, as delineated in the section on VSD with regard to Eisenmenger's syndrome.

Helpful Tests

The ECG is usually normal in the patient with small PDA, reflects left ventricular volume overload with left atrial enlargement and left ventricular hypertrophy if the shunt is moderate to large, and shows right ventricular hypertrophy with a classic "strain" pattern in patients with reversed shunt caused by Eisenmenger's physiology. The chest radiograph is also usually normal if the shunt is small, demonstrates cardiomegaly with

"shunt vascularity" in moderate-sized PDA, and displays findings similar to those of patients with large VSD and reversed shunt if Eisenmenger's syndrome exists. Occasionally, calcification of the ductus may be observed on chest radiographs in adults. Transthoracic echocardiography is sensitive and specific for the detection of even small PDAs in the adult. Although the ductus itself is not visualized, a high-velocity, continuous, "aliased" flow abnormality is evident in the main pulmonary artery near the take-off of the left pulmonary artery branch (Fig. 36.9). Pulmonary artery systolic pressure can be estimated with the modified Bernoulli equation by subtracting the product of 4 times the square of the peak velocity across the duct from the patient's systolic blood pressure measured by sphygmomanometer. In very rare cases, patients with larger PDAs may develop an aneurysm of the ductus, which can be seen on chest radiographs or by magnetic resonance imaging or computed tomography.

Differential Diagnosis

The differential diagnosis of PDA is the same as that of the continuous cardiac murmur and includes coronary artery–to–pulmonary artery fistula, ruptured sinus of Valsalva, and bronchial systemic–to–pulmonary artery collateral vessels. The diagnosis is usually easily made by transthoracic echocardiography.

Complications

Even in patients with small PDAs, infective endarteritis is infrequent, occurring in only 2 of 270 patients over 33 years in Sweden in the modern endocarditis prophylaxis era (53). In patients with moderate to large PDAs, the major risk is of developing progressive pulmonary vascular obstructive disease with right-sided heart failure and complications of cyanosis associated with Eisenmenger's syndrome. In rare cases, a large aneurysm of the ductus may form and rupture, causing hemoptysis and death.

Therapy

"Silent" PDA necessitates no specific therapy, although some authors suggest that endocarditis

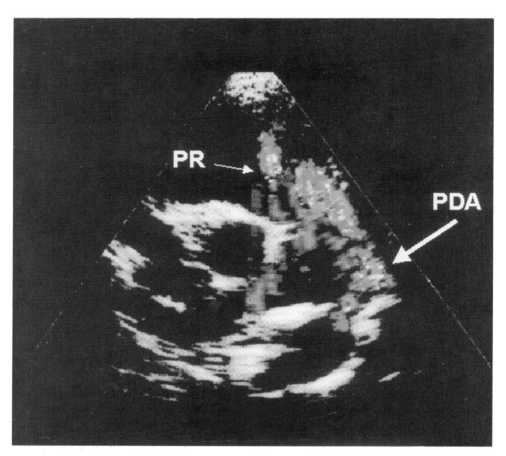

FIG. 36.9. Transthoracic echocardiogram in the parasternal short-axis view at the level of the great arteries of a small patent ductus arteriosus (PDA). A dilated pulmonary artery is noted. Two jets are apparent in diastole on the color-flow Doppler echocardiogram. The first, at the level of the pulmonic valve, is from pulmonic regurgitation (PR). The second high-velocity turbulent jet entering the main pulmonary artery near the left pulmonary artery branch at the bifurcation is from left-to-right flow from the descending thoracic aorta to the pulmonary artery through the PDA.

prophylaxis is prudent. Surgical closure of PDA has high immediate success rates, an operative mortality rate of 1.0% to 3.5% in adults, and associated potential bleeding risks (54). Percutaneous transcatheter closure of PDA with a variety of devices (Gianturco coil and Grifka-Gianturco vascular occluder, Cook, Inc., Bloomington, Indiana; AMPLATZER Ductal Occluder, AGA Medical, Golden Valley, Minnesota; and CardioSEAL Occluder, NMT Corporation, Boston, Massachusetts) has been shown to be highly effective in the short and long term and is very safe in patients with PDAs smaller than 8 mm

(55–57). Thus, percutaneous closure of PDA should be considered the procedure of choice in all patients with PDA diameter of less than 8 mm, regardless of symptoms, at centers with appropriate experience. The rates of morbidity and mortality with percutaneous closure are exceedingly low; therefore, many centers recommend that even small PDAs be closed, to obviate the need for continued antibiotic endocarditis prophylaxis, which is usually stopped 6 months after complete ductal closure. Endocarditis prophylaxis is recommended for patients with small PDAs and a murmur, but the role for prophylaxis in patients with "silent" PDA is unclear. Six months after successful closure of PDA, endocarditis prophylaxis may be discontinued.

Prognosis and Follow-up

Life expectancy is normal in patients with small PDAs and those that were closed before the development of pulmonary hypertension. In the patient with small PDA, endocarditis prophylaxis is recommended if the patient or physician chooses not to have the PDA closed percutaneously. In 117 adults with PDA, 39% of those whose PDAs were not closed had died by a mean follow-up time of 36 years (58). Only 34% of nonsurgically managed survivors were asymptomatic at follow-up. Patients who do not have small PDAs closed should be monitored periodically by auscultation and possibly echocardiography. Whether patients who have undergone percutaneous closure of PDA require continued follow-up is not known at this time. It is probably prudent to assess these patients some time after the procedure to ensure continued closure of the duct.

TETRALOGY OF FALLOT

The cardiac malformations that constitute the classic tetralogy of Fallot (TOF) include (a) a large subaortic VSD, (b) right ventricular outflow tract obstruction (infundibular, pulmonary valvular, supravalvular, or in the branch pulmonary arteries), (c) aortic override caused by anterior deviation of the interventricular septum, and (d) compensatory right ventricular hypertrophy. If an ASD is present (10% of patients with TOF), the condition is described as pentalogy of Fallot. A right-sided aortic arch is present in 10% to 25% of patients with simple TOF and in 30% to 40% of patients with the TOF variant pulmonary atresia. Coronary artery anomalies–most often an enlarged conus branch of the right coronary artery or origin of the left anterior descending artery from the right coronary artery–occur in 10% of patients with TOF. Because right ventricular outflow obstruction limits pulmonary blood flow, and thus oxygenation, and mandates a right-to-left shunt across the VSD, these patients are often cyanotic in early life and only infrequently sur-

vive to adulthood (survival rate, approximately 3% at age 40) if the TOF remains unrepaired (59).

Presenting Symptoms and Signs

In rare cases, an adult presents with unrepaired and unpalliated TOF. These unusual individuals typically have little right ventricular outflow tract obstruction in childhood, and thus the dominant hemodynamic lesion until adolescence or adulthood is the VSD with left-to-right shunt. Symptoms of volume overload, including dyspnea and exercise intolerance, are present and the patient is acyanotic; this scenario is the so-called pink tetralogy. Right ventricular outflow tract obstruction invariably progresses as the patient ages, with eventual shunt reversal. Adults with uncorrected TOF have severe exercise intolerance and cyanosis, and many suffer stroke, endocarditis, supraventricular arrhythmias, brain abscess, and left ventricular failure from progressive aortic insufficiency. Physical examination findings in these patients are remarkable for peripheral cyanosis and clubbing of fingers and toes. The jugular venous pressure is elevated with prominent a and V waves. A right ventricular heave is palpated, sometimes in association with a systolic thrill caused by turbulent flow across the stenotic outflow tract. The first heart sound is normal, and the second heart sound is loud and single because of absence of the pulmonic component. An ejection click from the dilated ascending aorta may be auscultated. A harsh systolic murmur of pulmonic obstruction is often heard. The intensity and duration of the murmur varies inversely with the severity of the obstruction. With severe pulmonary obstruction, blood is diverted across the VSD out the aorta, and the murmur becomes shorter and softer. As patients age, a diastolic blowing murmur of aortic insufficiency occurs more commonly.

Most adults with TOF have undergone a palliative procedure in childhood to provide blood flow to the pulmonary arteries: classically, implantation of a Blalock-Taussig shunt from the subclavian to the pulmonary artery or a central shunt (Waterston, between the ascending aorta and right pulmonary artery, or Potts, between the descending aorta and left pulmonary artery), followed by intracardiac repair in late childhood, adolescence, or adulthood. Current practice is to perform primary intracardiac repair in infancy or very early childhood; these patients have not yet grown to be adults. Occasionally, an adult who has undergone palliative shunting without repair presents either with cyanosis from progressive outflow tract obstruction or with the development of pulmonary hypertension or left ventricular failure from long-standing left-to-right shunting. In most of these patients, repair was not performed, initially because of multiple levels of right ventricular outflow tract obstruction or other intracardiac defects. Physical examination findings in these patients are similar to those of the uncorrected TOF, except that a continuous murmur may be heard in the chest, especially over the shunt. Also, pulse and blood pressure are diminished in the arm in which the subclavian artery was used in patients with a Blalock-Taussig shunt. If pulmonary resistance is low, the patient may not be cyanotic. If pulmonary hypertension has developed, the murmur from the palliative shunt may be present only in systole, and the patient exhibits varying degrees of cyanosis and clubbing. If no murmur is heard, the shunt can be assumed to be closed.

More than 85% of adults who have undergone intracardiac repair are asymptomatic on follow-up. The remaining adults present with symptoms related to hemodynamic residua (e.g., pulmonary obstruction with cyanosis and dyspnea) or long-term sequelae of the operation. Palpitations, usually from atrial tachyarrhythmias, are common. Syncope, although rare, may signal serious arrhythmias, including ventricular tachycardia, or heart block. Progressive pulmonary insufficiency with right ventricular dilation may produce symptoms of right-sided heart failure, including lower extremity edema. Aortic dilation may result in aortic insufficiency with symptoms of left ventricular failure and, occasionally, aneurysm with dissection or rupture. Physical examination findings reflect these residua and sequelae. In the patient with pulmonic obstruction, the S2 is soft and delayed or single, and a pulmonary flow murmur is heard. In the patient with right ventricular enlargement, a parasternal lift may be palpated and associated with a diastolic murmur of pulmonic insufficiency and right-sided S3 or S4. In the patient with VSD patch leak, a holosystolic murmur is heard. A blowing diastolic murmur of aortic insufficiency may be auscultated and, if severe, is associated with a widened pulse pressure and left-sided S3.

Helpful Tests

The ECG typically shows right axis deviation and right ventricular hypertrophy in the patient with unrepaired TOF. The ECG in patients with repaired TOF characteristically shows right bundle branch block, often with a very wide QRS complex, which correlates with the degree of right ventricular dilation (Fig. 36.10). In patients with palliative shunts, the ECG may display a prominent R wave in leads V5 and V6, which represents left ventricular hypertrophy. In some patients, ambulatory or continuous-loop monitoring may establish the presence and identity of atrial or ventricular dysrhythmias.

The chest radiograph of uncorrected TOF in the adult shows a normal heart size with right ventricular hypertrophy in the lateral view. The classic finding of *coeur en sabot,* or small, boot-shaped heart with rounded apex lifted off the left hemidiaphragm, is much less common in adults with unrepaired TOF than in children with unrepaired TOF. In the patient with unrepaired TOF, the pulmonary vessels are diminished. After Blalock-Taussig shunt implantation, the patient may have increased pulmonary vascularity with rib notching on the side of the shunt. The chest radiograph of the patient with corrected TOF may show cardiomegaly from right ventricular dilation or left ventricular dilation and a dilated ascending aorta (Fig. 36.11). Chest radiographs in each of these groups of patients show a right aortic arch in approximately 25%.

Transthoracic echocardiography is compulsory for the initial diagnosis and serial evaluation of adults with TOF. In the patient with unrepaired TOF, the level and severity of right ventricular outflow tract obstruction can be established, and the location and degree of shunting across the VSD can be determined. Flow across peripheral and central shunts may be assessed, and pulmonary artery and right ventricular systolic pressures may be estimated.

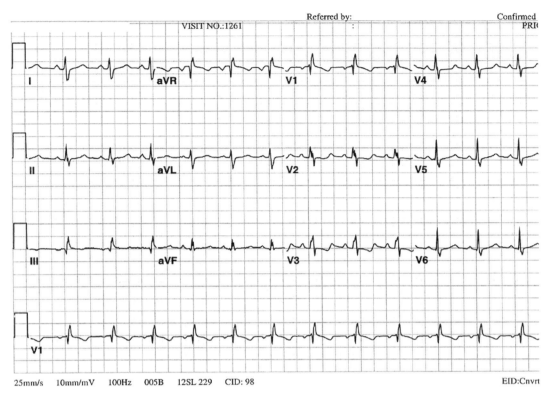

FIG. 36.10. Electrocardiogram of a patient after correction of tetralogy of Fallot, which shows incomplete right bundle branch lock and right axis deviation.

Thorough evaluation of the patient with corrected TOF involves echocardiography to evaluate for right ventricular outflow tract obstruction, right ventricular patch aneurysm, pulmonary insufficiency, right and left ventricular systolic function, VSD patch leak, and aortic dilation and aortic insufficiency. Occasionally, postoperative transthoracic imaging can be difficult in adults. In these patients, transesophageal echocardiography or cine magnetic resonance imaging may be helpful. When patients are being considered for reoperation, cardiac catheterization with hemodynamic pressure measurement, estimation of pulmonary artery size and vascular resistance, ventriculography or aortography, and determination of coronary anatomy may be necessary.

Differential Diagnosis

Many congenital cardiac anomalies other than TOF can cause cyanosis and systolic murmur in adults and should be considered in the differential diagnosis of the adult who presents with these findings. These anomalies include severe pulmonic stenosis, pulmonic atresia, Ebstein's anomaly, uncorrected atrioventricular canal, single-ventricle states, congenitally corrected transposition of the great arteries, double-chamber right ventricle, and other congenital cardiac conditions associated with Eisenmenger's syndrome such as VSD and PDA. Physical examination in conjunction with ECG, chest radiography, and echocardiography establish the diagnosis in the majority of cases.

Complications

The course of the patient with uncorrected TOF is marked by the consequences of right ventricular strain, chronic cyanosis, and erythrocytosis. Right ventricular failure occurs in the fourth and fifth decades of life in the rare adult who

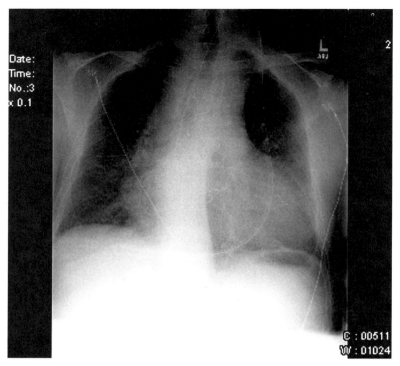

FIG. 36.11. Chest radiograph of the patient in Fig. 36.10, which shows only sternal wires and mild cardiomegaly.

survives to this point. Endocarditis with septic embolization is not uncommon. Complications of erythrocytosis include hyperviscosity syndrome, stroke, gout, cholelithiasis, and sudden death. Endocarditis frequently develops in patients with systemic–to–pulmonary artery shunts related to the high-velocity jet.

The clinical course of the repaired TOF is related to the residua and sequelae of the surgery. Arrhythmias are the most common and troubling problem after TOF repair. In one study of 53 patients after primary repair, sinus node dysfunction was identified in 19 patients (36%), 4 of whom required pacemaker implantation; atrial tachyarrhythmias were identified in 18 patients (34%); and nonsustained ventricular tachycardia was identified in 10 patients (19%) (60). In a retrospective cohort study of 242 patients after TOF repair, sustained atrial tachyarrhythmias occurred in 29 patients (12%) and were associated with significant morbidity, including congestive heart failure, subsequent ventricular tachycardia,

reoperation, stroke, and death, in 69% (61). Sudden death has been reported in 3% of adults late after repair and usually occurs in patients with prior arrhythmias (62). Inducible sustained ventricular tachycardia and sudden death correlate with prolonged QRS duration (63). The incidence of ventricular arrhythmias was lower in patients in whom the transatrial operative approach was used than in patients who underwent repair with the transventricular method with no higher risk of atrial arrhythmias in one study (64). Progressive pulmonary regurgitation with consequent right ventricular dilation and dysfunction occurs and may necessitate reoperation (65,66). The presence of progressive pulmonary insufficiency is the most common hemodynamic lesion in patients with ventricular tachycardia, whereas tricuspid regurgitation occurs most frequently in patients with atrial arrhythmias (67). Other reasons for reoperation include VSD patch leak, recurrent right ventricular outflow tract obstruction, peripheral pulmonary artery obstruction, repair of patch aneurysm, tricuspid regurgitation, aortic insufficiency, and aneurysm of the ascending aorta.

Therapy

Surgical intracardiac repair is recommended for all adults who have previously unrepaired TOF or who have undergone palliative shunting without repair of TOF, even those older than 40 years. The operative mortality rate is similar to that of pediatric patients (2.5% vs. 3%), although bleeding complications are common because of erythrocytosis and coagulation defects and necessitated reexploration in 15% of patients in one series (68,69). In one study of 30 adults who underwent repair between the ages of 40 and 60, 93% achieved pulmonary–to–systemic arterial pressure ratios of less than 0.65, and the survival rate was 73% at 9.2 years of follow-up (70). Preoperatively, 57% of patients had New York Heart Association function Class III or IV disease; 21 of 22 survivors had functional Class I or II disease at follow-up. Reoperation after repair of TOF is required most frequently for severe pulmonary regurgitation with compromise of right ventricular function (38% of reoperations), pulmonary conduit revision (22%), ventricular septal patch leak (10%), and tricuspid regurgitation (5%) (71). Studies suggest that right ventricular function deteriorates if pulmonary valve replacement for pulmonary regurgitation is not performed before right ventricular ejection fraction decreases to 40% (72). Pulmonary valve replacement in conjunction with intraoperative cryoablation reduced the incidence of preexisting atrial and ventricular arrhythmias in 70 patients who underwent valve replacement late after repair (73).

Prognosis and Follow-up

As noted previously, the long-term outlook for the patient with unrepaired TOF is dismal, with survival rates of 3% by age 40. Fortunately, despite potential complications of intracardiac repair, patients do quite well many years after repair. Survival 32 years after surgery was 86% vs. 96% in age-matched controls without congenital heart disease (74). Among 162 patients who underwent operation before 1967, the cumulative 25-year postoperative survival rate was 94.4% (75). Among 658 patients who underwent correction of TOF, actuarial survival rates were 97%, 94%, 89%, and 85% at 10, 20, 30, and 36 years, respectively (62). Multivariate correlates of impaired long-term survival were earlier operation, preoperative polycythemia, and use of a right ventricular outflow tract patch. Patients without polycythemia and a right ventricular outflow tract patch had a life expectancy of 36 additional years after surgery.

Patients who have undergone surgical TOF correction may be repaired, but they are not cured. Endocarditis prophylaxis is required for life. Patients should be evaluated at least every 1 to 2 years by a cardiologist experienced in the care of this condition and monitored for progressive pulmonary insufficiency, atrial and ventricular arrhythmias, and other sequelae of the repair.

PRACTICAL POINTS

- Closure of ASD is recommended for all symptomatic adults with secundum ASD and a Qp/Qs of 1.5:1 or higher, for asymptomatic adults with a Qp/Qs of 1.5:1 or higher and right-sided heart enlargement, and probably for adults older than 40 years with a Qp/Qs of 1.7:1 or higher who do not have fixed pulmonary hypertension.

- Surgical closure of VSD is recommended for adults with a Qp/Qs of 1.5:1 or higher who are symptomatic or who have reversible pulmonary hypertension or left ventricular enlargement or dysfunction and for asymptomatic adults with normal pulmonary artery pressure if the Qp/Qs is 2:1 or higher.

(continued)

- Coarctation of the aorta is associated with significant morbidity and mortality at fairly young ages from aortic rupture; complications related to bicuspid aortic valve, including endocarditis; ruptured cerebral aneurysm; and myocardial infarction.

- Percutaneous closure of PDA at experienced centers is probably the preferred method for PDAs smaller than 8 mm in diameter.

- Patients with corrected TOF are repaired but not cured. Serial follow-up is imperative with early intervention for severe pulmonary regurgitation and right ventricular dysfunction.

- Serial follow-up by cardiologists experienced in the care of adults with congenital heart disease is required for most adults with repaired or unrepaired congenital heart disease.

- The only congenital cardiac lesions that do not require bacterial endocarditis prophylaxis are secundum and sinus venosus ASD, before and 6 months after repair; VSD, 6 months after documented complete closure; and PDA, 6 months after documented closure.

REFERENCES

1. Care of the adult with congenital heart disease. 32nd Bethesda Conference. *J Am Coll Cardiol* 2001;37:1162–1187.

2. O'Toole JD, Reddy PS, Curtiss EI, et al. The mechanism of splitting of the second heart sound in atrial septal defect. *Circulation* 1977;56:1047–1053.

3. Hamilton WT, Haffajee CI, Dalen JE, et al. Atrial septal defect secundum: clinical profile with physiologic correlates. In: Roberts WC, ed. *Adult congenital heart disease*. Philadelphia: FA Davis, 1987:395–407.

4. Spitz HB. The roentgenology of atrial septal defect in the adult. *Semin Roentgenol* 1966;1:67–86.

5. Kronzon I, Tunick PA, Freedberg RS, et al. Transesophageal echocardiography is superior to transthoracic echocardiography in the diagnosis of sinus venosus atrial septal defect. *J Am Coll Cardiol* 1991;17:537–542.

6. Pascoe RD, Oh JK, Warnes CA, et al. Diagnosis of sinus venosus atrial septal defect with transesophageal echocardiography. *Circulation* 1996;94:1049–1055.

7. Beerbaum P, Kerperich H, Barth P, et al. Noninvasive quantitation of left-to-right shunt in pediatric patients: phase-contrast cine magnetic resonance imaging compared with invasive oximetry. *Circulation* 2001;103:2476–2482.

8. Perloff JK. Ostium secundum atrial septal defect: Survival 87–94 years. *Am J Cardiol* 1984;53:388–389.

9. Mendelson MA. Pregnancy in the woman with congenital heart disease. *Am J Card Imaging* 1995;9:44–52.

10. Gatzoulis MA, Freeman MA, Siu SC, et al. Atrial arrhythmia after surgical closure of atrial septal defects in adults. *N Engl J Med* 1999;340:839–846.

11. Konstantinides S, Geibel A, Oschewski M, et al. A comparison of surgical and medical therapy for atrial septal defect in adults. *N Engl J Med* 1995;333:469–473.

12. Vogel M, Berger F, Kramer A, et al. Incidence of secondary pulmonary hypertension in adults with atrial septal or sinus venosus defects. *Heart* 1999;82:30–33.

13. Attie F, Rosas M, Granados N, et al. Surgical treatment for secundum atrial septal defects in patients > 40 years old. *J Am Coll Cardiol* 2001;38:2035–2042.

14. Helber U, Baumann R, Seboldt H, et al. Atrial septal defect in adults: Cardiopulmonary exercise capacity before and 4 months and 10 years after defect closure. *J Am Coll Cardiol* 1997;29:1345–1350.

15. Shah D, Azhar M, Oakley CM, et al. Natural history of secundum atrial septal defect in adults after medical or surgical treatment: A historical prospective study. *Br Heart J* 1994;71:224–228.

16. Zamora R, Rao PS, Lloyd TR, et al. Intermediate-term results of Phase I Food and Drug Administration Trials of buttoned device occlusion of secundum atrial septal defects. *J Am Coll Cardiol* 1998;31:674–676.

17. Berger F, Vogel M, Alexi-Meskishvili V, et al. Comparison of results and complications of surgical and Amplatzer device closure of atrial septal defects. *J Thorac Cardiovasc Surg* 1999;118:674–678.

18. Rao PS, Berger F, Rey C, et al. Results of transvenous occlusion of secundum atrial septal defects with the fourth generation buttoned device: Comparison with first, second, and third generation devices. *J Am Coll Cardiol* 2000;36:583–592.

19. Cowley CG, Lloyd TR, Bove, et al. Comparison of results of closure of secundum atrial septal defect by surgery versus Amplatzer setptal occluder. *Am J Cardiol* 2001;88:589–591.

20. Hijazi ZM, Du ZD, Mahony L, et al. Comparison of transcatheter Amplatzer device and surgical closure of atrial septal defect : a multi-center con-randomized controlled study. *Circulation* 2001;104(Suppl II):II-780.

21. Carminati M, Giusti S, Hausdorf G, et al. A European multicentric experience using the CardioSeal and Starflex double umbrella devices to close interatrial communications holes within the oval fossa. *Cardiol Young* 2000;10:519–526.

22. Byrne JG, Adams DH, Mitchell ME, et al. Minimally invasive direct access for repair of atrial septal defect in adults. *Am J Cardiol* 1999;84:919–922.

23. El-Najdawi EK, Driscoll DJ, Puga FJ, et al. Operation for partial atrioventricular septal defect: a forty-year review. *J Thorac Cardiovasc Surg* 2000;119:880–889.

24. Murphy JG, Gersh BJ, McGoon MD, et al. Long-term

outcome after surgical repair of isolated atrial septal defect. Follow-up at 27 to 32 years. *N Engl J Med* 1990;323:1645–1650.

25. Alpert BS, Cook DH, Varghese PG, et al. Spontaneous closure of small ventricular septal defects: Ten year follow-up. *Pediatrics* 1979;63:204–206.

26. Gersony WM, Hayes CJ, Driscoll DJ, et al. Bacterial endocarditis in patients with aortic stenosis, pulmonary stenosis or ventricular septal defect. *Circulation* 1993;87:I-121–I-126.

27. Neumayer U, Stone S, Somerville J. Small ventricular septal defects in adults. *Eur Heart J* 1998;19:1573–1582

28. Gleicher N, Midwall J, Hochberger D, et al. Eisenmenger's syndrome and pregnancy. *Obstet Gynecol Survey* 1070;34:721–741.

29. Corone P, Doyon F, Gaudeau JS, et al. Natural history of ventricular septal defect: A study involving 790 cases. *Circulation* 1977;55:908–915.

30. Lun K, Li H, Leung MP, et al. Analysis of indications for surgical closure of subarterial ventricular septal defect without associated aortic cusp prolapse and aortic regurgitation. *Am J Cardiol* 2001;87:1266–1270.

31. Kidd L, Driscoll DJ, Gersony WM, et al. The second natural history study of congenital heart disease: Results of treatment of patients with ventricular septal defect. *Circulation* 1993;87(Suppl 2):138–151.

32. Kalra GS, Verma PK, Dhall A, et al. Transcatheter device closure of ventricular septal defects: immediate results and intermediate-term follow-up. *Am Heart J* 1999;138(2, Pt 1):339–344.

33. Janorkar S, Goh T, Wilkinson J. Transcatheter closure of ventricular septal defects using the Rashkind device: initial experience. *Catheter Cardiovasc Interv* 1999;46:43–48.

34. Lin PJ, Chang CH, Chu JJ, et al. Minimally invasive cardiac surgical techniques in the closure of ventricular septal defect: an alternative approach. *Ann Thorac Surg* 1998;65:165–169.

35. Rosenzweig EB, Kerstein D, Barst RJ. Long-term prostacyclin for pulmonary hypertension with associated congenital heart defects. *Circulation* 1999;99:1858–1865.

36. Aeba R, Griffith BP, Hardesty RL, et al. Isolated lung transplantation for patients with Eisenmenger's syndrome. *Circulation* 1993;88:452–455.

37. Lupinetti FM, Bolling SF, Bove EL, et al. Selective lung or heart-lung transplantation for pulmonary hypertension associated with congenital cardiac anomalies. *Ann Thorac Surg* 1994;57:1545–1548.

38. Daliento L, Somerville J, Prebitero P, et al. Eisenmenger syndrome: Factors relating to deterioration and death. *Eur Heart J* 1998;19:1845–1855.

39. Moller JH, Patton C, Varco RL, et al. Late results (30 to 25 years) after operative closure of isolated ventricular septal defect from 1954–1960. *Am J Cardiol* 1991; 68:1491–1497.

40. Houyel L, Vaksmann G, Fournier A, et al. Ventricular arrhythmias after correction of ventricular septal defects: importance of surgical approach. *J Am Coll Cardiol* 1990;16:1224–1228.

41. Campbell M. Natural history of coarctation of the aorta. *Br Heart J* 1970;32:633–640.

42. Liberthson RR, Pennington DG, Jacobs ML, et al.

Coarctation of the aorta: Review of 234 patients and clarification of management problems. *Am J Cardiol* 1979;43:835–840.

43. Behl PR, Sante P, Blesovsky A. Isolated coarctation of the aorta: surgical treatment and late results: Eighteen years' experience. *J Cardiovasc Surg* 1988;29:509–517.

44. de Giovanni JV, Lip YH, Osman K, et al. Percutaneous balloon dilatation of aortic coarctation in adults. *Am J Cardiol* 1996;77:435–439.

45. Fletcher SE, Nihill MR, Grifka RG, et al. Balloon angioplasty of native coarctation of the aorta: midterm follow-up and prognostic factors. *J Am Coll Cardiol* 1995;25:730–734.

46. Suarez de Lezo J, Pan M, Romero M, et al. Immediate and follow-up findings after stent treatment for severe coarctation of the aorta. *Am J Cardiol* 1999;83:400–406.

47. Harrison D, McLaughlin P, Lazzam C, et al. Endovascular stents in the management of coarctation of the aorta in the adolescent and adult: one-year follow-up. *Heart* 2001;85:561–566.

48. Perloff JK. Survival patterns without cardiac surgery or interventional catheterization: a narrowing base. In: Perloff JK, Childs JS, eds. *Congenital heart disease in adults*, 2nd ed. Philadelphia: WB Saunders, 1998:15–53.

49. Cohen M, Fuster V, Steele PM, et al. Coarctation of the aorta. Long-term follow-up and prediction of outcome after surgical correction. *Circulation* 1989;80:840–845.

50. Bhat MA, Neelakandhan KS, Unnikrishnan M, et al. Fate of hypertension after repair of coarctation of the aorta in adults. *Br J Surg* 2001;88:536–538.

51. Thierren J, Thorne SA, Wright A, et al. Repaired coarctation: a "cost-effective" approach to identify complications in adults. *J Am Coll Cardiol* 2000;35:997–1002.

52. Knyshov GV, Sitar LL, Glagola MD, et al. Aortic aneurysms at the site of the repair of coarctation of the aorta: a review of 48 patients. *Ann Thorac Surg* 1996;61:935–939.

53. Thilen U, Astrom-Olsson K. Does the risk of infective endarteritis justify routine patent ductus arteriosus closure? *Eur Heart J* 1997;18:503–506.

54. Sorenson KE, Kristensen B, Hansen OK. Frequency of occurrence of residual ductal flow after surgical ligation by color-flow mapping. *Am J Cardiol* 1991;67:653–654.

55. Goyal VS, Fulwani MC, Ramakantan R, et al. Follow-up after coil closure of patent ductus arteriosus. *Am J Cardiol* 1999;83:463–466.

56. Magee AG, Huggon IC, Seed PT, et al. Transcatheter coil occlusion of the arterial duct: Results of the European registry. *Eur Heart J* 2001;22:1817–1822.

57. Bilkis AA, Alwi M, Hasri S, et al. The Amplatz duct occluder: experience in 209 patients. *J Am Coll Cardiol* 2001;37:258–261.

58. Fisher RG, Moodie DS, Sterba R, et al. Patent ductus arteriosus in adults–long-term follow-up: Nonsurgical versus surgical treatment. *J Am Coll Cardiol* 1986;8:280–284.

59. Bertranou EG, Blackstone EH, Hazelrig JB, et al. Life expectancy without surgery in tetralogy of Fallot. *Am J Cardiol* 1978;42:458–466.

60. Roos-Hesselink J, Perlroth MG, McGhie J, et al. Atrial arrhythmias in adults after repair of tetralogy of Fallot. Correlations with clinical, exercise, and echocardiographic findings. *Circulation* 1995;91:2214–2219.

61. Harrison DA, Siu SC, Hussain F, et al. Sustained atrial arrhythmias in adults late after repair of tetralogy of Fallot. *Am J Cardiol* 2001;87:584–588.

62. Nollert G, Fischlein T, Bouterwek S, et al. Long-term survival in patients with repair of tetralogy of Fallot: 36-year follow-up of 490 survivors of the first year after repair. *J Am Coll Cardiol* 1997;30:1374–1383.

63. Balaji S, Lau YR, Case CL, et al. QRS prolongation is associated with inducible ventricular tachycardia after repair of tetralogy of Fallot. *Am J Cardiol* 1997;80:160–163.

64. Dietl CA, Cazzaniga ME, Dubner SJ, et al. Life-threatening arrhythmias and right ventricular dysfunction after surgical repair of tetralogy of Fallot: comparison between transventricular and transatrial approaches. *Circulation* 1994;90:7–12.

65. Uretzky G, Puga FJ, Danielson GK, et al. Reoperation after correction of tetralogy of Fallot. *Circulation* 1982;66:202–208.

66. Waien SA, Liu PP, Ross BL, et al. Serial follow-up of adults with repaired tetralogy of Fallot. *J Am Coll Cardiol* 1992;20:295–300.

67. Gatzoulis MA, Balaji S, Webber SA, et al. Risk factors for arrhythmia and sudden cardiac death late after repair of tetralogy of Fallot: a multicentre study. *Lancet* 2000;356:975–981.

68. John S, Mani GK, Abraham KA, et al. Intracardiac repair of tetralogy of Fallot in adults. *J Cardiovasc Surg* 1979;20:145–149.

69. Presbitero P, DeMarie D, Aruta E, et al. Results of total correction of tetralogy of Allot performed in adults. *Ann Thorac Surg* 1988;46:297–301.

70. Hu DCK, Seward JB, Puga FJ, et al. Total correction of tetralogy of Fallot at age 40 years or older: Long-term follow-up. *J Am Coll Cardiol* 1985;5:40–44.

71. Oechslin EN, Harrison DA, Harris L, et al. Reoperation in adults with repair of tetralogy of Fallot: indications and outcomes. *J Thorac Cardiovasc Surg* 1999;245–251.

72. Therrien J, Siu SC, McLaughlin PR, et al. Pulmonary valve replacement in adults late after repair of tetralogy of Fallot: Are we operating too late? *J Am Coll Cardiol* 2000;36:1670–1675.

73. Thierren J, Siu SC, Harris L, et al. Impact of pulmonary valve replacement on arrhythmia propensity late after repair of tetralogy of Fallot. *Circulation* 2001;103:2489–2494.

74. Murphy JG, Gersh BJ, Mair DD, et al. Long-term outcomes in patients undergoing surgical repair of tetralogy of Fallot. *N Engl J Med* 1993;329:593–599.

75. Rosenthal A, Behrendt D, Sloah H, et al. Long-term prognosis (15 to 26 years) after repair of tetralogy of Fallot. I. Survival and symptomatic status. *Ann Thorac Surg* 1984;38:151–156.

37

Management of Chronic Anticoagulation

William P. Fay and John A. Santinga

MECHANISM OF ACTION OF WARFARIN

Several new antithrombotic drugs have been introduced into clinical practice since 1990. However, warfarin remains the drug of choice in many clinical situations for chronically suppressing the blood coagulation system. Warfarin disrupts the normal metabolism of vitamin K. Vitamin K is a cofactor for gamma carboxylase, a hepatic enzyme that adds a carboxyl group to specific glutamic acid residues located in the amino-terminal region of vitamin K–dependent clotting factors. Table 37.1 lists the vitamin K–dependent coagulation factors. Gamma carboxylation of these factors is necessary for them to bind to phospholipid membranes. Warfarin inhibits vitamin K epoxide reductase, the enzyme responsible for generating the reduced form of vitamin K, which is a required cofactor for gamma carboxylase. In the presence of warfarin, clotting factors are produced; however, their conversion to functional forms by gamma carboxylase is inhibited, thereby producing an anticoagulant effect.

INITIATION AND MONITORING OF WARFARIN

Because warfarin does not inhibit circulating clotting factors present when the drug is started, it typically takes 4 to 5 days for an adequate anticoagulant effect to be achieved. If necessary, heparin is usually used to achieve anticoagulation in the patient during the first several days of warfarin therapy. In general, patients should receive heparin for at least 4 days after starting warfarin, and many experts recommend continuing heparin for an additional 1 to 2 days after therapeutic warfarin anticoagulation is achieved. Loading doses of warfarin should

be avoided, because they increase the frequency of excessive anticoagulation, which can result in bleeding (1). Loading doses also cause greater reductions in plasma levels of protein C, an endogenous anticoagulant, which may precipitate thrombotic complications. A typical initial dose of warfarin for an adult is 5 mg daily. 2.5 mg a day should be used in the elderly. Lower doses should be considered in elderly patients, in those taking other drugs known to potentiate warfarin (e.g., amiodarone), and in patients with reduced vitamin K intake.

Warfarin therapy must be monitored carefully because its anticoagulant effect can vary considerably among individuals. The laboratory test used to monitor warfarin is the prothrombin time (PT), because it is sensitive to reductions in factors II (prothrombin), VII, and X. The PT is obtained by adding calcium chloride and a thromboplastin to citrated plasma and then measuring the times required for a clot to form. The results of the PT can vary significantly depending on the type of thromboplastin that is used. Because different clinical laboratories may use different thromboplastins, a formula was introduced to transform the PT to an index that allows results from different laboratories to be meaningfully compared. This index, the International Normalized Ratio (INR), is routinely used to report PT results. A normal INR (i.e., from a healthy individual not receiving anticoagulant therapy) is approximately 1.0. Warfarin therapy prolongs the PT and increases the INR. The target intensity of anticoagulation for most individuals receiving warfarin is an INR of 2.5 (range, 2.0 to 3.0). For individuals at a higher risk of thrombosis (e.g., a mechanical heart valve in the mitral position), a target INR of 3.0 (range, 2.5 to 3.5) is appropriate. During the first week of warfarin therapy, the

571

TABLE 37.1. *Vitamin K–dependent factors*

Procoagulant
   Factor II (prothrombin)
   Factor VII
   Factor IX
   Factor X
Anticoagulant
   Protein C
   Protein S
   Protein Z

INR should be checked at least twice. Depending on the rapidity and stability of the anticoagulant response, the time interval between INR determinations is gradually increased. In the chronic phase of therapy, the INR should be checked at least monthly. Common indications for warfarin and the recommended intensity of anticoagulation are listed in Table 37.2.

INSTRUCTIONS FOR PATIENTS TAKING WARFARIN

Warfarin is a medication with a narrow therapeutic index and the potential to cause major, potentially fatal complications. Therefore, it is essential that all patients taking warfarin are thoroughly educated about this medication and that the educational process is properly documented.

Points to emphasize include the following:

1. Patients must be able to recognize symptoms and signs of bleeding (including internal bleeding), and they must report them immediately if noted.
2. Patients must play an active role in their anticoagulation management. They need to take the warfarin properly and to undergo laboratory testing as instructed.
3. Good communication between the patient and health care provider is essential. Mechanisms must be established to ensure that all laboratory results and warfarin dosing changes are promptly and accurately reported to the patient. This is best accomplished by using an anticoagulation management service, if available, which is usually staffed by nurses or pharmacists, or both, under the direction of a physician.
4. Women with potential for pregnancy who are undergoing anticoagulation must be aware of the potential teratogenic effects of warfarin.
5. Patients must know that many medications can interact with warfarin to either inhibit or potentiate its anticoagulant effect (Table 37.3). They must promptly report any changes in their other medications so that

TABLE 37.2. *Warfarin: common indications and recommended intensity of anticoagulation*

Indication	Target INR	INR range
Deep venous thrombosis (DVT) or pulmonary embolism	2.5	2.0–3.0
DVT prophylaxis for high risk surgery (e.g., total hip replacement)	2.5	2.0–3.0
Prevention of cardioembolism	2.5	2.0–3.0
Atrial fibrillation		
Intracardiac thrombus		
After myocardial infarction		
Cardiomyopathy		
Native valvular heart disease (e.g., severe mitral stenosis) or bioprosthetic cardiac valve		
Prevention of cerebrovascular or peripheral vascular thrombosis	2.5	2.0–3.0
Mechanical prosthetic cardiac valve		
Bileaflet or tilting disk		
Aortic position[a]	2.5	2.0–3.0
Mitral position	3.0	2.5–3.5
Caged ball or disk	3.0 + aspirin, 81 mg	3–4
Lupus anticoagulant/antiphospholipid syndrome with history of thrombosis	3.0[b]	2.5–3.5

INR, International Normalized Ratio.
[a]Provided patient is in sinus rhythm with normal left atrial and left ventricular size/function. If not, a target of 3.0 and a range of 2.5–3.5 should be used.
[b]Some experts recommend more intense anticoagulation.

TABLE 37.3. *Medications commonly used in cardiovascular patients that are reported to increase or decrease warfarin's anticoagulant effect*

Increase PT/INR	Can increase or decrease PT/INR	Decrease PT/INR
Acetaminophen	Cholestyramine	Spironolactone
Amiodarone	Prednisone	Vitamin C
Antibiotics (many, but not all)		(high doses)
Aspirin		
Fluvastatin		
Gemfibrozil		
Heparin		
Lovastatin		
Methyldopa		
Propafenone		
Propranolol		
Quinidine		
Simvastatin		
Ticlopidine		
Vitamin E		

PT, prothrombin time; INR, International Normalized Ratio.

laboratory testing can be ordered and warfarin dose adjustments, if indicated, can be made.

6. Significant changes in diet (i.e., vitamin K intake) can adversely affect anticoagulation management. Patients must know which foods are high in vitamin K content. Although patients can consume high–vitamin K foods (e.g., spinach) while taking warfarin, their weekly intake should not vary substantially.

7. Patients must report significant changes in their general medical status. For example, exacerbation of congestive heart failure can cause hepatic congestion, which can decrease clotting factor synthesis and cause excessive anticoagulation. If patients recognize and report appropriate symptoms, hemorrhagic and thrombotic complications can be reduced.

MANAGEMENT OF EXCESSIVE ANTICOAGULATION

Despite careful monitoring, excessive anticoagulation occasionally occurs in patients taking warfarin. The risk of bleeding increases substantially as the INR climbs above 4.0. Patients with significantly increased INRs should be evaluated for symptoms and signs of bleeding. If these are present, interventions to rapidly reverse excessive anticoagulation should be considered. The interventions include parenteral administration of vitamin K and infusion of functional clotting factors in the form of fresh-frozen plasma or factor concentrates. In most cases, however, increased INR values are not associated with bleeding. If there is no bleeding and the degree of INR increase is moderate (i.e., INR of 5.0 to 9.0), withholding warfarin 1 or 2 days, instructing the patient to consume vitamin K–rich foods (e.g., spinach, broccoli), and resuming warfarin at a decreased maintenance dosage are usually sufficient. However, if the patient is at increased risk of bleeding complications, vitamin K should be prescribed. Vitamin K should be administered to all patients with an INR higher than 9.0, even in the absence of bleeding. If the INR is less than 9.0, relatively small doses of oral vitamin K (i.e., 1.25 to 2.5 mg) can return the INR to the therapeutic range in approximately 24 hours in most patients (2). Higher doses of oral vitamin K (3 to 5 mg) are recommended for nonbleeding patients with an INR of more than 9.0.

An attempt should always be made to determine the cause of excessive anticoagulation. Common clinical scenarios include the addition of a new medication that potentiates warfarin (e.g., trimethoprim-sulfamethoxazole), dietary changes that result in decreased vitamin K intake, and exacerbation of underlying disease processes, such as congestive heart failure and liver disease.

COMPLICATIONS OF WARFARIN

Bleeding is the most common complication of warfarin therapy. Even with optimal anticoagulant management, the overall incidence of major bleeding in patients receiving warfarin is approximately 1.0 to 1.5 per 100 patient-years. However, individual bleeding risk may vary considerably, depending on underlying patient characteristics and the indication for anticoagulation (3). Risk factors for major bleeding are listed in Table 37.4. Internal bleeding, such as a retroperitoneal hematoma, can be difficult to diagnose. Therefore, the index of suspicion must be high, and appropriate diagnostic modalities

TABLE 37.4. *Risk factors for bleeding complications during warfarin therapy*

Age >65 years
Female gender
Prior stroke or myocardial infarction
History of gastrointestinal bleeding
Malignancy
Anemia, diabetes mellitus, renal insufficiency

From Beyth RJ, Quinn LM, Landefeld CS. Prospective evaluation of an index for predicting the risk of major bleeding in outpatients treated with warfarin. *Am J Med* 1998;105:91–99.

(e.g., computed tomography) should be utilized, if indicated. Warfarin-induced skin necrosis is an uncommon but important complication of anticoagulant therapy. This disorder is caused by suppression of protein C, an endogenous anticoagulant, during the initiation of warfarin therapy. Initiating warfarin at the estimated daily maintenance dose (i.e., avoiding loading doses) is probably the best way to prevent warfarin-induced skin necrosis. If a patient with known protein C deficiency requires initiation of warfarin therapy, therapeutic anticoagulation with heparin should be achieved before warfarin is started and should be continued until the INR enters the therapeutic range. Warfarin is a teratogen. Characteristic abnormalities associated with warfarin embryopathy include nasal bridge deformities and abnormal bone formation. Fetal risk from exposure to warfarin is greatest during weeks 6 to 12 of gestation. All women with potential for pregnancy should be advised of warfarin's potential teratogenic effects and instructed to contact their health care provider immediately if they believe they may be pregnant. If anticoagulation must be maintained during pregnancy, subcutaneous heparin (either unfractionated or low molecular weight) can be used. Less frequent complications of warfarin include the blue toes syndrome, alopecia, and urticaria.

TEMPORARY INTERRUPTION OF WARFARIN FOR INVASIVE OR SURGICAL PROCEDURES

It may be necessary to temporarily discontinue warfarin when a patient is scheduled for an invasive procedure associated with significant bleeding risk. When interruption of warfarin is necessary, the patient's risks of bleeding and thrombosis must be considered in order to determine appropriate management (4). If the bleeding risk is sufficiently low (e.g., for many routine dental procedures, including tooth extraction), interruption of warfarin is unnecessary. If there is significant bleeding risk but the risk of thrombosis is low, the most appropriate intervention in many cases is simply to discontinue warfarin approximately 4 days before the procedure and to resume it as soon as possible afterwards. Surgical procedures can be performed safely if the INR is less than 1.5, and the patient still receives some protection against thromboembolism when the INR is 1.5 to 2.0. Therefore, it is estimated that the approach of simply withholding warfarin for several days exposes the patient to the equivalent thromboembolic risk of 2 days without any anticoagulation, which may be very low. For example, a patient with a bileaflet mechanical valve in the aortic position, normal sinus rhythm, and a normal left atrium and left ventricle appears to have an annual rate of thromboembolism of less than 3% in the absence of warfarin. The corresponding thrombotic risk involved in withholding warfarin 4 days before an invasive procedure and restarting it immediately afterwards is estimated to be less than 0.02% (i.e., less than 1 in 5,000 chance). The INR should be checked the day before the invasive procedure. If it is higher than 1.7, a small dose of vitamin K (e.g., 1 mg) can be administered orally. If the risk of thrombosis while warfarin is withheld is considered high (e.g., deep venous thrombosis diagnosed less than 1 month earlier; mechanical mitral valve prosthesis in a patient with atrial fibrillation), then heparin should be administered while the INR is subtherapeutic. Low molecular weight heparin appears to be ideally suited for this purpose, because it can be self-administered by the patient by once or twice daily by subcutaneous injection, thereby avoiding hospitalization solely for heparin administration. Heparin should be discontinued for 6 hours (unfractionated heparin) to 12 to 24 hours (low molecular weight heparin) before the procedure and restarted afterwards when considered safe. Because its anticoagulant effect is delayed, warfarin should be resumed as soon as possible after the procedure, usually on the same day.

PRACTICAL POINTS

- When warfarin therapy is started, the physician should (a) consider the patient's age, general medical condition, and other medications when selecting the initial daily dose; (b) avoid loading doses; and (c) perform and document patient education regarding anticoagulation.

- During the first week of warfarin therapy, the INR should be checked at least twice.

- In the chronic phase of therapy, the INR should be checked at least monthly.

- Most asymptomatic episodes of moderate overanticoagulation (i.e., INR of 4 to 9) can be managed by temporarily withholding warfarin and, if necessary, by small doses (1.25 to 2.5 mg) of oral vitamin K.

- The physician should consider bleeding and thrombosis risks when deciding on anticoagulation management before and after elective invasive procedures. Discontinuation of warfarin is usually, but not always, necessary. Use of periprocedure heparin is often, but not always, necessary.

REFERENCES

1. Harrison L, Johnston M, Massicotte MP, et al. Comparison of 5-mg and 10-mg loading doses in initiation of warfarin therapy. *Ann Intern Med* 1997;126:133–136.
2. Weibert RT, Le DT, Kayser SR, et al. Correction of excessive anticoagulation with low-dose oral vitamin K1. *Ann Intern Med* 1997;126:959–962.
3. Beyth RJ, Quinn LM, Landefeld CS. Prospective evaluation of an index for predicting the risk of major bleeding in outpatients treated with warfarin. *Am J Med* 1998;105:91–99.
4. Kearon C, Hirsh J. Management of anticoagulation before and after elective surgery. *New Engl J Med* 1997;336:1506–1511.

RECOMMENDED READING

Sixth ACCP Consensus Conference on Antithrombotic Therapy. *Chest* 2001;119(Suppl):1S–370S.

Ansell JE, Oertel LB, Wittkowsky AK, eds. *Managing oral anticoagulation therapy.* Gaithersburg, MD: Aspen Publishers, 2000.

38

Assessing and Minimizing Cardiac Risk of Noncardiac Surgery

Rajendra H. Mehta, Eduardo Bossone, and Kim A. Eagle

The aging patient population and advances in surgical and anesthetic techniques have resulted in the performance of an increasing number of complex surgical procedures in greater number of patients with higher likelihood of significant cardiovascular disease (1). Thus, it is not surprising that coronary artery disease (CAD) accounts for most deaths in patients undergoing noncardiac surgery (2). Because of the magnitude of this problem, strategies for perioperative risk assessment are designed to estimate the risk of perioperative complications and to intervene in order to minimize adverse events in a rational manner. Approximately 5% of the elderly population in United States undergo noncardiac surgery each year, and about one third of these patients are at risk for CAD; in-hospital and long-term complications are estimated to occur in 1.5 million patients (2). Wide variability exists in how physicians approach preoperative risk assessment for cardiac events in patients undergoing noncardiac surgery (3). This chapter outlines a simplistic approach for assessing and modifying risk for patients undergoing a wide variety of noncardiac surgical procedures.

RISK OF PERIOPERATIVE CARDIAC EVENTS DURING NONCARDIAC SURGERY

Underlying CAD (often unrecognized before noncardiac surgery) plays an important role in the pathophysiologic processes of perioperative myocardial infarction (MI). Patients with no history of MI have a low risk of perioperative MI (0.1% to 0.6%); those with a history of prior MI are at significantly higher risk (2.8% to 7%) (4–7); and the highest risk is in patients who sustained

MI within 3 months before noncardiac surgery (6). The majority of perioperative MIs are known to occur in the first 3 days after surgery, with peak incidence on day 2 (5,7). The lack of classic symptoms of chest pain and, instead, an atypical presentation with new-onset congestive heart failure, hypotension, arrhythmias, nausea, or altered mental status makes the clinical diagnosis challenging. Perioperative MI is associated with high mortality rates, ranging from 26% to 70% (1–7). Therefore, it is imperative to identify patients who are at risk for untoward outcomes after surgery by using a systematic stepwise strategic preoperative evaluation, such as that put forward in the guidelines of the American College of Cardiology/American Heart Association (ACC/AHA) Task Force on Practice Guidelines (8–11).

ASSESSING PERIOPERATIVE CARDIAC RISK FOR PATIENTS UNDERGOING NONCARDIAC SURGERY (8–10)

A stepwise approach for assessing risk for patients undergoing noncardiac surgery should address the following questions:

1. Is noncardiac surgery urgently required?
2. Has the patient undergone recent coronary revascularization?
3. Has the patient been evaluated for CAD in the past 2 years?
4. Is the patient at risk for adverse cardiac events?
5. What is the patient's functional capacity?
6. What is the probability of cardiac complications for the patient according to the type of surgery and the institutional experience?

7. Is stress testing or another diagnostic test necessary?
8. Do the benefits of operation outweigh the posttest probability of cardiac complications after surgery?
9. What is needed in terms of modifying preoperative, intraoperative, and postoperative care to reduce the probability of cardiac complications after surgery?
10. What long-term risk stratification and management strategies should be implemented?

Is Noncardiac Surgery Urgently Required?

The urgency of surgery is dictated by patient- or surgery-specific factors, and in some instances, there may not be time for further cardiac assessment. Recommendations should be provided for perioperative medical management and surveillance in such instances. Selected patients, at high risk for long-term coronary events, should undergo risk stratification after their recovery from surgery (8–10).

Has the Patient Undergone Recent Revascularization?

A complete revascularization, in the form of coronary artery bypass grafting (CABG) in previous 5 years or percutaneous transluminal coronary angioplasty in the previous 6 months to 5 years in a functionally active patient who is otherwise free of clinical symptoms of ischemia, is associated with a low likelihood of perioperative cardiac events (8–11). Usually, such patients may proceed to surgery without further cardiac testing.

Has the Patient Been Evaluated for Coronary Artery Disease in the Past Two Years?

In the patients who have been evaluated in the past 2 years with either invasive or noninvasive techniques with favorable findings, no further cardiac workup is generally necessary if they have been free of cardiac symptoms after the test. Patients with changing symptoms or signs of ischemia should be considered for further evaluation (8–10).

Is Patient at Risk for Adverse Cardiac Events?

A baseline history, physical examination, and electrocardiogram (ECG) provide important data with which to estimate cardiac risk. Table 38.1 lists clinical predictors of adverse cardiac outcomes that are based on prior studies (9,11–15). These studies have combined various clinical features associated with poor prognosis into composite clinical risk scores to help quantitate the risk of postoperative events (9,11–15). More recent studies have used more simplistic algorithms (8,16). If a patient has a major clinical predictor as listed in Table 38.1 and is scheduled for elective surgery, it is usually best to postpone surgery until the cardiac problem is clarified (sometimes by coronary arteriography) and treated appropriately (8–10). Patients with

TABLE 38.1. *Clinical predictors of increased perioperative cardiovascular risk (myocardial infarction, congestive heart failure, death)*

Major
Unstable or severe angina (Canadian Cardiovascular Society Class III or IV)
Recent myocardial infarction (>7 days but ≤30 days) with evidence of important ischemic risk by clinical symptoms or noninvasive testing
Decompensated CHF
Symptomatic arrhythmias, including high-grade atrioventricular block, symptomatic ventricular arrhythmia in presence of underlying heart disease, and supraventricular arrhythmias with uncontrolled ventricular rate
Intermediate
Mild angina (Canadian Cardiovascular Society Classes I and II)
Prior myocardial infarction documented by history or ECG
Compensated or prior CHF
Diabetes mellitus
Renal insufficiency (creatinine, ≥2.0 mg/dL)
Minor
Advanced age
Abnormal ECG (left ventricular hypertrophy, left bundle branch block, ST-T abnormalities)
Rhythm other than sinus (e.g., atrial fibrillation)
Low functional capacity
History of stroke
Uncontrolled systemic hypertension

CHF, congestive heart failure; ECG, electrocardiogram.
From "Guidelines for perioperative evaluation for noncardiac surgery"[9]; Goldman et al.[14]; and Cooperman et al.[15]

TABLE 38.2. *Surgery-specific cardiac risk (combined risk of cardiac death and nonfatal myocardial infarction)*

High (reported cardiac risk, often >5%)
Emergency major operation, particularly in elderly
Aortic and other major vascular
Peripheral vascular
Anticipated prolonged surgical procedures associated
    with large fluid shifts and/or blood loss
Intermediate (reported cardiac risk, generally <5%)
Intrathoracic
Intraperitoneal
Carotid endarterectomy
Head and neck
Orthopedic
Prostate
Low (reported cardiac risk, generally <1%)
Endoscopic procedures
Superficial procedures
Cataract
Breast

From "Guidelines for perioperative evaluation for non-cardiac surgery"[9]; Goldman et al.[14]; Eagle et al.[16]; and Mangano et al.[20]

TABLE 38.3. *Functional capacity assessment from clinical history*

Excellent (activities requiring >7 METs)
Carry 24 lb. up eight steps
Carry objects that weight 80 lb.
Outdoor work (shovel snow, spade soil)
Recreation (ski, basketball, squash, handball, jog/walk
    5 mph)
Moderate (activities requiring >4 but <7 METs)
Have sexual intercourse without stopping
Walk at 4 mph on level ground
Outdoor work (garden, rake, weed)
Recreation (rollerskate, dance, foxtrot)
Poor (Activities requiring <4 METs)
Shower/dress without stopping, strip and make bed,
    dust, wash dishes
Walk at 2.5 mph on level ground
Outdoor work (clean windows)
Recreation (play golf, bowl)

MET, metabolic equivalent.
From Paul and Eagle[8]; "Guidelines for periopera-tive evaluation for noncardiac surgery"[9]; Mehta and Eagle[10]; Hiatky et al.[18]; Fiercher et al.[19]

moderate or excellent functional capacity and one or more intermediate predictors of clinical risk can normally undergo low- and intermediate-risk surgery (Table 38.2) with low perioperative cardiac risk. On the other hand, patients with poor functional capacity or a combination of high-risk surgery, moderate functional capacity, and intermediate clinical predictors of cardiac risk (especially two or more) should be evaluated by further noninvasive cardiac testing. In general, patients with minor or no clinical predictors of risk and with moderate or excellent functional capacity [less than four to six metabolic equivalents (METs)] can safely undergo most types of noncardiac surgery with low risk of cardiac complications (8–10).

What Is the Patient's Functional Capacity?

Functional status is reliably predictive of future cardiac events (17) and should be assessed by history in all preoperative patients. Functional capacity (usually expressed as MET levels) may be classified as excellent (more than seven METs), moderate (four to seven METs), poor (fewer than four METs) or unknown. Table 38.3 represents a sample of activities that characterizes each functional class (8,18,19). Poor functional capacity is

a marker for increased risk of perioperative and long-term cardiac events, and patients with poor functional capacity should be considered for non-invasive cardiac risk assessment before elective cardiac surgery, depending on the type of surgery and presence of clinical risk predictors as discussed previously. Patients with moderate or excellent functional capacity and few or no clinical predictors of risk, or patients with a combination of intermediate predictors of cardiac risk, low- or intermediate-risk surgery, and preserved functional capacity, can generally proceed to elective surgery without undergoing further cardiac workup. Patients with poor functional capacity facing intermediate- or high-risk surgery should be considered for cardiac noninvasive evaluation risk preoperatively (8–10).

What Is the Probability of Cardiac Complications for a Patient According to the Type of Surgery and the Institutional Experience?

Specific type of surgery also affects the pretest probability of cardiac complications, as depicted in Table 38.2 (9). Emergency surgery is associated with a fourfold to fivefold increase in risk in comparison with elective surgery (14). In addition, patients undergoing aortic, peripheral arterial, and other major vascular surgery or operations associated with large fluid shifts or blood loss have a relatively high probability (nearly twofold to threefold increase) of cardiac complications. Risk classification of various surgical procedures should be considered along with the predictors of clinical risk and functional capacity in properly risk-stratifying patients before noncardiac surgery (9,14,16,20).

Is Stress Testing or Another Diagnostic Test Necessary?

Simple strategies for preoperative noninvasive testing, proposed by Eagle et al. and other investigators, has been reiterated in current ACC/AHA task force recommendations (8,9,16). Patients classified as being at low clinical risk generally do not need any further risk stratification. Those with major predictors of high clinical risk have a high probability of left main artery or triple-vessel disease and need consideration for a more aggressive approach, including, in selected patients, preoperative coronary angiography and coronary revascularization. The patients at intermediate clinical risk may benefit from noninvasive testing, especially those with poor functional capacity (21). Noninvasive testing is aimed at identifying the degree of ischemic burden or inducible arrhythmias and, in some instances, helps quantify functional capacity and left ventricular function of a patient.

Current Evidence for Diagnostic Testing in Perioperative Risk Assessment

Exercise Electrocardiogram:

The role of exercise stress testing in preoperative assessment has been evaluated in numerous studies (22–29). McPhail et al. (28) reported using preoperative exercise testing in 100 patients undergoing vascular surgery and that the highest cardiac complication rate (33%) was evident in patients with exercise-induced ischemia and low workload achieved. Cutler et al. (24) documented that the ability to attain 75% to 85% of maximum age-predicted heart rate was predictive of

a low rate of perioperative cardiac events. Poor functional capacity associated with ischemia indicated high risk for perioperative cardiac events (30). Ischemia in patients with excellent functional capacity appeared to confer a small increase in risk (8). However, in many patients, the presence of baseline ECG abnormalities and their inability to exercise secondary to comorbid conditions limits the widespread use of exercise ECG for risk assessment.

Pharmacologic Stress Test and Myocardial Perfusion Imaging

The utility of preoperative dipyridamole-thallium imaging for risk stratification was first reported by Boucher et al. (31) in 1985 and has since been validated in numerous investigations (16,32–37). The positive predictive value has been consistently low, between 4% and 20%. This is attributed in part to the fact that stress testing results are now used for risk modification in the form of preoperative coronary revascularization, adjustment of medical management, aggressive monitoring, selection of a different surgical or anesthetic approach, and, for certain patients, cancellation of elective surgery (8–10). On the other hand, most studies have reported a consistently high negative predictive value (more than 95%). The presence of thallium redistribution, especially in increasing numbers of myocardial segments, identifies patients at high risk of perioperative cardiac complications (32,36), whereas the presence of fixed defects identifies patients at intermediate risk, particularly for late cardiac events (35).

Dobutamine Stress Echocardiography. Dobutamine stress echocardiography has been less extensively studied than dipyridamole-thallium imaging. Available data support its utility and safety (36–40). The number of myocardial segments demonstrating wall motion abnormalities or wall motion changes at low infusion rates of dobutamine identified patients at high risk. The positive predictive value and negative predictive value for hard end points (MI and death) were comparable to those of dipyridamole-thallium testing (positive predictive value, 7% to 23%; negative predictive value, 93% to 100%).

Ambulatory Electrocardiographic Monitoring

Studies using preoperative ambulatory ECG monitoring have demonstrated a predictive value similar to that of dipyridamole thallium (41,42,43). However, current evidence does not support its sole use for identifying patients to be referred for coronary angiography (9).

Coronary Angiography in Perioperative Evaluation for Patients Undergoing Noncardiac Surgery

Recommendations for coronary angiography are similar to those for patients with suspected or known CAD in general and should conform to the ACC/AHA guidelines for coronary angiography (45). This procedure should be considered for patients who have unstable angina, angina refractory to medical treatment, high-risk results on noninvasive testing, or a nondiagnostic test in patients at high risk undergoing high-risk noncardiac surgery. It should be considered on an individual basis for occasional patients with intermediate-risk results during noninvasive testing, for patients at low risk undergoing high-risk surgery with nondiagnostic test results, for patients convalescing from MI who needs urgent noncardiac surgery, and for patients with perioperative MI (9,45).

Do the Benefits of Operation Outweigh the Posttest Probability of Cardiac Complications after Surgery?

All information obtained from such a systematic stepwise approach for preoperative cardiac risk assessment for noncardiac surgery should then be used to decide whether the risk of perioperative cardiac events is sufficiently low to proceed with surgery. For patients identified at high cardiac risk who are not candidates for coronary revascularization, this may result in a decision to perform a less extensive procedure or to cancel the surgery. Once a decision is made to proceed with noncardiac surgery, the next goal is to attempt to modify cardiac risk by additional therapies, including coronary revascularization

in individuals at high risk. The periprocedural complication rate with coronary revascularization must be carefully weighed against the risk of cardiac complications after noncardiac surgery in such individuals (8–10).

What Is Needed in Terms of Modifying Preoperative, Intraoperative, and Postoperative Care to Reduce the Probability of Cardiac Complications after Surgery?

Role of Preoperative Coronary Artery Bypass Surgery

Retrospective observational studies have suggested a protective effect of prior CABG against postoperative cardiac complications after noncardiac surgery (12,13,46–48). Eagle et al. (49) examined the value of CABG on patients undergoing noncardiac surgery among the patients enrolled in the Coronary Artery Surgery Study (CASS) registry. Patients with known CAD who were being managed medically and undergoing high-risk surgery such as abdominal, vascular, thoracic, and head and neck surgery had a combined MI/death rate of greater than 4% for each procedure. In patients who have undergone prior CABG, reduced incidences of postoperative death (1.7% vs. 3.3%; $p = 0.03$) and MIs (0.8% vs. 2.7%; $p = 0.002$) were observed in comparison with the medical treatment group. Patients undergoing low-risk procedures, such as urologic, orthopedic, breast, and skin operations, had a low mortality rate (less than 1%) regardless of prior revascularization. Prior CABG was found to be especially protective in patients with more severe angina or multivessel CAD or both (49).

Patients who have undergone prior CABG within 5 years of noncardiac surgery usually require no further preoperative testing unless they have developed new coronary symptoms (6–8). Indications for CABG in patients undergoing noncardiac surgery include acceptable coronary revascularization risk and viable myocardium with left main artery disease, three-vessel disease in conjunction with left ventricular dysfunction, two-vessel disease with proximal left anterior descending arterial stenosis, and angina refractory to maximal medical management (50).

Role of Preoperative Coronary Angioplasty

Percutaneous coronary interventions (PCIs) have been increasingly used to treat patients with CAD undergoing noncardiac surgery. However, randomized trials addressing the issue of perioperative cardiac risk reduction with the use of preoperative PCI are lacking. A selected group of symptomatic patients facing high-risk surgery may benefit from PCI; this recommendation is based on retrospective series with small numbers of patients (51–54). A study by Kaluza et al. (55) suggested that coronary stent implantation may be actually harmful if performed in the immediate preoperative period. Of 40 patients who had coronary stent implantation within 6 weeks before noncardiac surgery, 7 had MI, 11 had major bleeding episodes, and 8 died. All Mis, all deaths, and most of the bleeding episodes occurred in patients who underwent coronary stent implantation less than 2 weeks before surgery. The authors speculated that the partial or complete interruption of antiplatelet therapy (which occurred in many patients preoperatively) led to the high incidence of perioperative stent thrombosis. In addition, the discontinuation of antiplatelet agents in the 1 to 2 days before surgery was insufficient to prevent excessive bleeding, and continuation of dual antiplatelet therapy perioperatively resulted in an increased risk of major bleeding. Thus, noncardiac surgery should probably be scheduled several weeks after PCI (preferably after 4 weeks). This is because arterial recoil and acute thrombosis may occur over the first 1 to 2 days after the procedure, the hypercoagulable state of surgery may increase the risk of coronary thrombosis (particularly in stent-implanted patients), and the antiplatelet therapy could lead to increased risk of bleeding during this period. In contrast, delaying surgery beyond 8 to 12 weeks after PCI increases the chance of restenosis. Also, because the incidence of coronary restenosis is reduced beyond 6 months, patients who are asymptomatic and physically very active between 6 months and 5 years after revascularization with PCI do not generally require further preoperative risk assessment before noncardiac surgery (8–10).

Whether revascularization with percutaneous techniques or CABG confers greater protection against perioperative events is unknown. The only study that addressed this issue to date is a retrospective analysis from the Bypass Angioplasty Revascularization Investigation (BARI) (56). In this study, patients with unstable angina and multivessel CAD with preserved left ventricular function that were suitable for either form of revascularization were assigned to undergo either PCI or CABG. During a mean follow-up of 7.7 years, a total of 501 patients underwent noncardiac surgery at a median of 29 months after their most recent revascularization. Rates of mortality and nonfatal MI within 30 days of noncardiac surgery were low (1.6% in both groups). Furthermore, the mean length of hospital stay and mean hospital cost were similar for patients undergoing PCI and CABG (56). Thus, at present, the choice of procedure should be guided by overall patient and coronary anatomic characteristics.

Role of Medical Therapy

Small studies have evaluated the use of perioperative beta blockers in reducing cardiac risk (57–59). Stone et al. (57), in a small, randomized trial of patients with mild hypertension, gave oral beta blockers 2 hours before the induction of anesthesia. The control group had a higher incidence of ischemia than did the patients who received beta blockers (28% vs. 2%). Similarly, perioperative ischemia and MI have been shown to be reduced by metoprolol (58,59). More recently, Mangano et al. showed that patients undergoing vascular surgery who were randomly assigned to receive atenolol (vs. placebo) had a reduced cardiac event rate over the first year or two after surgery (60,61). Similarly, Froehlich et al. (62) reported protection against cardiac death after vascular surgery in patients treated with beta blockers in a large observational study. Finally, Poldermans et al. (63) studied 112 patients undergoing high-risk vascular procedures. Those with one or more clinical markers of risk and ischemia demonstrated by dobutamine stress echocardiography were randomly assigned to receive the beta blocker bisoprolol (titrated to a heart rate of 60 beats per minute) or standard care before surgery. The incidence of death in the bisoprolol recipients was 3.4%, in contrast to 17% in the patients receiving standard care. Furthermore, there were no nonfatal MIs in the bisoprolol recipients, in contrast to a 17% incidence in the standard care recipients. Overall, treatment with bisoprolol was associated with a 90% reduction in the composite end point of nonfatal MI and death. Further analysis of the data from this study suggested that in patients at low clinical risk receiving beta blockers in the perioperative period, the additional predictive value of dobutamine stress echocardiography was limited (64). However, among patients at intermediate and high risk receiving beta blockers, dobutamine stress echocardiography can identify those who would potentially benefit from revascularization before noncardiac surgery (64).

Thus, in patients with strong suspicion of or at risk for CAD, beta blockers should be given in the perioperative period, starting at least 24 hours before the procedure and titrated rapidly to a heart rate of 60 beats per minute. Few data exist to support the use of calcium channel blockers and nitroglycerin. Whether this strategy of beta blockade is superior, similar, or inferior to revascularization is currently unknown. Results of a large randomized Department of Veterans Affairs Cooperative Trial [the Coronary Artery Revascularization Prophylaxis (CARP) Trial] will help address the role of revascularization before noncardiac versus aggressive medical treatment for reducing perioperative risk (65). Currently, these are recommended for all patients at high risk and for those who have active signs of myocardial ischemia without hypotension (9).

Other Strategies for Reducing Perioperative Risk

Pain management in the perioperative period is crucial for reducing cardiac risk. Adequate pain control reduces catecholamine surges, which are probably responsible for increasing myocardial oxygen demand, induction of coronary vasospasm, increasing the tendency for plaque rupture, and development of a hypercoagulable state. A hematocrit of more than 10 mg/dL and an oxygen tension higher than 60 facilitate tissue oxygenation and help decrease myocardial necrosis. Pulmonary artery catheters are indicated for patients with limited ventricular reserve who are undergoing procedures that are likely to cause major hemodynamic shifts (66). There is little to recommend their use for monitoring for ischemia (9). The routine use of intraoperative transesophageal echocardiography is not recommended for monitoring and guiding therapy during noncardiac surgery, because of lack of robust data. Literature supporting intraoperative ST segment monitoring via telemetry or ambulatory monitoring in patients at high risk is limited.

Monitoring for Perioperative Myocardial Infarction

Few studies have examined the optimal strategy for the diagnosis of perioperative MI (67). A protocol involving an ECG immediately after surgery and on the first and second postoperative days has the highest sensitivity, whereas routine measurements of serial creatine kinase and myocardial band fraction had higher false positive rates and did not increase the sensitivity. Higher levels of creatine kinase and myocardial band fraction elevation have been associated with worse survival rates (68). The newer myocardium-specific biomarkers such as troponin I and troponin T have similarly been shown to be associated with increased risk of cardiac events if their levels are found elevated in the postoperative period (69–71). Current recommendations favor monitoring for signs of cardiac dysfunction in patients with evidence of CAD. In such patients undergoing surgical procedures associated with high cardiac risk, ECG at baseline, immediately after surgery and on the first 2 days postoperatively, should be obtained. Measurement of cardiac biomarkers should be reserved for patients at high risk and for those who demonstrate clinical, ECG, or hemodynamic evidence of cardiovascular dysfunction (8).

What Long-Term Risk Stratification and Management Strategies Should Be Implemented?

Postoperative patient care involves assessment and treatment of modifiable cardiac risk factors, including hypertension, hyperlipidemia, smoking, obesity, hyperglycemia, and physical inactivity. Patients who sustain a perioperative MI or develop evidence of ischemia should be carefully investigated, because they are at substantial cardiac risk over the subsequent 5 to 10 years. Noninvasive testing to assess left ventricular function and inducible ischemia should be undertaken to identify patients who may benefit from revascularization or optimization of medical therapy (8–10).

NONCARDIAC SURGERY IN PATIENTS WITH SPECIFIC CARDIOVASCULAR CONDITIONS

Valvular Heart Disease

Severe aortic stenosis poses a higher risk in noncardiac surgery (14). Patients with severe symptomatic aortic stenosis should undergo aortic valve replacement before noncardiac surgery. In rare instances, balloon aortic valvuloplasty may be justified before elective noncardiac surgery. A retrospective study suggested that selected patients with asymptomatic severe aortic stenosis could safely undergo noncardiac surgery with careful hemodynamic monitoring (72).

Heart rate should be controlled to ensure sufficient diastolic filling period and avoid pulmonary congestion in patients with mild to moderate mitral stenosis. Patients with severe mitral stenosis benefit from balloon mitral valvuloplasty or surgical repair before high-risk surgery.

Patients with aortic or mitral regurgitation benefit from volume control and afterload reduction. A slow heart rate increases diastolic filling per minute and can exacerbate left ventricular volume overload, owing to aortic regurgitation. Faster heart rates are better tolerated in this particular condition.

In patients with a mechanical valve prosthesis, the prothrombin time should be reduced briefly to low or subtherapeutic range for minor procedures such as dental work and superficial biopsies, and anticoagulation should be resumed immediately after the procedure. Patients at high risk of bleeding while taking oral anticoagulants and those at high risk of thrombotic complications when not taking them should receive perioperative heparin. Patients between these two extremes should undergo individual assessment for the risk and benefit of reduced anticoagulation with warfarin versus perioperative heparin initiation and brief interruption surrounding surgery. Patients with valvular heart disease require appropriate antibiotic prophylaxis for endocarditis.

Arrhythmias and Conduction Defect

Cardiac arrhythmias in the perioperative period are common and are usually indicative of underlying cardiopulmonary disease, drug toxicity, or metabolic disturbances (14). Third-degree atrioventricular block can increase operative risk and necessitates pacing (9).

Congestive Heart Failure and Left Ventricular Dysfunction

Congestive heart failure (CHF) has been identified as significant marker of cardiac risk for noncardiac surgery (73). Every effort should be made to identify the etiology of CHF. Patients should be appropriately treated for the cause of CHF before noncardiac surgery. Close monitoring of the volume status is needed to avoid perioperative decompensation. Use of intravenous inotropic agents, vasodilators, or both for a short duration in the perioperative period is often useful to prevent and/or treat CHF.

Hypertrophic Cardiomyopathy

A decreased preload (large amount of blood or fluid loss or tachycardia caused by pain that reduces diastolic filling), a reduced afterload, and an increase in contractility (caused by inotropic agents) is poorly tolerated by patients with hypertrophic cardiomyopathy. These conditions should be avoided in such patients undergoing noncardiac surgery. Patients with hypertrophic cardiomyopathy are at significant risk for developing perioperative hypotension, CHF, and arrhythmias and should be monitored closely (74).

Congenital Heart Disease

Studies have demonstrated that patients with left-to-right cardiac shunts have residual hemodynamic abnormalities even after surgical repair, including decreased cardiac output response to exercise (75,76). Vigorous treatment of CHF is required for such patients before noncardiac surgery. Patients with a large left-to-right shunt but only a slight increase in pulmonary artery resistance should undergo cardiac repair before noncardiac surgery. Patients with irreversible pulmonary artery hypertension have an extremely high risk associated with nonsurgical procedures and should not undergo elective procedures unless there is absolutely no alternative.

Patients with prior repair of coarctation of the aorta have a significant frequency of sudden death during follow-up (77,78), caused by residual cardiac defects with CHF, rupture of a major vessel, dissecting aneurysm, or complications arising from severe atherosclerosis. Such patients also have a high incidence of residual hypertension. Therefore, these patients require appropriate preoperative assessment and close hemodynamic monitoring during the intraoperative and postoperative periods.

Patients with tetralogy of Fallot are also prone to sudden cardiac death (79). Monitoring and treatment of life-threatening arrhythmias such as ventricular tachycardia or atrioventricular block is recommended for such patients in the perioperative period.

Surgery in patients with cyanotic congenital heart disease with right-to-left shunts poses several unique problems. Most cyanotic patients are polycythemic and therefore are prone to thrombotic complications. Use of diuretics should be avoided in such patients, because dehydration may increase the blood viscosity and, in turn, increase the tendency for thrombosis, particularly cerebral thrombosis. Patients with a hematocrit greater than 70% should be considered for plasmapheresis before noncardiac surgery. Phlebotomy is not advisable in this circumstance, because this can decrease intravascular blood volume and thus increase cyanosis. Patients with a hematocrit between 55% and 65% should receive intravenous fluids starting the night before the surgery. Patients with congenital heart disease should also receive appropriate prophylaxis for bacterial endocarditis. One retrospective report suggested that, with careful monitoring and precautions as outlined previously, patients with right-to-left shunts could undergo noncardiac surgery with relatively few complications (80).

PRACTICAL POINTS

- CAD accounts for most deaths in patients undergoing noncardiac surgery.
- The majority of perioperative MIs are known to occur in the first 3 days after surgery; the incidence peaks on day 2.
- Perioperative MI is associated with high mortality rates.
- Functional status is reliably predictive of future cardiac events and should be assessed by documenting the history in all preoperative patients. Functional capacity (usually expressed as MET levels) may be classified as excellent (more than seven METs), moderate (four to seven METs), poor (fewer than four METs), or unknown.
- All information obtained from a systematic stepwise approach for preoperative cardiac risk assessment for noncardiac surgery should then be used to decide whether the risk of perioperative cardiac events is sufficiently low to proceed with surgery.
- In patients with strong suspicion or at risk for CAD, beta blockers should be given in perioperative period, starting at least 24 hours before the procedure and titrated

(continued)

rapidly to a heart rate of 60 beats per minute.

- Besides perioperative beta blockers, other strategies found useful in reducing the perioperative risk include pain management, maintaining hematocrit at more than 30 mg/dL, and avoiding excessive fluid repletion. Pain management in the perioperative period is crucial for reducing cardiac risk. Adequate pain control reduces catecholamine surges, which are probably responsible for increasing myocardial oxygen demand, induction of

coronary vasospasm, increasing the tendency for plaque rupture, and development of a hypercoagulable state.

- Postoperative patient care involves assessment and treatment of modifiable cardiac risk factors, including hypertension, hyperlipidemia, smoking, obesity, hyperglycemia, and physical inactivity.
- Patients who sustain a perioperative MI or develop evidence of ischemia should be carefully investigated because they are at substantial cardiac risk over the subsequent 5 to 10 years.

REFERENCES

1. Dudley JC, Brandenburg JA, Hartley JA, et al. Last minute pre-operative cardiology consultations: epidemiology and impact. *Am Heart J* 1996;131:245–249.
2. Mangano DT. Perioperative cardiac morbidity. *Anesthesiology* 1990;72:153–184.
3. Brener S, Cohen MC, Talley JD, et al. Striking hospital to hospital variation in pre-operative cardiac work-up for patients referred for major non-cardiac surgery. *Circulation* 1995;92:I-679(abst).
4. Topkins MJ, Artusio JF. Myocardial infarction and surgery. *Anesth Analg* 1964;43:716–720.
5. Tarhan S, Moffitt EA, Taylor WF, et al. Myocardial infarction after general anesthesia. *JAMA* 1972;220:1451–1454.
6. Steen PA, Tinker JH, Tarhan S. Myocardial reinfarction after anesthesia and surgery. *JAMA* 1978;239:2566–2570.
7. Von Knorring J. Postoperative myocardial infarction: a prospective study in a risk group of surgical patients. *Surgery* 1981;90:55–60.
8. Paul SD, Eagle KA. A stepwise strategy for coronary risk assessment for noncardiac surgery. *Med Clin North Am* 1995;79:1241–1262.
9. Guidelines for perioperative evaluation for noncardiac surgery. Report of the American College of Cardiology/American Heart Association Task Force on Practice Guidelines (Committee on Perioperative Cardiovascular Evaluation for Noncardiac Surgery). *J Am Coll Cardiol* 1996;27:910–948.
10. Mehta RH, Eagle KA. How to assess cardiac risk before noncardiac surgery?. *Int Med* 1998;19:27–39.
11. Mahar LJ, Steen PA, Tinker JH, et al. Perioperative myocardial infarction in patients with coronary artery disease with and without aorta-coronary bypass grafts. *J Thorac Cardiovasc Surg* 1978;76:533–537.
12. Hertzer NR, Beven EG, Young JR, et al. Coronary artery disease in peripheral vascular patients: a classification of 1000 coronary angiograms and results of surgical management. *Ann Surg* 1984;199:223–233.
13. Hertzer NR, Young JR, Beven EG, et al. Late results of coronary bypass in patients with peripheral vascular dis-

ease, II: five-year survival according to sex, hypertension, and diabetes. *Cleve Clin J Med* 1987;54:15–23.
14. Goldman L, Caldera DL, Nussbaum SR, et al. Multifactorial index of cardiac risk in noncardiac surgical procedures. *N Engl J Med* 1977;297:845–850.
15. Cooperman M, Pflung B, Martin EW Jr, et al. Cardiovascular risk factor in patients with peripheral vascular disease. *Surgery* 1978;84:505–509.
16. Eagle KA, Coley CM, Newell JB, et al. Combining clinical and thallium data optimizes perioperative assessment of cardiac risk before major vascular surgery. *Ann Intern Med* 1989;110:859–866.
17. Weiner DA, Ryan TJ, McCabe CH, et al. Prognostic importance of clinical profile and exercise test in medically treated patients with coronary artery disease. *J Am Coll Cardiol* 1984;3:772–779.
18. Hlatky MA, Boineau RE, Higginbotham MB, et al. A brief self administered questionnaire to determine functional capacity (the Duke Activity Status Index). *Am J Cardiol* 1989;64:651–654.
19. Fletcher GF, Balady G, Froelicher VF, et al. Exercise standard: a statement for health professionals from the American Heart Association: Writing Group. *Circulation* 1995;91:580–615.
20. Mangano DT, Browner WS, Hollenberg M, et al. Association of perioperative myocardial ischemia with cardiac morbidity and mortality in men undergoing noncardiac surgery: the Study of Perioperative Ischemia Group. *N Engl J Med* 1990;323:1781–1788.
21. L'Italien GJ, Cambria RP, Cutler BS, et al. Comparative early and late cardiac morbidity among patients requiring different vascular surgery procedures. *J Vasc Surg* 1995;21:935–944.
22. Arous EJ, Baum PL, Cutler BS. The ischemic exercise test in patients with peripheral vascular disease: implications for management. *Arch Surg* 1984;119:780–783.
23. Carliner NH, Fisher ML, Plotnick GD, et al. Routine preoperative exercise testing in patients undergoing major noncardiac surgery. *Am J Cardiol* 1985;56:51–58.
24. Cutler BS, Wheeler HB, Paraskos JA, et al. Applicability and interpretation of electrocardiographic stress testing

in patients with peripheral vascular disease. *Am J Surg* 1981;141:501–506.

25. Gardine RL, McBride K, Greenberg H, et al. The value of cardiac monitoring during peripheral arterial stress testing in surgical management of peripheral vascular disease. *J Cardiovasc Surg* 1985;26:258–261.

26. Gerson MC, Hurst JM, Hertzberg VS, et al. Prediction of cardiac and pulmonary complications related to elective abdominal and noncardiac thoracic surgery in geriatric patients. *Am J Med* 1990;88:101–107.

27. Leppo J, Plaja J, Gionet M, et al. Noninvasive evaluation of cardiac risk before elective vascular surgery. *J Am Coll Cardiol* 1987;9:269–276.

28. McPhail N, Calvin JE, Shariatmadar A, et al. The use of preoperative exercise testing to predict cardiac complications after arterial reconstruction. *J Vasc Surg* 1988;11:70–74.

29. Von Knorring J, Lepantalo M. Prediction of postoperative cardiac complications by electrocardiographic monitoring during treadmill exercise testing before peripheral vascular surgery. *Surgery* 1986;99:610–613.

30. Morris CK, Ueshima K, Kawaguchi T, et al. The prognostic value of exercise capacity: a review of literature. *Am Heart J* 1991;122:1423–1431.

31. Boucher CA, Brewster DC, Darling RC, et al. Determination of cardiac risk by dipyridamole-thallium imaging before peripheral vascular surgery. *N Engl J Med* 1985;312:389–394.

32. Lette J, Waters D, Cerino M, et al. Coronary artery disease risk stratification based on dipyridamole imaging and a simple three-step, three-segment model for patients undergoing noncardiac vascular surgery or major general surgery. *Am J Cardiol* 1992;70:1243–1249.

33. McEnroe CS, O'Donell RF, Yeager A, et al. Comparison of ejection fraction and Goldman risk factor analysis of dipyridamole–thallium-201 studies in the evaluation of cardiac morbidity after aortic aneurysm surgery. *J Vasc Surg* 1990;11:497–504.

34. Baron JF, Mundler O, Bertrand M, et al. Dipyridamole-thallium scintigraphy and gated radionuclide angiography to assess cardiac risk before abdominal aortic surgery. *N Engl J Med* 1994;330:663–669.

35. Coley CM, Field TS, Abraham SA, et al. Usefulness of dipyridamole-thallium scanning for preoperative evaluation of cardiac risk for nonvascular surgery. *Am J Cardiol* 1992;69:1280–1285.

36. Hendel RC, Whitfield SS, Villegas BJ, et al. Prediction of late cardiac events by dipyridamole-thallium imaging in patients undergoing elective vascular surgery. *Am J Cardiol* 1992;70:1243–1249.

37. Shaw L, Miller DD, Kong BA, et al. Determination of perioperative cardiac risk by adenosine thallium-201 myocardial imaging. *Am Heart J* 1992;124:861–869.

38. Lane RT, Sawada SG, Segar DS, et al. Dobutamine stress echocardiography for the assessment of cardiac risk before noncardiac surgery. *Am J Cardiol* 1991;68:976–977.

39. Lalka SG, Sawada SG, Dalsing MC, et al. Dobutamine stress echocardiography as a predictor of cardiac events associated with aortic surgery. *J Vasc Surg* 1992;15:831–840.

40. Eichelberger JP, Schwarz KQ, Black ER, et al. Predictive value of dobutamine echocardiography just before noncardiac vascular surgery. *Am J Cardiol* 1993;72:602–607.

41. Langan EM III, Youkey JR, Franklin DP, et al. Dobutamine stress echocardiography for cardiac risk assessment before aortic surgery. *J Vasc Surg* 1993;18:905–911.

42. Davila-Roman VG, Waggoner AD, Sicard GA, et al. Dobutamine stress echocardiography predicts surgical outcome in patients with aortic aneurysm and peripheral vascular disease. *J Am Coll Cardiol* 1993;21:957–963.

43. McPhail NV, Ruddy TD, Barber GG, et al. Cardiac risk stratification using dipyridamole myocardial perfusion imaging and ambulatory ECG monitoring prior to vascular surgery. *Eur J Vasc Surg* 1993;7:151–155.

44. Fleisher LA, Rosenbaum SH, Nelson NH, et al. Preoperative dipyridamole thallium imaging and Holter monitoring as predictor of perioperative cardiac events and long term outcome. *Anesthesiology* 1995;83:906–917.

45. Guidelines for coronary angiography. A report of the American College of Cardiology/American Heart Association Task Force on Assessment of Diagnostic and Therapeutic Cardiovascular procedures (Subcommittee on Coronary Angiography). *J Am Coll Cardiol* 1987;10:935–950.

46. Diehl JT, Cali RF, Hertzer NR, et al. Complications of abdominal aortic reconstruction: an analysis of perioperative risk factors in 557 patients. *Ann Surg* 1983;197:49–56.

47. Nielsen JL, Page CP, Mann C, et al. Risk of major elective operation after myocardial revascularization. *Am J Surg* 1992;164:423–426.

48. Rihal CS, Eagle KA, Mickel MC, et al. Surgical therapy of coronary artery disease among patients with combined coronary and peripheral vascular disease. *Circulation* 1995;91:46–53.

49. Eagle KA, Rihal CS, Mickel MC, et al, for CASS Investigators and University of Michigan Heart Care Program. Cardiac risk of noncardiac surgery: influence of coronary artery disease and type of surgery in 3368 operations. *Circulation* 1997;96:1882–1887.

50. Guidelines and indications for coronary artery bypass graft surgery: a report of the American College of Cardiology/American Heart Association Task Force on Assessment of Diagnostic and Therapeutic Cardiovascular Procedures (Subcommittee on Coronary Artery Bypass Graft Surgery). *J Am Coll Cardiol* 1991;17:543–589.

51. Huber KC, Evans MA, Bresnahan JF, et al. Outcome of noncardiac operations in patients with severe coronary artery disease successfully treated preoperatively with coronary angioplasty. *Mayo Clin Proc* 1992;67:15–21.

52. Elmore JR, Hallett JW, Gibbons RJ, et al. Myocardial revascularization before abdominal aortic aneurysmorrhaphy: effect of coronary angioplasty. *Mayo Clin Proc* 1993;68:637–641.

53. Allen JR, Helling TS, Hartzler GO. Operative procedures not involving the heart after percutaneous transluminal coronary angioplasty. *Surg Gynecol Obstet* 1991;173:285–288.

54. Gottlieb A, Banoub M, Sprung J, et al. Perioperative cardiovascular morbidity in patients with coronary artery disease undergoing vascular surgery after percutaneous transluminal coronary angioplasty. *J Cardiothorac Vasc Anesth* 1998;12:501–506.

55. Kaluza GL, Joseph J, Lee JR, et al. Catastrophic outcomes of noncardiac surgery soon after coronary stenting. *J Am Coll Cardiol* 2000;35:1288–1294.

56. Hassan SA, Hlatky MA, Boothroyd DB, et al. Outcomes of noncardiac surgery after coronary artery bypass surgery or coronary angioplasty in the Bypass Angioplasty Revascularization Investigation (BARI). *Am J Med* 2001;110:260–266.

57. Stone JG, Foex P, Sear JW, et al. Myocardial ischemia in untreated hypertensive patients: effect of a single small oral dose of beta-adrenergic blocking agent. *Anesthesiology* 1988;68:495–500.

58. Pasternack PF, Grossi EA, Baumann FG, et al. Beta blockade to decrease silent myocardial ischemia during peripheral vascular surgery. *Am J Surg* 1989;158:113–116.

59. Pasternack PF, Imparto AM, Baumann FG, et al. The hemodynamics of beta-blockade in patients undergoing abdominal aneurysm repair. *Circulation* 1987;76(Suppl III):III-1–III-7.

60. Mangano DT, Layug EL, Wallace A, et al. Effect of atenolol on mortality and cardiovascular morbidity after noncardiac surgery. Multicenter Study of Perioperative Ischemia research Group. *N Engl J Med* 1996;335:1713–1720.

61. Eagle KA, Froehlich JB. Reducing cardiovascular risk in patients undergoing noncardiac surgery [Editorial; comment]. *N Engl J Med* 1996;335:1761–1763.

62. Froehlich JB, L'Italien G, Paul S, et al. Improved cardiovascular mortality with perioperative beta blockade in patients undergoing major vascular surgery. *J Am Coll Cardiol* 1997;29:219A.

63. Poldermans D, Boersma E, Bax JJ, et al. The effect of bisoprolol on perioperative mortality and myocardial infarction in high-risk patients undergoing vascular surgery. Dutch Echocardiographic Cardiac Risk Evaluation Applying Stress Echocardiography Study Group. *N Engl J Med* 1999;341:1789–1794.

64. Boersma E, Poldermans D, Bax JJ, et al. Predictors of cardiac events after major vascular surgery: role of clinical echocardiography and beta-blocker therapy. *JAMA* 2001;285:1865–1873.

65. McFalls EO, Ward HB, Krupski WC, et al. Prophylactic coronary artery revascularization for elective vascular surgery: study design. Veterans Affairs Cooperative Study Group on Coronary Artery Revascularization Prophylaxis for Elective Vascular Surgery. *Control Clin Trials* 1999;20(3):297–308.

66. Practice guidelines for pulmonary artery catheterization: A report by the American Society of Anesthesiologists Task Force on Pulmonary Artery Catheterization. *Anesthesiology* 1993;78:380–394.

67. Charlson ME, MacKenzie CR, Ales K, et al. Surveillance for post operative myocardial infarction after noncardiac operations. *Surg Gyn Obstet* 1988;167:404–414.

68. Rettke SR, Shub C, Naessen JM, et al. Significance of mildly elevated creatine kinase (myocardial band) activity after elective abdominal aneurysmectomy. *J Cardiovasc Vasc Anesth* 1991;56:20–23.

69. Lee TH, Thomas EJ, Ludwig LE, et al. Troponin T as a marker for myocardial ischemia in patients undergoing major noncardiac surgery. *Am J Cardiol* 1996;77:1031–1036.

70. Lopez-Jimenez F, Goldman L, Sacks DB, et al. Prognostic value of cardiac troponin T after noncardiac surgery: 6-month follow-up data. *J Am Coll Cardiol* 1997;29:1241–1245.

71. Metzler H, Gries M, Rehak P, et al. Perioperative myocardial cell injury: the role of troponins. *Br J Anesth* 1997;78:386–390.

72. O'Keefe JH, Shub C, Rettke SR. Risk of noncardiac surgical procedures in patients with aortic stenosis. *Mayo Clin Proc* 1989;64:400–407.

73. Detsky AS, Abrams HB, McLaughlin JR, et al. Predicting cardiac complications in patients undergoing noncardiac surgery. *J Gen Intern Med* 1986;41:42–50.

74. Thompson RC, Liberthson RR, Lowenstein E. Perioperative anesthetic risk of noncardiac surgery in hypertrophic obstructive cardiomyopathy. *JAMA* 1985;254:2419–2421.

75. Tikoff G, Keith TB, Nelson RM, et al. Clinical and hemodynamic observations after closure of large atrial septal defects complicated by heart failure. *Am J Cardiol* 1969;23:810–817.

76. Lueker RD, Vogel JH, Blount SG Jr. Cardiovascular abnormalities following surgery for left to right shunts: observations in atrial septal defects, ventricular septal defects and patent ductus arteriosus. *Circulation* 1969;40:785–801.

77. Maron BJ, Humphries JO, Rowe RD, et al. Prognosis of surgically corrected coarctation of the aorta: a 20-year postoperative appraisal. *Circulation* 1973;47:119–126.

78. Simon AB, Zloto AE. Coarctation of aorta: longitudinal assessment of operated patients. *Circulation* 1974;50:456–464.

79. James FW, Kaplan S, Swartz DC, et al. Response to exercise in patients after total surgical correction of tetralogy of Fallot. *Circulation* 1976;54:671–679.

80. Ammash NM, Connolly HM, Abel MD, et al. Noncardiac surgery in Eisenmenger syndrome. *J Am Coll Cardiol* 1999;33:222–227

39

Management of the Cardiac Surgery Patient

David B. S. Dyke, Richard L. Prager, and Kim A. Eagle

THE EVOLUTION OF PROCEDURES, CARE SYSTEMS, TECHNOLOGY, AND EXPECTATIONS

The history of coronary artery revascularization dates back to the pre–World War I era. Alexis Carrel developed a canine model of aortocoronary anastomosis, using carotid arteries as conduit, work for which he was ultimately awarded the Nobel Prize (1). In an address to the American Surgical Association, Carrel spoke of some of the difficulties he encountered:

> "In certain cases of angina pectoris, when the mouth of the coronary is calcified, it would be useful to establish a complementary circulation for the lower part of the arteries. I attempted to perform an indirect anastomosis between the descending aorta and the left coronary. It was, for many reasons, a difficult operation. On account of continuous motion of the heart it was not easy to dissect and to suture the artery. In one case, I implanted one end of a long carotid artery, preserved in cold storage, on the descending aorta. The other end was passed through the pericardium and anastomosed to the peripheral end of the coronary, near the pulmonary artery. Unfortunately, the operation was too slow. Three minutes after the interruption of the circulation [by caval occlusion], fibrillatory contractions appeared, but the anastomosis took five minutes. By massage of the heart, the dog was kept alive. But he died less than two hours afterwards. It shows that the anastomosis must be done in less than three minutes."

It was not until the advent of cardiopulmonary bypass technology that this surgical technique could be applied to human heart surgery. Up until that time, surgical techniques aimed at myocardial revascularization had met with only limited success. The Vineberg procedure (2), in which the internal mammary artery was implanted into the myocardium with subsequent collateralization, was one such technique.

The first successful use of full cardiopulmonary bypass occurred in 1953. Dr. John Gibbon used this technology to close an atrial septal defect (3). The clinical use of this early "heart-lung machine" ushered in a new era in cardiac surgery. Soon to follow was the evolution of different types of conduits. Carotid arteries, were quickly replaced first by the use of internal mammary arteries and later by saphenous veins. Not until years later were the benefits of arterial over venous conduits recognized.

The advent of modern cardiac surgery led to a new paradigm for patient care. The physicians charged with such responsibility, the equivalent of the modern-day "intensivist," developed techniques to deal with the multisystem issues that arose as a consequence of cardiopulmonary bypass and cardiac surgery. One of the most useful developments of this era, the intensive care unit, is now widely used across the various surgical and medical subspecialties.

The role of new technologies, such as off-pump and minimally invasive techniques, total arterial revascularization, and percutaneous and laser approaches to coronary revascularization, continue to push the boundaries of cardiovascular medicine. Today, physicians have entered a true surgical and medical cardiac revascularization renaissance. Because of ever-increasing options, the process of determining which procedure or technique is correct for a patient is becoming increasingly more challenging. With this challenge, physicians find themselves in the process of relying on yet another tool: outcomes research.

The accumulation of large databases of information relating to medical and surgical

588

treatment of coronary artery disease provides "benchmarks" to which new therapies can be compared. This allows us to rigorously determine which therapies hold promise and which therapies hold less appeal. The development of new technologies and therapies requires us to hold ourselves accountable, both medically and financially, for the direction that these technologies and therapies take us. Outcomes research allows us to do this with impressive results.

From a humanistic standpoint, outcomes research related to cardiovascular disease also allows us to better understand the limitations of our therapeutic options. It allows us to accurately communicate our expectations to patients and their families. This allows patients and families to compare their expectations with the reality of what the therapy and health care system can provide. This chapter was written with the benefit of data derived from meticulously performed outcomes research.

ROLE OF THE CARDIOLOGIST AND INTENSIVIST

The skill of the cardiothoracic surgeon is the cornerstone of successful outcomes for patients undergoing cardiac surgery, although it is becoming increasingly difficult for surgeons to provide the minute-to-minute bedside care required by these patients. Therefore, a collaborative effort between cardiac surgeons and specialists with backgrounds across several disciplines is increasing. The team at our institution consists of the surgical staff, perfusionists, anesthesiologists, critical care physicians, cardiologists, and nurses with a specialization in cardiac care. Of all the physicians involved, the cardiologist has the unique privilege of observing the entire process: the initial referral, the diagnosis and workup phase, the surgical and recovery phase, and ultimately the return to and maintenance of health.

Cardiac surgical procedures create major physiologic challenges that are imposed on patients, many of whom have multiple underlying systems dysfunction. The understanding and anticipation of these alterations in physiology are imperative, and the time course required for return to baseline function should also be understood. With the evolution and expansion of off-pump techniques for operative revascularization, additional benefits and limitations of these techniques and the population best served by them are becoming better understood. At the present time, it remains more common to utilize full cardiopulmonary bypass support for the majority of coronary artery surgical and all other intracardiac procedures. Therefore, this chapter focuses on the management of patients undergoing fully supported cardiac surgery.

PHYSIOLOGY OF CARDIOPULMONARY BYPASS

Cardiopulmonary bypass allows for continued systemic perfusion while the heart is arrested during the surgical procedure. It has been recognized as both a magnificent facilitator as well as a nonphysiologic and disruptive support system. It is well understood that systemic inflammatory responses are created by exposure to the extracorporeal circuits and nonpulsatile flow that define modern-day cardiopulmonary bypass. This response in and of itself alters clotting ability and membrane stability and creates the potential for fluid accumulation. Nonpulsatile flow further disrupts regulatory feedback loops found within certain organ systems, such as the kidneys and brain, which are responsive to normal pulsatile flow.

During the period of cardiopulmonary bypass, the body is subjected to an altered hemodynamic milieu. Pulsatile blood flow is replaced by continuous blood flow at a mean pressure that is frequently lower than a normal mean arterial pressure. In order to tolerate this state of relative low-pressure circulation, the body is cooled to a temperature of approximately 28°C to 32°C. During certain procedures in which a cross clamp cannot be applied to the aorta, exemplified by aortic arch repair, this process is taken to an extreme in which circulation, with the exception of antegrade arterial and retrograde venous cerebral perfusion, is completely arrested.

During the period of cardiopulmonary bypass, platelets are activated, and a general systemic inflammatory state ensues. This can result in lung injury, which in most cases is subtle but may lead to the acute respiratory distress syndrome. Renal injury is common, usually manifesting as a mild elevation in serum creatinine levels. Acute tubular necrosis, necessitating temporary or permanent renal replacement therapy, occurs uncommonly. Other consequences of cardiopulmonary bypass include relative transient gut ischemia that can manifest as temporarily altered motility. In severe cases, such as in patients with occult mesenteric vascular occlusive disease, altered gut perfusion can lead to effective loss of the mucosal barrier, which may allow for transmigration of intestinal flora with resultant bacterial sepsis, but this is only rarely seen clinically. Neurologic injury may also occur. This topic is covered in more detail later in this chapter.

PREOPERATIVE EVALUATION

Estimation of Risk

One of the most important factors contributing to successful outcomes in cardiac surgery is the decision-making phase. Deciding whether long-term benefits will be achieved with an operative procedure, particularly in view of advances in medical therapy as well as in percutaneous interventions, has become a difficult task. Integral in making a sound decision is the ability to consider all of the comorbid conditions particular to an individual patient that influence operative outcomes. Issues such as age, gender, obesity, and the presence of renal, pulmonary, neurologic, and other disease processes such as diabetes all factor into assessing the appropriateness, the predictive risks, and the expected benefits of cardiac surgery. Experience has enabled the development of predictive indices that improve the understanding of risk and allow individual estimation of perioperative risk.

Simple bedside tools, based on prediction models of these indices, make it easier for physicians, patients, and patients' families to make clear, informed decisions when weighing all the possible therapeutic options. These tools also allow for more realistic expectations, particularly when questions of postoperative complications arise. A full discussion of this topic is beyond the scope of this chapter; however, there are several resources that provide a comprehensive review of this subject. The American College of Cardiology/American Heart Association guidelines for coronary artery bypass graft surgery (4) contain many useful resources for preoperative risk prediction (See Tables 39.1, 39.2). These resources are based on data derived from thousands of patients who underwent cardiac surgery between 1987 and 1995. From these risk prediction tools, the likelihood of mortality, cerebrovascular accident, and mediastinitis can be estimated with data encompassing basic demographics, ejection fraction, and the presence of chronic obstructive pulmonary disease, diabetes, peripheral vascular occlusive disease, renal dysfunction, and procedural urgency. The risk of postoperative renal dysfunction can similarly be predicted with basic preoperative data.

Prevention of Complications

Of every $10 spent on surgical treatment of coronary disease, $1 is related to complications (5). Because of the importance of preventing postoperative complications, it is imperative to be mindful of simple interventions that can improve outcomes. In the preoperative phase, several steps can be taken to minimize the likelihood of postoperative complications.

Prevention of neurologic injury, primarily by reduction of atheroembolic episodes related to aortic manipulation, can be achieved by the use of epiaortic imaging. This technique allows a surgeon to carefully select the locations for cross clamp application, aortic cannulation, and proximal conduit anastomosis. If extreme aortic disease is identified, no-clamp fibrillatory arrest and off-pump techniques may be used in order to avoid aortic manipulation.

From a medical perspective, adverse neurologic outcome can be minimized by identification of chronic atrial fibrillation that has not previously been treated by anticoagulation. Adequate anticoagulation for 3 to 4 weeks allows for resolution or organization, or both, of left atrial clot. The same treatment should be considered for patients who have recently suffered from an extensive anterior wall myocardial infarction, because these patients are at high risk for developing left ventricular mural thrombus.

Adverse neurologic outcomes may also be avoided by appropriate screening for cerebrovascular occlusive disease. Any patient with an audible cervical bruit or a history of left main disease, transient ischemic attack, or stroke should undergo noninvasive carotid imaging. The presence of significant disease (more than 75% stenosis in asymptomatic patients) may necessitate a staged procedure or combined carotid artery endarterectomy and coronary artery surgery.

In addition to these protective measures, appropriate management of diabetes-associated hyperglycemia may also help reduce the degree of cognitive neurologic injury that occurs during cardiac surgery (6).

Minimizing postoperative infection begins in the preoperative period. Guidelines for standard clinical practice have been extensively reviewed in the American College of Cardiology/American Heart Association practice guidelines on coronary artery bypass graft (4). In general, preoperative antibiotics should be given routinely to any patient undergoing cardiac surgery. Antibiotics should be adequate at the tissue level during the entire procedure, which requires administration 30 to 60 minutes before skin incision. If the surgical duration exceeds 3 hours, antibiotics should be readministered appropriately. The cephalosporin class of antimicrobials is generally used unless a true penicillin allergy exists, in which case vancomycin can be substituted. Unless clinically indicated by the presence of infection, antibiotics should be continued for only 1 day postoperatively.

Postoperative atrial fibrillation (see treatment of this entity later in this chapter) can potentially be avoided by preoperative administration of either beta-adrenergic blocking agents or amiodarone (7,8). Likewise, postoperative withdrawal of previously prescribed beta-adrenergic blocking agents should be avoided, because this considerably increases the risk of postoperative atrial fibrillation.

Finally, a good general physical examination and routine laboratory studies, including chest radiography, should be performed on all patients before they undergo cardiac surgery. Medical conditions such as hypertension, anemia, diabetes, thyroid dysfunction, and chronic obstructive pulmonary disease should be thoroughly evaluated and optimally treated if feasible before any cardiac surgical procedures.

THE EARLY POSTOPERATIVE PERIOD

Hemodynamic Monitoring

The physiologic changes that occur as a result of cardiac surgery include rapid fluid and electrolyte shifts, transient depression of myocardial function, and rapid fluctuations in vascular tone. Because of this dynamic process, hemodynamic monitoring is mandatory. Hemodynamic monitoring is used to ensure cardiovascular integrity and adequate oxygen delivery to the periphery. Oxygen delivery is determined by the following equation:

$$O_2 \text{ delivery} = \text{cardiac output} \\ \times \text{ hemoglobin concentration} \\ \times \text{ arterial oxygen saturation.}$$

The typical method for accurate and continuous measurement of systemic blood pressure and O_2 delivery is by cannulation of the radial artery. The femoral or axillary artery can also be used. Arterial lines are useful for continuous blood pressure monitoring and for sampling of arterial blood for blood gas and electrolyte analysis.

Central hemodynamics are monitored with a pulmonary artery (Swan-Ganz) catheter. This device allows for determination of intracardiac and central venous pressures, periodic or continuous cardiac output, and mixed-venous saturation. In this patient population, the ability to correctly interpret the data is essential. Understanding potential inaccuracies and pitfalls in data interpretation is also essential. Various patterns of hemodynamic derangements that are encountered in the patient after cardiac surgery are discussed in more detail later.

Early removal of invasive lines, if the patient is stable enough for this to occur, is an important step in the recovery process because it decreases the risk of complications such as thrombosis and infection. Early removal also facilitates increased patient mobility.

TABLE 39.1. *Preoperative estimation of risk of mortality, cerebrovascular accident, and mediastinitis*

For use only in isolated CABG surgery
Directions: Locate outcome of interest, e.g., mortality. Use the score in that column for each relevant
 preoperative variable, then sum these scores to get the total score. Take the total score and look up the
 approximate preoperative risk in the table below.

Patient or disease characteristic	Mortality score	CVA score	Mediastinitis score
Age 60–69	2	3.5	—
Age 70–79	3	5	—
Age ≥80	5	6	—
Female sex	1.5	—	—
EF <40%	1.5	1.5	2
Urgent surgery	2	1.5	1.5
Emergency surgery	5	2	3.5
Prior CABG	5	1.5	—
PVD	2	2	—
Diabetes	—	—	1.5
Dialysis or creatinine ≥2	4	2	2.5
COPD	1.5	—	3.5
Obesity (BMI 31–36)	—	—	2.5
Severe obesity (BMI ≥37)	—	—	3.5
Total Score			
Perioperative risk			

Total score	Mortality (%)	CVA (%)	Mediastinitis (%)
0	0.4	0.3	0.4
1	0.5	0.4	0.5
2	0.7	0.7	0.6
3	0.9	0.9	0.7
4	1.3	1.1	1.1
5	1.7	1.5	1.5
6	2.2	1.9	1.9
7	3.3	2.8	3.0
8	3.9	3.5	3.5
9	6.1	4.5	5.8
10	7.7	≥6.5	≥6.5
11	10.6	—	—
12	13.7	—	—
13	17.7	—	—
14	≥28.3	—	—

Calculation of mortality risk: An 80-year-old woman with an EF <40% who is having elective CABG surgery has
 had no prior CABG surgery and has no other risk factors. Her total score = 5 (age ≥80) + 1.5 (female) <1.5
 (EF <40%) = 8. Because her total score = 8, her predicted risk of mortality = 3.9%.
Definitions:
EF <40% (left ventricular ejection fraction): the patient's current EF is less than 40%.
Urgent: medical factors require patient to stay in hospital to have operation before discharge. The risk of
 immediate morbidity and death is believed to be low.
Emergency: patient's cardiac disease dictates that surgery should be performed within hours to avoid
 unnecessary morbidity or death.
PVD (peripheral vascular disease): cerebrovascular disease, including prior CVA, prior TIA, prior carotid surgery,
 carotid stenosis shown by history or radiographic studies, or carotid bruit; lower-extremity disease, including
 claudication, amputation, prior lower-extremity bypass, absent pedal pulses, or lower-extremity ulcers.
Diabetes: currently treated with oral medications or insulin.
Dialysis or creatinine ≥2: Peritoneal or hemodialysis-dependent renal failure or creatinine ≥2 mg/dL.

(continued)

TABLE 39.1. *(Continued)*

COPD (chronic obstructive pulmonary disease): treated with bronchodilators or steroids.
Obesity: Find the approximate height and weight in the table below to classify the person as obese or severely obese. Obesity: BMI 31–36; severe obesity: BMI ≥37.
Example: A patient 5 feet, 7 inches tall and weighing 200 lb. is classified as obese. If the patient weighted 236 lbs or more, he or she would be classified as severely obese.

Height (feet and inches)	Weight (lbs)		Height (feet and inches)	Weight (lbs)	
	Obesity BMI 31–36	Severe Obesity BMI ≥37		Obesity BMI 31–36	Severe Obesity BMI ≥37
5'0″	158–184	≥189	5'8″	203–236	≥244
5'1″	164–190	≥195	5'9″	209–243	≥250
5'2″	169–196	≥202	5'10″	215–250	≥258
5'3″	175–203	≥208	5'11″	222–258	≥265
5'4″	180–209	≥215	6'0″	228–265	≥272
5'5″	186–217	≥222	6'1″	235–273	≥280
5'6″	191–222	≥228	6'2″	241–280	≥287
5'7″	198–229	≥236	6'3″	248–288	≥296

Data set and definitions for dependent variables:
The regression models that generated the scores for these prediction rules were based on 7,290 patients receiving isolated CABG surgery between 1996 and 1998. The dependent variables and observed event rates are as follows: In-hospital mortality, 2.93%; cerebrovascular accident, defined as a new focal neurologic event persisting at least 24 hours, 1.58%; and mediastinitis during the index admission, defined by positive deep culture and/or Gram vs stain and/or radiographic findings indicating infection and necessitating reoperation, 1.19%.
From Northern New England Cardiovascular Disease Study Group, June 1999.
BMI, body mass index; CABG, coronary artery bypassgraft; CVA, cardiovascular accident; EF, ejection fraction; TIA, transient ischemic attack.

TABLE 39.2.

No. of risk factors	Combinations of preoperative risk factors for PRD				Risk of PRD in Various Clinical Strata Depending on Risk Factors and Age		
	CHF	Reop	DM	Creat>1.4 mo/dL	<70 yr	70–79 yr	≥80 yr
0	−	−	−	−	1.9% (n = 909)	7.0% (n = 330)	11.8% (n = 68)
1	−	−	−	+	5.0% (n = 80)	18.4% (n = 76)	12.5% (n = 16)
	−	−	+	−	5.9% (n = 68)	4.8% (n = 81)	0.0% (n = 1)
	−	+	−	−	6.2% (n = 130)	14.3% (n = 56)	25.0% (n = 4)
	+	−	−	−	7.6% (n = 144)	12.3% (n = 73)	29.4% (n = 17)
2	−	−	+	+	22.2% (n = 9)	0% (n = 7)	0% (n = 0)
	−	+	−	+	20.0% (n = 25)	30.8% (n = 13)	0% (n = 0)
	−	+	+	−	37.6% (n = 8)	33.3% (n = 3)	0% (n = 1)
	+	−	−	+	47.4% (n = 19)	7.7% (n = 26)	44.4% (n = 9)
	+	−	+	−	25.9% (n = 27)	18.2% (n = 11)	0% (n = 0)
	+	+	−	−	31.6% (n = 19)	7.1% (n = 14)	100.0% (n = 1)
3	−	+	+	+	100% (n = 1)	100% (n = 1)	0% (n = 0)
	+	−	+	+	8.3% (n = 12)	25% (n = 4)	0% (n = 1)
	+	+	−	+	0.0% (n = 2)	33.3% (n = 9)	0% (n = 2)
	+	+	+	−	33.3% (n = 3)	0% (n = 0)	0% (n = 0)
4	+	+	+	+	50.0% (n = 2)	0% (n = 0)	0% (n = 0)

CHD, prior congestive heart disease; Creat, preoperative serum creatinine level; DM, type I diabetes mellitus; PRD, preoperative risk prediction; Reop, repeat coronary bypass operation; −, risk factor absent; +, risk factor present.
From Managano CM, Diamondstone LS, Ramsay JG, et al. Renal dysfunction after myocardial revascularization: risk factors, adverse outcomes, and hospital resource utilization: the Multicenter Study of Perioperative Ischemia Research Group. *Ann Intern Med.* 1998;128:194.

A relatively new addition to the tools used in the post–cardiac surgery intensive care unit is transesophageal echocardiography. The placement of bandages, the location of chest tubes, and the presence of residual intrathoracic air frequently limits standard transthoracic echocardiography. Transesophageal echocardiography, albeit more invasive, is frequently more useful. Global and regional wall motion, valvular anatomy, and the presence of external compression of the heart by pericardial clot or blood are relatively easy to visualize with transesophageal echocardiography. This mode of cardiac imaging is frequently used intraoperatively; therefore, its use in surgical intensive care units is a logical extension of this technology in selected patients with hemodynamic compromise.

Postoperative Hemodynamic Changes

After cardiac surgery, patients undergo the process of rewarming. A frequent consequence of rewarming is systemic vasodilation, which leads to redistribution of blood volume to the periphery as well as to a drop in systemic blood pressure. This process is usually complete after several hours; however, in order to maintain adequate mean arterial pressure during this time, vasoconstricting agents are frequently required. Standard vasopressors include dopamine, norepinephrine, epinephrine, phenylephrine, and, in extreme cases, arginine vasopressin.

Patients who undergo cardiac surgery may also develop a transient increase in pulmonary vascular resistance. This is largely secondary to platelet activation and administration of protamine and blood products when required. If it is severe enough to compromise right ventricular function, pulmonary arterial vasodilators such as milrinone, nitroglycerin, and, occasionally, inhaled nitric oxide are employed.

Transient right ventricular dysfunction may also develop as a consequence of relative inadequacy of standard myocardial preservation techniques. Because the right ventricle is an anterior structure, topical hypothermia induced with ice slush is less effective over this structure than it is around the left ventricle, which lies in a well created by the marsupialized open pericardium.

The combination of relative right ventricular dysfunction and elevated pulmonary vascular resistance can lead to cardiogenic shock with an underfilled left ventricle.

Equally important to right ventricular dysfunction is transient left ventricular dysfunction, which can be multifactorial in origin. This topic is also considered in greater detail later in this chapter.

Management of Intravascular Volume

In addition to the fluid redistribution that occurs with systemic vasodilation, a potential consequence of cardiopulmonary bypass is a generalized capillary leak syndrome that results in excessive third-spacing of intravascular volume. This results in a state of both total-body fluid overload and relative intravascular depletion. As a consequence, cardiac chamber filling pressures can fall below normal, with a resultant decrease in cardiac output and mean arterial pressure.

In the presence of adequate hemodynamic monitoring, this situation is easily recognized and corrected by volume expansion. Appropriate fluid replacement is guided by many factors such as the patient's hematocrit and the level of hemodynamic alteration, both of which affect oxygen delivery. Early postoperative fluid replacement may include residual blood products, specifically red blood cells, which are recovered from the cardiopulmonary bypass circuit. Blood product allogenic transfusion is also common in the first day after surgery. However, the use of homologous blood products is associated with a dose-related increased risk for viral and bacterial infections secondary to an immunosuppressive, immunomodulatory effect (9). The use of various leukodepletion strategies as well as avoidance of transfusions, unless absolutely necessary, can attenuate these effects (10). Volume expansion can also be accomplished with the use of crystalloid or colloid solutions or both.

It should be expected that third-spaced fluid accumulation is eventually redistributed back into the vascular compartment. This occurs once the general capillary leak syndrome brought upon by cardiopulmonary bypass ceases, frequently after the first 48 hours. At this point in the recovery process, hemodynamic monitoring catheters have frequently been removed. Judging a patient's intravascular volume status becomes much more dependent on the ability to perform an accurate physical examination. Even in the presence of excellent bedside examination skills, clinical examination results are frequently misleading. Many patients have residual pleural effusions and rales despite normal pulmonary artery and left atrial pressures. Edema, usually diffuse at first, can redistribute to the lower extremities as the patient spends more time in an upright position. When severe, lower extremity edema can jeopardize the healing of the saphenous vein harvest site wound.

Helpful clues include a careful examination for elevation in jugular venous pressure and respiratory rate. On the rare occasion that intravascular volume status cannot be accurately determined from clinical signs and symptoms, reinstitution of a pulmonary artery catheter can be safer than a clinician's best guess, particularly in the patient with tenuous renal and pulmonary function.

Most patients begin to "autodiurese" sometime between postoperative days one and three. Despite this, many require the addition of a loop diuretic in order to facilitate diuresis. This should be administered cautiously, avoiding intravascular depletion, because renal function may still be compromised as a lingering effect of cardiopulmonary bypass support.

Unless the index hospitalization has been prolonged, the best estimate of a patient's true dry weight is the preoperative weight. By the time a patient is approaching discharge, his or her weight should at least approximate the preoperative weight. Once diuresis to the preoperative weight has been achieved, loop diuretics are generally discontinued.

Postoperative Shock and Circulatory Support

Evaluation of the adequacy of cardiac performance after cardiac surgery requires an understanding of the patient's preoperative cardiac function, the operative procedure, and physiologic performance expectations. For example,

some patients, particularly those with a prior diagnosis of heart failure, may have baseline hemodynamics that are abnormal. Expecting a full return to normal in such a patient may be unrealistic.

On occasion, a postcardiotomy patient has hemodynamic parameters consistent with cardiogenic shock, the hallmark of which is low cardiac output or index. Pulmonary artery catheters and arterial lines are invaluable sources of information in this situation. The best way to manage such a patient is with a well-rehearsed algorithm. Two questions should be asked: (a) What was the hemodynamic profile before initiation of general anesthesia or cardiopulmonary bypass? and (b) What are the right and left ventricular filling pressures and cardiac output?

A high left ventricular filling pressure (more accurately, its surrogate: a high pulmonary capillary wedge pressure) is a sign of poor left ventricular performance. Correctible causes should be aggressively sought from standard clinical and biochemical information. Imbalances in acid-base status, particularly acidemia, can cause profound impairment in left ventricular function. Respiratory acidosis is easily corrected by increasing effective ventilation (by increasing the tidal volume or ventilation rate). If ventilatory compliance is low, other sources of decreased effective ventilation, such as pneumothorax/hemothorax, malpositioned endotracheal tube, or gastric overdistention, should be sought. Standard chest radiography is helpful for identifying these correctible causes. Other potential causes of impaired left ventricular function include cardiac ischemia secondary to vein graft closure or arterial graft spasm. A 12-lead electrocardiogram is frequently helpful in excluding or confirming this diagnosis, particularly in a sedated patient who cannot complain of anginal chest discomfort.

If the cardiac index is less than 2.0 L/minute/m^2 after optimization of such factors as heart rate and rhythm, volume status, and an adequate hemoglobin concentration (at least 10 g/dL), and if there is confidence that no technical factors are causing the compromise (e.g., tamponade, ischemia), pharmacologic or nonpharmacologic or both approaches to improve contractility and effective cardiac output become necessary.

Various inotropic agents are available, including epinephrine and norepinephrine, both $beta_1$-adrenergic agonists; dopamine, which has $beta_1$-adrenergic action at lower doses and alpha-adrenergic effects at doses higher than 10 μg/kg/minute; and dobutamine, which has effects similar to those of dopamine with less vasoconstriction and a reduction in left ventricular preload and afterload (11). Milrinone is a phosphodiesterase inhibitor that increases cardiac output by slowing degradation of cyclic adenosine monophosphate (12) and lowers pulmonary and systemic vascular resistances. Because of its ability to lower pulmonary vascular resistance, milrinone is often administered in situations that involve right ventricular dysfunction.

In addition to inotropic support, calcium supplementation should be considered, particularly if serum ionized calcium levels are low. Calcium plays an important role in cardiac contractility and the excitation-contraction coupling of myocardial cells. Bolus injections of calcium have been shown to create brief hemodynamic improvements in critically ill patients (13).

Despite best attempts at support, there are situations of severe left ventricular dysfunction in which pharmacologic support proves inadequate. In this situation, mechanical support must be used to facilitate improved hemodynamics while cardiac recovery occurs.

The most commonly used device is the intraaortic balloon pump, which was introduced into clinical practice in 1968 by Adrian Kantrowitz (14). The balloon is usually placed through the common femoral artery and is timed to inflate during diastole and deflate with the onset of systole. An intraaortic balloon pump functions to improve coronary perfusion during diastole and diminish afterload by deflating with the onset of systole. Contraindications for intraaortic balloon counterpulsation include the presence of severe iliofemoral occlusive disease, abdominal or thoracic aortic aneurysm, and severe aortic stenosis or regurgitation.

More aggressive forms of mechanical support are occasionally necessary. Short-term support with a temporary external ventricular assist device, such as the Abiomed BVS 5000, is the most clinically available. This device can be configured to provide univentricular or biventricular support. It functions by gravity drainage of the appropriate cardiac chamber, usually the atria, followed by pneumatically driven pulsatile blood delivery into either the pulmonary artery or the aorta. Weaning from this short-term external ventricular assist device is attempted if the cardiac index can be maintained at greater than 2 L/minute/m^2 with low support device flow and if there is echocardiographic evidence of improving ventricular function.

In the absence of the ability to be weaned from short-term mechanical support, more durable long-term support can be achieved with an internal left ventricular assist device (LVAD). Examples include the Thoratec HeartMate LVAD and the Worldheart Novacor LVAD. There are advantages and disadvantages with each system. A full discussion of this topic is beyond the scope of this chapter, but it is well reviewed elsewhere (15). At present, these more long-term internal devices are best suited for bridging to eventual transplantation, although the HeartMate device has been demonstrated to be a viable, albeit expensive, alternative to transplantation for patients who are not transplantation candidates (16).

On occasion, left ventricular filling pressure may be inadequate, whereas right ventricular filling pressure, as assessed by the right atrial or central venous pressure, is excessive. This is the hallmark of right ventricular failure, which is a particularly challenging problem. This is usually present in conjunction with an elevated pulmonary vascular resistance.

When present with relatively normal pulmonary vascular resistance, this indicates near-total right ventricular failure. Flow across the pulmonary vascular bed becomes essentially passive. Preoperative right ventricular infarction is a risk factor for this occurrence. If cardiac output is inadequate, and if therapy with inotropic agents does not adequately improve right-to-left flow, then a short-term right ventricular assist device (such as the Abiomed BVS 5000) should be considered.

If, on the other hand, pulmonary vascular resistance is elevated, which can be seen in cases with long duration of cardiopulmonary bypass or a high requirement for blood products, particularly platelets, therapy is also aimed at lowering this resistance. Pulmonary hypertension may be present, depending on the degree of right ventricular failure. Primary treatment is to reduce pulmonary vascular resistance with the use of agents that are active pulmonary artery vasodilators. Milrinone is particularly helpful. Dobutamine and isoproterenol are also helpful. These agents are additionally useful in that they are positive inotropic agents and can help improve right ventricular function. Another therapeutic maneuver is pacing. If, despite the therapeutic maneuvers just mentioned, heart rate remains low, increased right ventricular delivery of blood across the pulmonary circuit can be achieved by dual-chamber pacing at a higher rate. In extreme cases, inhaled nitric oxide can be extraordinarily useful. This agent is the most effective vasodilator of the pulmonary vascular bed. An added benefit of inhaled nitric oxide is that it is rapidly metabolized by red blood cells and therefore does not cause a drop in systemic blood pressure. One potential difficulty with inhaled nitric oxide is that it is not universally available.

If, despite these therapies, cardiac output remains inadequate, a short-term right ventricular assist device should be considered. Right ventricular dysfunction and elevations in pulmonary vascular resistance in the postoperative setting are usually transient, and more permanent forms of artificial support are rarely needed.

Tamponade

Despite the fact that the pericardium is rarely reapproximated completely and that there frequently exists a communication between the pericardium and the pleural spaces, postoperative tamponade may nonetheless occur. Tamponade should be in the differential diagnosis for any patient with a low cardiac output, impaired perfusion, or both.

The classical presentation of pericardial tamponade is that of dyspnea, jugular venous distention, and low blood pressure—the so-called Beck triad. Although this may be seen in the postcardiotomy patient, the presentation is not usually classic. A patient who is ventilated and sedated is not likely to display dyspnea. Whereas blood or pericardial fluid usually surrounds the heart,

causing equal constriction in classic tamponade, postoperative constriction may be caused by either blood or clot, which can manifest as focal chamber compression. For example, if a large hematoma primarily compresses the left ventricle, the typical diastolic collapse of the right-sided chambers with standard surface echocardiography might not be seen. A pulsus paradoxus also may not be present.

The diagnosis of postoperative tamponade is considered when a patient's hemodynamics are more impaired than expected. Diagnosis of tamponade is made more readily with appropriate hemodynamic monitoring. High pressures proximal to the chamber that is being compressed may indicate the presence of focal tamponade. Definitive diagnosis is aided by use of echocardiography. Because chest tubes, sternal bandages, and residual mediastinal air significantly impair the quality of images obtained from the surface, transesophageal echocardiography is a much more sensitive tool for the diagnosis of postcardiotomy tamponade. Echocardiography is not fool proof, and if clinical suspicion is high enough, the patient should return to the operating room for exploration.

Postoperative Hypertension

Hypertension is a risk factor for cardiovascular disease. Therefore, it is not surprising that hypertension is a common occurrence after cardiac surgery. Treatment of hypertension is aimed at the source of the hypertension. In the majority of cases, essential hypertension is the underlying mechanism. Nonetheless, a careful search for other causes of hypertension is important. Inadequate pain control can significantly contribute to postoperative hypertension. Fluid overload, a common occurrence after heart surgery, also contributes to postoperative hypertension.

In the early phases after cardiac surgery, treatment with intravenous agents allows for easier titration of effect, particularly while hemodynamic status is in a rapid state of flux. Agents most commonly used include intravenous nitroglycerin, nitroprusside, beta blockers, calcium channel blockers, and hydralazine. Nitroglycerin and calcium channel blockers have the added effect of preventing graft artery spasm, and beta blockers have the added effect of preventing post-operative atrial fibrillation (see later discussions). Loop diuretics are also used to help reduce over-all body sodium and water overload.

When the patient is able to take oral medication, the agents of choice are similar to those recommended at the sixth meeting of the Joint National Commission (17), which emphasized initial treatment with diuretics and beta blockers. Calcium channel blocking agents and long-acting nitrates are used as described previously. Goal blood pressures in the predischarge phase should be less than 140 mm HG for systolic pressures and less than 85 mm HG for diastolic pressures.

Modification of the renin-angiotensin-aldosterone axis with angiotensin-converting enzyme (ACE) inhibitors deserves special consideration. There is no question that therapy with this class of medication decreases mortality rates among patients with left ventricular dysfunction (18–23). There is now even more evidence that ACE inhibitors decrease overall rates of cardiovascular morbidity and mortality. A large multicenter study demonstrated a decrease in rates of cardiovascular morbidity and mortality in populations at risk for cardiovascular disease (24). Therefore, there is little question that patients who undergo cardiac surgery should benefit from judicious use of ACE inhibitors. The best timing of use is, however, less clearly defined. Because ACE inhibitors cause constriction of renal afferent vessels, it is conceivable that ACE inhibitors could be detrimental in the *early* post–cardiopulmonary bypass period, particularly if there is any degree of renal instability.

Because many patients who have undergone coronary revascularization have concomitant peripheral vascular occlusive disease, occult renal artery stenosis must also be suspected. Of course, known bilateral renal artery stenosis is an absolute contraindication to the use of ACE inhibitors.

Postoperative Hemostasis

Understanding a patient's coagulation status after cardiac surgery requires an understanding of the patient's preoperative status, the type and ex-

tent of the operative procedure, and appropriate expectations after the operation.

Treatment of postoperative bleeding requires an understanding of the patient's preoperative coagulation profile. This is accomplished with a proper history and physical examination in conjunction with laboratory testing aimed at defining a patient's coagulation status. Specifically, this includes laboratory assessment of a patient's prothrombin time, partial thromboplastin time, and platelet count. Because renal failure and cirrhosis predispose to bleeding complications, assessment of serum creatinine level and liver function tests are warranted as well.

Knowledge of a patient's use of antiplatelet agents, glycoprotein IIb/IIIa inhibitors, or warfarin is essential. Although most patients take aspirin up until the day of surgery, as is appropriate in the setting of acute, recent, or high-risk coronary anatomy, the use of aspirin is associated with increased intraoperative and postoperative bleeding. Despite this, asprin should be continued up until the day of surgery. Other antiplatelet agents such as ticlopidine and clopidogrel may cause significant intraoperative and postoperative bleeding. Although the use of these medications should not preclude emergency cardiac surgery, many surgeons may wish to have these medications discontinued before surgery for elective cases.

The use of glycoprotein IIb/IIIa inhibitors poses additional risks for postoperative bleeding, and a working knowledge of the agents commonly used is essential. Abciximab irreversibly binds to the glycoprotein IIb/IIIa receptor, which inhibits platelet aggregation for the life of the platelet. Because of this, abciximab can cause significant bleeding problems. Tirofiban and eptifibatide are competitive antagonists of the glycoprotein IIb/IIIa receptor that rapidly dissociate. Platelet function returns to normal within 2 to 4 hours of discontinuance of these agents, and bleeding is therefore less of a risk.

For patients taking warfarin before surgery, a strategy of either switching to heparin or reversing the effects of warfarin with vitamin K or fresh-frozen plasma, or both, is appropriate.

Other strategies for decreasing intraoperative and postoperative bleeding involve either prehospitalization autologous blood donation and pre–cardiopulmonary bypass blood donation. Autotransfusion of scavenged mediastinal blood can decrease the need for allogeneic blood transfusion as well, but it may be associated with continued stimulation of fibrinolysis greater than that of the strategies previously described.

Antifibrinolytics are commonly used to decrease intraoperative and postoperative bleeding. Lysine analogues (epsilon-aminocaproic acid and tranexamic acid) and serine protease inhibitors (aprotinin) constitute this class of drugs. The lysine analogues are most commonly used, particularly in first-time operations. Advantages to the use of these agents include relatively low cost for what is usually an adequate effect. When these agents are used intraoperatively, they are usually continued for approximately 4 hours into the postoperative period. Aprotinin, which is more effective at promoting hemostasis, is considerably more expensive. It is also associated with severe hypersensitivity reactions upon reexposure. For these reasons, the use of aprotinin is generally restricted to patients undergoing repeat cardiac procedures, those with expected prolonged cardiopulmonary bypass periods, those with renal dysfunction and secondary platelet dysfunction, and those with known bleeding tendencies or factor deficiencies. Aprotinin has a long half-life, and administration is usually completed in the operating room.

It is well documented that cardiopulmonary bypass activates platelets, produces thrombocytopenia (25), creates fibrinolysis (26), and reduces circulating factor levels. This scenario promotes the potential for postoperative bleeding. Technical operative site bleeding can complicate this. Evaluation of the patient in the first 6 postoperative hours includes attentive observation of mediastinal and chest tube drainage. Excessive bleeding can be defined as 500 mL/hour in the first hour, 400 mL/hour during the first 2 hours, 300 mL/hour during the first 3 hours, or 200 mL/hour during the first 6 hours (27). If this occurs, early assessment and correction of reversible causes and prompt treatment are imperative. Assessment includes accurate measurement of coagulation factors, including prothrombin time, partial thromboplastin time, activated clotting time, platelet count, and fibrinogen. If excessive bleeding persists, early surgical reexploration is warranted while the coagulation profile is corrected.

There is a phenomenon of heparin rebound. This refers to the reappearance of heparin effect after neutralization with protamine. This can occur because of the differential elimination of protamine versus heparin and because of inadequate or nonuniform rewarming. Because the activated clotting time and partial thromboplastin time are prolonged by numerous factors other than residual heparin, protamine titration assays occasionally provide valuable additional information. Note should also be made of the syndrome of heparin-induced thrombocytopenia. This complication, which is caused by circulating antiplatelet antibodies, can lead to profound thrombocytopenia. Antiplatelet antibodies can form when there has been prior exposure to heparin. The treatment is meticulous elimination of all heparin from a patient's medical regimen (including heparinized intravenous flush solutions).

When bleeding persists and hemodynamic compromise occurs, evaluation for the potential of tamponade is appropriate. This includes clinical evaluation of tissue perfusion and hemodynamic evaluation, including assessment of central venous, pulmonary arterial, and pulmonary capillary wedge pressures, as well as cardiac output. An enlarging cardiac silhouette on chest radiograph is suggestive of this complication, and transesophageal echocardiography may help clarify whether mediastinal clot or ventricular dysfunction or both are the causes of the hemodynamic instability. Operative reexploration is imperative if tamponade is suspected or confirmed.

The complexities of the topic of intraoperative and postoperative hemostasis are beyond the scope of this text but are well reviewed elsewhere (28).

Graft Patency

Both early and late compromise of conduit graft patency can have catastrophic effects. It is well established that revascularization with the *in situ* internal mammary artery, also referred to as the internal thoracic artery, yields long-term results superior to those from saphenous vein grafts (29). Greater saphenous vein grafts are prone to progressive intimal proliferation and early atherosclerotic changes, probably because these vessels are subjected to systemic, as opposed to the typical venous, pressures. In comparison, internal mammary grafts are not subjected to pressures that are different from those seen in the unharvested vessel. At 1 year, internal mammary grafts have patency rates similar to those of saphenous grafts. However, at 5 and 10 years, the patency rates for internal mammary grafts are 88% and 83%, respectively, whereas the 5- and 10-year patency rates for saphenous grafts are only 74% and 41% (29). Internal mammary grafts are associated with lower rates of recurrent angina, myocardial infarction, and need for revascularization and with improved survival. Because of these findings, the routine use of internal mammary grafts, usually the left internal mammary artery as a conduit to the left anterior descending artery, is now considered standard of care. It is therefore imperative that the routine preoperative physical examination include careful auscultation for bruits, particularly those located in the region of the left clavicle. Grafting with a left internal mammary artery in the presence of left subclavian stenosis can result in a situation in which native coronary flow is diverted to the left arm via the grafted left internal mammary artery. This creates a subclavian steal phenomenon.

Because of the success noted with the use of the internal mammary artery as a conduit, many surgeons have begun using other arterial conduits. The right internal mammary artery is occasionally used as either an *in situ* or free graft. The gastroepiploic artery has been similarly used. Radial free grafts are also being used with increasing frequency.

The use of bilateral internal mammary arteries in coronary artery surgery appears to offer even greater clinical benefit than the use of unilateral internal mammary arteries. However, there is a higher rate of complications associated with bilateral internal mammary artery use. The most notable complication is that of sternal wound infection secondary to poor residual blood flow to the healing tissues. Sternal wound infections are associated with a much lower rate of survival, and the use of bilateral internal mammary arteries is therefore best avoided in patients at high risk for this complication. Such patients include those who are obese or have diabetes.

The radial artery may be prone to postoperative spasm. Because of this, all patients who undergo revascularization with this type of conduit should receive a calcium channel blocker, or a long-acting nitrate if a calcium channel blocker is contraindicated. The appropriate duration of therapy is unknown. The use of the radial artery as a graft may be associated with hand ischemia. Because of this, a careful preoperative Allen test to ensure adequate blood flow to the palmar arch (via the ulnar artery) is essential. Several groups have used radial artery duplex studies as well. The use of the radial artery as a graft is also associated with forearm dysesthesia that is usually transient.

The use of preserved homologous and synthetic grafts is associated with unacceptably high graft attrition rates. The use of such conduits should be considered only if no other is available.

Postoperative vascular spasm can occur, both in the native coronary arteries (grafted and ungrafted) and in conduit vessels (arterial more common than venous). This can lead to catastrophic perioperative myocardial infarction, ventricular arrhythmias, and death. Mechanical manipulation or exposure to high levels of circulating catecholamines may cause this complication. In many instances, no obvious cause may be found. Because of this, vessel spasm should be suspected, particularly for patients with unexplained poor ventricular function or ventricular arrhythmias. Diagnosis is usually made by electrocardiogram, with follow-up echocardiography if warranted to note wall motion abnormalities. Aggressive treatment with nitroglycerin, calcium channel blockers, or both is frequently effective for alleviating vascular spasm. If they are unsuccessful, emergency cardiac catheterization with direct infusion of nitroglycerin or papaverine is warranted. Emergency reexploration may become necessary with regrafting with venous conduit.

Graft patency, particularly for saphenous vein conduits, is best maintained by early administration of low-dose aspirin (325 mg per day) (30,31). This benefit is lost when aspirin is started more than 48 hours after surgery (32). For this reason, a mechanism for ensuring early aspirin use is imperative.

For patients with true aspirin sensitivity, a thienopyridine (ticlopidine or clopidogrel) should be used. Ticlopidine is associated with life-threatening neutropenia; therefore, frequent complete blood cell counts should be performed, particularly in the early months of use. Because of this serious side effect, clopidogrel appears to be a better option.

It is well known that a subset of patients appear to be "aspirin resistant," as defined by the lack of significant, detectable platelet inhibition after ingesting aspirin (33). Because of this fact, studies have been performed to compare the effects of aspirin versus clopidogrel for patients who have cardiovascular disease. Preliminary results indicate that clopidogrel may be more effective for patients undergoing coronary artery surgery (34). Clopidogrel is significantly more expensive than aspirin, and studies are still only preliminary. For these reasons, aspirin remains the antiplatelet agent of choice, at least until more definitive studies have been performed. In the future, the most cost-effective strategy may involve screening individuals for aspirin resistance and modifying clinical practice accordingly.

The use of warfarin has not been associated with an improved graft patency rate. Warfarin should therefore be used in individuals with other indications for more complete anticoagulation. Such patients include those with atrial fibrillation, those with mechanical valves, and those who have sustained recent significant anterior myocardial infarctions.

Epicardial Pacing Electrodes

Epicardial electrodes are frequently, although not universally, placed during cardiac surgery. The location and number of the electrodes varies depending on type of procedure and surgeon preference. Placement of two atrial electrodes allows for bipolar atrial pacing and electrogram recording. Bipolar pacing usually requires less energy output from the external pacemaker, reducing the incidence of capture of the diaphragm (via the phrenic nerve), chest wall muscles, and ventricles. Bipolar recording of an atrial electrogram can help identify specific atrial arrhythmias, specifically atrial flutter. In order to record an atrial electrogram, the individual atrial wires are attached to the right and left arm leads of a multichannel electrocardiograph machine or monitor. The electrogram should be clearly recognizable in the lead I position of the graph. Recording of an atrial electrogram can be performed during ventricular pacing. The presence of two atrial electrodes also allows for rapid atrial pacing for termination of atrial flutter and multisite atrial pacing, which may help prevent atrial arrhythmias (see later discussion).

One or two ventricular wires are also placed on the right ventricular free wall. When two wires are placed, similar electrograms can be obtained from the ventricles. When obtained simultaneously with an atrial electrogram, this may allow for differentiation between ventricular tachycardia and aberrant ventricular conduction in the setting of atrial flutter.

Atrial electrodes usually exit though the right side of the chest, and ventricular electrodes exit to the left. This pattern allows for fast recognition in the situation when an external pacemaker needs to be rapidly employed. In addition to atrial and ventricular electrodes, a ground, or indifferent, electrode is occasionally placed in the subcutaneous tissue and usually exits to the far left of other leads.

The mechanism for removal of these wires varies. Most wires are simply removed by gentle traction, inasmuch as they are only loosely attached to the heart with small dissolvable clips or loosely placed sutures. On occasion, the wires are cut at the level of the skin. Although it is a rare complication, bacteria can ascend these wires, causing a foreign body infection and necessitating electrode removal.

Atrial Arrhythmias

Postoperative atrial arrhythmias can significantly increase the length of stay, the cost of hospitalization, and the risk for postoperative stroke (35–37). Atrial fibrillation and, less commonly, atrial flutter are the most common postoperative arrhythmias, occurring in up to 43% of patients. These entities are more common after valvular procedures and in the presence of postoperative pericardial effusion. The incidence of atrial fibrillation peaks on the second or third postoperative day. Preoperative predictors for atrial fibrillation include advanced age, male gender, history of atrial arrhythmia or congestive heart failure, beta blocker withdrawal, and a signal-averaged P wave duration greater than 155 milliseconds (38).

Episodes are frequently paroxysmal and self-limited, rarely lasting more than 4 to 6 weeks. As discussed previously, the best way to prevent postoperative atrial arrhythmias, particularly atrial fibrillation, is by preoperative and early postoperative use of beta blockers or amiodarone. Early and aggressive weaning from sympathomimetic agents, when required in the postoperative setting, should be attempted as soon as is feasible. Early recognition and treatment of hypomagnesemia, which occurs frequently after cardiac surgery, may prevent atrial arrhythmias. Serum magnesium levels should be maintained above 2.0 mg/dL. In addition to these measures, the use various modes of atrial pacing have been investigated, with mixed results. There may be a synergistic antiarrhythmic effect when atrial pacing is combined with beta blocker use.

Management of atrial fibrillation and atrial flutter is based on three goals: control of ventricular response, restoration of normal sinus rhythm, and prevention of thromboembolism. In a patient who develops severe hemodynamic compromise secondary to the atrial arrhythmia, synchronized direct-current cardioversion should be performed immediately. In all other patients, the focus should be on controlling the ventricular response. This is best accomplished with the use of beta blocking agents. If a contraindication to beta blocker use exists, rate control can be achieved with diltiazem or verapamil. Because high circulating catecholamine levels that overwhelm the vagotonic properties of digoxin are frequently encountered in the postoperative patient, digoxin is only minimally effective in controlling the ventricular response in this population. An electrocardiogram should be performed on all patients with the first episode of an atrial arrhythmia in order to rule out active ischemia as the cause.

The second goal of therapy, restoration and maintenance of normal sinus rhythm, can be achieved by several different means. With a few minor differences, atrial fibrillation and atrial flutter are treated similarly. Once the rate has been controlled, one of several antiarrhythmic agents can be used. Procainamide can be administered in a loading dose of 20 mg/minute until termination of the arrhythmia or until a total of 17 mg/kg has been given. A continuous infusion of 1-4 mg/minute can be used after the initial load. Restoration of normal sinus rhythm is usually seen within the first 24 hours. If the rhythm has not converted to normal sinus rhythm by that time, use of a different drug or direct-current cardioversion should be considered. Procainamide should not be used unless electrolyte imbalances have been corrected, because this drug can have proarrhythmic effects. Significant QT prolongation should impel discontinuation of this drug, as torsades de pointes may result. If a continuous infusion is used, daily drug levels should be performed, particularly in the presence of renal failure. Procainamide can enhance conduction through the atrioventricular node; therefore, rate control is essential before initiation of the loading dose. An increase in the ventricular response, with potential hemodynamic compromise, can be observed in the presence of inadequate rate control. Note should also be made that mild hypotension is relatively common with infusion of a loading dose.

Ibutilide, a new Vaughn Williams class III agent, is relatively effective for treatment of both atrial fibrillation and atrial flutter. It is given in a bolus dose of 1 mg over 10 minutes and may be repeated one time 10 minutes after the first dose. Ibutilide has a relatively short half-life, and effects are usually seen rapidly after administration of the drug. In contrast to procainamide, hypotension is rare with ibutilide. The major limitation of ibutilide is a relatively high incidence of proarrhythmia, including torsades de pointes (around 2%). Incidence of proarrhythmia is higher in the presence of electrolyte abnormalities or impaired left ventricular function. For this reason, continuous arrhythmia monitoring for 4 to 6 hours after administration of the dose is mandatory.

Amiodarone, a complex drug with effects on sodium, potassium, and calcium channels as well as alpha- and beta-adrenergic blocking properties, is becoming the agent of choice at our institution. It is administered in a 150-mg bolus over 10 minutes, followed by 1 mg/minute for 6 hours and then 0.5 mg/minute for 18 hours. Supplementary infusions of 150 mg can be given for refractory arrhythmias up to a total daily dose of 2 g. Amiodarone acts as an effective rate-controlling agent as well, making the concomitant use of other rate-controlling agents unnecessary. Benefits of amiodarone include high efficacy and a relatively low incidence of proarrhythmia. Amiodarone is the preferred agent for patients with impaired ventricular function. A relative disadvantage of intravenous amiodarone is its high cost.

A special note should be made about the treatment of atrial flutter. Because a macro-reentry circuit within the right atrium causes this rhythm, overdrive pacing (via the epicardial pacing electrodes attached to the atria) can be used to terminate it. By pacing at a rate slightly faster than the flutter rate (not the ventricular rate), which is usually approximately 300 beats per minute, followed by cessation of pacing, atrial flutter can be successfully terminated. The advantage of using this method is that it is simple, requires no additional pharmacologic manipulation, and is easily tolerated by the patient. The disadvantages are that efficacy is limited and that, in some cases, atrial fibrillation may be induced. In the case that rapid atrial pacing is unsuccessful, the same pharmacologic maneuvers used for atrial fibrillation can be employed. Rate control before procainamide use is particularly important. Procainamide can slow the rate of the atrial flutter while simultaneously improving conduction through the atrioventricular node. This creates a milieu in which 1:1 conduction is possible, which can cause rapid hemodynamic collapse and induction of ventricular fibrillation.

This risk is avoided if amiodarone is used rather than procainamide. As with atrial fibrillation, direct-current cardioversion can be particularly effective and easy to perform in the patient who is still sedated and ventilated.

The third goal of therapy is the prevention of thromboembolic events. If atrial fibrillation persists longer than 48 hours, anticoagulation is generally recommended unless a realistic, postoperative bleeding risk is present. Anticoagulation is usually initiated with intravenous heparin, because this can be rapidly reversed with protamine sulfate, should the need arise. Once atrial fibrillation or flutter has been converted to normal sinus rhythm, there still remains a relative electromechanical dissociation that can result in noncontractile atria. This usually resolves within days to weeks. For this reason, conversion from heparin to warfarin for 4 weeks (International Normalized Ratio of 2 to 3) after the arrhythmia has been terminated is standard if the duration of the atrial arrhythmia exceeds 48 hours. There is a trend toward the use of low molecular weight heparins to serve as a "bridge" from the initial use of unfractionated heparin to adequate anticoagulation with warfarin. Low molecular weight heparins can be administered at home, which facilitates earlier discharge from the hospital and lowers overall cost.

Other atrial arrhythmias, such as atrial tachycardia and various forms of reentrant supraventricular or atrioventricular nodal tachycardias are occasionally observed in the postoperative patient. Many of the drugs used for atrial fibrillation and flutter are useful in the management of these arrhythmias. Reentrant tachycardias involving the atrioventricular node (atrioventricular nodal reentrant tachycardia and tachycardias that involve an accessory pathway) can also be terminated with adenosine. Adenosine is given in an injection of 6 mg intravenous push, followed by a 20-mL saline flush. If that is unsuccessful, a 12-mg intravenous push may be used. The use of adenosine is relatively safe but the drug can cause transient flushing, dyspnea, and chest pain. Certain patients may have a very slow ventricular escape rhythm after administration of adenosine. In this setting, backup epicardial pacing (if available) or transcutaneous pacing may be necessary. In rare circumstances, adenosine can cause atrial fibrillation.

Ventricular Arrhythmias

Sustained ventricular arrhythmias can cause acute hemodynamic compromise and are associated with a significant mortality rate. For this reason, an up-to-date working knowledge of basic and advanced cardiac life support (ACLS) is mandatory for any physician with primary responsibilities for patients after cardiac surgery.

Sustained ventricular arrhythmias are associated with prior myocardial infarction, severe congestive heart failure, and acute graft closure (in up to 25% of cases). In addition, patients with nonsustained ventricular tachycardia associated with a left ventricular ejection fraction of less than 40% are at higher risk of sudden death.

Appropriate treatment of ventricular arrhythmias is reviewed in the ACLS protocols. Guidelines for both basic life support and ACLS have been updated (39). A full description of these algorithms is beyond the scope of this article; however, a few of the changes are highlighted here. Ventricular fibrillation and sustained ventricular tachycardia with severe hemodynamic compromise should be treated initially and rapidly with defibrillation. Chest compressions should be performed until defibrillation is performed, unless hemodynamics makes this unnecessary. If the arrhythmia persists despite three defibrillation attempts, epinephrine (1-mg intravenous push) or vasopressin (40-U intravenous push, single dose only) are the initial drugs used. This is followed by a repeat attempt at defibrillation. If defibrillation is still not successful, antiarrhythmic agents are used. Of the antiarrhythmics available, amiodarone is now the drug of choice for treatment of ventricular fibrillation and ventricular tachycardia with hemodynamic compromise. Amiodarone is administered in a 300-mg intravenous push, followed by an infusion, as discussed earlier in this chapter. Additional bolus doses of 150 mg can be given as needed. Lidocaine, although no longer the drug of choice, can also be used (1.0 to 1.5 mg/kg intravenous push every 3 to 5 minutes, up to a total dose of 3.0 mg/kg). Pro-

cainamide is no longer recommended because of prolonged administration time. Bretylium is also no longer recommended, because its efficacy is marginal and its availability is no longer universal. Magnesium sulfate (1 to 2 g intravenously) should be considered in polymorphic ventricular tachycardia or suspected hypomagnesemia.

Any occurrence of ventricular arrhythmia should prompt a search for a correctable cause. Serum electrolyte levels should be obtained, with particular attention to maintaining potassium levels in the upper normal range. Serum hypomagnesemia is another correctible cause of ventricular arrhythmias; however, it should be noted that serum magnesium levels do not necessarily reflect intracellular magnesium stores. Patients who have received long-term diuretics before surgery are at particular risk for low intracellular magnesium levels. Serum calcium and, more important, ionized calcium levels should be kept within normal ranges. Hypoxia and impaired ventilation should be corrected. An electrocardiogram should be obtained as soon as possible, because this may help to identify QT prolongation, which is indicative of drug toxicity, or ST segment elevation that results from acute graft closure or native artery spasm.

Sustained ventricular tachycardia without significant hemodynamic compromise can be treated more conservatively. On occasion, a wide–QRS complex tachycardia may be the result of a supraventricular tachycardia in the background of a bundle branch block or aberrant conduction. Accurate diagnosis of wide–QRS complex tachycardias is critical to development of effective treatment strategies.

Nonsustained ventricular tachycardia in a patient with normal left ventricular function necessitates no particular treatment other than correction of potential underlying causes, such as ischemia or electrolyte or metabolic disturbances. Nonsustained ventricular tachycardia that occurs in patients with ischemic cardiomyopathy and an ejection fraction of 40% or less should prompt electrophysiologic testing. Inducible sustained monomorphic tachycardia in this population is predictive of a high rate of sudden cardiac death and should be treated with an implantable cardioverter-defibrillator (40).

Occasionally, catheter-based ablation can be performed if the inducible arrhythmia is slow enough to be hemodynamically stable during the mapping and ablation procedures. Electrophysiologic testing in similar patients with nonischemic cardiomyopathy is not usually helpful in predicting who is at risk for sudden cardiac death. At our institution, these patients are usually treated with either an implantable cardioverter-defibrillator or amiodarone.

Conduction Disturbances

Postoperative conduction disturbances are relatively common after cardiac surgery. Right bundle branch block is the most frequently observed conduction abnormality. Other abnormalities observed include sinus node dysfunction; first-, second-, or third degree block; and incomplete or complete left bundle branch block. Conduction disturbances are associated with the use of cold-blood cardioplegia and valvular procedures.

Management of conduction disturbances includes epicardial or transvenous pacing, when necessary, and removal of drugs that suppress conduction, such as digitalis glycosides, beta blockers, and calcium channel blockers. In the event that conservative management fails to improve high-grade blocks, implantation of a permanent pacemaker is occasionally required.

Neurologic Injury

It is well known that neurologic complications occur after cardiac surgery and range from permanent cerebrovascular accidents, with a rate of 1% to 4% after standard cardiopulmonary bypass coronary procedures, to cognitive decline, which occurs in up to 50% to 80% of patients at the time of discharge (41,42). Adverse cerebral outcomes have been divided into two types: Type 1 deficits are those associated with major focal neurologic deficits, and type 2 deficits are characterized by deterioration in cognitive function or memory. Both types of neurologic injury are associated with excessive mortality, increased length of hospital stay, and increased likelihood of discharge to a nursing home (43).

Preoperative predictors of type 1 neurologic dysfunction have been identified. The most predictive risk factor is the presence of aortic atherosclerosis. Other predictors include a history of previous neurologic disease; the presence of carotid bruit, hypertension, or diabetes mellitus; increasing age; duration of cardiopulmonary bypass; preoperative use of an intraaortic balloon pump; and a history of unstable angina (43–46). Postoperative atrial arrhythmias are also a cause of type 1 neurologic dysfunction. Treatment of these arrhythmias is covered in detail earlier in this chapter.

Preoperative predictors of type 2 neurologic dysfunction include a history of alcohol consumption; the presence of preoperative arrhythmia, hypertension, peripheral vascular disease, or congestive heart failure; and a history of prior open-heart procedures. The incidence of neurobehavioral dysfunction is thought to be similar for both coronary artery and valve surgery (47).

Preoperative and intraoperative strategies aimed at reducing neurologic risk focus largely on the presence and degree of aortic atherosclerosis and cerebrovascular disease, as well as on intracardiac sources of emboli. From the purely cardiac surgical perspective, attempts have been made to lessen aortic manipulation during cardiopulmonary bypass, including the single-clamp technique and the use of off-pump coronary revascularization procedures when deemed feasible. Studies suggest that the risk of cerebrovascular accident can be reduced from 4.6% to 2.5% when off-pump approaches are used (41). Ongoing efforts continue to evaluate the role of off-pump in comparison with on-pump approaches. Issues surrounding screening for cerebrovascular disease, treatment strategies for this entity, and intracardiac sources of embolism are covered in detail earlier in this chapter. Further studies of postoperative cognitive deficits and methods to lessen these occurrences in patients noted to have increased risk continue to evolve.

The presence of type 2 neurologic injury should prompt a search for toxic, pharmacologic, or metabolic causes. Electrolyte and acid-base status should be normalized. The presence of uremia, thyroid derangements, and adrenal insufficiency (particularly in patients taking steroids preoperatively) should be ruled out. The use of narcotics, benzodiazepines, anticholinergics, and other sedating drugs should be minimized. The sleep-wake cycle should be preserved whenever possible. Alcohol withdrawal is probably underdiagnosed in postoperative patients and should always be considered, as should withdrawal from other addictive substances such as benzodiazepines or tobacco.

Neurologic injury related to cardiac surgery not only occurs in the central nervous system but can also affect the peripheral nervous system. These injuries are usually the result of the mechanical compression and thermal injury inherent in cardiac surgery. Brachial plexus injuries can occur secondary to sternal retraction, particularly in patients with cervical ribs and in obese patients. Radial or ulnar nerve compression may occur from positioning or compression. Vocal cord paralysis resulting from injury to the recurrent laryngeal nerve can occur if the operative procedure involves extensive manipulation of the aortic arch, as in arch repair. More common is injury to the phrenic nerve. Nerve division (particularly in the case of redo procedures), thermal injury (secondary to the ice slush commonly used for topical cardiac hypothermia or Bovie use near the nerve), or loss of blood supply (caused by division of the pericardiophrenic branch of the internal mammary artery) can cause phrenic nerve injury. Phrenic nerve injury can result in diaphragmatic paresis or paralysis that can impair separation from mechanical ventilation and contribute to postoperative reduction in pulmonary function, manifested clinically by dyspnea. A chest radiograph usually shows elevation of a hemidiaphragm. The fluoroscopic "sniff test" is the simplest way to confirm presence of this entity. It is most commonly seen on the left side secondary to left internal mammary harvest. Other peripheral nerve injuries include paresthesias of the chest wall, the thigh, and the lower extremity secondary to division of intercostal, femoral, and other cutaneous nerves during vascular conduit harvest and vascular compartment dissection.

Infectious Complications

Because of the invasive nature of cardiac surgery, the percutaneous lines and drains, the need for temporary mechanical ventilation, and the underlying preoperative illness that occur in these patients, infectious complications may occur. A majority of patients develop low-grade fevers within the first several days of surgery. Most such fevers resolve spontaneously; however, an aggressive strategy for identification of pathogens should be adopted. Aerobic and anaerobic cultures of blood, urine, and sputum should be performed before institution of antimicrobial agents.

Soft tissue infections are usually caused by *Staphylococcus aureus* or *Staphylococcus epidermidis*. These infections can usually be treated easily. Serious infections, such as gram-negative wound, blood, or pulmonary infections are more common in patients with prolonged intensive care unit stays and are somewhat more difficult to treat.

Deep sternal wound infections and mediastinitis are dreaded complications of cardiac surgery. These infections are associated with a twofold to threefold increase in the incidence of death, as well as increased morbidity, cost, and length of hospital stay. Predisposing risk factors include obesity, chronic obstructive pulmonary disease, redo procedures, a history of tobacco use, and the use of bilateral internal mammary arteries for coronary conduits. The most important risk factor is the presence of diabetes, particularly when perioperative glucose control is suboptimal. Tight glucose control has been shown to greatly reduce the incidence of deep sternal wound infections in diabetic patients undergoing cardiac surgery (48).

Once a deep sternal wound infection has been diagnosed, appropriate treatment includes the use of aggressive antimicrobial agents as well as aggressive surgical dèbridement and early muscle flap coverage. Sternal rewiring continues to play a role, but is associated with a high rate of failure (48).

THE LATE POSTOPERATIVE PERIOD

Dyslipidemia

The majority of adults who undergo cardiac surgery have coronary artery disease. Although coronary artery surgery decreases symptoms and, in some cases, improves survival, it does nothing to alter the actual disease burden or the natural history of atherosclerotic disease. On the other hand, methods for secondary prevention have consistently demonstrated benefit. For this reason, secondary prevention is of paramount importance for patients who have undergone coronary artery revascularization procedures.

Serum lipid levels may be affected by the surgical intervention, at least in the short term. For this reason, it is advisable that a fasting lipid profile be obtained preoperatively if not obtained in the prior 3 months. Therapy that is in place preoperatively should be reinitiated as soon as a patient is able to take oral medication.

Therapy aimed at modifying serum cholesterol levels for the purpose of reducing future cardiovascular events is cost effective and can be accomplished best with the use of easy-to-follow guidelines. Although there is no uniform agreement as to exact therapeutic interventions, guidelines based on evidence-based medicine have been put forth by expert panels. Perhaps the most widely used guide is the National Cholesterol Education Program (NCEP) Expert Panel on Detection, Evaluation, and Treatment of High Blood Cholesterol in Adults. The most recent recommendations—the Adult Treatment Panel III (ATP-III), which was published in May of 2001—has revised guidelines for certain groups at high risk, such as diabetic patients (49) The focus of the NCEP ATP-III recommendations is on therapeutic lifestyle changes (TLCs) and low-density lipoprotein (LDL) goals.

Patients with established coronary artery disease should be monitored to ensure that LDL levels remain below 100 mg/dL. If LDL levels are above this goal, therapy based on TLC and drug therapy is appropriate. Most patients with established coronary artery disease require drug therapy in order to achieve a LDL of 100 mg/dL or less. The most common class of drugs used for this goal is the 3-hydroxy-3-methylglutaryl coenzyme A reductase inhibitors, better known as "statins." Currently available statins include atorvastatin, fluvastatin, lovastatin, pravastatin, and simvastatin. Other medications that are known to lower LDL include nicotinic acid, bile acid sequestrants, and fibric acids. Although their ability to decrease LDL is,

in general, not as strong as that of the statins, they do play an important role, particularly for patients with severe elevations in LDL, coexistant low levels of high-density lipoprotein, or hypertriglyceridemia. Other therapeutic options include the use of plant stanols/sterols (available in several preparations found in grocery stores), and optimal daily recommended fiber intake (20 to 30 g/day).

Despite the fact that LDL goals can usually be met with the use of drug therapy, TLC is of equal importance. Dietary modification should include a reduction in intake of saturated fats to less than 7% of caloric intake and a reduction in intake of cholesterol to less than 200 mg/day. Emphasis on weight reduction for patients who are obese, smoking cessation, optimal physical activity, and adequate blood glucose control for those with diabetes also contributes to optimization of serum lipid levels.

Patients who undergo noncoronary cardiac surgery (valvular or congenital repairs) should be managed in accordance with the NCEP ATP-III guidelines as well, even though their risk for atherosclerotic cardiovascular events may be much lower than that of patients who undergo coronary surgery.

There are other interventions that can be considered, such as assessment and treatment of serum homocysteine and lipoprotein(a) levels, which may also be of benefit. However, evidence-based data is not yet available to institute universal guidelines. A complete discussion of this topic is beyond the scope of this chapter but is well covered in Chapter 8.

Diet

Cardiac surgery imposes a significant physiologic burden on patients. In order to optimize wound healing, adequate nutritional status must be ensured. Adequate caloric intake is often somewhat difficult to obtain in the first days to weeks after surgery. Because of this, many physicians allow certain level of dietary indiscretion in order to stimulate adequate caloric intake. Although this may be appropriate at first, patients should rapidly resume a "heart-smart" approach to nutrition. In fact, an excellent opportunity for dietary teaching exists while a patient is still hospitalized. Methods for teaching range from easy-to-read written literature to videotaped information sessions that can be designed to be patient-driven in the last days of hospitalization. Scheduled visits with nutritionists are also helpful. Ultimately, adherence with guidelines set forth by the American Heart Association is a very cost-effective method for reducing future cardiovascular events. Further discussion of this topic is presented in Chapters 7 and 8.

Smoking Cessation

Smoking is the number one modifiable risk factor for the prevention of cardiovascular events. For this reason, the time period surrounding cardiovascular surgery is an excellent opportunity to modify this behavior.

If at all possible, patients who smoke should be encouraged to discontinue at least 1 week before surgery. This facilitates extubation and decreases the rate of postoperative pulmonary complications such as pneumonia. When time permits, the use of an incentive spirometer in the preoperative period also is helpful in achieving these goals, particularly for smokers. Preoperative incentive spirometry also allows a patient to learn proper technique before the incisional discomfort that will be present in the immediate postoperative period.

Patients who smoke should be offered interventions in the postoperative period. Patients should be exposed to teaching and information tools and, when available, should be seen by smoking-cessation counselors. Occasionally, drug therapy should be considered. Nicotine replacement therapy should probably be avoided in the immediate postoperative period because of the potential for inducing vasospasm and impairing wound healing. Other agents, such as bupropion (Wellbutrin, Zyban), may be very beneficial for patients with refractory habits.

The psychologic trauma that is imposed by a major surgical procedure is frequently severe enough to elevate a patient's motivation to the level required for effective lifestyle modification. Because of this fact, the perioperative period is an opportunity to facilitate lifestyle changes.

Anticoagulation

Many patients who undergo cardiac surgery require long-term postoperative anticoagulation with warfarin (Coumadin). Valvular procedures (particularly if mechanical prosthetic valves are used), atrial fibrillation or atrial flutter, and recent significant anterior wall myocardial infarction are common indications for anticoagulation.

The timing for initiation of warfarin depends on the patient, the procedure, and the presence or absence of postoperative bleeding complications. In general, if there is concern for excessive bleeding, anticoagulation should be initiated with heparin, as this is readily reversed with protamine sulfate, should the need arise. Warfarin can usually be safely started once invasive lines are removed, usually after the first postoperative day. The level of desired anticoagulation depends on the indication. A complete discussion of this topic is beyond the scope of this chapter but is well covered in Chapter 37.

Follow-up

Patients who undergo cardiac surgery should have early follow-up. In general, an office visit for a formal wound check should occur within the first 2 to 4 weeks after discharge. Further follow-up is tailored to the needs of the patient. As soon as surgical issues are well on the way to resolution, responsibility for follow-up care can be transferred from surgeon to cardiologist and ultimately to the patient's primary care provider. Well before surgical issues are resolved, a strategy for effective secondary prevention should be initiated. Appropriate follow-up should reflect this.

Cardiac Rehabilitation

Cardiac rehabilitation begins with the first postoperative step. Ambulation should be encouraged early in the postoperative course. Upon discharge, a patient should be given instructions as to what forms of activity should be undertaken in an individualized manner. In general, light ambulation around the house for the first few days followed by short walks outside is a reasonable expectation. As a patient regains strength, the length and duration of the walks are gradually increased and should be guided by fatigue level. A certain amount of fatigue should be expected, but excessive fatigue should be avoided for the first several weeks.

A formal program of cardiac rehabilitation should be initiated 4 to 8 weeks after coronary artery surgery. This should consist of three-times-weekly exercise sessions that are performed in a monitored setting at first. Routine graded exercise treadmill tests are frequently used in order to determine the best exercise prescription for each patient. Entry and exit graded exercise treadmill tests also allow patients to gauge their progress. Three months is the usual amount of time prescribed. Under ideal circumstances, cardiac rehabilitation programs should also provide teaching in other topics, such as nutrition and weight loss. Cardiac rehabilitation should also include family education and sexual and emotional counseling.

Postpericardotomy Syndrome

Approximately 10% to 40% percent of patients who undergo open cardiac procedures develop postpericardiotomy syndrome (50). This syndrome is identified by the presence of fever, pericarditis, and pleuritis that occur more than 1 week after surgery. Other features can include leukocytosis, elevated sedimentation rate, and noncardiac pulmonary edema. Clinical findings include pericardial and pleural friction rubs, although it should be noted that these are frequently heard in the first few postoperative days as well. Other clinical findings include pleural effusions, nonspecific ST segment and T wave abnormalities, pulmonary infiltrates, and, occasionally, cardiac tamponade (50). Echocardiography is helpful in determining the size of pericardial fluid collections. This syndrome is similar to post–myocardial infarction Dressler's syndrome.

The origin of this syndrome appears to be autoimmune in nature, as some patients develop antiheart antibodies in the setting of the postpericardiotomy syndrome. The clinical course is usually self-limited; however, it can be quite disabling and can recur. Treatment includes the use of liberal nonsteroidal antiinflammatory agents and, occasionally, corticosteroids. A relationship may exist between the postpericardiotomy syndrome and chronic constrictive pericarditis (50).

PRACTICAL POINTS

- With risk prediction tools, the likelihood of mortality, cerebrovascular accident, and mediastinitis can be estimated from data encompassing basic demographics, ejection fraction, and the presence of chronic obstructive pulmonary disease, diabetes, peripheral vascular occlusive disease, renal dysfunction, and procedural urgency.
- The risk of postoperative renal dysfunction can be predicted with basic preoperative data.
- Perioperative neurologic injury and infection can be minimized with thorough preoperative evaluation.
- Hemodynamic monitoring is mandatory after surgery because this period is accompanied by rapid fluid and electrolyte shifts, transient depression of myocardial function, and rapid fluctuations in vascular tone.
- Understanding a patient's coagulation status after cardiac surgery requires an understanding of the patient's preoperative status, the type and extent of the operative procedure, and appropriate expectations after the operation.
- Postoperative atrial arrhythmias can significantly increase the length of hospital stay, the cost of hospitalization, and the risk for postoperative stroke.

(continued)

- Sustained ventricular arrhythmias can cause acute hemodynamic compromise and are associated with a significant mortality rate. For this reason, an up-to-date working knowledge of ACLS is mandatory for any physician with primary responsibilities for patients after cardiac surgery.
- Neurologic complications occur after cardiac surgery and range from permanent cerebrovascular accidents, with a rate of 1% to 4% after standard cardiopulmonary bypass coronary procedures, to cognitive decline, which occurs in up to 50% to 80% at the time of discharge.
- Secondary prevention is of paramount importance for patients who have undergone coronary artery revascularization procedures, because these measures have consistently demonstrated benefit.

- Cardiac surgery imposes a significant physiologic burden on patients. In order to optimize wound healing, adequate nutritional status must be ensured.
- Patients who undergo cardiac surgery should have early follow-up. In general, an office visit for a formal wound check should occur within the first 2 to 4 weeks after discharge.
- Cardiac rehabilitation begins with the first postoperative step. Ambulation should be encouraged early in the postoperative course. A formal program of cardiac rehabilitation should be initiated 4 to 8 weeks after coronary artery surgery.
- Approximately 10% to 40% percent of patients who undergo open cardiac procedures develop postpericardiotomy syndrome.

REFERENCES

1. Shumaker HB. *The evolution of cardiac surgery.* Bloomington, IN: Indiana University Press, 1992.
2. Vineberg AM, Miller G. Internal mammary coronary anastomosis in the surgical treatment of coronary artery insufficiency. *Can Med Assoc J* 1951;64:204.
3. Gibbon JH. The development of the heart-lung apparatus. *Am J Surg* 1978;135:608–619.
4. Eagle KA, Guyton RA, Davidoff R, et al. ACC/AHA guidelines for coronary artery bypass graft surgery: a report of the American College of Cardiology/American Heart Association Task Force on Practice Guidelines (Committee to Revise the 1991 Guidelines for Coronary Artery Bypass Graft Surgery). *J Am Coll Cardiol* 1999;34:1262–1347.
5. Mangano DT. Cardiovascular morbidity and CABG surgery: a perspective: epidemiology, costs, and potential therapeutic solutions. *J Card Surg* 10:366–368.
6. Guyton RA, Mellitt RJ, Weintraub WS. A critical assessment of neurological risk during warm heart surgery. *J Card Surg* 1995;10:488–492.
7. Lamb RK, Prabhakar G, Thorpe JA. The use of atenolol in the prevention of supraventricular arrhythmias following coronary artery surgery. *Eur Heart J* 1988;9:32–36.
8. Daoud EG, Strickberger SA, Man KC, et al. Preoperative amiodarone as prophylaxis against atrial fibrillation after heart surgery. *N Engl J Med* 1997;337:1785–1791.
9. Murphy PJ, Connery C, Hicks GL, et al. Homologous blood transfusion as a risk factor for postoperative infection after coronary artery bypass graft operations. *J Thorac Cardiovasc Surg* 1992;104:1092–1099.
10. van de Watering LM, Hermans J, Houbiers JG, et al. Beneficial effects of leukocyte depletion of transfused blood on postoperative complications in patients undergoing cardiac surgery: a randomized clinical trial. *Circulation* 1998;97:562–568.
11. DiSesa VJ, Brown E, Mudge GH. Hemodynamic comparison of dopamine and dobutamine in the postoperative volume loaded, pressure loaded and normal ventricle. *J Thorac Cardiavasc Surg* 1982;83:256.
12. Alonsi AA, Stankus GP, Stuart JC. Characterization of cardiothoracic effects of milrinone. *J Clin Pharmacol* 1983;5:804.
13. Shapira N, Schaff HV, White RD, et al. Hemodynamic effects of calcium chloride injections following cardiopulmonary bypass. *Ann Thorac Surg* 1984;37:133–140.
14. Kantrowitz A, Tjonaeland S, Freed PS, et al. Initial clinical experience with intraaortic balloon pumping in cardiogenic shock. *JAMA* 1968;203:113.
15. Dyke DB, Pagani FD, Aaronson KD. Circulatory assist devices—2000: an update. *Congest Heart Fail* 2000;6:259–271.
16. Rose EA, Gelijns AC, Moskowitz AJ, et al. The Randomized Evaluation of Mechanical Assistance for the Treatment of Congestive Heart Failure (REMATCH) Study Group. Long-term use of a left ventricular assist device for end-stage heart failure. *N Engl J Med* 2001;345:1435–1443.
17. The sixth report of the Joint National Committee on Prevention, Detection, Evaluation, and Treatment of High Blood Pressure. *Arch Intern Med* 1997;157:2413–2446.
18. Cohn JN, Archibald DG, Ziesche S, et al. Effect of vasodilator therapy on mortality in chronic congestive heart failure. Results of a Veterans Administration Cooperative Study. *N Engl J Med* 1986;314:1547–1552.
19. CONSENSUS Trial Study Group. Effects of enalapril in

mortality in severe congestive heart failure. *N Engl J Med* 1987;316:1429–1435.

20. SOLVD Investigators. Effect of enalapril in survival in patients with reduced left ventricular ejection fractions and congestive heart failure. *N Engl J Med* 1991;325:293–302.

21. SOLVD Investigators. Effect of enalapril in mortality and the development of heart failure in asymptomatic patients with reduced left ventricular ejection fractions. *N Engl J Med* 1992;327:685–691.

22. Pfeffer MA, Braunwald E, Moye LA, et al. Effect of captopril on mortality and morbidity in patients with left ventricular dysfunction after myocardial infarction. Results of the Survival and Ventricular Enlargement trial. The SAVE Investigators. *N Engl J Med* 1992;327;669–677.

23. Acute Infarction Ramipril Efficacy (AIRE) Study Investigators. Effect of ramipril on mortality and morbidity of survivors of acute myocardial infarction with clinical evidence of heart failure. *Lancet* 1993;3423:821–828.

24. Yusuf S, Sleight P, Pogue J, et al. Effects of an angiotensin-converting-enzyme inhibitor, ramipril, on cardiovascular events in high-risk patients. The Heart Outcomes Prevention Evaluation Study Investigators. *N Engl J Med* 2000;342:145–153. [Errata, *N Engl J Med* 2000;342:1376 and 2000;342:748.]

25. Weerosinghe A, Taylor K. The platelet in cardiopulmonary bypass. *Ann Thorac Surg,* 1998;66:2145–2152.

26. Khuri SF, Wolfe JA, Jos M, et al. Hematologic changes during and after cardiopulmonary bypass and their relationship to the bleeding time and non surgical blood loss. *J Thorac Cardiovasc Surg* 1992;104:94.

27. VanderSal T, Stohl R. Early postoperative care. In: Edmunds LH Jr, ed. *Cardiac surgery in the adult.* New York: McGraw-Hill, 1997:339.

28. Milas BL, Jobes DR, Gorman RC. Management of bleeding and coagulopathy after heart surgery. *Semin Thorac Cardiovasc Surg* 2000;12(4):326–336.

29. Barner HB, Standeven JW, Reese J. Twelve-year experience with internal mammary artery for coronary artery bypass. *J Thorac Cardiovasc Surg* 1985;90:668–675.

30. Chesebro JH, Fuster V, Elveback LR, et al. Effect of dipyridamole and aspirin on late vein-graft patency after coronary bypass operations. *N Engl J Med* 1984;310:209–214.

31. Lorenz RL, Schacky CV, Weber M, et al. Improved aortocoronary bypass patency by low-dose aspirin (100 mg daily): effects on platelet aggregation and thromboxane formation. *Lancet* 1984;1:1261–1264.

32. Sharma GV, Khuri SF, Josa M, et al. The effect of antiplatelet therapy on saphenous vein coronary artery bypass graft patency. *Circulation* 1983;68(Suppl II):II-218–II-21.

33. Poggio ED, Kottke-Marchant K, Welsh PA, et al. The prevalence of aspirin resistance in cardiac patients as measured by platelet aggregation and the PFA-100. *J Am Coll Cardiol* 1999;33:254A(abst).

34. Bhatt DL, Chew DP, Hirsch AT, et al. Superiority of clopidogrel versus aspirin in patients with prior cardiac surgery. *Circulation* 2001;103:363–368.

35. Aranki SF, Shaw DP, Adams DH, et al. Predictors of atrial fibrillation after coronary artery surgery: current trends and impact on hospital resources. *Circulation* 1996;94:390–397.

36. Almassi GH, Schowalter T, Nicolosi AC, et al. Atrial fibrillation after cardiac surgery: a major morbid event? *Ann Surg* 1997;226:501–511.

37. Mathew JP, Parks R, Savino JS, et al. Atrial fibrillation following coronary artery bypass graft surgery: predictors, outcomes, and resource utilization: Multi-Center Study of Perioperative Ischemia Research Group. *JAMA* 1996;276:300–306.

38. Steinberg JS, Aelenkofske S, Wong S, et al. Value of the P-wave signal-averaged ECG for predicting atrial fibrillation after cardiac surgery. *Circulation* 1993;88:2618–2622.

39. Guidelines 2000 for cardiopulmonary resuscitation and emergency cardiovascular care. The American Heart Association in collaboration with the International Liaison Committee on Resuscitation. *Circulation* 2000;102(8, Suppl):I-1–I-370.

40. Buxton AE, Lee KL, DiCarlo L, et al. Electrophysiologic testing to identify patients with coronary artery disease who are at risk for sudden death. *N Engl J Med* 2000;342:1937–1945.

41. Cleveland J, Shroyer L, Chen A, et al. Off-pump coronary artery bypass grafting decreases risk adjusted mortality and morbidity. *Ann Thorac Surg* 2001;7282–7289.

42. Newman M, Kirchner J, Phillips-Bute B, et al. Longitudinal assessment of neurocognitive function after coronary artery bypass surgery. *N Engl J Med* 2001;344:395–402.

43. Roach GW, Kanchuger M, Mangano CM, et al. Adverse cerebral outcomes after coronary bypass surgery: Multicenter Study of Perioperative Ischemia Research Group and the Ischemia Research and Education Foundation Investigators. *N Engl J Med* 1996;335:1857–1863.

44. McKhann G, Goldsborough M, Borowicz L, et al. Predictors of stroke risk in coronary artery bypass patients. *Ann Thorac Surg* 1997;63:516–521.

45. Lynn GM, Stefanko K, Reed JF, et al. Risk factors for stroke after coronary artery bypass. *J Thorac Cardiovasc Surg* 1992;104:1518–1523.

46. Duda AM, Letwin LB, Sutter FP, et al. Does routine use of aortic ultrasonography decrease the stroke rate in coronary artery bypass surgery? *J Vasc Surg* 1995;21:98–107.

47. Neville M, Butterworth J, James R, et al. Similar neurobehavioral outcome after valve or coronary artery operations despite differing carotid embolic counts. *J Thorac Cardiov Surg* 2001;121:125–136.

48. Furnary AP, Zerr KJ, Grunkemeier GL, et al. Continuous intravenous insulin infusion reduces the incidence of deep sternal wound infection in diabetic patients after cardiac surgical procedures. *Ann Thorac Surg* 1999;67:352–362.

49. Expert Panel on Detection, Evaluation, and Treatment of High Blood Cholesterol in Adults. Executive summary of the third report of the National Cholesterol Education Program (NCEP) Expert Panel on Detection, Evaluation, and Treatment of High Blood Cholesterol in Adults (Adult Treatment Panel III). *JAMA* 2001;285:2486–2497.

50. Braunwald E, ed. *Heart disease: a textbook of cardiovascular medicine,* 5th ed. Philadelphia: WB Saunders, 1997.

40

Common Drugs in Cardiovascular Care: Doses, Side Effects, & Key Interactions

Mike Shea, Marshal Shlafer

TABLE 40.1. *Diuretics*

Drug	Indication(s), typical dosages (oral administration unless noted otherwise)	Key side effects	Comments
Thiazide and thiazide-like agents (potassium-wasting)			
		For all: hypokalemia, hypercalcemia, elevations of serum lipids, hyperglycemia (reduced sensitivity of parenchymal cells to insulin), hyponatremia and excessive diuresis (risk slight if used alone); flat dose-response curve: when maximum recommended dosages fail to cause effect(s) of desired intensity, do not increase dosage: doing so is likely only to increase risk and severity of side effects; instead, switch to diuretic of another class (e.g., loop) or add potassium-sparing diuretic if that approach seems fruitful	Generally the preferred diuretic class when clinical goal is monotherapy or adjunctive management of HTN; loop diuretic (described later) usually chosen when main goal is managing edema, especially if significant or refractory, or when rapid effects are needed
Bendroflumethiazide (Naturetin)	Edema: 5 mg once daily to start; typical maintenance dosage, 2.5–5 mg/day HTN: 5–20 mg/day to start; maintenance dosage, typically 2.5–15 mg/day	—	—
Benzthiazide (Exna)	Edema: 50–200 mg to start, with doses >100 mg given in two equal divided doses; maintenance dosage, typically 25–200 mg/day as single dose or in two equal divided doses if total dose/day >100 mg HTN: 25 or 50 mg twice daily, with breakfast and lunch; maximum effective maintenance dosage is 200 mg/day	—	—
Chlorothiazide (Diuril)	Edema: 0.5–1 g twice daily orally or IV if oral route cannot be used HTN: 0.5–1 g/day orally in single or two equal divided doses; infants and children: 22 mg/kg/day; infants <6 months old may need up to 33 mg/kg/day	—	Only thiazide available in parenteral formulation; loop diuretic generally preferred when parenteral therapy desired or needed
Chlorthalidone (Hygroton, Thalitone)	Edema: 50–100 mg once daily to start (30–60 mg if using Thalitone) or 100 mg (60 mg of Thalitone) every other day; some patients may require 150–200 mg/day (90–120 mg Thalitone) HTN: 12.5–25 mg once daily (15 mg of Thalitone); titrate as needed to 50 mg/day (30–15 mg Thalitone)	Clinically significant bioequivalence differences: do not substitute Hygroton and Thalitone haphazardly on a mg-for-mg basis	—

(continued)

TABLE 40.1. (*Continued*)

Drug	Indication(s), typical dosages (oral administration unless noted otherwise)	Key side effects	Comments
Hydrochlorothiazide (Esidrix, HydroDIURIL)	Edema: 25–200 mg/day to start; typical maintenance dosage, 25–100 mg once daily; HTN: 12.5–50 mg once daily; for infants and children, 2.2 mg/kg/day in two equal divided doses	—	—
Hydroflumethiazide (Diucardin, Saluron)	Edema: 50 mg once or twice a day to start; maintenance dosage, 25–200 mg/day, given in two equal divided doses if total daily dose > 100 mg; HTN: 50–100 mg/day up to maximum of 200 mg/day	—	—
Indapamide (Lozol)	Edema: 2.5 or 5 mg each morning; HTN: 1.25 mg to start; maintenance dosage, up to maximum of 5 mg/day	—	Allegedly lower incidence of hyperuricemia than thiazides, thiazide-like agents
Methyclothiazide (Aquatensen, Enduron)	Edema: 2.5–10 mg once daily; HTN: 2.5–5 mg once daily	—	—
Metolazone (Mykrox, Zaroxolyn)	Edema: Zaroxolyn, 5–20 mg once daily; HTN: if using Zaroxolyn, 2.5–5 mg once daily; if using Mykrox, 0.5 mg once daily, 1 mg if needed	Mykrox and Zaroxolyn are not bioequivalent or therapeutically equivalent on a mg-for-mg basis; do not interchange or substitute	—
Polythiazide (Renese)	Edema: 1–4 mg once daily; HTN: 2–4 mg once daily	—	—
Quinethazone (Hydromox)	Edema or HTN: 50–100 mg once daily	—	—
Trichlormethiazide (Metahydrin, Naqua)	Edema or HTN: 2–4 mg once daily	—	—
Loop diuretics (potassium-wasting; also known as "high-		For all: most are qualitatively similar to those at thiazides but quantitatively greater, thereby posing greater risks, especially from excessive sodium, fluid retention, hypochloremia, and metabolic alkalosis; drugs increase calcium, magnesium excretion; are ototoxic (mainly hearing loss, which may or may not be reversible, especially prevalent with ethacrynic acid)	

Bumetanide (Bumex)	Edema: 0.5–2 mg once daily, up to maximum daily maintenance dosage of 10 mg; IM or IV (use only when oral route not practical or GI absorption is compromised): 0.5–1 mg (infuse IV slowly over 1–2 min); repeat at 2- to 3-hr intervals as needed to maximum of 10 mg/day	—	—	Steep dose-response curve makes it relatively easy to cause excessive effects; hypokalemia due to loop diuretics, given concomitantly with digoxin for CHF, is most common cause of digoxin toxicity
Ethacrynic acid (Edecrin), ethacrynate sodium (Edecrin Sodium)	Edema, acute pulmonary edema, ascites: 50–200 mg daily; some patients with severe refractory edema may require more; children: start with 25 mg IV (ethacrynate sodium), 50 mg, or 0.5–1 mg/kg, infused over several minutes	—	—	
Furosemide (Lasix)	Edema: 20–80 mg once daily; titrate at intervals not <6–8 hr to achieve desired diuresis; or give in two equal divided doses, up to maximum of 600 mg/day; IV or IM: 20–40 mg; if given IV, infuse slowly over 1–2 min; high-dose parenteral therapy can also be achieved by continuous IV infusion ≤4 mg/min Acute pulmonary edema (adjunct): 40 mg IV to start (infuse over 1–2 min) for adults, 1 mg/kg IM or IV for children CHF with chronic renal failure: typically 2–2.5 g/day IV; oral dosage of 2–2.5 g may be needed, is often well tolerated HTN: 40 mg twice daily, titrated as needed; if furosemide is being added to regimen involving other antihypertensive medications, decrease dose of other agent(s) by >50% at time furosemide is started HTN in infants and children: 2 mg/kg to start, increase by 1 or 2 mg/kg at 6- to 8-hr intervals if needed; usual maintenance dosage, 0.5–2 mg/kg			
Torsemide (Demadex)	CHF: Initially 10 or 20 mg once daily, orally or IV Chronic renal failure: 20 mg once daily, orally or IV Hepatic cirrhosis: 5 or 10 mg once daily, orally or IV HTN: start with 5 mg once daily; maintenance dosage, up to 10 mg once daily; if greater reduction of BP is required, cautiously add another class of antihypertensive drug rather than increasing torsemide dose	—		

(continued)

TABLE 40.1. (*Continued*)

Drug	Indication(s), typical dosages (oral administration unless noted otherwise)	Key side effects	Comments
Potassium-sparing diuretics			
		For all: hyperkalemia, especially if used with oral potassium supplements or potassium-containing drugs (avoid combined use); otherwise, side effects are largely similar, qualitatively and quantitatively, to those noted for thiazides	
Amiloride (Midamor)	When used alone or as adjunct, start with 5 mg once daily, increase to 10 mg (usual maintenance) if needed; some patients may require 15 or 20 mg/day	—	Blocks distal sodium channels that normally reabsorb sodium, secrete potassium
Spironolactone (Aldactone)	Diagnosis of primary hyperaldosteronism: 400 mg/day for 4 days, 3–4 wk Maintenance therapy for hyperaldosteronism: 100–400 g/day for several days preoperatively or continuously if surgery cannot be performed for definitive treatment Edema (as from CHF, nephrotic syndrome, hepatic cirrhosis): start with 25–200 mg/day, titrate to maximum response; if this response is insufficient, continue spironolactone at current dose and add thiazide or loop diuretic (for children, give 3.3 mg/kg/day as single daily dose or in two equal divided doses HTN: 50–100 mg/day as single dose or in two equal divided doses, alone or in combination with a thiazide (for children, 1–2 mg/kg/day as single dose or in two divided doses Prevention of hypokalemia (e.g., diuretic-induced) or management of mild, asymptomatic diuretic-induced hypokalemia	Acne, deepening of the voice, gynecomastia in men, due to antiandrogen-like effects of the drug; other side effects: see general comments for potassium-sparing diuretics	Competitive blockade of aldosterone receptors, rather than interference with specific renal tubular transporters or ion channels, is mechanism of action
Triamterene (Dyrenium)	Edema or HTN: alone or as adjunct: usually 100 mg twice daily after meals; do not exceed 300 mg/day	—	Amiloride-like mechanism; may cause photosensitivity, bluish discoloration of urine

BP, blood pressure; CHF, congestive heart failure; GI, gastrointestinal; HTN, hypertension; IM, intramuscularly; IV, intravenously.

616

TABLE 40.2. *Beta-adrenergic blockers for hypertension and selected other indications*

Drug	Indication(s), typical dosages (oral administration unless noted otherwise)	Key side effects	Comments
	Only "cardiovascular" uses are listed here. Some agents (e.g., propranolol for prophylaxis of migraine, topical timolol for glaucoma) have other uses. When any beta blocker is used for any of these other indications, even via the topical ophthalmic route, their potential cardiac/cardiovascular impact should be considered; beta blockers, along with thiazide/thiazide-like diuretics, calcium channel blockers, and ACE inhibitors/angiotensin receptor blockers), are the "big 4" drug groups for starting therapy for essential HTN in most patients (depending on, e.g., individual patient profiles, comorbid conditions)	Side effects are varied, affecting virtually all organ systems; all have the potential to cause hypotension (especially if administered with other antihypertensives) and/or excessive cardiac depression (contractility, rate, and conduction, especially if administered with other cardiac depressants such as nondihydropyridine-type calcium channel blockers such as verapamil or diltiazem); highly lipid soluble beta blockers such as propranolol are associated with higher incidence of CNS side effects (somnolence, drowsiness, fatigue, altered libido and sexual performance); nonselective beta blockers are generally contraindicated for patients with asthma (risk of fatal bronchospasm) and poorly controlled diabetes mellitus (type I or II; risk of hypoglycemia, delayed recovery from hypoglycemia); severely reduced LV ejection fractions; AV block ≥2nd degree; bradycardia; "cardioselective" (beta$_1$) beta blockers may pose a lower risk, but risk of serious adverse responses persists nonetheless and is highly dose-dependent (cardioselectivity is lost at higher dosages); sympathomimetics with alpha agonist (vasoconstrictor) activity, including OTC agents, pose risk of serious hypertensive responses in patients taking any beta blocker	
Acebutolol hydrochloride (Sectral)	HTN: 400 mg once daily or 200 mg twice daily; maintenance dose, usually 200–1,200 mg/day in two divided doses Ventricular arrhythmias (premature beats): usually 200 mg to start; maintenance dosage, 300–600 mg twice daily; dosages for either indication require adjustment down with either reduced renal or reduced hepatic function	See general side effects	Cardioselective; like propranolol, causes considerable prolongation of effective refractory period of AV node, greatest slowing of AV nodal conduction velocity
Atenolol (Tenormin)	HTN or chronic stable angina: 50 mg once daily; maximum recommended maintenance dosage, 100 mg/day	See general side effects	Cardioselective at low dosages

(continued)

TABLE 40.2. (Continued)

Drug	Indication(s), typical dosages (oral administration unless noted otherwise)	Key side effects	Comments
	Acute MI: if possible, give IV infusion of 5 mg over 5 min, repeat 10 min later; if patient tolerates full 10-mg IV dose, start 50 mg orally 10 min after last IV dose, give 50 mg 12 hr later, then give 50 mg twice daily or 100 mg once a day for 6–9 days; oral therapy may be started directly, without IV administration, if there are concerns about IV administration of the drug		
Betaxolol hydrochloride (Kerlone)	HTN: typically, 10 mg once daily; usual maintenance dosage, 10–20 mg/day	See general side effects	Cardioselective at low dosages
Bisoprolol fumarate (Zebeta)	HTN: initially, 5 mg once daily; maintenance dosage, 2.5–20 mg once daily	See general side effects	Cardioselective at low dosages
Carteolol hydrochloride (Cartrol)	HTN: 2.5 mg once daily, then 5 mg or 10 mg once daily if needed; usual maintenance dosage, 2.5–5 mg once daily; reduce dosage interval with increasing degrees of renal impairment	See general side effects	Nonselective (beta$_1$ and beta$_2$) blockade, has ISA
Carvedilol (Coreg)	HTN: Initially, 6.25 mg twice daily; if tolerated and needed, increase after 1–2 weeks to 12.5 mg twice daily; further weekly/biweekly increases to maximum of 50 mg/day in two divided doses may be necessary	See general side effects	Has both alpha- and beta-blocking activity
	CHF: Usually 3.125 mg twice daily for 2 weeks; if tolerated and needed, double dosage every 2 weeks to maximum of 25 mg twice daily for patients <85 kg or 50 mg twice daily for heavier patients		
Esmolol hydrochloride (Brevibloc)	Supraventricular tachycardia: IV: usually start with 500 μg/kg/min for 1 min to load, maintain with 50 μg/kg/min for 4 min. If needed, repeat loading dose, increase maintenance infusion by 50 μg/kg/min each time	See general side effects	—
Labetalol hydrochloride (Normodyne, Trandate)	HTN: oral: usually 100 mg twice daily alone or with diuretic; maintenance dosage, usually 200–400 mg twice daily; IV: initially, 20 mg (or approximately 0.25 mg/kg) injected over 2 min; Slow IV infusion: infuse 1 mg/mL solution at 2 mg/min	See general side effects	Has both alpha- and beta-blocking activity Labetalol is not compatible with or stable in alkaline media, including 5% sodium bicarbonate injection or fluids containing furosemide
Metoprolol (Lopressor, Toprol XL)	HTN: Usually 100 mg/day of immediate-release formulation in single daily or two equal divided doses (extended-release tablets: 50–100 mg/day once daily)	See general side effects	Cardioselective at low dosages; bioavailability, and hence effects, increased when taken with food (avoid)
	Angina: 100 mg/day in two divided doses (or 100 mg of extended-release formulation once daily); usual effective dosage, 100–400 mg/day in single or divided doses		
	Early post-MI cardioprotection: three IV boluses of 5 mg each at about 2-min intervals as soon as patient is hemodynamically stable; if patient tolerates full IV regimen, switch to oral, 50 mg every 6 hr, then transfer to maintenance oral dosage of 100 mg twice daily		

Drug	Dosage	Side effects	Comments
Nadolol (Corgard)	HTN or angina: Usually 40 mg once daily to start; maintenance doses, typically 40–80 mg once daily; prolong dose interval with decreasing renal function	See general side effects	Nonselective beta blockade; noteworthy as undergoing virtually no hepatic metabolism; elimination totally dependent on renal function
Penbutolol sulfate (Levatol)	HTN: Typically, 20 mg once daily to start and maintain	See general side effects	Nonselective; high lipid solubility and propensity for more CNS effects
Pindolol (Visken)	HTN: Usually 5 mg twice daily to start; if needed, increase in 10-mg/day increments every 3–4 weeks to maximum of 60 mg/day, given in two equal divided doses	—	Has intrinsic sympathomimetic activity; nonselective
Propranolol hydrochloride (Inderal)	HTN: 40 mg of immediate-release formulation (or 80 mg of sustained-release preparation) to start; maintenance dosage, 120–240 mg/day in two to three equal divided doses (120–160 mg of sustained-release preparation once daily) Angina: initially, 80–320 mg two, three, or four times daily (or 80 mg of sustained-release preparation once daily); maintenance dosage, typically 160 mg of sustained-release preparation once daily Post-MI cardioprotection: 180–240 mg/day in three or four divided doses Idiopathic hypertrophic subaortic stenosis: 20–40 mg three or four times a day or 80–160 mg of sustained-release preparation once daily Pheochromocytoma: 30 mg/day in divided doses for inoperable tumors/symptom control, 60 mg/day for 3 days after pheochromocytoma surgery Migraine prophylaxis: 80 mg/day once daily of sustained-release preparation or same dose of immediate-release form in divided doses; usual maintenance dosage, 160–240 mg/day of immediate-release preparation or same dose of sustained-release preparation once daily	See general side effects	Nonselective; very high lipid solubility, propensity for CNS side effects; significant effects on AV nodal refractory periods and conduction velocity; bioavailability increased by food (avoid); undergoes extensive first-pass hepatic metabolism when dosing is started
Sotalol hydrochloride (Betapace)	Maintenance of normal sinus rhythm in patients with symptomatic atrial fibrillation/flutter in patients already in normal sinus rhythm: 80 mg twice daily if creatinine clearance >60 mL/min; reduce dosage and/or dose interval with lower creatinine clearance; maintenance dosage and dosage interval dependent on QT interval (corrected), QRS duration, and other factors	See general side effects	—
Timolol maleate (Blocadren)	HTN: 10 mg twice daily to start; maintenance, typically 20–40 mg/day in two equal divided doses MI, oral long-term prophylaxis: 10 mg twice daily after recovery from acute post-MI phase	See general side effects	—

ACE, angiotensin-converting enzyme; AV, atrioventricular; CHF, congestive heart failure; CNS, central nervous system; HTN, hypertension; ISA, intrinsic sympathomimetic activity; IV, intravenously; LV, left ventricular; MI, myocardial infarction; OTC, over-the-counter.

TABLE 40.3. *Antihypertensive drugs: peripheral alpha-adrenergic blockers*

Drug	Indication(s), typical dosages (oral administration unless noted otherwise)	Key side effects	Comments
	For all oral agents except phenoxybenzamine: management of essential hypertension, usually second line after beta blocker, ACE inhibitor, calcium channel blocker, and diuretic (alone or in combination); adjunctive management of pheochromocytoma (i.e., with beta blocker)	All oral agents except phenoxybenzamine act by selectively blocking alpha$_1$ adrenergic receptors (postsynaptic). Side effects include risk of orthostatic/postural hypotension, including and especially symptomatic hypotension after first dose or after first dose of an increase when titrating up (allegedly most prevalent with prazosin); reflex tachycardia, usually slight; rhinorrhea, excessive lacrimation, urinary frequency; peripheral edema; poor vision in dim/low light (miosis); compensatory renal sodium and water retention in response to BP fall may warrant adding diuretic	
Oral agents			
Doxazosin mesylate (Cardura)	1 mg once daily to start; maintenance dosage, typically 1–16 mg once daily; doses >4 mg/day likely to cause excessive postural hypotension and related signs/symptoms/side effects	See general side effects	—
Phenoxybenzamine (Dibenzyline)	Adjunctive management (with beta blocker) of pheochromocytoma: 5–10 mg twice daily to start; increase every other day as needed to usual maintenance dosage of 20–40 mg two to three times daily	Significant orthostatic hypotension and reflex tachycardia (hence adjunctive use with beta blocker); potentially greatest risk of hypotension-tachycardia- related myocardial ischemia; start therapy with alpha blocker before initiating beta blocker (agents above or phenoxybenzamine) to avoid inducing acute heart failure and hypertensive crisis from excessive catecholamine levels	Nonselective (alpha$_1$ and alpha$_2$) alpha blocker (phentolamine-like)

Agent	Dosage	Comments	
Prazosin hydrochloride (Minipress)	Initially, 1 mg two or three times daily; typical maintenance dosage, 6–15 mg/day in divided doses; when adding other antihypertensives, decrease prazosin dosage to 1–2 mg three times daily, then retitrate upward as needed	See general side effects	Allegedly highest incidence of "first-dose syncope" effect; administer first dose at bedtime and forewarn patient about syncope, what to do about it
Terazosin hydrochloride (Hytrin)	1 mg at bedtime to start; maintenance dosage, 1–5 mg/day; if hypotensive response is inadequate at end of dosing interval, consider either increasing the dosage or administering the total daily dose in two equal divided doses	See above	—
Parenteral agents Phentolamine mesylate (Regitine)	Prophylaxis or management of hypertensive episodes in pheochromocytoma patients (e.g., as triggered by stress, surgery) and/or during preoperative preparation: IV or IM: 5 mg (1 mg for children) 1–2 hr before surgery, repeated as needed before/during surgery. Unlabeled uses include management of hypertensive episodes associated with beta blocker or clonidine withdrawal, monoamine oxidase–sympathomimetic interactions, or overdoses with alpha agonist vasoconstrictors (e.g., phenylephrine)	Much greater reflex tachycardia/cardiac stimulation, and consequences thereof, than with selective alpha blockers; may require pharmacologic control	Nonselective (alpha$_1$ alpha$_2$) blocker
Tolazoline hydrochloride (Priscoline HCl)	IV for persistent pulmonary HTN in newborns: 1–2 mg/kg initially, then infuse 1–2 mg/kg/hr (usually for no more than 36–48 hr) to achieve desired arterial oxygen saturation	See description for phentolamine; adjunctive diuretic may be needed if compensatory renal sodium and water retention becomes problematic	—

ACE, angiotensin-converting enzyme; BP, blood pressure; HTN, hypertension; IM, intramuscularly; IV, intravenously.

TABLE 40.4. *Other (miscellaneous) antihypertensive drugs*

Drug	Indication(s), typical dosages (oral administration unless noted otherwise)	Key side effects	Comments
	None is generally considered "first line" for managing essential hypertension, for which a diuretic, ACE inhibitor, beta blocker, or calcium channel blocker is usually preferred, depending on patient profile (see methyldopa, however, in context of managing hypertension during pregnancy); some are indicated only for parenteral intervention in hypertensive urgencies/emergencies	For all: overdoses cause dose-dependent hypotension and consequences thereof (e.g., myocardial and cerebral ischemia); BP-lowering effect may trigger compensatory renal sodium and water retention, necessitating adding diuretic if one is not being given already	
Clonidine hydrochloride (Catapres)	HTN (usually that which is not responsive to traditional first-line oral antihypertensives, alone or in combination): initially, 100 μg twice daily; increase by 100 μg/day at weekly intervals to desired response (usually 200–600 μg/day in divided doses. Transdermal: start with one 0.1-mg/24-hr delivery system applied each day; increase to total of 0.2 mg/24 hr after 1–2 weeks if necessary; efficacy is not increased by use of more than two 0.3-mg/24-hr systems	Prototypic centrally acting antihypertensive; somnolence, impaired ejaculatory function, dry mouth; mechanism of action may concomitantly cause slight reduction of sympathetic tone of heart (rate, contractility), which tends to blunt reflex cardiac stimulation; compensatory renal sodium and water retention may necessitate adding thiazide	Discontinue gradually to avoid significant, severe rebound hypertension and potential abrupt hypertensive crisis
Diazoxide (Hyperstat)	Severe HTN, urgent hypertensive crisis, particularly when other drugs (e.g., parenteral labetalol, nitroprusside) are not available or cannot be used for other reasons: IV: rapidly infuse (over <30 sec) 1–3 mg/kg up to maximum of 150 mg; may repeat at 5- to 15-min intervals until BP is at desired level; then switch to oral antihypertensive	Renal sodium and water retention may necessitate diuretic, which provides additive lowering of BP; direct cardiac stimulation plus reflex cardiac stimulation from vasodilation may cause tachycardia; other consequences, including ischemia, often warrant pharmacologic control of cardiac response; hyperglycemia may occur	Evidence suggests that bolus administration is not necessary and rapid IV infusion usually suffices
Fenoldopam mesylate (Corlopam)	In-hospital emergency control of hypertension: IV: typically 0.05- to 0.1-mg/kg/min infusion	Headache, flushing, nausea, and hypotension are most common; renal and reflex cardiac responses may necessitate adjunctive control with diuretic, beta blocker, or nondihydropyridine calcium channel blocker	—
Guanabenz citrate (Wytensin)	HTN (usually that which is not responsive to traditional first-line oral antihypertensives, alone or in combination): initially, 4 mg twice daily; if needed, increase at 1- to 2-wk intervals by 4–8 mg/day; maximum dosage studied, 32 mg twice daily, rarely needed	Clonidine-like centrally acting antihypertensive; see clonidine description	—

Drug	Indications and Dosage	Comments	
Guanadrel sulfate (Hylorel)	HTN (usually that which is not responsive to traditional first-line oral antihypertensives, alone or in combination): usually 5 mg twice daily; typical maintenance dosage (with normal renal function), 20–75 mg/day in two equal divided doses; maintenance dosage, >75 mg/day, should be divided in three to four equal doses	Catecholamine depletor (reserpine-like) causes orthostatic hypotension, parasympathetic predominance (e.g., lacrimation, salivation, diarrhea)	—
Guanethidine monosulfate (Ismelin)	Moderate-severe HTN in ambulatory patients: initially, 100 mg/day; for hospitalized adults, 25–50 mg/day or every other day to start; loading dose protocol involves giving dose three times a day at 6-hr intervals over 1–3 days; for children, typically 0.2 mg/kg/24 hr (or 6 mg/square meter of body surface area/24 hr) as single daily oral dose	Paradoxical worsening of HTN (due to initial catecholamine release) upon start of therapy; later, hypotension (especially orthostatic) and cardiac depression; severe parasympathetic predominance manifested as diarrhea, urinary frequency, excessive lacrimation, salivation	Use as afterload reducer in severe CHF, aortic insufficiency, or after value replacement surgery; anticipate need for diuretic as adjunct to control renal sodium and water retention
Guanfacine hydrochloride (Tenex)	HTN (usually that which is not responsive to traditional first-line oral antihypertensives, alone or in combination): initially, 1 mg/day at bedtime; assess response over 3–4 wk before increasing dosage to 2 mg/day; usual daily maximum, 3 mg	Clonidine-like centrally acting antihypertensive; see description for clonidine	
Hydralazine hydrochloride (Apresoline)	HTN, especially if moderate to severe, usually as adjunct to diuretic and drug to control reflex cardiac stimulation (e.g., beta blocker or nondihydropyridine calcium channel blocker (e.g., diltiazem, verapamil): oral: 10 mg four times daily to start for first 4 days; increase to 25 mg four times daily for remainder of week, then increase as needed to 50 mg 2–4 times a day Severe essential HTN when oral therapy is impractical, and for eclampsia: IV or IM: 20–40 mg; for children, 0.1–0.2 mg/kg every 4–6 hr, repeated as necessary	Lupus-like syndrome possible; peripheral neuritis, managed or prevented with oral vitamin B_6 (pyridoxine); renal sodium and water retention usually necessitate adjunctive management with diuretic; vasodilation may trigger reflex tachycardia and myocardial ischemia, necessitating control with beta blocker or nondihydropyridine calcium channel blocker	Do not use as afterload reducer in severe CHF, in aortic insufficiency, or after value replacement surgery (constitutes unlabeled use); HTN due to eclampsia is relieved with delivery of the fetus
Mecamylamine hydrochloride (Inversine)	Moderate to severe HTN and uncomplicated malignant HTN: 2.5 mg twice daily to start, increase as needed over intervals of 2- or more days; average daily dosage, 25 mg in three divided doses	Ganglionic blocker associated with significant orthostatic hypotension, compensatory renal sodium and water retention (may necessitate diuretic); discontinue gradually to avoid episode of significant rebound HTN	—

(continued)

623

TABLE 40.4. (Continued)

Drug	Indication(s), typical dosages (oral administration unless noted otherwise)	Key side effects	Comments
Methyldopa (Aldomet)	Usually 250 mg two to three time a day for first 48 hr; increase, if needed, at intervals of ≥2 days, to maintenance dosage of 500 mg: 2 g daily in two to four divided doses	Hepatotoxicity (rare, but monitor); Coombs' test + (monitor), although incidence of hemolytic anemia is low	A preferred drug for managing HTN (other than that due to preeclampsia-eclampsia) during pregnancy
Methyldopate hydrochloride	Hypertensive crisis: IV: 250–500 mg every 6 hr, diluted to 10 mg/mL in 5% dextrose in water, infused over 30–60 min; as soon as BP is controlled, switch to oral dosing at same dosage schedule as for parenteral administration	See description for methyldopa	Is soluble ester of methyldopa
Minoxidil (Loniten)	Severe, refractory HTN with evidence of end-organ damage not manageable with diuretic plus two other antihypertensives: Patients ≥12 yr: start with 5 mg once daily; typical maintenance dosage, 10–40 mg/day. Children <12 yr: 0.2 mg/kg/day as single dose; typical maintenance dosage, 0.25–1 mg/kg/day	Vasodilation triggers renal sodium and water retention, often necessitating adjunctive diuretic; reflex tachyardia and consequences thereof, which usually necessitate pharmacologic control; hirsutism; pericardial effusion progressing to tamponade is most serious adverse effect	—
Papaverine hydrochloride (Pavabid Plateau Caps, Pavagen TD)	Myocardial ischemia complicated by arrhythmias, relief of cerebral and peripheral ischemia associated with arterial spasm: 150 mg every 12 hr; 150 mg every 8 hr or 300 mg every 12 hr may be needed	Large doses may depress cardiac function (especially AV conduction), leading to ventricular ectopy, premature beats, and so Forth; may decrease control of Parkinson's disease by levodopa	—
Reserpine	HTN (usually that which is not responsive to traditional first-line oral antihypertensives, alone or in combination): initially, 0.5 mg/day for 1–2 wk; usual maintenance dosage, 0.1–0.25 mg/day	Hypotension (especially orthostatic), cardiac depression; parasympathetic predominance, manifested as diarrhea, urinary frequency, excessive lacrimation, salivation; psychiatric depression and/or exacerbation of signs/symptoms of Parkinson's disease may occur, the former rarely at usual antihypertensive doses	Available in many fixed-dose combination products (e.g., with diuretic, hydralazine)

ACE, angiotensin-converting enzyme; AV, atrioventricular; BP, blood pressure; CHF, congestive heart failure; HTN, hypertension; IM, intramuscularly; IV, intravenously.

TABLE 40.5. Angiotensin-converting enzyme inhibitors and angiotensin II receptor blockers

Drug	Indication(s), typical doses (oral administration)	Key side effects	Comments
ACE Inhibitors	General dosing strategy for use of ACE inhibitors as antihypertensives: if patient is already taking a diuretic, discontinue the diuretic 2–3 days before starting ACE inhibitor, to avoid excessive hypotension; if that is not practical or possible, use half the recommended starting dose of the ACE inhibitor listed as follows. ACE inhibitors vary in their dependence on renal function or hepatic metabolism for clearance; always consult package insert for each agent you plan to prescribe, and obtain baseline laboratory measurements for renal and hepatic function	Decreases of renal function prolong half-lives of all ACE inhibitors; the effects may be clinically significant for all except fosinopril unless dosage is reduced	All are contraindicated in pregnancy (especially during second and third trimesters) and should be avoided in women with childbearing potential if possible
Benazepril hydrochloride (Lotensin)	HTN: 10 mg once daily; typical maintenance dosage, 20–40 mg as single dose or in two equal divided doses	Hypotension, especially if added to current diuretic regimen or if patient is sodium- or volume-depleted for any other reason; hyperkalemia if not used with potassium-wasting (thiazide, thiazide-like, or loop) diuretic; cough	Extensive plasma protein binding; significant hepatic metabolism with only trace excreted unchanged in urine; food significantly reduces absorption
Captopril (Capoten)	HTN: typically, 7.5–30 mg as single daily dose or in two equal divided doses	Rash is most common side effect; incidence of cough, often attributed to this drug, is actually low (< 1%)	Shortest half-life (<2 hr) of all ACE inhibitors; excreted unchanged in urine; should be taken 1 hr before meals, because food significantly reduces absorption
Enalapril maleate (Vasotec)	HTN: initially, 5 mg once daily; typical maintenance dosage, 10–40 mg/day in single or two equal divided doses Heart failure or asymptomatic LV dysfunction: 2.5 mg twice daily to start; titrate to typical maintenance dosage of 10 mg twice daily	Hypotension and dizziness are most common side effects	50% of administered dose excreted unchanged
Fosinopril sodium (Monopril)	HTN or heart failure: 10 mg once daily to start; typical maintenance dosage 20–40 mg	See above; dizziness and cough are most common side effects	Half-life prolonged with decreasing renal function but with apparently negligible clinical effect; virtually complete hepatic metabolism to active metabolite
Lisinopril (Prinivil, Zestril)	HTN: 10 mg once daily; typical maintenance dosage, 20–40 mg once daily Heart failure: 5 mg once daily (usually as adjunct to digoxin) Acute MI: if patient is hemodynamically stable within 24 hr of symptom onset, give 2.5 or 5 mg twice at 24-hr intervals; increase gradually to 10 mg once daily for 6 weeks	See above; dizziness is most common side effect	Only ACE inhibitor with no active hepatic metabolite; nearly 100% of absorbed dose excreted unchanged in urine

(continued)

625

TABLE 40.5. *(Continued)*

Drug	Indication(s), typical doses (oral administration)	Key side effects	Comments
Moexipril (Univasc)	HTN: 2.5 mg once daily, then 5 mg or 10 mg once daily if needed; usual maintenance dosage, 2.5–5 mg once daily; reduce dosage interval with increasing degrees of renal impairment	See above; cough is most common side effect	Food markedly reduces absorption; should be taken 1 hr before meal
Perindopril erbumine (Aceon)	HTN: 4 mg once daily to start; usual daily maintenance dosage, 4–8 mg as single dose or in two equal divided doses	See above	—
Quinapril hydrochloride (Accupril)	HTN: usually 10–20 mg once daily to start; maintenance dosage, usually 20–80 mg once daily or (often preferred) 10–40 mg twice daily Heart failure: usually 5 mg twice daily to start; maintenance dosage, usually 20–40 mg/day in two equal divided doses	See above; headache, dizziness are most common side effects	—
Ramipril (Altace)	HTN and (reduction of risk from MI, stroke or other cardiovascular mortality: 2.5 mg once daily to start; typical maintenance dosage, 2.5–20 mg in single or two equally divided daily doses	See above; headache and cough are most common side effects	Longest half-life of all ACE inhibitors: 13–17 hrs
Trandolapril (Mavik)	HTN and heart failure/left ventricular dysfunction after MI: 1 mg/day (2 mg/day recommended for black patients if patient is *not* receiving diuretic; typical maintenance dosage, 2–4 mg/day; with creatinine clearances <30 mL/min or with hepatic cirrhosis, start with 0.5 mg/day	See dizziness reported in up to 20% of patients, cough in up to 35%; syncope incidence, about 5%— more common than with other ACE inhibitors; "highest" incidence of angioedema of all ACE inhibitors, but actual incidence is around 0.1%	—

Angiotensin II receptor blockers for HTN

		Most common general adverse response to this group of drugs is upper respiratory tract infection	For most AT-II receptor blockers, if maximum maintenance dose listed provides inadequate BP control, the usual recommendation is not to increase the dose further but to cautiously add a diuretic (e.g., thiazide); pregnancy-related warning noted for ACE inhibitors applies to these drugs; risk of hypotension in sodium- and/or volume-depleted patients, noted for ACE inhibitors, applies also
Candesartan cilexetil (Atacand)	Usually, 16 mg once daily to start; typical maintenance dosage, 8–32 mg as single dose or in two equal divided doses	See above; most common side effects are upper respiratory tract infection, muscle pain,	—
Eprosartan mesylate (Teveten)	Usually, 600 mg/day to start; maintenance dosage, 400–800/day in single or two equal divided doses	See above	—
Irbesartan (Avapro)	150–300 mg/day	See above	—
Losartan potassium (Cozaar)	Usually, 50 mg to start; maintenance dosage, 25–100 mg/day in single dose or two equal divided doses	See above	—
Telmisartan (Micardis)	40 mg once daily to start; daily maintenance dosage, typically 20–80 mg	See above	—
Valsartan (Diovan)	Usually 80 mg/day	See general side effects	Significantly decreased bioavailability if taken with food; negligible hepatic metabolism

ACE, angiotensin-converting enzyme; AT-II, angiotension II; BP, blood pressure; LV, left ventricular; MI, myocardial infarction.

TABLE 40.6. *Calcium channel blockers for angina, hypertension, and selected other indications*

Drug	Indication(s), typical doses (oral administration unless noted otherwise)	Key side effects	Comments
		Calcium channel blockers are generally well tolerated at usual therapeutic dosages when used alone, causing relatively infrequent and mild cardiovascular, GI, and CNS side effects except as noted	
Amlodipine (Norvasc)	HTN: Usually 5 mg once daily, up to maximum of 10 mg/day; start with 2.5 mg once daily in patients with hepatic insufficiency or patients already taking antihypertensive medication Chronic stable or vasospastic angina: 5 mg once daily to start; usual maintenance dosage, 10 mg once daily	Headache, fatigue, and lethargy are most common minor side effects; high incidence of peripheral edema due to significant fall of peripheral vascular resistance	Use cautiously in patients with CHF
Bepridil (Vascor)	Chronic stable angina: 200 mg/day to start (usually the minimum effective dosage); typical maintenance dosage, 300 mg/day	High incidence of headache, dizziness, lightheadedness; highest incidence of nausea (5%–25%) Significant depression of AV nodal conduction	Renal excretion; use with care in patients with decreased renal function Prototypic nondihydropyridine calcium channel blocker (along with verapamil): causes both peripheral vascular calcium channel blockade (leading to vasodilation) and cardiac (depressant) effects on rate, contractility, and conduction; use cautiously in patients with CHF
Diltiazem hydrochloride (Cardizem, Tiamate, Dilacor, Tiazac, Cartia)	Chronic stable or vasospastic angina: 30 mg of immediate-release formulation, three times daily, to start; increase gradually to 180–360 mg/day, given in three to four divided doses, or 120 mg sustained-release formulation once daily HTN (sustained-release formulations only): 180–240 mg once daily; if needed, after about 14 days adjust to typical optimum dosages of 240–360 mg for Cardizem CD, up to 480 mg for Dilacor XR, given once daily Atrial fibrillation, flutter, paroxysmal supraventricular tachycardia: IV bolus of 0.25 mg/kg (or 20 mg total) given over 2 min; if needed, 15 min later give bolus of 0.35 mg/kg (or 25 mg total); after administering bolus(es), if needed, infuse at 10 mg/hr, increasing to 15 mg/hr as needed; infuse for no longer than 24 hours		
Felodipine (Plendil)	HTN: Start with 5 mg once daily; increase or decrease as needed at intervals of >2 wk; usual maintenance dosage, 2.5–10 mg once daily	Headache is most common side effect (about 20% incidence)	Use cautiously in patients with CHF

Drug	Dosage	Side effects	Comments
Isradipine (DynaCirc, DynaCirc CR)	HTN: 2.5 mg twice daily; dosages >10 mg/day usually do not increase symptom relief, do increase number/severity of side effects	Peripheral edema, headache, dizziness, and lightheadedness are most common side effects; significant decreases of peripheral vascular resistance	Use cautiously in patients with CHF
Nicardipine hydrochloride (Cardene, Cardene SR)	HTN: Start with 20 mg (range, 20–40 mg) three times daily (immediate-release) or 30 mg twice daily (sustained-release formulation); IV for hypertensive urgencies: monitor BP and other vital signs while infusing 0.1-mg/mL solution to titrate to desired response if patient is not taking nicardipine already, up to usual maximum of 2.5 mg/hr	5%–10% incidence of headache, peripheral edema; significant decreases of peripheral vascular resistance, rise in cardiac output	Despite hemodynamic effects, cautious use in patients with CHF still warranted
Nifedipine (Adalat, Procardia, various immediate-release and sustained-release formulations)	Chronic stable angina (immediate-release formulations only): 20–40 mg three times daily HTN (sustained-release formulations only): 30–60 mg once daily Chronic stable or vasospastic angina (immediate- or sustained-release): 10 mg four times daily to start, but some patients with coronary spasm may need 20–30 mg three or four times a day; titrate to higher doses if needed at 1- to 2-week intervals up to a total daily dose of 120 mg given in three to four divided doses	Headache in 10%–20% of patients; dizziness, lightheadedness in about 25%; significant fall in peripheral vascular resistance, rise in cardiac output; associated with highest incidence of peripheral edema as side effect; dose-dependent hypotension and reflex cardiac stimulation may counteract desired antianginal effects	Prototypic dihydropyridine calcium channel blocker: peripheral vasodilator action, no direct cardiac depressant activity; tends to trigger reflex tachycardia and other manifestations of reflex cardiac stimulation that may be unwanted or dangerous; contents of nifedipine capsules should never be removed or administered sublingually, in attempt to urgently lower BP; doing so may cause inadequate or excessive and rapid lowering of BP, profound reflex cardiac stimulation, and potentially fatal myocardial ischemic events
Nimodipine (Nimotop)	Subarachnoid hemorrhage: 60 mg every 4 hours for 21 days	Highest overall incidence of hypotension	—
Nisoldipine (Sular)	HTN: 20 mg once daily to start; increase by 10 mg/day at weekly or longer intervals as needed; usual maintenance dosage, 20–40 mg once daily	Peripheral edema, headache, dizziness, lightheadedness	Tends to cause significant fall in peripheral vascular resistance

(continued)

TABLE 40.6. (*Continued*)

Drug	Indication(s), typical doses (oral administration unless noted otherwise)	Key side effects	Comments
Verapamil hydrochloride (Calan, Isoptin, others, both immediate-release and systained-release formulations)	Chronic stable or vasospastic angina: typically 80–120 mg three times daily to start, but some patients may respond to or need as little as 30 mg three times daily HTN: 80 mg of immediate-release formulation three times daily to start, titrate upward as needed; no evidence that daily doses >360 mg have added BP-lowering effect; sustained-release dosage form: 240 mg, with food, every morning; titration may necessitate 240 mg mornings and 120 mg at bedtime Control of ventricular rate in chronic atrial fibrillation/flutter: 240–320 mg/day of immediate-release form in three or four divided doses. Prophylaxis against PSVT: 240–480 mg/day in three or four divided doses	Causes greatest suppression of AV nodal conduction; highest incidence of constipation (although diarrhea infrequently occurs)	Use cautiously in patients with CHF; slow-release/extended-release dosage forms are approved only for managing HTN

AV, atrioventricular; BP, blood pressure; CHF, congestive heart failure; CNS, central nervous system; GI, gastrointestinal; HTN, hypertension; IV, intravenously; PSVT, paroxysmal supraventricular tachycardia.

TABLE 40.7. *Nitrovasodilators for angina*

Drug	Indication(s), administration route(s), typical doses	Key side effects	Comments
	For self-administration by patient, only sublingual dosage forms (e.g., nitroglycerin) are suitable for acute prophylaxis or symptom relief; patients taking any other formulation as "primary therapy" should always have a sublingual preparation available for use	For all nitrovasodilators: key side effects arise directly or indirectly from peripheral vasodilation (and tolerance develops to some): headache; facial flushing; lightheadedness/dizziness; tachycardia; palpitations; are most problematic with short-rapid-acting drugs (e.g., sublingual nitroglycerin), less so with long-acting oral or topical formulations; cardiac responses may necessitate control with adjunctive beta blocker or verapamil-/diltiazem-like calcium channel blocker, provided there are no contraindications	
Isosorbide mononitrate (Imdur, others)	Angina: oral: 20 mg twice daily (immediate-release tablets); 30 mg once daily to start; maintenance dosage, typically 120 mg/day for extended-release tablets	—	Oral formulations are not indicated for acute prophylaxis or symptom relief; patients taking these formulations should always carry sublingual form
Isosorbide dinitrate (Isordil, Sorbitrate, others)	Angina: oral, for acute prophylaxis, sublingual or chewable tablets: usually 2.5–5 mg for sublingual tablets, 5 mg for chewable tablets (or 5–10 mg of either dosage form) every 2–3 hr	—	—
Isosorbide dinitrate (Isordil Titradose, others)	Angina: oral, for chronic prophylaxis, immediate-release tabs: usually 5–20 mg every 6 hr; maintenance dosage, typically 10–40 mg; sustained-release formulation: 40 mg to start, every 8–12 hr; maintenance dosage, typically 40 or 80 mg every 8–12 hr	—	—
Nitroglycerin, sublingual	Angina, acute or prophylaxis, sublingual/translingual: typically, 0.3–0.6 mg for acute symptoms, repeated every 5 min to maximum of no more than 3 tablets (or sprays) in 15 min; transmucosal or buccal tablets: usually 1–3 mg every 3–5 hours during waking hours; oral sustained-/timed-release (for prophylaxis only): Usually 2.5–2.6 mg three to four times daily to start; increase gradually as needed over days or weeks to achieve lowest effective dosage when taken three to four times daily	—	Failure of three doses of sublingual nitroglycerin to completely relieve discomfort is good indication of ongoing MI; emergency medical assistance should be sought at once (i.e., patient should call 911); administration of additional doses in uncontrolled setting may cause profound hypotension, stroke, exacerbation of myocardial ischemia, death

(continued)

TABLE 40.7. (Continued)

Drug	Indication(s), administration route(s), typical doses	Key side effects	Comments
Nitroglycerin, transdermal (Nitrodisc, Nitro-Dur, Transderm-Nitro, others)	Angina prophylaxis: start with delivery system releasing 0.2–0.4 m/hr, worn 12–14 hr per 24-hr period; nitroglycerin ointment: start with 0.5 inch (12.5 mm) every 8 hr; typical maintenance dosage, 1–2 inches applied every 8 hr	—	Wearing transdermal delivery systems around the clock (24 hr, 7 days/week) not advised, as it probably leads to tolerance to drug and tolerance to rapidly acting nitrates when acute symptom relief is needed; patients using a transdermal formulation should always have ready access to sublingual form for acute prophylaxis or symptom relief
Nitroglycerin (Nitro-Bid IV, others)	Perioperative BP control, congestive heart failure with acute MI, and angina refractory to other organic nitrovasodilators, beta blockers, or other antianginals: typically 5 μg/min IV to start, titrate upwards gradually (e.g., 5-μg/min increments every 3–5 min) to desired BP or other clinical end points	—	—

BP, blood pressure; IV, intravenously; MI, myocardial infarction.

TABLE 40.8. Drugs for dyslipidemias

Drug	Indication(s), typical doses; oral administration	Key side effects	Comments
HMG-CoA reducatase inhibitors ("statins")			For all statins: initial dose varies, depending on desired degree of lowering LDL-C; lower doses are generally indicated when used with other lipid-lowering drugs; combined therapy with other classes of lipid-lowering drugs may control multiple dyslipidemias but generally increases risk of statin-induced myositis, myopathy, and rhabdomyolysis
Atorvastatin calcium (Lipitor)	Start with 10 mg once daily at any time of day, with or without meals; maintenance dosage, 10–80 mg once daily	Headache and diarrhea are most common, but overall occur with <10% incidence	Approved for primary hypercholesterolemia, mixed dyslipidemias, hypertriglyceridemia, primary dysbetalipoproteinemia, homozygous familial hyperlipidemia
Fluvastatin sodium (Lescol, Lescol XL)	40 mg of immediate-release capsules or 80 mg of extended-release tablets, as single dose in evening, or 40 mg of immediate-release capsules twice daily	Dyspepsia; highest incidence of upper respiratory tract infections of all the statins	Approved for primary hypercholesterolemia, mixed dyslipidemias, secondary prevention of cardiovascular events associated with dyslipidemias, CHD
Lovastatin (Mevacor)	Initially, 20 mg/day with evening meal; usual maintenance dosage, 10–80 mg/day as single daily dose or in two equal divided doses	Headache, various (and usually minor) GI symptoms (e.g., upset, dyspepsia) are the most common	Approved for primary hypercholesterolemia, primary or secondary prevention of cardiovascular events, CHD
Pravastatin sodium (Pravachol)	10–40 mg/day, once daily at any time without regard to meals	Same as for lovastatin	Approved for primary hypercholesterolemia, mixed dyslipidemias, hypertriglyceridemia, primary dysbetalipoproteinemia, primary or secondary prevention of cardiovascular events, CHD
Simvastatin (Zocor)	20 mg once daily to start; maintenance dosage, 5–80 mg/day	Same as for lovastatin	Approved for homozygous familial hyperlipidemia, secondary prevention of cardiovascular events
Fibric Acid Derivatives		For all fibrates, various GI complaints (especially dyspepsia, sometimes severe) are most common side effects; abnormal elevations of liver function measurements (AST, ALT) are most common reason for discontinuing drug; all tend to pose increased risk of cholelithiasis, myositis, and renal function impairment, additive to that associated with statins	

(continued)

633

TABLE 40.8. *(Continued)*

Drug	Indication(s), typical doses; oral administration	Key side effects	Comments
Clofibrate (Atromid-S)	Primary dysbetalipoproteinemia, hyperlipidemias: 2 g daily in divided doses		Malignancy risk
Gemfibrozil (Lopid)	600 mg 30 min before morning and evening meals	Diarrhea, dyspepsia, abdominal pain most common	—
Fenofibrate (Tricor)	67–200 mg/day	Abnormal liver function measurements (e.g., increased AST, ALT) most common vs. placebo	—
Ezetemibe (Zetia)	Monotherapy of primary hypercholesterolemia, combination therapy with HMG-CoA reductase inhibitors, homozygous familial hypercholesterolemia, homozygous sitosteralemia: 10 mg/day.	—	Avoid in patients with moderate-severe hepatic insufficiency; insufficient data on coadministration fibrates: may interact with cyclosporin.
Bile acid–binding resins (sequestrants)		For all bile acid sequestrants, the most common side effect is constipation, which at times may be severe and lead to fecal impaction; all tend to bind to, interfere with absorption (bioavailability) of many other orally administered drugs; general recommendation is to space administration of other agents by at least 2 hr	
Cholestyramine resin (LoCholest, Questran)	4 g one to two times a day		—
Colesevelam hydrochloride (WelChol)	3 tablets (625 mg each) twice daily or 6 tablets once daily, with meals		—
Colestipol hydrochloride (Colestid)	5–30 g given once daily or in divided doses	—	
Nicotinic acid (niacin)			
Nicotinic acid (Niacor)	Hypertriglyceridemia associated with other dyslipidemias (adjunct), extended-release form: 500 mg at bedtime for 1–4 wk, then 1 g at bedtime for another 1–4 weeks; maintenance dosage, generally 1.5–2 g/day; immediate-release form: start with 250 mg once daily with evening meal, titrate upward as needed every 4–7 days to typical maintenance dosage of 1–2 g twice or three times a day	GI upset; cutaneous/facial flushing and headache from vasodilation (incidence and severity may be reduced by using extended-release formulation, dividing doses of immediate-release formulation, or aspirin pretreatment if not contraindicated)	—

ALT, alanine aminotransferase; AST, aspartate aminotransferase; CHD, coronary heart disease;
GI, gastrointestinal; HMG-CoA, 3-hydroxy-3-methylglutaryl coenzyme A; LDL-C, low-density lipoprotein cholesterol.

TABLE 40.9. *Antiplatelet agents*

Drug	Indications and dose	Drug interactions	Key side effects	Contraindications
Aggregation inhibitors				
Cilostazol (Pletal)	Intermittent claudication 50–100 mg b.i.d.	Macrolides and diltiazem drug effect (CYP3A4) interaction	—	Congestive heart failure
Clopidogrel bisulfate (Plavix)	Atherosclerotic events 75 mg/d	—	—	Active bleeding
Ticlopidine hydrochloride (Ticlid)	Stroke 250 mg b.i.d. with food	Antacids increase plasma levels, cimetidine decreases clearance levels Phenytoin levels increased	—	Active bleeding, neutropenia, thrombocytopenia, history of thrombotic thrombocytopenic purpura
Dipyridamole (Persantine)	Thromboembolic complications 75–100 mg q.i.d.	—	—	Bleeding with NSAIDs and anticoagulants
Dipyridamole and aspirin (Aggrenox)	Stroke 200 mg/25 mg b.i.d.	—	Bleeding	—
Aspirin	Atherosclerotic events 75–325 mg/d	—	Bleeding	—
Glycoprotein IIB/IIIA inhibitors				
Abciximab (ReoPro)	Acute coronary syndromes 2-mg bolus, 10 g/min for 12 hr	—	Bleeding, hypotension, allergic reactions	Active bleeding, stroke <2 yrs, Thrombocytopenia < (100,000)
Eptifibatide (Integrilin)	180-μg/kg bolus, 2 μg/kg/min infusion for 72 hr	—	Bleeding	Active bleeding
Tirofiban hydrochloride (Aggrastat)	0.4 μg/kg/min × 30 min initially, then 0.1 μg/kg/min for 48 to 108 hr with heparin or 12–24 hr after angioplasty For CrCl <30 mL/min, halve maintenance dosage	—	Bleeding	Active bleeding

CrCl, creatinine clearance rate; NSAID, nonsteroidal antiinflammatory drug.

635

TABLE 40.10. *Anticoagulants: Low-molecular-weight heparins*

Drug	Indications and dose	Drug interactions	Key side effects	Contraindications
Heparin				
Heparin sodium	Thrombosis, embolism prevention 60-U/kg- load IV, followed by 12 U/kg/hr to maintain aPTT at 1.5–2 times control level (50–70 sec)	Platelet inhibitors/anticoagulants, penicillins/cephalosporins may increase bleeding risk	Bleeding	Active major bleeding, heparin-associated thrombocytopenia
Dalteparin sodium (Fragmin)	Acute coronary syndromes, DVT 120 IU/kg SC b.i.d. (not to exceed 10,000 U) with aspirin for DVT	Use care with concomitant anticoagulants/antiplatelet drugs	Bleeding	—
Enoxaparin sodium (Lovenox)	Acute coronary syndromes, DVT mg/kg SC b.i.d. with aspirin for UAP/DVT	Use care with concomitant anticoagulants/antiplatelet drugs	Bleeding	Active major bleeding, heparin-associated thrombocytopenia
Tinzaparin sodium (Innohep)	DVT 175 U/kg SC q.d.	Use care with concomitant anticoagulants/antiplatelet drugs	Bleeding	Active major bleeding, heparin-associated thrombocytopenia
Thrombin Inhibitors				
Lepirudin (Refludan)	Heparin-induced thrombocytopenia 0.4-mg/kg IV bolus over 20 sec; maintenance, 0.15 mg/kg/hr if body weight is <110 kg (reduce if CrCl < 60 mL/min	Increased risk of bleeding with thrombolytics or warfarin	—	—
Bivalirudin (Angiomax)	Unstable angina Bolus 1 mg/kg, initial 4 hr infusion 2.5 mg/h, and maintenance infusion, all weight adjusted	Use care with concomitant anticoagulants/antiplatelet drugs	Bleeding	Active major bleeding, heparin-associated thrombocytopenia
Warfarin sodium (Coumadin, generics)	Prophylaxis and treatment of atrial fibrillation, flutter, and thromboembolism 5–10 mg/d for 2–4 days, adjust to INR (lower doses in elderly)	Multiple potential drug interactions may increase or decrease anticoagulant effect; dietary changes may also be important	Bleeding	Active bleeding risk or internal bleeding (e.g., carcinoma), severe hepatic/renal diseases, fall risk

aPTT, activated partial thromboplastin time; CrCl, creatine clearance rate; DVT, deep venous thrombosis; INR, International Normalized Ratio; IV, intravenously; SC, subcutaneously; UAP, unstable angina pectoris.

41

Complementary and Alternative Medicine

Mauro Moscucci, Sara L. Warber, and Keith Aaronson

Complementary and alternative medical (CAM) therapies can be defined as medical interventions that are currently not an integral part of conventional medicine and that, as such, are not taught widely in United States medical schools and are generally unavailable at U.S. hospitals (1). Since 1990, documentation by several surveys of the widespread and increasing use by consumers of CAM therapies has brought the attention of the health care community, employers and insurers to the importance of this form of therapies. In 1998 Eisenberg et al. reported that 43% of Americans used at least one form of CAM therapy in 1997 (2) and that there had been a 25% increase in the number of users and a 43% increase in visits to CAM practitioners since 1990 (1). Eighteen percent of patients taking prescription drugs were also using herbal remedies, and the estimated market for CAM therapy was $21 billion annually. More recently, a survey from the Josiah Macy, Jr., Foundation showed that in the year 2001, more than 50% of Americans were using CAM therapies (3). An estimated 600 million visits per year were made to CAM practitioners, with an estimated market of $30 billion annually. In that survey, the estimated market for herbal remedies was $10 billion, with a growing market share estimated at 20% to 30% per year. In addition, as shown by another survey of 376 consecutive patients undergoing preoperative or postoperative cardiac surgery evaluation at Columbia Presbyterian Medical Center in New York, many patients use some form of alternative medicine but do not or do not want to discuss its use with their physicians (4). Among patients surveyed, 75% admitted the use of alternative medical therapy (44% without prayers and vitamins), but only 17% had discussed this use with their physicians, and 48% did not want to discuss it with

their physicians. Thus, it is increasingly important for practitioners to gain familiarity with various forms of CAM and to specifically elicit and document a history of use of CAM from patients.

CLASSIFICATION OF COMPLEMENTARY AND ALTERNATIVE MEDICAL THERAPIES

CAM therapies can be categorized in five major groups [National Institutes of Health classification (5)]: (a) alternative medical systems, (b) mind-body interventions, (c) manipulative and body-based methods, (d) energy therapies, and (e) biologically based treatments.

Alternative Medical Systems

Alternative medical systems can be defined as complete systems of theory and practice of medicine that have evolved independently and often before the conventional medical system (5). Examples of alternative medical systems include Asian medical practices, homeopathic and naturopathic medicine, Ayurveda medicine, and other traditional medical systems developed by Native American, Aboriginal, African, Middle-Eastern, Tibetan, and Central and South American cultures. The characteristics and principles of several systems are summarized in Table 41.1.

In contraposition to conventional allopathic medicine, alternative medical systems are generally characterized by the recognition that mind, body, and spirit are integrated and interconnected and that treatment of illnesses should be aimed toward reestablishment of lost balances and promotion of self-healing processes. As outlined in Table 41.1, many alternative medical systems include the use of herbal therapies. Herbal

TABLE 41.1. *Alternative medical systems*

Medical system	Region developed	Principle
Asian medical systems		
Traditional Chinese medicine	China	Integrated system based on the central concept of Qi, the vital force that connects body, mind, and spirit. It includes acupuncture, Chinese herbs, massage, breathing and moving exercises, food therapy, and lifestyle modification.
Acupressure	China	System based on the principle that illness is the results of stressors that challenge the homeostatic mechanism of the body. Pressing on key points on the skin aligned on meridians or pathways along which the energy flows stimulates the body's self-healing abilities.
Acupuncture	China	Similar to acupressure. The anatomic points are stimulated by needles rather than by touch. Over several centuries, numerous subsystems have evolved in different cultures.
Tai chi (Taiji and Taijiquan)	China	System based on the principle of Y in (receptive, dark, negative, closed, empty) and Yang (creative, bright, positive, open, full). The smooth alteration of the two during movements results in harmony and balance. It includes movements with coordinated and timed breathing, round motion, and alignment of joints.
Qi Gong	China	System based on integration of mind, body, and breathing through meditation, movements, self-massage, and special healing techniques. It is one of the major branches of traditional Chinese medicine, and it relies on the principles of Qi, yin/yang, meridians, and pathogenesis of disease.
Ayurveda	India	Traditional medical system of India based on the principle that diseases are caused by lack of harmony of the individual with the environment. It includes herbs, meditation, exercise, massage, exposure to sunlight, and breathing exercises.
Western medical systems		
Homeopathy	Germany	Empirical system of medicine based on the principle "Similia similibus curantur"—i.e., drugs that produce symptoms in a healthy person will treat the same symptoms in a disease state—and each individual has a self-healing capacity. The system is based on the laws of similars, of single dose (one dose will stimulate the body), of minimal or lowest possible dose, and of dilution (the more the medication is diluted, the stronger the effect).
Naturopathic medicine	Western world	Natural approach to health and healing based on the principle of treating diseases by stimulating the inherent healing capacity of the individual. Its fundamentals includes the healing power of nature, the treatment of the whole person, the identification and treatment of the cause, the "do no harm" principle, prevention as the best cure, and the role of physician as an educator for patients. Standard diagnostic procedures are integrated with herbal medicine, homeopathy, physical medicine, hydrotherapy, clinical nutrition, minor surgery, and mind-body connections.

therapies commonly used in cardiovascular care are discussed later in this chapter, in the section on herbal remedies.

Mind-Body Interventions

Mind-body interventions can be defined as interventions aimed toward promoting the ability of the mind to affect body functions and symptoms (5). Examples of mind-body interventions include art therapy, biofeedback, dance and movements, hypnotherapy, interactive guided therapy, meditation, music therapy, neurolinguistic therapy, poetry therapy, relaxation therapies, spiritual healing and prayer, yoga, and cognitive-behavioral approaches.

There is now extensive evidence supporting the importance of mind-body interactions on the development of cardiovascular disease. In particular, type A behavior, hostility, stress, and low physical activity have been identified as important correlates of the development of cardiovascular disease (6,7). On the basis of these premises, it is conceivable that mind-body interventions could have an important impact on the natural history of cardiovascular disease. This hypothesis has been confirmed by the results of a metaanalysis of 23 randomized clinical trials evaluating the addition to conventional therapy of interventions addressing emotional and psychosocial issues (8). In that analysis, the addition of mind-body interventions was found to significantly reduce morbidity and mortality rates. More recently, an extensive review of various mind-body interventions, including social supports, yoga, religious attendance, imagery, and meditation in the treatment of cardiovascular diseases, revealed that many interventions used as complementary or stand-alone therapy might have beneficial effects on disease progression and on long-term outcomes (9). Scientific evidence of efficacy based on randomized clinical trials is still limited. However, the lack of significant adverse effects and the anecdotal and, in some instances, scientific evidence of effectiveness supports a potential role of mind-body interventions as complementary therapy for cardiovascular disease.

Manipulative and Body-Based Methods

These therapies are based on manipulation of the body and movements and include chiropractic, massage therapy, and osteopathic medicine.

Chiropractic is based on the relationship between body and function and on the foundation of facilitating the body's own healing power. The aims of this therapy are to alter local tissue stresses, to reduce mechanical stimulation, and to allow the organism to recover. The most common and best-known chiropractic treatment is spinal manipulation. However, chiropractic also includes lifestyle counseling, nutrition management, rehabilitation, and other physiotherapeutic modalities. The beneficial effects of chiropractic have been documented in several clinical trials, and it is now considered an effective treatment modality for spine and related disorders (10). It is important to note that spinal manipulation is not completely risk free and that there have been several reports of stroke and of vertebral and carotid artery dissection during manipulation of the cervical spine. Thus, extreme caution is advisable particularly for patients with cerebrovascular disease. Hypertension is the only cardiovascular disease listed among conditions treated relatively often by chiropractors (11).

Massage therapy is one of the oldest health care practices; its origin can be traced back to China in 2000 B.C. It can be divided in five major categories: traditional European; contemporary Western; Asian (acupressure, shiatsu, tuina, AMMA therapy, jin shin do); energetic; and structural, functional, and movement integration. Each of these categories is based on different principles, but the common denominator is promotion of the body's ability to heal itself.

Energy Therapies

Energy therapies are based on the concept of healing through manipulation of energy fields originating within the body (biofields) or through application of energy fields from other sources (electromagnetic fields) (5).

Examples of biofields therapies include polarity therapy, Qi gong, reiki, and therapeutic touch. Polarity therapy was developed by Randolph Stone, and it incorporates in its philosophy healing based on the flow or disruption of electromagnetic fields in the human body. Qi gong is based on the integration of mind, body, and breathing through meditation, movements, self-massage, and special healing techniques. It is one of the major branches of traditional Chinese medicine, and it relies on the same principles of *Qi*, the vital force that connects body, mind and spirit, and on the principle of yin/yang and meridians in the pathogenesis of disease. Reiki can be traced back to Tibet (3000 B.C.). It was later developed and practiced in Japan in the mid-1800s. Reiki is a touch healing system ("laying on of hands") that promotes healing on the physical, mental, emotional and spiritual levels. The practitioner, by laying his or her hands on the patient's body, channels the healing energy of the "universal life-force energy." The skills of the practitioner are acquired through training from a reiki master or teacher who has the ability to connect the student to the reiki energy. At this time, there is lack of objective evidence to support the medical use of any of these modalities.

Biologically Based Treatments

Biologically based treatments are practices, interventions, and products aimed toward modification of biologic functions and processes (5). They include herbal, dietary, enzyme, and orthomolecular therapies. Chelation therapy and special diet therapies such as those proposed by Drs. Robert C. Atkins, Dean Ornish, Nathan Pritikin, and Andrew Weil are also part of this group.

ACUPUNCTURE

Acupuncture has been extensively used in Western countries for the treatment of numerous conditions, including chronic pain, postoperative pain, asthma, drug addiction, headache, nausea, osteoarthritis, fibromyalgia, allergies, and gastrointestinal motility disorders. An extensive review of available evidence by a National Institutes of Health (NIH) panel of the effectiveness of acupuncture brought consensus that acupuncture is effective for pain control and for the treatment of nausea. It might also be promising in other conditions, including asthma, myocardial infarction, bronchitis, and rehabilitation from stroke (12).

However, data on the use of acupuncture for the treatment of cardiovascular disease are currently limited. In Russia and in China, acupuncture has been used for the treatment of hypertension, congestive heart failure, and myocardial ischemia. However, these uses have not yet been tested in randomized clinical trials. In spontaneously hypertensive rats, acupuncturelike electrical stimulation activates central opioid pathways, which leads to a decrease in sympathetic activity and in blood pressure. Thus, there appears to be a pharmacologic basis for the use of acupuncture in essential hypertension and in

other conditions such as congestive heart failure, in which sympathetic activation plays an important role. An NIH-sponsored randomized clinical trial is currently recruiting patients with hypertension to determine the effectiveness of acupuncture in essential hypertension (13).

HERBAL REMEDIES

An herb is a plant or part of a plant that produces and contains chemical substances that can exert a biologic or pharmacologic effect. According to the Dietary Supplement Health and Education Act of 1994, herbal remedies or botanicals are currently not regulated by the U.S. Food and Drug Administration if sold as dietary supplements. Therefore, they are not regulated for purity, potency, standardization, and formulation. The lack of regulation for potency and composition implies that there might be significant batch-to-batch variability and that there are often many active ingredients in the same preparation. The current regulations allow marketing with statements explaining their reported effect on the structure or function of the human body or the role in promoting general well-being, but not for diagnosis, treatment, cure, or prevention of diseases. Table 41.2 lists the most common herbal remedies used for cardiovascular care.

Garlic

The medicinal use of garlic (*Allium sativum*) dates back to early Egyptian times, and it has been advocated for the treatment and prevention of several diseases. The active ingredient is allicin, an odorous sulfurous compound that has been shown to exert several pharmacologic effects, including inhibitions of platelet aggregation (possibly irreversible), lowering of cholesterol and triglyceride levels, and lowering of blood pressure. In animal models, garlic has an antiatherosclerotic effect, as evidenced by a reduction of the development of new atheromatous lesions and a slowing in the progression of existing lesions. Garlic is currently available as fresh cloves, extracts, powders, and tablets. Several studies have suggested that at least ½ garlic clove per day (14,15) is required for a

TABLE 41.2. *Herbal products and orthomolecular therapies commonly used in cardiovascular care*

Herbal product	Active compound	Mechanism of action	Indication	Clinical evidence
Garlic	Allicin	Inhibition of platelet aggregation, antilipemic effect, antihypertensive effect	Hypertension Hypercholesterolemia	Limited
Soy protein	Soy protein	Phytoestrogenic effect, decreased cholesterol absorption	Hypercholesterolemia	Limited
Cholestin ("red rice yeast")	Statin compounds	Inhibition of HMG CoA reductase	Hypercholesterolemia	Supportive
Guggul gum	Gugulipid	Cholesterol lowering	Hypercholesterolemia	Supportive
Ginkgo biloba	Ginkgo flavone glycosides and terpenoids	Antiplatelet effect, antioxidant effect, vasodilatation (NO mediated)	Dementia Cognitive dysfunction	Supportive
Hawthorn	Poliphenolic compounds (flavonoids and glycosides) and triterpene acids	Positive inotropic effect, vasodilatation, antioxidant and antiinflammatory effects	Congestive heart failure	Study currently ongoing
Coenzyme Q-10	Coenzyme Q-10	Antioxidant effect (obligatory component of mitochondrial electron transport chain)	Congestive heart failure CAD	None
Vitamin E	—	Antioxidant effect on lipoprotein metabolism, antiplatelet effect	Prevention of CAD	None
Vitamin C	—	Antioxidant effect	Prevention of CAD	None
Vitamin A	—	Antioxidant effect	Prevention of CAD	None
Lutein	—	Antioxidant effect	Prevention of CAD	Animal data
Folic acid	—	Pivotal role in DNA synthesis	Prevention of CAD Prevention of restenosis after percutaneous coronary intervention	Supportive

CAD, coronary artery disease; HMG CoA, 3-hydroxy-3-methylglutaryl coenzyme A; NO, nitric oxide.

pharmacologic effect. Dried powders and tablets appear to be more practical formulations, but doses of the active ingredient are often inadequate. Several studies have assessed the effect of garlic on serum lipids and blood pressure control. Two recent metaanalyses showed that garlic administration resulted in a 9% to 12% reduction in total cholesterol, a modest reduction in triglyceride levels, and no significant changes in high-density lipoprotein levels (14,15). A metaanalysis of eight antihypertensive trials showed on average an 11–mm HG reduction in systolic blood pressure and a 6.5–mm HG reduction in diastolic blood pressure (Silagy CA, Neil HA. A meta-analysis of the effect of garlic on blood pressure. *Journal of Hypertension* 1994). Another well-designed randomized clinical trial evaluating the effect of garlic on claudication secondary to peripheral vascular disease showed no significant effect on pain-free walking distance or on ankle/brachial index. In yet another double-blind, randomized, placebo-controlled clinical trial evaluating the effect of garlic oil on serum lipoprotein levels and potential mechanisms of action, no significant effects on serum lipoproteins, cholesterol absorption, or cholesterol synthesis were identified (16). Variation in the concentration of the active compound in formulations may explain some of the differences between the results of clinical trials. The most common adverse effects of garlic are on the gastrointestinal system and include flatulence, esophageal pain, and abdominal pain. A significant interaction between garlic and an antiretroviral agent has been reported. This interaction results in marked reduction of blood levels of the anti–human immunodeficiency virus drug saquinavir in patients taking garlic supplements (17).

Soy Protein

Soy protein has been shown to be effective in lowering cholesterol through a decrease of cholesterol absorption, a decrease in bile reabsorption in the gut, and a phytoestrogenic effect. A metaanalysis of 22 trials showed a 9% decrease in total cholesterol levels, a 13% decrease in low-density lipoprotein (LDL) levels, and a 10% decrease in triglyceride levels (18). A more recent study has shown that the lipid-lowering effect is present both in normocholesterolemic and in hypercholesterolemic men. The health claim for soy protein at a dose of 25 g per day has been approved by the Food and Drug Administration.

Cholestin (Red Rice Yeast)

Cholestin is a fermented product of rice on which red yeast is grown, and it has been used for centuries in China. It contains starch, proteins, fiber, and at least eight statin compounds which function as 3-hydroxy-3-methylglutaryl coenzyme A reductase inhibitors. Chinese studies have shown that total cholesterol reduction after cholestin administration varies from 11% to 32%. A more recent randomized clinical trial showed a 15% reduction in total cholesterol and a 22% reduction in LDL cholesterol (19). Because cholestin contains several statinlike compounds, its use requires the same precautions as with prescription statins.

Gugulipid (Guggul Gum)

Gugulipid is an extract from the natural resin (gum guggula) of the mukul myrrh tree. It has been used in India to lower cholesterol, and it has been evaluated in well-designed clinical trials performed in India (20–22). These studies have shown that gugulipid administration results in a reduction of total cholesterol levels ranging from 11% to 22% and a reduction of triglyceride levels ranging from 12% to 25%. One study showed a 12% reduction of LDL. Gugulipid is inexpensive, and it does not have any significant adverse effects. The suggested dose is 75 mg per day (up to 500 mg).

Ginkgo Biloba

Ginkgo biloba has been used for memory loss and to improve circulation. The EGB 761 extract of ginkgo biloba is highly standardized, and it is currently widely used in Europe. There are at least three active compounds in ginkgo biloba: ginkgo flavone, glycosides, and terpenoids. Ginkgo biloba has an antiplatelet and antioxidant effect, it reduces platelet-activating factors, and it reduces production of thromboxane A_2 (23). It has also been shown to enhance endothelial cell derived nitric oxide through either an increase in nitric oxide synthase activity or a decrease breakdown of nitric oxide mediated by its antioxidant effect. Ginkgo biloba has been approved in Europe for treatment of dementia. In a study involving 202 patients, ginkgo biloba was found to decrease the Alzheimer's Disease Assessment Scale–Cognitive subscale score better than did placebo (24). There were no significant differences in the incidence of adverse reactions.

Overall, ginkgo biloba is considered a safe supplement; the most common adverse effects are headache and gastrointestinal. However, cases of subdural hematomas and bleeding have been described (25–27). It is currently believed that the increase in bleeding risk is due to ginkgolide B, an important inhibitor of platelet-activating factor. Thus, the use of ginkgo biloba is currently not recommended for patients receiving anticoagulants, aspirin, or nonsteroidal anti-inflammatory agents or for patients undergoing surgical procedures.

Hawthorn (*Crataegus*)

The use of hawthorn as a cardiac medication can be traced back to Roman physicians in the first century A.D. Since then, it has been used for the treatment of congestive heart failure. Hawthorn is derived from a small, fruit-bearing tree that grows throughout the world in woodlands. It has been used in Japanese, Chinese, European, and Native American traditional medicine and by American herbalists. The active components include two groups of polyphenolic derivatives that are present in the leaf and the flower, and, at a lower concentration, in the berries. The polyphenolic compounds include flavonoids and their glycoside and oligomeric proanthocyanidins. Triterpene acids are additional active components (28). The pharmacologic effects of hawthorn include a positive inotropic effect, coronary and peripheral vasodilation and antioxidant and antiinflammatory effects, resulting in an overall cardioprotective activity. Hawthorn has been evaluated in several clinical trials enrolling a total of 1,500 patients. In these studies, administration of hawthorn was found to improve exercise efficiency, to increase duration of exercise to anaerobic threshold, to increase left ventricular function, and to result in beneficial hemodynamic changes, which include a decrease of systemic blood pressure, a decrease in heart rate, an increase in cardiac output, a decrease in pulmonary artery pressure and pulmonary wedge pressure, and an overall decrease in systemic vascular resistance. These study are limited in that some were unblinded and uncontrolled, they were largely limited to New York Heart Association Class II patients, and background therapy usually included only diuretics and possibly digoxin. The place of hawthorn in the contemporary management of chronic congestive heart failure is being investigated in two ongoing randomized, placebo-controlled clinical trials, both using *Crataegus* special extract WS1442 (Willmar Schwabe Pharmaceuticals, Karlsruhe, Germany). The Hawthorn Extract Randomized Blinded Chronic Heart Failure (HERB CHF) study plans to enroll 120 patients to evaluate changes in exercise capacity, left ventricular function, quality of life, neurohormonal profile, and oxidative stress. The Study of Prognosis in Congestive Heart Failure (SPICE) will study 2,400 patients to examine effects on mortality and hospitalization. Both studies require background ther-apy with an angiotensin-converting enzyme inhibitor, if tolerated. The HERB CHF study also includes a beta blocker as standard background therapy.

ORTHOMOLECULAR THERAPIES

Orthomolecular therapies are based on the theory that restoring the optimal amount of substances normally present in the body can cure diseases and, in particular, mental illnesses (29). Their aim is to treat diseases with varying concentrations of chemicals, such as magnesium, zinc, selenium, melatonin, coenzymes, and megadoses of vitamins.

Coenzyme Q-10 (Ubiquinone)

Coenzyme Q-10, also known as ubiquinone, is a powerful antioxidant. The alternative name of ubiquinone is derived from the word *ubiquitous,* and it can be translated as "everywhere." Coenzyme Q-10 is a mitochondrial coenzyme that is present in every cell, and it is derived by endogenous synthesis from acetyl-coenzyme A and phenylalanine. The most common medicinal use of coenzyme Q-10 is for systolic congestive heart failure. Coenzyme Q-10 is also used for the treatment of coronary artery disease, diastolic heart failure, and hypertension and to prevent myocardial toxic effects of chemotherapeutic agents (30).

The rationale for use of coenzyme Q-10 for congestive heart failure is related to the fact that heart failure is characterized by chronic myocardial energy depletion and increased oxidative stress. Because coenzyme Q-10 is an obligatory component of the electron transport chain, and because it is essential for adenosine triphosphate generation during oxidative phosphorylation, dietary supplement could facilitate adenosine triphosphate generation and restore myocardial energy deposits. In addition, it has been proposed that, as a potent lipid soluble antioxidant, coenzyme Q-10 can act as free radical scavenger, thus counteracting the increased oxidative stress that characterizes congestive heart failure. Finally, a membrane-stabilizing property may also have a role in preventing arrhythmic death.

More than 30 studies that have suggested that coenzyme Q-10 can improve symptoms, quality of life, left ventricular function, and prognosis of patients with systolic congestive heart failure. Unfortunately, these studies have been limited by small sample size, lack of controls, suboptimal study design (no randomization or blinding), and inadequate measures of left ventricle systolic function.

More recently, Watson et al. (31) reported the result of a double-blind, randomized trial of 30 patients with congestive heart failure and who had an ejection fraction of less than 35%. Coenzyme Q-10, at a dose of 33 mg three times daily, or placebo was administered for 3 months. There were no significant differences in congestive heart failure–related quality of life and no improvement in left ventricular ejection fraction despite a more than twofold increase in serum levels of coenzyme Q-10. In addition, no changes in baseline left ventricular ejection fraction, peak exercise oxygen consumption, or exercise duration were reported from another double-blind placebo-controlled clinical trial in which 55 patients were randomly assigned to receive either placebo or coenzyme Q-10 at a dose of 200 mg daily and were monitored for 6 months (32). Thus, according to the results of these two well-designed randomized clinical trials, it does not appear that coenzyme Q-10 is effective in the treatment of congestive heart failure.

Vitamin E

Vitamin E includes at least eight compounds, of which alpha-tocopherol is the most active. The potential beneficial effect of alpha-tocopherol on the risk of coronary artery disease is related to its antioxidant effect on the metabolism of LDL. In addition, vitamin E has an antiplatelet effect (33), and it inhibits smooth muscle cell proliferation (34). Available dietary supplements contain 200 to 800 IU, a dose that is significantly higher than the current recommended daily allowance (RDA) of 30 IU and significantly higher than the dose that could be achieved with diet alone. The data concerning the effect of vitamin E on the risk of coronary artery disease are conflicting; some studies show a beneficial effect, and some studies show no effect. Part of the conflicting results might be related to dosing, to study design, to duration of clinical follow-up, and to its use for "primary prevention" versus "secondary prevention." In the Nurses' Health Study, women in the fifth quintile of daily intake diet of vitamin E supplements had significant reductions in age- and smoking-adjusted risk of major adverse cardiac events, including myocardial infarction and cardiovascular death (relative risk, 0.66; 95% confidence interval, 0.50 to 0.87). The median dose of vitamin E in this group was 208 IU/day, and the total follow-up time was 679,485 person-years (35). In another large prospective study of 39,910 men with 139,883 person-years of follow-up, men in the highest quintile had a significant reduction in major adverse cardiac events in comparison with men in the lowest quintile of dietary vitamin E intake (relative risk, 0.60; 95% confidence interval, 0.44 to 0.81) (36). Both studies evaluated patients who were free of cardiovascular disease at the time of the enrollment. A third nonrandomized prospective study also showed an inverse relationship between dietary intake of vitamin E and the risk of death from coronary disease in 34,486 postmenopausal women, from lowest quintile of less than 5.68 IU/day to the highest quintile of >35.59 IU/day. In that study, no additional benefit from vitamin E supplement was identified. However, no information was available on the duration of dietary supplements use, and only 12.9% of women reported a supplemental intake of more than 100 IU/day (37).

Several randomized controlled clinical trials have evaluated the use of vitamin E for secondary prevention. In the Heart Outcome Prevention Evaluation, patients with existing coronary artery disease or at high risk of coronary events because of a history of diabetes and other risk factors were randomly assigned to receive placebo or to vitamin E, 400 IU/day, and to ramipril or matching placebo. Treatment with vitamin E for a mean of 4.5 years did not result in a reduction of cardiovascular events (38). Also, no significant effect of vitamin E supplement on the incidence of major cardiac events was reported by the Gruppo Italiano per lo Studio della Soprav-vivenza nell'Infarto Miocardico (39). However, in that study, a reduction in deaths from cardiac causes was observed.

The Cambridge Heart Antioxidant Study randomly assigned 2,002 patients with coronary atherosclerosis to receive either vitamin E (400 or 800 IU per day) or placebo (40). At a median follow-up of 1.4 years, there was a significant reduction in the incidence of nonfatal myocardial infarction in the vitamin E recipients in comparison with the placebo recipients (relative risk, 0.53), but there was no significant difference in rates of mortality from cardiovascular causes. A small number of events and differences in baseline clinical characteristics were potential limitations of that study. In another randomized clinical trial of primary prevention, no significant effects were observed in patients at high risk (41).

In summary, although vitamin E, particularly long-term high dietary intake of vitamin E, might have a role in primary prevention of coronary artery disease, current available data do not support short-term use of vitamin E supplements for secondary prevention.

Vitamin C

Available data do not support the use of vitamin C supplements for the prevention of coronary artery disease (42). Some studies have suggested an inverse relationship between dietary intake of vitamin C and the risk of coronary disease and of stomach cancer. Except for one study that did not adjust for supplemental intake of vitamin E, no study has so far shown a benefit from higher dietary or supplemental intake. Tissue saturation at high level of intake may explain the lack of effect observed with supplements (43). The current recommended dietary allowance is 60 mg/day.

Vitamin A and Carotenoids

The generic term *vitamin A* is used to denote a family of fat-soluble compounds that have the same biologic properties as retinol, the most active form of vitamin A. The observation that vitamin A content in plants varies with the degree of pigmentation led to the discovery of carotenoids

(provitamin A) (44). The group of carotenoids includes beta-carotene, alpha-carotene, lycopene, lutein, and zeaxanthin. Beta-carotene and alpha-carotene are important sources of vitamin A; the other carotenoids cannot be converted into retinol but nonetheless have important antioxidant effects. Vitamin A plays an essential role in the function of the retina, has an antioxidant effect, and regulates cell differentiation (44). In view of these effects, several investigators have assessed the relationship between vitamin A intake and the risks of cancer and coronary artery disease. Unfortunately, although observational studies have suggested an inverse relationship between carotenoid intake and the risk of coronary artery disease (45), randomized clinical trials have consistently failed to demonstrate a beneficial effect of supplemental doses of beta-carotene on the risk of cancer or of coronary artery disease (46–50). It has been suggested that this discrepancy between observational studies and clinical trials might be due to the fact that clinical trials have used beta-carotene as a supplement, but the effect of dietary intake of vitamin A might be attributable to other carotenoids (42,51).

Lutein

Lutein is a carotenoid found in dark green leafy vegetables and in egg yolks. In one study, an inverse relationship was found between lutein concentration and progression of intima-media thickness of the carotid artery in 480 middle-aged men and women who were monitored for 18 months (52). In that study, just one portion of dark green leafy vegetables a day increased plasma concentration of lutein to the highest level. *In vitro* experiments showed inhibition by lutein of LDL-induced migration of monocytes in arterial walls, and in apolipoprotein E–null and in LDL receptor–null mice, addition of lutein in the diet decreased the development of atherosclerotic lesions (52). Although, as in other observational studies, a direct causal relationship between lutein levels and the observed progression of intima-media thickness cannot be inferred, these results are promising and support the need for further investigation of carotenoids other than beta-carotene in the prevention of atherosclerotic vascular disease.

Folic Acid

The term *folate* was coined by Mitchell and coworkers in 1941 after its isolation from leafy vegetables. *Folic acid* refers to the synthetic form of this vitamin. The folate-cobalamin (vitamin B_{12}) interaction plays a pivotal role for the normal synthesis of purines, pyrimidines, and deoxyribonucleic acid. Folate deficiency has been unquestionably associated in a causative relationship with the development of neural tube defects and of megaloblastic anemia, and folic acid supplementation has been shown in randomized clinical trials to reduce the incidence of neural tube defects by up to 70% (53). In addition, there is now substantial evidence linking a low intake of folic acid to an increase risk of cancer and of coronary artery disease. The relationship between folate and risk of coronary disease is further strengthened by the identification of high homocysteine levels as a risk factor for coronary artery disease. High folate intake has been shown to be associated with lower homocysteine levels (54). In addition, randomized clinical trials have shown that folic acid administration in patients with high pretreatment homocysteine levels results in a 25% reduction of plasma homocysteine levels. The addition of vitamin B_{12} results in an additional 7% reduction (55). The absolute reduction is related to pretreatment homocysteine levels; higher reductions are observed in patients with higher levels. The current Recommended Daily Allowance of folate is 400 μg/day. This dose is adequate for reducing plasma homocysteine levels in most patients, but higher doses might be required. Thus, daily dosages of 1 mg of folate and of 0.5 mg of vitamin B_{12} have been suggested for patients with persistently elevated homocysteine levels (56). Because the estimated daily intake of folate with the average diet is 200 μg/day, routine folate supplementation with at least the RDA appears advisable.

More recently, high plasma homocysteine levels have been found to be associated with a higher risk of restenosis after coronary angioplasty (57). As a follow-up of this finding, a ran-

domized placebo-controlled clinical trial showed that administration of a combination of folic acid (1 mg/day), vitamin B_{12} (400 μg/day), and pyridoxine (10 mg/day) significantly reduced homocysteine levels, and decreased restenosis and the need of target lesion revascularization in patients undergoing percutaneous transluminal angioplasty (58).

CHELATION THERAPY

The concept of chelation as a way to sequester metal ions into chemical structures was developed initially by Alfred Werner, who received the Nobel Prize in 1913. G.T. Morgan coined the term *chelation* in 1920 from the Greek word *chela,* or "claw." Natural chelators such as tartrate and citrate were used between the 1920s and 1950s to treat iron overload, treat lead poisoning, and reduce the toxicity of antiparasitic agents containing antimonium. During the same period, synthetic chelators were developed to treat lead poisoning [ethylenediaminetetraacetic acid (EDTA)], arsenic poisoning (dimercaprol or British antilewisite) and iron overload (deferoxamine).

EDTA is a synthetic chelator that exists in two forms: a sodium salt (Na_2 EDTA) and a calcium salt ($CaNa_2$ EDTA). The activity and the toxicity of the chelating agent depend on the affinity of the metal ion for the chelator. Na_2 EDTA binds calcium and can cause hypocalcemic tetany, whereas $CaNa_2$ EDTA can be used to treat poisoning by metal ions that have higher affinity than calcium for the chelating agents. EDTA was introduced in the early 1950s for the treatment of lead poisoning, and since then it has been used as an analytical tool and to treat a series of conditions, including hypercalcemia, digoxin toxicity, and radiation toxicity from plutonium. A reduction in the frequency of angina during EDTA therapy in patients with coronary disease was anecdotally reported in 1955 by Clarke et al. (59). Since then, there have been at least 22 case reports and small case series and five clinical trials suggesting a marked benefit of chelation therapy in patients with coronary or peripheral vascular disease. Unfortunately, the reported case series and clinical trials have been flawed by lack of blinding of patients and of investigators, lack of standardization of medical therapy, nonuniformity in applied clinical end points within the same study, and insufficient sample size. Thus, although in the United States chelation therapy is advocated for the treatment of coronary artery disease and peripheral vascular disease, there is currently no solid scientific evidence to support such use.

The proposed mechanism of action of chelation therapy includes chelation of calcium directly from atherosclerotic plaque, induction of parathyroid hormone secretion, a reduction in serum cholesterol through an unknown mechanism, chelation of transitional metals with consequent reduction in free radical formation, and inhibition of platelet aggregation. Current chelation therapy protocols involve repeated intravenous administration of EDTA, usually in combination with vitamins, trace elements, and iron supplementation, and the standardized regimen includes two treatments per week, 20 to 30 or more treatments total.

Chelation therapy is associated with significant adverse effects (Table 41.3), and several deaths clearly related to chelation have been reported. However, in studies in which the recommended standardized regimen is not exceeded, no deaths have been reported, and the adverse events are rare.

Chelation therapy is popular, with a currently estimated $40 million annual market in the United States alone. This popularity despite the lack of solid scientific evidence, and the questions raised by the numerous case reports and small case series, has led the NIH to sponsor a large, well-designed randomized clinical trial

TABLE 41.3. *Adverse effects of chelation therapy*

Renal failure
Arrhythmias
Tetany
Hypocalcemia
Hypoglycemia
Hypotension
Bone marrow depression
Prolonged bleeding time
Seizures
Respiratory arrest

(13). It is hoped that the results of this study will answer the question about the true effectiveness of this treatment modality.

ADVERSE EFFECTS OF HERBAL SUPPLEMENTS AND ORTHOMOLECULAR THERAPIES COMMONLY USED IN CARDIOVASCULAR CASES

Many medicinal herbs have biologically active compounds that can have toxic effects and can interact with commonly used drugs. As stated before, herbal supplements are currently not regulated for purity, potency, standardization, and formulation. Thus, there might be significant variability in efficacy between different manufactures but also within batches from the same manufacturer (60). Labeling of products may also not reflect their content. For example, cases of nephrotoxicity from a weight loss preparation initially attributed to fang-ji (*Stephania tetrandra*) were later found to be caused by the presence in the preparation of guang-fang-ji (*Aristolochia fangchi*), an herb that contains a known nephrotoxin. The confusion in that case was attributed to the similarity between the two names (61). The importance of variability among products has been well documented by a study of St. John's wort products that was commissioned by the *Los Angeles Times* (62). The result of the study showed that there were significant differences between the potency of the product and the claims on labels. Other potential problems related to herbal products include contamination with heavy metals in several Asian herbal products and the addition of pharmaceutical compounds, including caffeine, acetaminophen, indomethacin, hydrochlorothiazide, and prednisolone to proprietary "herbal" Chinese products (60,63).

Adverse effects and herb-drug interactions for the most commonly used herbal products are listed in Table 41.4 (17,26,64–81).

CONCLUSION

CAM therapies are commonly used by patients with cardiovascular diseases treated by conventionally trained physicians. It is therefore

TABLE 41.4. *Herb-drug interactions for the ten most popular herbs in 1998*

Herbal product	Use	Adverse events	Drug class	Drug interaction	Evidence
Ginkgo biloba	—	—	Antidiabetic agents	Possible increased risk of hypoglycemia	Theoretical
			Aspirin[26,64]	Possible increased risk of bleeding due to decreased platelet aggregation	Case report
			Nonsteroidal antiinflammatory drugs	Possible increased risk of bleeding due to decreased platelet aggregation	Theoretical
			Trazodone[65]	Increased risk of sedation	Case report
St. John's wort	—	—	Warfarin[66]	Increased risk of bleeding	
			Cyclosporine[67–69]	Cyclosporine levels may be reduced, resulting in a decrease in efficacy (e.g., possible organ rejection)	Case report
			Digoxin[70–72]	Decreased plasma levels and clinical efficacy of digoxin	Controlled study in healthy volunteers
			Iron	Decreased iron absorption	Theoretical
			Oral contraceptives[73]	Possible decreased efficacy of the oral contraceptive due to increased hepatic metabolism	Case report
			Protease inhibitors[74,75]	Decreased plasma levels and efficacy of protease inhibitor	Open-label study
			Serotonin reuptake inhibitors[76,77]	Possible increased sedative effects or serotonin syndrome	Case report
			Theophylline	Decreased plasma levels and efficacy of theophylline	Case report
			Tricyclic antidepressants	Decreased plasma levels and efficacy of tricyclic antidepressants	Open-label study
			Warfarin	Anticoagulant effect may be decreased	Case report
Ginseng	—	—	Loop diuretics	Decrease in pharmacologic effect of the loop diuretic	Case report
			Monoamine oxidase inhibitors	Insomnia, irritability, visual hallucinations, and headache	Case report
			Antidiabetics[78,79]	Hypoglycemia	
			Warfarin[80]	Anticoagulant effect may be decreased	Case report
Garlic	—	—	Warfarin	Possible increased risk of bleeding	Theoretical
			Antiretrovirals[17]	Decreased plasma concentration	Clinical study
Echinacea	—	—	Corticosteroids; cyclosporine	Possible interference with immunosuppressive effect of the drug	Theoretical
Saw palmetto	—	—	Estrogens and oral contraceptives	Possible increased risk of adverse effects	Theoretical
			Iron	Decreased iron absorption	Theoretical
Kava kava	—	—	Alprazolam[81]	Possible additive or synergistic CNS effects, leading to lethargy	Case report
Pycnogenol and grape seed[a]	—	—	No documented interactions	N/A	N/A
Cranberry	—	—	No documented interactions	N/A	N/A
Valerian	—	—	Barbiturates; benzodiazepines; opiates	Possible prolongation of sleep or sedative effects	Theoretical
			Iron	Decreased iron absorption	Theoretical

CNS, central nervous system; N/A, not available.

important for practitioners to be familiar with CAM therapies, with their proposed mechanism of action and effectiveness, and with the potential risks of adverse effects and drug interactions. It is likely that the rising interest of the medical community and of regulatory and funding agencies in CAM therapies will soon lead to a better understanding of their role in cardiovascular care.

PRACTICAL POINTS

- CAM therapies are commonly used by patients with cardiovascular diseases treated by conventionally trained physicians.
- Major domains of CAM therapy include (a) alternative medical systems, (b) mind-body interventions, (c) manipulative and body-based methods, (d) energy therapies, and (e) biologically based treatments.
- Data on the effect of garlic or garlic supplements have been conflicting. Variation in the concentration of the active compound in formulations may explain some of the differences between clinical trials.
- Cholestin (red rice yeast) has been shown in a randomized clinical trial to be effective in reducing total cholesterol (15% reduction) and LDL cholesterol (22% reduction). Because cholestin contains several statinlike compounds, its use requires the same precautions as with prescription statins.
- According to the results of two well-designed randomized clinical trials, it does not appear that coenzyme Q-10 is effective in the treatment of congestive heart failure.
- Hawthorn contains several active components that appear beneficial in patients with congestive heart failure. Two randomized clinical trials investigating its effectiveness in congestive heart failure (the HERB CHF study and the SPICE trial) are currently ongoing.
- Soy protein has been shown to be effective in lowering lipids (mild reduction).
- Vitamin E, particularly long-term high dietary intake of vitamin E, might have a role in primary prevention of coronary artery disease. However, available data do not support short-term use of vitamin E supplements for secondary prevention.
- Randomized clinical trials have failed to demonstrate a beneficial effect of supplemental dosages of beta-carotene and vitamin A on the risk of cancer or of coronary artery disease.
- There is substantial evidence linking a low intake of folic acid to an increase risk of cancer and of coronary artery disease. In addition, a randomized placebo-controlled clinical trial showed that administration of a combination of folic acid, vitamin B_{12}, and pyridoxine significantly reduced homocysteine levels and decreased restenosis and the need of target lesion revascularization in patients undergoing percutaneous transluminal angioplasty.
- Because the estimated daily intake of folate with the average diet is 200 μg/day, routine folate supplementation with at least the RDA appears advisable.
- Lutein is a carotenoid found in dark green leafy vegetables and in egg yolks. Preliminary results support the need for further investigation of lutein and of carotenoids other than beta-carotene in the prevention of atherosclerotic vascular disease.
- Chelation therapy is advocated in the United States for the treatment of coronary artery disease and peripheral vascular disease. However, there is currently no solid scientific evidence to support such use.

(continued)

> - Herbal supplements are not regulated for purity, potency, standardization, and formulation. Thus, there might be significant variability in efficacy between different manufacturers and within batches from the same manufacturer.
> - Many medicinal herbs have biologically active compounds that can have toxic effects and can interact with commonly used drugs.

REFERENCES

1. Eisenberg DM, Kessler RC, Foster C, et al. Unconventional medicine in the United States. *N Engl J Med* 1993; 328:246–252.
2. Eisenberg DM, Davis RB, Ettner SL, et al. Trends in alternative medicine use in the United States, 1990–1997. *JAMA* 1998;280:1569–1575.
3. Hager M, ed. *Chairman's Summary of the Conference Education of Health Professionals in Complementary/Alternative Medicine,* Fishman AP, Chair. New York: Josiah Macy, Jr. Foundation, 2001.
4. Liu EH, Turner LM, Lin SH, et al. Use of alternative medicine by patients undergoing cardiac surgery. *J Thorac Cardiovasc Surg* 2000;120:335–341.
5. http://nccam.nih.gov/
6. Hemingway H, Marmot M. Evidence based cardiology: psychosocial factors in the aetiology and prognosis of coronary heart disease. Systematic review of prospective cohort studies. *BMJ* 1999;318:1460–1467.
7. Grunbaum JA, Vernon SW, Clasen CM. The association between anger and hostility and risk factors for coronary heart disease in children and adolescents: a review. *Ann Behav Med* 1997;19:179–189.
8. Linden W, Stossel C, Maurice J. Psychosocial interventions for patients with coronary artery disease: a meta-analysis. *Arch Intern Med* 1996;156:745–752.
9. Luskin FM, Newell KA, Griffith M, et al. A review of mind-body therapies in the treatment of cardiovascular disease: part 1; implication for the elderly. *Altern Ther Health Med* 1998;3:46–52.
10. van Tudler MW, Koes BW, Bouter LM. Conservative treatment for acute and chronic non-specific low back pain: a systematic review of randomized controlled trials of the most common interventions. *Spine* 1997:22:2128–2156.
11. Sandefur R, Coulter ID. Licensure and legal scope of practice. In: Cherkin DC, Mootz RD, eds. *Chiropractic in the United States: training, practice and research.* Rockville, MD: U.S. Department of Health and Human Services, Agency for Health Care Policy and Research, 1997;AHCPR Pub. No. 98-N002
12. http://nccam.nih.gov/health/acupuncture/
13. http://nccam.nih.gov/clinical-trials/accupuncture.htm
14. Warshafsky S, Kamer RS, Sivak SL. Effect of garlic on total serum cholesterol: a meta-analysis. *Ann Intern Med* 1993;119:599–605.
15. Silagy C, Neil A. Garlic as a lipid lowering agent—a meta-analysis. *J Roy Coll Phys Lond* 1994;28:39–45.
16. Berthold HK, Sudhop T, von Bergmann K. Effect of a garlic oil preparation on serum lipoproteins and cholesterol metabolism: a randomized controlled trial. *JAMA* 1998;279:1900–1902.
17. Piscitelli SC, Burstein AH, Welden N, et al. The effect of garlic supplements on the pharmacokinetics of saquinavir. *Clin Infect Dis* 2002;34:234–238.
18. Anderson JW, Johnstone BM, Cook-Newell ME. Meta-analysis of the effects of soy protein intake on serum lipids. *N Engl J Med* 1995;333:276–282.
19. Heber D, Yip I, Ashley JM, et al. Cholesterol-lowering effects of a proprietary Chinese red-yeast-rice dietary supplement. *Am J Clin Nutr* 1999;69:231–236.
20. Singh RB, Niaz MA, Ghosh S. Hypolipidemic and antioxidant effects of *Commiphora mukul* as an adjunct to dietary therapy in patients with hypercholesterolemia. *Cardiovasc Drugs Ther* 1994;8:659–664.
21. Ararwal RC, Singh SP, Saran RK, et al. Clinical trial of gugulipid—a new hypolipidemic agent of plant origin in primary hyperlipidemia. *Indian J Med Res* 1986;84:626–634.
22. Verma SK, Bordia A. Effect of *Commiphora mukul* (gum guggula) in patients with hyperlipidemia with special reference to HDL-cholesterol. *Indian J Med Res* 1988;87:356–360.
23. Chung KF, Dent G, McCusker M, et al. Effect of a ginkgolide mixture (BN 52063) in antagonising skin and platelet responses to platelet activating factor in man. *Lancet* 1987;1:248–251.
24. Le Bars PL, Katz M, Berman N, et al. A placebo controlled, double blind, randomized trial of an extract of ginkgo biloba for dementia. *JAMA* 1997;278:1327–1332.
25. Rowin J, Lewis SL. Spontaneous bilateral subdural hematomas associated with chronic ginkgo biloba ingestion. *Neurology* 1996;46:1775–1776.
26. Vale S. Subarachnoid haemorrhage associated with ginkgo biloba [Letter]. *Lancet* 1998;352:36.
27. Benjamin J, Muir T, Briggs K, et al. A case of cerebral haemorrhage—can ginkgo biloba be implicated?. *Postgrad Med J* 2001;77:112–113.
28. Rigelsky JM, Sweet BV. Hawthorn: pharmacology and therapeutic uses. *Am J Health Syst Pharm* 2002;59:417–422.
29. http://www.healthplusweb.com
30. Tran MT, Mitchell TM, Kennedy DT, et al. Role of coenzyme Q10 in chronic heart failure, angina, and hypertension. *Pharmacotherapy* 2001;21:797–806.
31. Watson PS, Scalia GM, Galbraith A, et al. Lack of effect of coenzyme Q on left ventricular function in patients with congestive heart failure. *J Am Coll Cardiol* 1999;33:1549–1552.
32. Khatta M, Alexander BS, Krichten CM, et al. The effect of coenzyme Q10 in patients with congestive heart failure. *Ann Intern Med* 2000;132:636–640.
33. Calzada C, Bruckdorfer KR, Rice-Evans CA. The

influence of antioxidant nutrients on platelet function in healthy volunteers. *Atherosclerosis* 1997;128:97.

34. Boscoboinik D, Szewczyk A, Hensey C, et al. Inhibition of cell proliferation by alpha-tocopherol: role of protein kinase C. *J Biol Chem* 1991;266:6188.

35. Stampfer MJ, Hennekens CH, Manson JE, et al: Vitamin E consumption and the risk of coronary disease in women. *N Engl J Med* 1993;328:1444.

36. Rimm EB, Stampfer MJ, Ascherio A, et al: Vitamin E consumption and the risk of coronary heart disease in men. *N Engl J Med* 1993;328:1450.

37. Kushi LH, Folsom AR, Prineas RJ, et al: Dietary antioxidant vitamins and death from coronary heart disease in postmenopausal women. *N Engl J Med* 1996;334:1156–1162.

38. The Heart Outcomes Prevention Evaluation Study Investigators. Vitamin E supplementation and cardiovascular events in high-risk patients. *N Engl J Med* 2000;342:154–160.

39. GISSI-Prevenzione Investigators (Gruppo Italiano perlo Studio della Sopravvivenza nell'Infarto Miocardico). Dietary supplementation with n-3 polyunsaturated fatty acids and vitamin E after myocardial infarction: results of the GISSI-Prevenzione trial. *Lancet* 1999;354:447–455. (Erratum, *Lancet* 2001;357:342.)

40. Stephens NG, Parsons A, Schofield PM, et al. Randomized controlled trial of vitamin E in patients with coronary disease: Cambridge Heart Antioxidant Study (CHAOS). *Lancet* 1996;347:781–786.

41. Collaborative Group of the Primary Prevention Project. Low dose aspirin and vitamin E in people at cardiovascular risk: a randomized trial in general practice. *Lancet* 2001;357:89–96.

42. Rimm EB, Stampfer MJ. Antioxidant for vascular disease. *Med Clin North Am* 2000;84:239–249.

43. Food and Nutrition Board, Institute of Medicine. *Dietary reference intake for vitamin C, vitamin E, selenium and carotenoids: a report of the Panel of Dietary Antioxidants and Related Compounds.* Washington, DC: National Academy Press, 2000:529.

44. Marcus R, Coulston AM. The vitamins. In: Gilman AG, Rall TW, Nies AS, et al., eds. *Goodman and Gilman's The pharmacological basis of therapeutics,* 8th ed. New York: Pergamon Press, 1990:1523–1571.

45. Kritchevsky SB: Beta-carotene, carotenoids and the prevention of coronary heart disease. *J Nutr* 1999;129:5.

46. Greenberg ER, Baron JA, Karagas MR, et al: Mortality associated with low plasma concentration of beta carotene and the effect of oral supplementation. *JAMA* 1996;275:699.

47. Hennekens CH, Buring JE, Manson JE, et al: Lack of effect of long-term supplementation with beta carotene on the incidence of malignant neoplasms and cardiovascular disease. *N Engl J Med* 1996;334:1145.

48. Omenn GS, Goodman GE, Thornquist MD, et al: Effects of a combination of beta carotene and vitamin A on lung cancer and cardiovascular disease. *N Engl J Med* 1996;334:1150.

49. Malila N, Virtamo J, Virtanen M, Pietinen P, Albanes D, Teppo L. Dietary and serum alpha-locopherol, beta-carotene and retinol, and risk for colorectal cancer in male smokers. [Clinical Trial. Journal Article. Randomized Controlled Trial] *European Journal of Clinical Nutrition.* 56(7):615–21, 2002 Jul.

50. The Alpha-Tocopherol Beta-Carotene Cancer Prevention Study Group: The effect of vitamin E and beta carotene on the incidence of lung cancer and other cancers in male smokers. *N Engl J Med* 1994;330:1029.

51. Kohlmeier L, Kark JD, Gomez-Gracia E, et al: Lycopene and myocardial infarction risk in the EURAMIC Study. *Am J Epidemiol* 1997;146:618.

52. Dwayer JH, Navab M, Dwyer KM, et al. Oxygenated carotenoid lutein and progression of early atherosclerosis. The Los Angeles Atherosclerosis Study. *Circulation* 2001;103:2922–2927.

53. MRC Vitamin Study R search Group. Prevention of neural tube defects: results of the Medical Research Council Vitamin Study. *Lancet* 1991;338:131–137.

54. Jacques PF, Selhub J, Bostom AG, et al. The effect of folic acid fortification on plasma folate and total homocysteine concentrations. *N Engl J Med* 1999;340:1449–1454.

55. Homocysteine Lowering Trialists' Collaboration. Lowering blood homocysteine with folic acid based supplements: meta-analysis of randomised trials. *BMJ* 1998; 316:894–898.

56. Tice JA, Ross E, Coxton PG, et al. Cost-effectiveness of vitamin therapy to lower plasma homocysteine levels for the prevention of coronary heart disease effect of grain fortification and beyond. *JAMA* 2001;286:936–943.

57. Schnyder G, Roffi M, Flammer Y, et al. Association of plasma homocysteine level with restenosis after percutaneous coronary angioplasty. *Eur Heart J* 2002;23:726–733.

58. Schnyder G, Roffi M, Pin R, et al. Decreased rate of coronary restenosis after lowering of plasma homocysteine levels. *N Engl J Med* 2001;345:1593–600.

59. Clarke NE, Clarke CN, Mosher RE. The *"in vivo"* dissolution of metastatic calcium. An approach to atherosclerosis. *Am J Med Sci* 1955;229:142–149.

60. Fugh-Berman A. Herb-drug interactions. *Lancet* 2000; 355:134–138.

61. But PP-H. Herbal poisoning caused by adulterants or erroneous substitutes. *J Trop Med Hyg* 1994;97:371–374.

62. Monmaney T. Remedy's U.S. sales zoom, but quality control lags. St. John's wort: regulatory vacuum leaves doubt about potency, effects of herb used for depression. *Los Angeles Times* 1998 Aug 31:xx(col xx).

63. Huang WF, Wen K-C, Hsiao M-L. Adulteration by synthetic therapeutic substances of traditional Chinese medicines in Taiwan. *J Clin Pharmacol* 1997;37:344–350.

64. Rowin J, Lewis SL. Spontaneous bilateral subdural hematomas associated with chronic ginkgo biloba ingestion. *Neurology* 1996;46:1775–1776.

65. Galluzzi S, Zanetti O, Binetti G, Trabucchi M, Prisoni GB. Coma in a patient with Alzheimer's disease taking low dose trazodone and gingko biloba. [Letter] *Journal of Neurology, Neurosurgery & Psychiatry.* 68(5):679–80, 2000 May.

66. Mohutsky MA, Elmer GW. *Inhibition of cytochrome P450 in vitro by the herbal product ginkgo biloba.* Presented at the 41st Annual Meeting of the American Society of Pharmacognosy, Seattle, WA, July 2000.

67. Breidenbach T, Kliem V, Burg M, et al. Profound drop of cyclosporin A whole blood trough levels caused by St. John's wort (*perforatum*). *Transplantation* 2000;69:2229–2230.

68. Breidenbach T, Hoffmann MW, Becker T, et al. Drug interaction of St John's wort with cyclosporin. *Lancet* 2000;355:1912.

69. Barone GW, Gurley BJ, Ketel BL, et al. Drug interaction between St. John's wort and cyclosporine. *Ann Pharmacother* 2000;34:1013–1016.

70. Durr D, Stieger B, Kullak-Ublick GA, et al. St. John's wort induces intestinal P glycoprotein/MDR1 and intestinal and hepatic CYP3A4. *Clin Pharmacol Ther* 2000;68:598–604.

71. Cheng TO. St. John's wort interaction with digoxin [Letter]. *Arch Intern Med* 2000;160:2548.

72. Johne A, Brockmoller J, Bauer S, et al. Pharmacokinetic interaction of digoxin with an herbal extract from St. John's wort (*Hypericum perforatum*). *Clin Pharmacol Ther* 1999;66:338–345.

73. Yue QY, Bergquist C, Gerden B. Safety of St John's wort (*Hypericum perforatum*). *Lancet* 2000;355:576–577.

74. Piscitelli SC, Burstein AH, Chaitt D, et al. Indinavir concentrations and St John's wort. *Lancet* 2000;355:547–548.

75. Lumpkin MM, Alpert S. *Risk of drug interactions with St. John's wort and indinavir and other drugs [Letter].* Washington, DC: U.S. Food and Drug Administration, Center for Drug Evaluation and Research, 2000 February 10 (www.fda.gov/cder/drug/advisory/stjwort.htm).

76. Gordon JB. SSRIs and St. John's wort: possible toxicity?. [Letter]. *Am Fam Physician* 1998;57:950,953.

77. Schneck C. St. John's wort and hypomania [Letter]. *J Clin Psychiat* 1998;59:689.

78. Vuksan V, Sievenpiper JL, Koo VY, et al. American ginseng (*Panax quinquefolius L*) reduces postprandial glycemia in nondiabetic subjects and subjects with type 2 diabetes mellitus. *Arch Intern Med* 2000;160:1009–1013.

79. Sotaniemi EA, Haapakoski E, Rautio A. Ginseng therapy in non-insulin-dependent diabetic patients. *Diabetes Care* 1995;18:1373–1375.

80. Janetzky K, Morreale AP. Probable interaction between warfarin and ginseng. *Am J Health Syst Pharm* 1997;54:692–693.

81. Almmeida JC, Grimsley EW. Coma from the health food store: interaction between kava and alprazolam [Letter]. *Ann Intern Med* 1996;125:940–941.

Keith Aaronson, MD and Sara Warber, MD are recipients of NIH grant P50AT00011 from the National Center for Complementary and Alternative Medicine, Bethesda, MD.

Subject Index

Page numbers followed by *f* denote figures. Page numbers followed by *t* denote tables.